# THE CRITICALLY ILL CARDIAC PATIENT
Multisystem Dysfunction and Management

# THE CRITICALLY ILL CARDIAC PATIENT
## Multisystem Dysfunction and Management

Editors

**Vladimir Kvetan, M.D.**
*Director, Critical Care Medicine*
*Associate Professor of Anesthesiology and Medicine*
*Albert Einstein College of Medicine*
*Montefiore Medical Center*
*Bronx, New York*

**David R. Dantzker, M.D.**
*President and C.E.O.*
*Long Island Jewish Medical Center*
*New Hyde Park, New York*

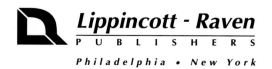

**Lippincott - Raven**
P U B L I S H E R S

*Philadelphia • New York*

Printed in the United States of America

9  8  7  6  5  4  3  2  1

---

**Library of Congress Cataloging-in-Publication Data**

The critically ill cardiac patient : multisystem dysfunction and management / editors,
   Vladimir Kvetan, David R. Dantzker.
      p.   cm.
   Includes bibliographical references and index.
   ISBN 0-397-51465-4
   1. Cardiac intensive care.   I. Kvetan, Vladimir.   II. Dantzker, David R.
   [DNLM:   1. Heart Diseases—complications.   2. Heart Diseases—therapy.
   3. Critical Care.   WG 210 C934 1996]
   RC684.I56C75   1996
   616.1'2028—dc20
   DNLM/DLC
   for Library of Congress                                          96-19018
                                                                         CIP

---

Care has been taken to confirm the accuracy of the information presented and to describe generally accepted practices. However, the authors, editors, and publisher are not responsible for errors or omissions or for any consequences from application of the information in this book and make no warranty, express or implied, with respect to the contents of the publication.

   The authors, editors, and publisher have exerted every effort to ensure that drug selection and dosage set forth in this text are in accordance with current recommendations and practice at the time of publication. However, in view of ongoing research, changes in government regulations, and the constant flow of information relating to drug therapy and drug reactions, the reader is urged to check the package insert for each drug for any change in indications and dosage and for added warnings and precautions. This is particularly important when the recommended agent is a new or infrequently employed drug.

   Some drugs and medical devices presented in this publication have Food and Drug Administration (FDA) clearance for limited use in restricted research settings. It is the responsibility of the health care provider to ascertain the FDA status of each drug or device planned for use in their clinical practice.

*To Cindy, Max, and Henry*
*whose patience and support*
*made it possible for me*
*to have great fun with my fellows and faculty.*

*Vladimir Kvetan, M.D.*


*To Jami and Marc Dantzker*
*whose inquisitive minds and passion for research*
*bode well for the future of science.*

*David R. Dantzker, M.D.*

# Contents

# Contributors

**Steven Ayres, M.D.**
*Director, International Health Programs*
*Medical College of Virginia*
*Box 843071*
*Richmond, Virginia 23284*


**Richard Barnett, M.D.**
*Director of Medicine Inpatient Services*
*University Hospital at Stony Brook*
*Attending Physician*
*VA Medical Center, Northport, New York*
*Division of Nephrology and Hypertension*
*Stony Brook Health Sciences Center*
*School of Medicine*
*State University of New York at Stony Brook*
*Stony Brook, New York 11794-8152*


**Richard C. Becker, M.D.**
*Associate Professor of Medicine*
*University of Massachusetts Medical School*
*Director, Coronary Care Unit*
*Director, Thrombosis Research Center*
*Clinical Trials Section*
*Laboratory for Vascular Biology Research*
*Anticoagulation Services*
*University of Massachusetts Medical Center*
*55 Lake Avenue North*
*Worcester, Massachusetts 01655*


**John F. Butterworth IV, M.D.**
*Associate Professor and Vice Chairman for*
  *Research*
*Department of Anesthesia*
*Bowman Gray School of Medicine of Wake*
  *Forest University*
*Medical Center Boulevard*
*Winston-Salem, North Carolina 27157*

**Peter M. Buttrick, M.D.**
*Director, Cardiology Fellowship Medicine*
*Division of Cardiology*
*Montefiore Medical Center*
*Albert Einstein College of Medicine*
*111 East 210th Street*
*Bronx, New York 10467*


**David B. Cotton, M.D.**
*Professor and Chairman*
*Department of Obstetrics and Gynecology*
*Detroit Medical Center*
*Wayne State University*
*4707 St. Antoine Boulevard*
*Detroit, Michigan 48201*


**David Crippen, M.D.**
*Clinical Professor of Anesthesiology*
*University of Pittsburgh*
*Director, Surgical Critical Care*
*Department of Critical Care Medicine*
*St. Francis Medical Center*
*Pittsburgh, Pennsylvania 15201*


**Jonathan F. Critchlow, M.D.**
*Assistant Professor of Surgery*
*Harvard Medical School*
*Department of Surgery and Multidisciplinary*
  *Critical Care Service*
*Beth Israel Hospital*
*330 Brookline Avenue*
*Boston, Massachusetts 02215*


**David R. Dantzker, M.D.**
*President and C.E.O.*
*Long Island Jewish Medical Center*
*270-05 76th Avenue*
*New Hyde Park, New York 11040*

**Kim A. Eagle, M.D.**
*Associate Professor of Internal Medicine*
*Department of Internal Medicine*
*University of Michigan Medical Center*
*3910 Taubman Center*
*Ann Arbor, Michigan 48103*

**Leonid A. Eidelman, M.D.**
*Attending Physician and Lecturer*
*Department of Anesthesiology and Critical*
*  Care*
*Hadassah University Hospital*
*Hebrew University Medical School*
*Kiryat Hadassah*
*P.O. Box 12000*
*Jerusalem, Israel 91120*

**N. Tony Eissa, M.D.**
*Senior Staff*
*Department of Pulmonary Critical Care*
*  Medicine*
*National Heart, Lung, and Blood Institute*
*National Institutes of Health*
*Building 10, Room 6D-03*
*Bethesda, Maryland 20892*

**Mitchell P. Fink, M.D.**
*Johnson & Johnson Professor of Surgery*
*Department of Surgery*
*Harvard Medical School*
*Surgeon-in-Chief*
*Beth Israel Hospital*
*330 Brookline Avenue*
*Boston, Massachusetts 02215*

**Bradley D. Freeman, M.D.**
*Department of Surgery*
*Washington University School of Medicine*
*Washington University Medical Center*
*660 South Euclid Avenue*
*St. Louis, Missouri 63110*

**William A. Gay, Jr. , M.D.**
*Professor of Surgery*
*Division of Cardiothoracic Surgery*
*Washington University School of Medicine*
*One Barnes Hospital Plaza*
*Queeny Tower, Suite 3108*
*St. Louis, Missouri 63110*

**Michael Geheb, M.D.**
*Professor of Medicine*
*Director of Health Systems*
*University of Alabama at Birmingham*
*701 20th Street South*
*Birmingham, Alabama 35294*

**Yehuda Ginosar, B.Sc., M.B.B.S.**
*Attending Physician and Instructor*
*Department of Anesthesiology and Critical Care*
*Hadassah University Hospital*
*Hebrew University Medical School*
*Kiryat Hadassah*
*P.O. Box 12000*
*Jerusalem, Israel 91120*

**Kenneth Greer, M.D.**
*Clinical Assistant Professor of Anesthesiology*
*Department of Critical Care*
*St. Francis Medical Center*
*University of Pittsburgh*
*400 45th Street*
*Pittsburgh, Pennsylvania 15201*

**Ake Grenvik, M.D., Ph.D.**
*Distinguished Service Professor of Critical*
*  Care Medicine*
*Director Multidisciplinary Critical Care*
*  Training Program*
*University of Pittsburgh School of Medicine*
*University of Pittsburgh Medical Center*
*Scaife Hall, Room 612*
*Pittsburgh, Pennsylvania  15213*

**Jiho J. Han, M.D.**
*Clinical Assistant Professor of Medicine*
*Department of Medicine*
*Division of Cardiology and Cardiopulmonary*
*  Labs and Research*
*Medical College of Virginia*
*Virginia Commonwealth University*
*MCV Station, Box 980281*
*Richmond ,Virginia 23298*

**Michael L. Hess, M.D.**
*Professor and Chairman*
*Department of Medicine*
*Division of Cardiology and Cardiopulmonary*
*  Labs and Research*
*Medical College of Virginia*
*Virginia Commonwealth University*
*MCV Station, Box 980281*
*Richmond, Virginia 23298*

**John Hoyt, M.D.**
*Clinical Professor, Anesthesiology and Critical*
*  Care*
*University of Pittsburgh*
*Chairman, Department of Critical Care*
*  Medicine*
*St. Francis Medical Center*
*400 45th Street ·*
*Pittsburgh, Pennsylvania 15201*

**Alexander G. Justicz, M.D.**
*Professor of Surgery*
*Department of Thoracic and Cardiovascular*
*Surgery*
*Piedmont Hospital*
*95 Collier Road, Suite 2055*
*Atlanta, Georgia 30309*

**Waheedullah Karzai, M.D.**
*Klinik für Anästhesiologie und Intensitherapie*
*Klinikum der Friedrich-Schiller-Universität*
*Jena*
*Bachstrasse 18*
*07740 Jena, Germany*

**David P. Katz, Ph.D.**
*Assistant Professor*
*Associate Director Research*
*Department of Anesthesiology*
*Montefiore Medical Center*
*Albert Einstein College of Medicine*
*111 East 210th Street*
*Bronx, New York 10467*

**Arfa Khan, M.D.**
*Professor of Radiology*
*Albert Einstein College of Medicine*
*Associate Chairman*
*Chief, Division of Thoracic Radiology*
*Long Island Jewish Medical Center*
*270-05 76th Avenue*
*New Hyde Park, New York 11040*

**Vladimir Kvetan, M.D.**
*Director, Critical Care Medicine*
*Associate Professor of Anesthesiology and*
*Medicine*
*Albert Einstein College of Medicine*
*Montefiore Medical Center*
*111 East 210th Street*
*Bronx, New York 10467*

**Ronald J. Lis, M.D.**
*Assistant Professor of Anesthesiology and*
*Medicine*
*Medical Director, Medical ICU*
*Associate Director, CCM Fellowship Program*
*Division of Critical Care*
*Albert Einstein College of Medicine*
*Montefiore Medical Center*
*111 East 210th Street*
*Bronx, New York 10467*

**Drew A. MacGregor, M.D.**
*Assistant Professor of Anesthesia and Medicine*
*Department of Anesthesia*
*Bowman Gray School of Medicine*
*of Wake Forest University*
*Medical Center Boulevard, Box 1009*
*Winston-Salem, North Carolina 27157*

**Sunil Mankad, M.D.**
*Cardiology Fellow*
*Department of Medicine*
*University of Pittsburgh*
*200 Lothrop Street*
*Pittsburgh, Pennsylvania 15213*

**G. Daniel Martich, M.D.**
*Assistant Professor of Anesthesiology/Critical*
*Care Medicine*
*Associate Director, Cardiothoracic Intensive*
*Care Unit*
*Medical Director, Critical Care Information*
*Systems Department*
*University of Pittsburgh*
*School of Medicine*
*Sciafe Hall, Suite 648*
*Pittsburgh, Pennsylvania 15201*

**Adelaida M. Miro, M.D.**
*Assistant Professor of Anesthesiology/Critical*
*Care Medicine*
*University of Pittsburgh Medical Center*
*Sciafe Hall, Suite 648*
*200 Lothrop Street*
*Pittsburgh, Pennsylvania 15201*

**Charles Natanson, M.D.**
*Senior Investigator*
*Critical Care Medicine Department*
*National Institutes of Health*
*9000 Rockville Pike, Building 10*
*Bethesda, Maryland 20892*

**Daniel Nyhan, M.D.**
*Associate Professor and Chief of Cardiac*
*Anesthesia*
*Department of Anesthesiology/Critical Care*
*Medicine*
*Division of Cardiac Anesthesia*
*The Johns Hopkins University School of*
*Medicine*
*600 North Wolfe Street, Tower 711*
*Baltimore, Maryland 21287*

**RoseMarie Pasmantier, M.D.**
*Director of Metabolic Clinic*
*Division of Endocrinology*
*Health Sciences Center*
*State University of New York*
*450 Clarkson Avenue*
*Brooklyn, New York 11203*

**Stephen McCarthy Pastores, M.D.**
*Assistant Professor of Anesthesiology and*
*  Medicine*
*Division of Critical Medicine*
*Albert Einstein College of Medicine*
*Montefiore Medical Center*
*111 East 210th Street*
*Bronx, New York 10467*

**Sumita D. Paul, M.D., M.P.H.**
*Clinical Fellow in Cardiology*
*Department of Medicine*
*Massachusetts General Hospital*
*Cardiac Unit, Ellison 908*
*Boston, Massachusetts 02114*

**David T. Porembka, D.O.**
*Associate Professor of Anesthesia and Surgery*
*Associate Director of Surgical Intensive Care*
*Department of Anesthesia*
*University of Cincinnati Medical Center*
*231 Bethesda Avenue, ML-531*
*Cincinnati, Ohio 45229*

**Richard C. Prielipp, M.D.**
*Associate Professor*
*Department of Anesthesia and Critical Care*
*  Medicine*
*Bowman Gray School of Medicine of Wake*
*  Forest University*
*Medical Center Boulevard*
*Winston-Salem, North Carolina 27157*

**David Rubinstein, M.D.**
*Fellow*
*Division of Cardiology*
*Montefiore Medical Center*
*Albert Einstein College of Medicine*
*111 East 210th Street*
*Bronx, New York 10467*

**Steven M. Scharf, M.D., Ph.D.**
*Director of Research*
*Division of Pulmonary and Critical Care*
*  Medicine*
*Department of Medicine*
*Long Island Jewish Medical Center*
*270-05 76th Avenue*
*New Hyde Park, New York 11042*

**Daniel F. Settle, M.D.**
*Chief Resident*
*Department of Radiology*
*Long Island Jewish Medical Center*
*270-05 76th Avenue*
*New Hyde Park, New York 11042*

**Charles L. Sprung, M.D., J.D.**
*Director of Respiratory Intensive Care Unit*
*Professor of Medicine*
*Department of Anesthesiology and Critical*
*  Care Medicine*
*Hadassah University Hospital*
*The Hebrew University of Jerusalem*
*Box 12000*
*Jerusalem, Israel 91120*

**Jay S. Steingrub, M.D.**
*Assistant Professor of Medicine and Surgery*
*Tufts University School of Medicine*
*Director, Adult Critical Care Division*
*Baystate Medical Center*
*759 Chestnut Street*
*Springfield, Massachusetts 01199*

**Panagiotis N. Symbas, M.D.**
*Professor of Cardiothoracic Surgery*
*Emory University School of Medicine*
*Director, Cardiothoracic Surgery Service*
*Grady Memorial Hospital*
*69 Butler Street*
*Atlanta, Georgia 30303*

**Daniel Teres, M.D.**
*Tufts University School of Medicine*
*Associate Professor of Medicine and Surgery*
*Director, Critical Care Division*
*Baystate Medical Center*
*759 Chestnut Street*
*Springfield, Massachusetts 01199*

**Richard J. Traystman, Ph.D.**
*Distinguished Research Professor*
*Vice Chairman for Research*
*Department of Anesthesiology/Critical Care*
  *Medicine*
*The Johns Hopkins University School of Medicine*
*600 North Wolfe Street, Blalock 1408*
*Baltimore, Maryland 21287*

**Stefan Wiese, M.D.**
*Research Fellow*
*Division of Critical Care Medicine*
*Department of Anesthesiology*
*Albert Einstein College of Medicine*
*Montefiore Medical Center*
*111 East 210th Street*
*Bronx, New York 10467*

**Janice E. Whitty, M.D.**
*Assistant Professor*
*Department of Obstetrics and Gynecology*
*Wayne State University*
*Director, Maternal Special Care Unit*
*Hutzel Hospital*
*4707 St. Antoine Boulevard*
*Detroit, Michigan 48201*

**Gary P. Zaloga, M.D.**
*Professor and Head of Section on Critical*
  *Care*
*Department of Anesthesia*
*Bowman Gray School of Medicine of Wake*
  *Forest University*
*Medical Center Boulevard*
*Winston-Salem, North Carolina 27157*

# Preface

Cardiologists have a crucial role in managing critical care resources in the United States. Critical care medicine consumes 10% of hospital beds, 30% of hospital costs, and 1% of the gross national product. Cardiologists have direct responsibility for coronary care units. They are intimately involved in cardiothoracic surgery units. They consult on the perioperative care patients in surgical intensive care units and on complex cardiac problems in medical intensive care units. While cardiology fellowship training guarantees expertise in cardiovascular intensive care management, it usually does not stress the multisystem critical care frequently required in patients with severe primary cardiac disease.

This book is directed at cardiologists in training and in practice and is meant to be a developing curriculum of critical care medicine for cardiologists. The goal is to offer a collaborative view of state-of-the-art multisystem management science. Among the contributing authors are academic cardiologists, cardiovascular and general surgeons, anesthesiologists, and pulmonary and nonpulmonary intensivists.

Among the major surgical issues covered are discussion of perioperative cardiac management of patients undergoing noncardiac surgery, abdominal crisis in patients with cardiac disease, cardiac trauma, cardiovascular complications of organ transplantations, and obstetric crises in patients with cardiac disease.

Major medical issues are discussed that are relevant to cardiologists involved in the management of critically ill cardiac patients. They include discussions of the different approaches to respiratory support in cardiac patients compared with patients with respiratory insufficiency due to primary pulmonary injury; management of oxygen metabolism; regional circulation abnormalities in critical illness; relevance of inflammatory mediators released during severe cardiac disease; metabolic and nutritional support; management of renal failure; sepsis; the central nervous system; and hematologic abnormalities.

Pharmacology issues are discussed both from the perspective of cardiac effects of noncardiac drugs and vice versa. Attention is devoted to cardiac toxicity of illicit and licit drugs.

Technical sections of this volume include discussions of selected aspects of cardiorespiratory monitoring, management of cardiac complications of procedures, and the finer points of intensive care radiology.

Since high-quality critical care is frequently delivered by qualified personnel in adverse environments outside of the ICU, attention is also devoted to transport of critically ill cardiac patients.

Finally, the use of scoring systems and outcome assessment of critical illness, both in medical and surgical settings, is reviewed from the perspective of an intensivist.

# Acknowledgments

We would like to gratefully acknowledge the contribution of Ms. Leida Colon without whose help this volume would not be possible.

*The Critically Ill Cardiac Patient,*
edited by V. Kvetan and D. R. Dantzker,
Lippincott-Raven Publishers, Philadelphia © 1996.

CHAPTER 1

# Pathophysiology of Cardiac Insufficiency and Failure

## Diagnosis and Management from a Critical Care Perspective

Jiho J. Han, Steven Ayres, and Michael L. Hess

The heart is an organ that resists change and is quite resilient in the face of stress. However, in the critically ill, cardiac insufficiency can play a central role in the patient with preexisting heart disease and in the patient with multisystem failure. Occult cardiac dysfunction often presents as "spells" in the intensive care unit (ICU) or as inability of a patient to wean from the ventilator. Spells are rapid unexplainable changes in mental status, oxygenation, and systemic and pulmonary arterial pressures in a patient who is critically ill. Myocardial dysfunction is familiar to the intensivist as a critical element of hyperdynamic septic shock (1). Combined with ischemic and valvular heart disease, the septic patient with heart diseases poses a diagnostic and management conundrum. Intubated patients do not have classical symptoms, and angina pectoris often masquerades as anxiety and agitation. This chapter addresses the major advances in diagnosis and therapy in the management of cardiac insufficiency and failure in the critically ill patient. Advances in the diagnosis of cardiac insufficiency have aided the intensivist to identify early cardiac dysfunction and treat cardiac failure in a timely manner.

Underlying cardiovascular disease is pervasive in our aging population. Cardiovascular mortality is the leading cause of death in patients over the age of 65, representing 83% of all cardiovascular deaths (2). Moreover, 13% of the population are elderly (age greater than 65), with this group projected to increase to 21%, or 35 million people

in 45 years. The oldest of the old (those over 85) are increasing at a faster rate, with an estimated 12 million people expected by the year 2010 (3). Thus identifying and treating coronary artery disease will be the rule rather than the exception in the critically ill elderly patient.

At the opposite spectrum, the increasing use of cocaine and recreational drugs implicates coronary artery disease in the young. Cocaine produces not only coronary vasospasm and acute thrombotic myocardial infarction (MI) but also accelerated atherosclerosis (4). In patients with an overdose and with history of drug abuse, the specter of coronary artery disease needs to be excluded, especially with the symptoms of chest discomfort and signs of hemodynamic instability.

### MYOCARDIAL FAILURE AND THE ICU

The ICU presents a unique setting for the study, diagnosis, and management of acute myocardial failure (Table 1). Both the common ICU syndromes of hypovolemic shock and gram-negative sepsis are associated with acute myocardial failure often seen in the setting of previously normal myocardial function. This can be complicated by the aggressive use of crystalloid solutions used to replace or expand intravascular volume. The common use of pulmonary artery catheters inserted to measure pulmonary capillary wedge (PCW) pressure has greatly facilitated the monitoring of left ventricular (LV) filling pressures and indirectly serves as an accurate measure of LV end-diastolic pressure in the absence of mitral valve obstruction or pulmonary venous obstruction. These data, taken together with the assessment of global myocardial function using

J.J. Han, S. Ayres, and M.L. Hess: Department of Medicine, Division of Cardiology and Cardiopulmonary Labs and Research, Medical College of Virginia, Virginia Commonwealth University, Richmond, Virginia 23219.

**TABLE 1.** *Shock classification with myocardial dysfunction.*

1. Cardiogenic shock
   Acute MI
     Pump failure
     Acute mitral regurgitation
     Acute papillary muscle rupture
     Acute ventricular septal defect
     Acute free wall rupture with tamponade
   Dilated CM
   Valvular–acute MR
     Aortic stenosis
     IHSS
   Arrhythmias
2. Obstructive
   Pericardial tamponade
   Constrictive pericarditis
   Pulmonary emboli
   Severe pulmonary hypertension
   Coraction
   Aortic dissection
   Tension pneumothorax
3. Oligemic
   Hemorrhage
   Burns
   Fluid depletion
4. Distributive
   Septic shock
   Anaphylaxis
   Neurogenic
   Endocrine—acute beriberi

Adapted from Dixon AC, Parrillo JE. Managing the cardiovascular effects of sepsis and septic shock. *J Crit Illness* 1991;6:1197.

MI, myocardial infarction; CM, cardiomyopathies; MR, mitral regurgitation; IHSS, idiopathic hypertrophic subaortic stenosis.

the two-dimensional echocardiogram can provide valuable information about the status of the heart during numerous pathophysiologic events.

It must be remembered that the heart of the patient in the acute care setting has the potential to be inundated with numerous negative inotropic agents. Acidosis is a direct negative inotrope and compounding the problem is the fact that, in the face of acidosis, positive inotropic agents will demonstrate a decreased effectiveness. Hyperkalemia and various circulating endogenous negative inotropic agents such as tumor necrosis factor, myocardial depressant factor(s), and gram-negative endotoxin all contribute to a depression of myocardial contractility. This problem can be compounded in the face of preexisting coronary artery disease in the elderly or in the patient with a preexistent cardiomyopathy due to such diverse etiologies as hypertension, alcohol, or valvular heart disease.

Thus the heart of the critically ill patient can be caught in a vicious circle of positive feedback where progressive myocardial depression results in a decrease in cardiac output and end-organ hypoperfusion. This in turn activates the sympathetic nervous system, increases the level of circulating catecholamines and antidiuretic hormone (vasopressin), and activates the renin-angiotensin system.

This physiologic response to a reduced cardiac output further increases total peripheral resistance, increases impedance to LV ejection, and further decreases cardiac output. The decrease in cardiac output further fuels this pathophysiologic cascade, decreasing cardiac output and organ perfusion.

The global myocardial dysfunction of the critically ill patient is thus best managed by optimizing the PCW pressure to between 15 and 20 mm Hg (optimizing preload) and the support of myocardial contractility with positive inotropic agents such as dobutamine, amrinone, or milrinone. The phosphodiesterase inhibitors amrinone and milrinone offer the additional advantage of being peripheral arteriolar vasodilators, thus reducing total peripheral resistance, decreasing impedance to LV ejection, and further increasing cardiac output while providing inotropic support to the myocardium.

## AGING POPULATION AND THE ICU

The vessels and the heart literally stiffen with age. Arteries remodel so that less elastic fibers and more collagen compose the media. Mean arterial pressure increases with an elevation of systolic pressure and widening of the pulse pressure. Aortic impedance and peripheral vascular resistance increase. Left ventricular wall thickness increases due to an increase in cell size. The heart mass usually increases with left atrial enlargement. Myocardial compliance decreases and the heart depends more on atrial contraction for adequate ventricular filling. The heart becomes increasingly preload dependent (5). Thus the normal physiology of aging is characterized by a hyperdynamic apical impulse, brisk carotid upstrokes, and a prominent S4. In addition, the heart become less responsive to adrenergic stimulation, as reflected by a 30% reduction in the maximal heart rate (HR) from age 20 to 80. In the octogenarian, there is an 85% reduction in the cells of the sinoatrial (SA) node and at the atrioventricular (AV) nodal junction. Under adrenergic stress, the elderly rely more on increasing preload than on increasing HR, as in the young (6)—thus the importance of adequate volume in critically ill elderly patients to achieve adequate heart function.

## IMPORTANCE OF NUTRITION IN THE CRITICALLY ILL PATIENTS

In 24 hours, the heart utilizes 35 kg of adenosine triphosphate (ATP) (100 times more than its own weight) and 10,000 times the amount that is stored (7). The heart achieves this tremendous transfer of energy with mitochondrial cell volume being 25% and specialized mitochondria that have more abundant cristae (the site of the respiratory chain enzymes) than mitochondria of other organs such as skeletal muscle or the brain (8). This significant increase in mitochondrial volume contributes to the statement that "the heart is an obligate aerobe" and is thus exquisitely sensitive to a decrease in coronary flow and oxygen delivery. In addition to its large energy expenditure, the heart requires substrate for synthesis and degradation for its constitutive proteins. Protein synthesis is impaired under stress and with myocardial ischemia (9). Although each protein has its half-life, the human heart regenerates itself completely over a period of 3 weeks at a rate of 4.8% per day (10). The specific conditions that affect synthesis and degradation myocardial protein are not yet understood. Acute volume overload appears to stimulate synthesis and chronic congestive failure appears to suppress degradation. In the critically ill patient who is nutritionally impaired, myocardial energetics and myocardial remodeling may be affected.

## MYOCARDIAL FUNCTION IN THE MECHANICALLY VENTILATED PATIENT

Mechanical ventilation imposes a constraint on both preload and afterload as well as autonomic regulation of the heart. Changes in intrapleural pressures affect not only intracardiac filling (preload) but also systemic resistance. Although many factors are responsible for respiratory hemodynamic variation, including changes in autonomic tone, mechanical factors such as lung volume and intrapleural pressures are the key components, as the heart is a pump within another muscular pump, the thorax. In a patient with cardiac insufficiency, small changes in lung volume and intrapleural pressures can have profound effects on systemic venous return and LV and right ventricular (RV) afterload.

Changes in intrapleural pressure affect venous return and LV ejection (afterload) independently of cardiac inotropic status. Negative intrapleural pressures as with spontaneous inspiration or forced inspiration against a closed glottis (Mueller maneuver) increase systemic venous return, thus increasing preload by increasing intrathoracic blood volume. For the left ventricle, a greater output needs to be generated against greater intrapleural pressure which impedes ventricular ejection and causes a reduction in stroke volume (SV). This physiology is exaggerated in the various conditions that cause pulsus paradoxus. Because the right and left ventricles are interdependent, within two to three cardiac cycles, these changes are offset.

Positive or increased intrapleural pressures, as with a positive-pressure mechanical inspiratory breath, delay right atrial venous return but augments LV emptying. Total intrathoracic blood volume decreases. These effects are exaggerated in a patient that requires high positive end-expiratory pressure (PEEP).

Precise studies of intrapleural pressures changes are hampered by the difficulties in measuring this potential space's pressure. Intraesophageal balloons estimate intrapleural pressure in the upright position but are unreliable in the supine position (11). The use of *intrathoracic pressure* has made it convenient to apply all background pressures for structures within the chest. Thus, respiratory changes in intrathoracic pressure should not impact on *right* ventricular afterload, since the lungs, pulmonary vasculature, and left atrium are within the chest. Changes in intrathoracic pressure do affect *left* ventricular afterload and systemic venous return into the heart, as the blood is being returned to and ejected from within the chest. However, because the pulmonary vascular bed has high capacitance, changes in RV stroke volume do not affect the LV stroke volume unless hypovolemia is present. The use of large tidal volumes (TVs) above the functional residual capacity, prolonged inspiratory times, or state of decreased vasomotor tone exaggerate this phenomenon.

Changes in TV do affect pulmonary vascular resistance. The alveolar vessels are sensitive to changes in TV and can be compressed when alveolar structures distend. This situation decreases alveolar blood and increases pulmonary vascular resistance. In addition to compressive forces, when TV or PEEP is excessive, higher alveolar pressure compared to intrapleural pressure directly causes an increase in pulmonary vascular resistance.

Acute rises in pulmonary vascular resistance impair RV ejection. Right cardiac output can be maintained by increased RV end-diastolic volume, especially with adequate volume loading (preload). Since the normal right ventricle can acutely generate up to 35 mm Hg, cor pulmonale results from acute elevation in RV afterload caused by excessive TV or PEEP. As the right ventricle fails, pulmonary venous return to the left ventricle is impaired and systemic hypotension results. This physiology is well observed in massive pulmonary embolism.

In critically ill patients with hypoxemia and pulmonary vasoconstriction, PEEP and higher TV can improve (lower) pulmonary vascular resistance by reversing hypoxic pulmonary vasoconstriction and restoring interstitial radial forces. Thus PEEP initially will improve RV cardiac output until excessive PEEP is applied.

Changes in TV (5 to 12 mL/kg) usually do not impact on RV performance if the heart is not impaired. In patients with RV ischemia and dilated cardiomyopathy, smaller changes in TV and the application of PEEP can influence cardiac output. Hemodynamic monitoring with the use of *PEEP-vs.-CI* curves and *TV-vs.-CI* curves can be a useful exercise in patients with impaired cardiac function.

Although PEEP improves oxygenation in patients with adult respiratory distress syndrome primarily through a reduction in intrapulmonary shunting as a result of redistribution of lung water from alveoli to the perivascular interstitial space, PEEP can increase right to left intracardiac shunting so that paradoxical hypoxemia can occur. In autopsy studies, 29% of the population have probe patent foramen ovale (up to 0.5 cm) and 6% have pencil patent foramen ovale (up to 1 cm), with the incidence increasing with age (12). Contrast study with agitated saline using two-dimensional transthoracic echocardiography (TTE) and especially transesophageal echocardiography (TEE) can be useful if paradoxical hypoxemia occurs.

## DIAGNOSTIC TECHNOLOGY

### The Assessment of Coronary Artery Disease: Cardiac Catheterization and Coronary Angiography

Coronary artery disease seems to be ubiquitous in our society and along with our aging population often represents a major underlying problem in the critically ill patient. The detection and identification of coronary artery disease becomes an important task in this patient population, and cardiac catheterization and coronary arteriography remain the gold standard for detecting critical coronary artery lesions. It can be safely performed in intubated patients as long as they are hemodynamically stable. In assessing coronary stenosis, the visual estimate of occlusion is still the best method of detecting potential ischemia. A reduction in *coronary flow* results in physiologic ischemia. Under resting conditions, there is no reduction in coronary flow until at least a 90% reduction in coronary diameter is reached (13). Under hyperemic states or vasodilatation (hyperemia), reduction in coronary flow occurs with less critical stenosis such as 50% to 60%. Thus, under conditions of rest in the critically ill patient, subcritical stenosis in a coronary vessel may not produce ischemia. But under stress, such as that of overwhelming sepsis or respiratory failure, subcritical stenosis can cause ischemia if the point of critical stenosis is reached.

In addition, it is important when interpreting angiograms that serial stenosis and the length of stenosis be considered. Diffusely diseased segments could represent a significant reduction in coronary flow but yet could be interpreted erroneously as noncritically disease of 50%, especially if the diseased segment is a particularly long segment (14).

Angiography is appropriate in evaluating critically ill patients who have high risk of incurring coronary disease and in patients who have rapidly evolving, life-threatening diseases with hemodynamic compromise. Often a leisurely, noninvasive approach is deleterious, exposes the patient to delayed harm, and has more long-term expense (15). Besides anatomic data, the hemodynamic information derived from cardiac catheterization can yield important clues to the critically ill patients with spells. Oximetry of the left and right sides of the heart can lead to the presence of intracardiac shunting that might be compromising oxygenation in the intubated patient with elevated right-sided heart pressures. The presence of constrictive pericarditis and restrictive cardiomyopathy manifests in the rapid filling and plateau of the RV and LV diastolic pressures. Aortic stenosis and dynamic intracavitary obstruction can be distinguished by the characteristic wave patterns of simultaneous aortic and LV pressures (16).

### Technology and Cardiac Function: Transesophageal Echocardiography and Transthoracic Echocardiography

Echocardiography is a powerful, portable, diagnostic and prognostic tool. Using high-frequency sound waves, it can image the structures of the heart and the great vessels and provide anatomic and physiologic information about myocardial performance. Because dilemmas in a critical care unit revolve around issues of hypotension and shock, echocardiography can differentiate cardiac and noncardiac causes of hypotension and provides a way to follow therapeutic interventions. In addition to anatomic information, through the use of Doppler and color flow imaging, important physiologic data about valvular and myocardial function may be obtained. Because studies can be performed at the bedside without significant risk to the patient, echocardiography is convenient, may be performed serially, and avoids the dangers of transporting critically ill patients to other departments.

In the mechanically ventilated patient or patients with chest wall trauma, TTE is unable to obtain satisfactory images. With the advent of TEE, exquisite detailed anatomy of the heart and the great vessels is available for review. With only mild sedation, TEE is a safe procedure to perform in critically ill patients with a major complication rate of less than 1 in 3,000 (17, 18). Transesophageal echocardiography is the procedure of choice in suspected aortic dissection with hemodynamic instability (19). In the critically ill hypotensive patients, TEE is probably underutilized. It provides rapid, valuable assessment of myocardial function as well as hemodynamic data (20). Volume status can be assessed from Doppler interrogation of pulmonary venous flow, and these data correlate with PCW or left atrial pressure (21, 22). Similarly, aortic and pulmonary systolic outflow velocities have the potential to correlate with thermodilution cardiac output measurements (23). Since TEE indirectly measures SV, cardiac output is calculated from the product of SV and HR (24, 25).

High-resolution images of the foramen ovale during venous phase injection of agitated saline can reveal the presence of shunts, especially in a patient with unexplained hypoxemia. Cardiac sources of emboli are readily evaluated, especially in a patient with stroke and coma (26). In the patient with a prosthetic valve and hemodynamic instability, TEE studies of the valve ring and proper function of the leaflets are critical. Ventilated brain-dead patients who are being considered for organ donation often require TEE to better evaluate cardiac status. Other applications of TEE include stress echocardiography where low-dose infusion of dobutamine can be used to assess myocardial ischemia and viability to future interventions (27).

## TECHNOLOGY AND PATHOPHYSIOLOGY

### Echocardiography and Ischemic Coronary Disease

Regional wall motion abnormalities develop in the left ventricle within seconds of coronary occlusion. The first change seen on two-dimensional echocardiography is diastolic dysfunction with bulging and thinning of the myocardium (28, 29). In a recent study of 180 patients presenting to the emergency department with chest pain, regional dysfunction on TTE identified patients with acute MI better than conventional assessment or electrocardiographic (ECG) criteria (30).

The presence of LV systolic dysfunction predicts a subset of patients that are at high risk during the hospital stay and beyond (31). One should realize, however, that regional wall motion abnormalities do not necessarily correlate with ischemic heart disease. Patients with idiopathic dilated cardiomyopathy, subarachnoid hemorrhage, and anorexia nervosa have been reported to have segmental LV wall motion abnormalities (32, 33).

Ischemic mitral regurgitation is a marker of adverse prognosis and is usually due to LV dysfunction rather than isolated papillary ischemia (34). Recognition of this entity is important because future management with angiotensin-converting enzyme (ACE) inhibitors and closer monitoring for heart failure may improve survival (35).

### The Clinical Laboratory and Ischemic Heart Disease

The patient's history is the key in suspecting ischemic heart disease and a luxury that an intensivist usually has to do without. Most episodes of myocardial ischemia occur without changes in heart rate or blood pressure and can present atypically in the critically ill and the elderly patient (36, 37). Although the mortality from heart disease is on the decline, there were over 450,000 deaths in 1990 due to primary heart disease. For acute MI, the fatality rate has declined in 6 years, from 7.7% to 5% in patients under 65 years. For patients over 65 years in 1990, the mortality from MI is still 17.6% (38). Most of the decline in mortality can be attributed to earlier detection of MI and aggressive medical therapy with successful thrombolysis reducing mortality by 25% to 50% (39). Thus early recognition of acute MI is vital for instituting prompt therapy and has been coined in the popular phrase "time is muscle."

The electrocardiogram is the foundation for diagnosing acute MI, but it is highly insensitive. Two-millimeter ST elevation in continuous anatomic leads has a sensitivity of 70% to 90% (40). However, the confounding variable is that the absence of acute ST elevation does not exclude the diagnosis of acute MI. A significant proportion of people (64%) with nonspecific ST-T changes develop MI (41). Other conditions can mimic MI even when ST elevation is present (Table 2). Computerized continuous ST-T segment monitors can detect ongoing myocardial ischemia, especially with clinically silent ischemia and in the intubated patient.

The myocardium has abundant macromolecules such as creatine kinase (CK), troponin T, and myosin light chains. Elevation in serum glutamic oxaloacetic transaminase (SGOT) was the first plasma enzymatic marker of acute MI (1954) (42). Creatine kinase isoenzymes were introduced in 1966 and have become the standard measure of MI. Creatine kinase MB is released into the circulation after 40 to 60 minutes of sustained ischemia; however, the *rate* of release is slow so that the total CK can be within the normal range for up to 8 to 10 hours. As the baseline CK levels vary among individuals, total CK-MB could double or triple without being elevated beyond statistical normals (43). Interest in rapid detection of MI has led to development of sensitive assays for CK isoforms and for troponin.

Creatine kinase MB represents 15% of all CK total in the heart (the rest being MM). Upon its release into the bloodstream, CK-MB (CK-MB$_2$) is altered to CK-MB$_1$ by lysine carboxypeptidase. Normally, these two isoforms, CK-MB$_2$ and CK-MB$_1$, are in equilibrium with each other with a ratio 1.0. With acute MI, the ratio of CK-MB$_2$ to CK-MB$_1$ increases to over 1.5, with absolute increase to greater than 1.0 IU/L. In 1110 patients, this rapid assay of (25 minutes) CK-MB subforms allowed discrimination of acute MI within 6 hours with a sensitivity of 95.7% (compared to 48% with CK-MB only in 6 hours) and a specificity of 96% (44). Most patients with acute MI had elevation in CK-MB subforms within 1.5

**TABLE 2.** *Differential of ST segment evaluation on the Electrocardiogram.*

AMI: slow ECG evolution with localization, concavity down, reciprocal ST-T changes, development of Q waves with QTc prolongation

Pericarditis: rapid ECG evolution with generalized, nonanatomic ST-T changes, concave up, with often normal QTc

LV aneurysm: chronic with no evolution, localized ST elevation with variable ST-T changes and often prolonged QTc

Vasospasm: rapid ECG evolution, localized ST-T elevation with normal Qtc

Early repolarization: variable ECG evolution with generalized ST-T changes with J-point elevation and upward concavity. T waves are often tall. QTc is normal.

Adapted from Califf RM. The diagnosis of acute myocardial infarction. *Chest* 1992;101:106S.

AMI, acute myocardial infarction; LV, left ventricular; ECG, electrocardiographic.

hours. False-positive elevations in CK-MB occur in the setting of extensive muscular damage, seizures, vigorous exercise, prostate cancer, collagen diseases, trauma to small intestines, and tongue, diaphragm, and myocarditis (Table 3).

Cardiac troponin T promises to be reliable and a more specific test for myocardial damage, especially in cases of false-positive CK-MB elevation (45). Cardiac troponin T is common for both skeletal and cardiac muscle; however, the skeletal and cardiac isoforms are encoded by different genes. Monoclonal antibodies against cardiac troponin form the basis for this assay and are commercially available (46). Cardiac troponin is released after 1 hour of coronary occlusion and remains elevated for up to 14 days and thus can be used to diagnose late MI (47).

### The Nuclear Medicine Laboratory and Diagnosis in the ICU

Technetium-99m pyrophosphate scanning can detect infarction within the 24- to 72-hour period with a sensitivity and specificity of 90%. Irreversible myocardial damage results in crystalline and subcrystalline calcium deposition, especially in the mitochondria (48). Technetium-99m pyrophosphate binds with calcium, and "hot" images are collected by planar or SPECT (single photon emission computed tomography) (49). With serial imaging, all infarcts greater than 3 g (planar) or 1 g (SPECT) of myocardium can be detected (50). After 2 to 3 days, the

**TABLE 3.** *Creatine phosphokinase (CPK) elevations.*

Total CK
  Muscular disorders
    Rhabdomyolysis
    Vigorous exercise
    Neuroleptic malignant syndrome
    Hypo- and hyperthermia
  Surgery
  Trauma
  Alcohol intoxication
  Seizures
  Pulmonary emboli
  Hypothyroidism
  Collagen vascular disorders
  Diabetes mellitus
CPK-MB
  Prostate cancer/surgery
  Uterine surgery/cancer
  Small intestine, tongue, or diaphragm trauma or surgery
  Vigorous exercise
  Cardiac surgery
  Myocarditis
  Subarachnoid hemorrhage
  Renal failure
False-negative CPK-MB
  Inadequate sampling time
  Collection time—prolonged time without processing > 1 hr

scintigram usually evolves to be negative, and the histology of older infarct (after 13 days) reveals disappearance of the crystalline mitochondrial calcium and wide zones of granulation tissue with few calcium deposits (51). In addition to detecting acute MI, technetium-99m pyrophosphate scintigraphy allows the location and sizing of the infarct. Because of the availability of serum markers and the limited time window, pyrophosphate scintigraphy is rarely used in critical practice.

Myocardial imaging with a potassium analogue, thallium-201, is useful in detecting ischemia and myocardial viability but has a limited role in detecting infarction. Thallium-201 is a monovalent cation with a half-life of 73 hours and an energy peak at the lower end of the resolution of the scintillation camera (80 keV). When injected into a patient, there is an initial uptake phase and then a continuous exchange with the blood pool that recirculates from the systemic compartment. Decreased flow to the myocardium results in initial delay in thallium uptake that is reversible when redistribution occurs. Uptake of thallium by the myocardium indicates that the region is viable. Scar or persistent filling defects usually correlate with infarction. The kinetics of thallium-201 uptake and redistribution is complex and dependent on metabolic conditions (52).

Thallium-201 imaging is probably underutilitzed in the critically ill patient. Although portable planar cameras are available, the difficulty in positioning the patient may preclude its use. In the more cooperative patient who can be transported to the nuclear medicine department, thallium scintigraphy is used to detect myocardial ischemia with a sensitivity and specificity of 90% (53). Thallium-201 coupled with pharmacologic stressors such as dipyridamole or dobutamine can be useful in differentiating chest pain and in assessing the physiologic significance of known coronary artery disease. In addition, it can serve for risk stratification for upcoming operative procedures in a patient at risk for coronary artery disease (54).

### MANAGEMENT OF CORONARY ARTERY DISEASE IN THE CRITICALLY ILL PATIENT

Since the first percutaneous transluminal coronary angioplasty (PTCA) by Gruentzig in 1977, PTCA has become an accepted modality of coronary revascularization (55). In 1992, over 325,000 procedures were performed, with a ratio of 3:2 for PTCA to coronary bypass surgery (56). In a critically ill patient with cardiogenic shock from acute MI, primary PTCA is the only modality of intervention that results in reduced mortality (57). Thrombolysis is ineffective in patients with acute MI and cardiogenic shock, with mortality approaching 80% (58). Primary angioplasty in the setting of cardiogenic shock reduces mortality from 80% to 40 (59, 60). Direct angioplasty compared to thrombolysis appears to be equally efficacious in restoring LV function and is associated with a lower rate of intracranial hemorrhage in centers that are proficient with PTCA (61). Primary PTCA was also associated with lower recurrent myocardial ischemia and higher patency than thrombolysis (62). In the 6-month follow-up of the Primary Angioplasty in Myocardial Infarction (PAMI) study, the angiographic restenosis rate was 45% with significant numbers of patients that were free from symptoms despite angiographic restenosis. Most patients with angiographic restenosis with symptoms were treated successfully with repeat PTCA (63). Logistical consideration and cost may prohibit this widespread application of primary PTCA despite its favorable outcome.

In patients with multisystem disease and in the elderly, the risks associated with coronary venous bypass grafting may be unacceptable. The elderly also have more diffuse and multivessel disease and may not be able tolerate antianginal medications. Recent data from the PTCA registries show that the elderly have 80% to 90% angiographic success rates without an excess of complications (64). In octogenarians, the 6-month restenosis rate was 31%, which is higher than in younger cohorts but acceptable given present technology (65).

High-risk PTCA has been analyzed by several centers. Ellis and colleagues retrospectively examined over 8,000 PTCA at Emory University. The primary cause of death was abrupt closure of the dilated vessel (41%), left main dissections (13%), multisystem failure after coronary venous bypass grafting (9%), and sudden cardiac death (18.8%) (66). Female gender, jeopardy score (myocardium at risk), and proximal right coronary artery dilations were independently predictive of mortality. Left ventricular ejection fraction was not, interestingly, predictive. The Mayo Clinic experience also supports that female gender, congestive heart failure, and age greater than 65 are predictors of a higher rate of abrupt closure and death (67). In nearly 9,000 patients at the Mid America Heart Institute, there was no difference in mortality in patients with LV ejection fraction less than 40% when compared to patients with LV ejection fractions greater than 40% (68).

Despite the fact that low LV ejection fraction may not be predictive of mortality, the physiologic consequence of ischemia to an already compromised heart can be devastating. Echocardiography has shown that regional hypokinesis occurs within 15 to 20 seconds of coronary occlusion and akinesis and dyskinesis occurs by 45 to 50 seconds (69). Ischemia results first in diastolic dysfunction and then in systolic dysfunction with congestive heart failure and hypotension as a result. In a compromised patient, severe angina, hypotension, malignant arrhythmias, and congestive heart failure can limit balloon angioplasty.

Intra-aortic balloon counterpulsation can limit potential adverse outcomes in patients with high-risk angioplasty and in patients with low LV ejection fraction.

Intra-aortic balloon counterpulsation has been used to support critically ill patients in cardiogenic shock, unstable angina, and perioperative LV failure. Optimizing SV and afterload results in increases in cardiac output of between 10% and 40% (70). By improving coronary blood flow in diastole, intra-aortic balloon counterpulsation may decrease the incidence of abrupt closure (71). The use of intra-aortic balloon counterpulsation is limited by vascular access and stable rhythm. It is ineffective in asystole, ventricular tachycardia, and with extremely low systemic pressures.

Percutaneous cardiopulmonary bypass support (CPS) has made PTCA available to clinically unstable patients with LV dysfunction, left main disease, and high jeopardy scores. Percutaneous cardiopulmonary bypass support system actively aspirates blood from the right atrial-inferior vena cava into an external unit that oxygenates the blood and returns it to the body in the distal aorta. Systemic perfusion of up to 5 L/min and reduction in preload occur (72). Because percutaneous cardiopulmonary bypass support requires 20 Fr vascular sheaths, it cannot be used in patients with prohibitive peripheral vascular disease. The national registry experience suggests that the use of percutaneous cardiopulmonary bypass support in PTCA of high-risk patients resulted in PTCA success in 95% with in-hospital mortality of 6% (73). Age greater than 70 years and left main disease were predictive of death. Left ventricular dysfunction was not predictive of mortality, but the prophylactic use of percutaneous cardiopulmonary bypass support in patients with LV ejection fraction less than 20% correlated with decreased mortality (74). Although percutaneous cardiopulmonary bypass support allows PTCA of left main stenosis to be feasible, it does not reduce the risk of catastrophic postprocedural closure (75). In the critically ill patient with left main disease, large myocardium at risk, or severe LV dysfunction, percutaneous cardiopulmonary bypass support may allow PTCA as a bridge to later definitive revascularization.

The proliferation of new devices and technology has expanded the scope of interventional cardiology. Despite newer devices, the success rate and restenosis rate are comparable. A lesion-specific approach is increasingly utilized (Table 4). The use of intracoronary stents is the only technology that has made an impact on restenosis, decreasing the rate from 32% to 22% (76). Because of the need for larger vascular access and mandated short-term anticoagulation, higher incidence of vascular complications (13% vs. 3%) and longer hospital stays occur in stented patients.

## MANAGEMENT OF SEPTIC SHOCK IN THE PATIENT WITH CARDIAC DYSFUNCTION

Sepsis syndrome is a multiorgan disorder with increased mortality when it progresses into shock. Acti-

**TABLE 4.** *Interventional devices for coronary revascularization: a lesion-specific approach.*

Directional coronary atherectomy—first new device for coronary revascularization after the balloon. Debulking atherosclerotic lesions, especially in eccentric lesions. Contraindications include small vessels and calcified lesions.

Percutaneous coronary rotational angioplasty (rotablator)—abrasive diamond-tipped burr welded to a long flexible drive shaft that ablates tissue. Specific use in calcified and long lesions. Effective in ostial or bifurcation lesions in reducing rate of restenosis.

Transluminal extraction-endarterectomy catheter—rotating flexible tube that has a distal wire-based motor-driven cutter that is attached to a vacuum system. Specific uses include ostial lesions, lesions with intraluminal thrombus, and degenerative saphenous graft lesions. Contraindicated in heavily calcified stenosis, eccentricity, dissections, small vessel (<2.5 mm).

Palmaz-Schatz stent—balloon-deployed stainless steel tubular mesh with midarticulation. Low initial thrombogenicity. Indication: de novo stenosis in native vessels.

Gianturco-Roubin stent—balloon-deployed monofilamentous surgical-steel-in-coil design. Indicated for acute and threatened closure.

Excimer laser angioplasty—pulsed "cold" laser that ablates tissue based on photochemical or direct bond-breaking effect. Uses limited to total occlusions and aorto-ostial stenosis.

Holmium–yttrium-aluminum-garnet laser—solid-state pulse laser based on the photochemical effect. Better with thrombus. Uses include total occlusions and balloon-resistant stenosis.

vation of pluripotent cytokines creates local and systemic cellular damage and maldistribution of blood flow with inappropriate vascular reactivity. Circulating myocardial depressant substance (MDS) (77) as well as other factors such as tumor necrosis factor alpha (78) and endothelin-1 (79) can cause direct cardiac depression. Both LV (80, 81) and RV ejection fraction (82) as measured by radionuclide cineangiography is impaired in sepsis. Ejection fraction undermines the extent of myocardial function because of compensatory increases in SV and dramatically lower afterload in septic patients. The large increase in cardiac output does not imply improved cardiac function but rather implies that the failing heart is in overtime as cardiac output is maintained at the expense of increased workload with tachycardia and larger SVs. As sepsis syndrome progresses, the hyperdynamic phase progresses to depressed cardiac index and irreversible cardiac dysfunction and intractable shock (83).

Earlier use of dobutamine in a patient with sepsis syndrome can improve cellular perfusion and reverse lactic acidosis. Especially in a patient with "normal" cardiac output, significant myocardial depression can contribute to cellular acidosis. Studies have demonstrated an improvement in tissue perfusion when dobutamine was

added to septic patients despite normal cardiac outputs (84). Especially in patients with a transiently dilated left ventricle, dobutamine's positive inotropic effect superseded its weak vasodilatory effect. Amrione has been used in septic syndrome and has resulted in improved myocardial performance. Because of its independent vasodilating capacity and potential thrombocytopenia, dobutamine is probably indicated if significant myocardial dysfunction is present. Two-dimensional transthoracic echocardiography can potentially be used to monitor the dosing of inotropes although no formal protocol studies currently exist. The early use of dobutamine may enable lower doses and rapid weaning of potent alpha pressors such as norepinephrine.

In the patient with ischemic heart disease who develops sepsis syndrome, invasive hemodynamic monitoring can guide the intensivist to optimal management. The initial lowered afterload can paradoxically improve myocardial performance in the beginning of sepsis. However, with the development of multisystem failure, often a combination of pump failure and inappropriate maldistribution of blood volume results in intractable shock. Myocardial ischemia is more of a problem as the sepsis syndrome improves and afterload normalizes. Transient hypoxemia in a patient recovering from pneumonia or adult respiratory distress syndrome can be secondary to pulmonary edema. When ischemia is suspected in a patient recovering from sepsis syndrome, early use of nitroglycerin and antiplatelet agents is warranted. When a patient is deteriorating hemodynamically or when other measures of sepsis syndrome have improved, myocardial ischemia should be suspected and imaging studies such as dobutamine stress echocardiography be considered.

Secondary correction of heart rate in the septic patient with known heart disease is often unfruitful. Despite the tremendous stress on the heart from tachycardia, the use of beta-blockers to lower heart rate can be detrimental if cardiac output is decreased. The septic heart is operating on the rightward corner of the Starling curve and is dependent on higher filling pressures (PCW) and a faster heart rate to maintain cardiac output.

As the patient recovers from sepsis syndrome and as afterload normalizes, the use of nitrovasodilators such as IV nitroglycerin can improve coronary perfusion in a patient with ischemic heart disease. In addition, if objective evidence of myocardial ischemia is found, the use of aspirin and intravenous (IV) heparin is useful, especially in the setting of positive CK-MB and non-Q MI. In patients with diabetes mellitus, episodes of ketoacidosis can be the trigger or secondary result of MI. In the patient with risk factors for coronary artery disease, it is important to not forget that the heart as the primary critical problem is resolving.

Sedation and comfort are paramount in the critically ill patient with heart disease. Mental stress has been a factor in the triggering of acute plaque rupture, coronary spasm, and abnormal coronary endothelium dependent relaxation. Fentanyl has been known to potentiate hypotension in sepsis in animals but appears to not make an impact in patients in our ICU. Fentanyl is used effectively in the cardiac catheterization laboratory during PTCA without significant hypotension. Anxiolytics such as Versed and lorazepam are used in addition. Continuous infusion of Versed appears to be well tolerated and without significant hypotension in this setting. Lorazepam as a continuous IV drip has also been used at a lower cost.

## CONCLUSIONS

Cardiopulmonary interaction is the rule rather than the exception in the modern ICU. Because the heart is a pump that resides within a larger pump, changes in intrathoracic pressures impact on preload and afterload. For the fragile heart weakened by myopathy, small changes in TV will impact on left and right ventricular filling pressures. Heart failure can be due to both preload overload but afterload mismatch as in the acutely hypertensive patients with supranormal ejection fraction.

The heart is often a target of injury in systemic illness, and myocardial dysfunction can contribute to poor oxygen delivery in the sepsis syndrome. As the elderly represent a disproportionate number of patients in the ICU, coronary artery disease is pervasive and myocardial ischemia can underlie many of the transient spells observed in patients. Advances in the diagnosis and detection of myocardial ischemia, especially with the advent of two-dimensional transthoracic and transesophageal echocardiography with sophisticated Doppler hemodynamic measurements, have enabled the heart-minded intensivist to visualize and treat the heart in distress. When obstructive coronary disease is discovered, advances in interventional cardiology have allowed critically ill patients to benefit from PTCA if coronary artery disease is hampering recovery. The heart is a resilient organ that should not be taken for granted, and further advances in cardiovascular imaging and therapeutics, such as three-dimensional echocardiography and intravascular ultrasound, will enable the intensivist to optimally manage the critically ill patient with cardiac insufficiency.

## REFERENCES

1. Parrillo JE, Parker MM, Nathanson C, et al. Septic shock in humans: advances in the understanding of pathogenesis, cardiovascular dysfunction and therapy. *Ann Intern Med* 1990;113:227.
2. Wenger NK. Cardiovascular disease in the elderly. *Curr Probl Cardiol* 1992;10:615.
3. National Center for Health Statistics. Advance report of final mortality statistics, 1988. *Monthly Vital Statistics Report* 1990;39(7, Suppl):1.
4. Minor RL, Scott BD, Winniford MD. Cocaine-induced myocardial infarction in patients with normal coronary arteries. *Ann Intern Med* 1991;115:797.
5. Lernfelt B, Wikstrand J, Svanborg A, et al. Aging and left ventricular function in elderly healthy people. *Am J Cardiol* 1988;65:1147.
6. Rodeheffer RJ, Gerstenblith G, Becker LC, et al. Exercise cardiac output is maintained with advancing age in healthy human subjects: cardiac dilation and increased stroke volume compensate for diminished heart rate. *Circulation* 1984;69:203.
7. Taegtmeyer H. Energy metabolism of the heart: from basic concepts to clinical applications. *Curr Probl Cardiol* 1994;2:54.
8. McNutt NS, Fawcett DW. Myocardial ultrastructure. In: Lauger G, Brady A, eds. *The mammalian myocardium.* New York: Wiley; 1974:1.
9. Lesch M, Taegtmeyer H, Peerson MB, Vernick R. Studies on the mechanism of the inhibition of myocardial protein synthesis during oxygen deprivation. *Am J Physiol* 1976;230:120.
10. Magid NM, Borer JS, Young MS, Wallerson DC, Demonteiro C. Suppression of protein degradation in progressive cardiac hypertrophy of chronic aortic regurgitation. *Circulation* 1993;87:1249.
11. Milic-Emili J, Mead J, Tuner JM. Improved method for assessing the validity of esophageal balloon technique. *Am Rev Respir Dis* 1982;126:5583
12. Hagen PT, Scholz D, Edwards WD. Incidence and size of patent foramen ovale during the first 10 decades of life: an autopsy study of 965 normal hearts. *Mayo Clin Proc* 1984;59:17.
13. Gould KL, Kirkeeiden RL, Buchii M. Coronary flow reserve as a physiologic measure of stenosis severity. *J Am Coll Cardiol* 1990;15:459.
14. Feldman RL, Nichols WW, Pepine CJ, Conti CR. Hemodynamic significance of the length of a coronary arterial narrowing. *Am J Cardiol* 1978;34:48.
15. Pauker SG, Kopelman RI. Invasive interventions. *N Engl J Med* 1994;331:601.
16. Kern MJ, Deligonul U. Intraventricular pressure gradients. In: Kern MJ, ed. *Hemodynamic rounds: interpretation of cardiac pathophysiology from pressure waveform analysis.* New York: Wiley-Liss; 1993:27.
17. Daniel WG, Erbel R, Kasper W, et al. Safety of transesophageal echocardiography: a multicenter survey of 10,419 examinations. *Circulation* 1993;83:817.
18. Pearson AC, Castello R, Labovitz AJ. Safety and utility of transesophageal echocardiography in the critically ill patient. *Am Heart J* 1990;119:1083.
19. Oh JK, Seward J, Khanderia B, et al. TEE in critically ill patients. *Am J Cardiol* 1990;66:1492.
20. Matsukzi M, Toma Y, Kusukawa R. Clinical applications of transesophageal echocardiography. *Circulation* 1990;82:709.
21. Kuecherer HF, Muhiudeen IA, Kusumoto FM, et al. Estimation of mean left atrial pressure from transesophageal pulsed doppler echocardiography of pulmonary venous flow. *Circulation* 1990;82:1127.
22. Rossvoll O, Hatle LK. Pulmonary venous flow velocities recorded by transthoracic doppler ultrasound: relation to left ventricular diastolic pressures. *J Am Coll Cardiol* 1993;21:1687.
23. Muhiudeeen IA, Kuecherer HF, Lee E, Cahalan MK, Schiller NB. Intraoperative estimation of cardiac output by transesophageal pulsed doppler echocardiography. *Anesthesiology* 1991;74:9.
24. Rafferty TD. Transesophageal two-dimensional echocardiography in the critically ill—Is the Swan-Ganz catheter redundant? *Yale J Biol Med* 1991;64:375.
25. Bouchard A, Blumlein S, Schiller NB, et al. Measurement of left ventricular stroke volume using continuous wave doppler echocardiography of the ascending aorta and M-mode echocardiography of the aortic valve. *J Am Coll Cardiol* 1987;9:75.
26. DeRook FA, Comes KA, Albers GW, Popp RL. Transesophageal echocardiography in the evaluation of stroke. *Ann Intern Med* 1992;117:922.
27. Baer FM, Voth E, Deutsch HJ, Schneider CA, Schicha H, Sechtem U. Assessment of viable myocardium by dobutamine transesophageal echocardiography and comparison with fluorine-18 flurodeoxyglucose positron emission tomography. *J Am Coll Cardiol* 1994;24:343.
28. Tennant R, Wiggers CJ. The effect of coronary occlusion on myocardial contraction. *Am J Physiol* 1935;112:351.
29. Pandian NG, Kerber RE. Two-dimensional echocardiography in experimental coronary stenosis: sensitivity and specificity in detecting transient myocardial dyskinesia: comparison with sonomicrometers. *Circulation* 1982;66:597.

30. Sabia P, Abbot RD, Afookteh A, et al. The importance of two-dimensional echocardiographic assessment of left ventricular systolic function in patients presenting to the emergency room with cardiac related symptoms. *Circulation* 1991;84:1615.

31. Kan G, Visser CA, Kooler JJ, Dunning AG. Short and long term predictive value of abnormal wall motion score in acute myocardial infarction: a cross sectional echocardiographic study of 345 patients. *Br Heart J* 1986;56:442.

32. Pollick C, Cuje B, Parker S, et al. Left ventricular wall motion abnormalities in subarachnoid hemorrhage: an echocardiographic study. *J Am Coll Cardiol* 1988;12:600.

33. Popp RL. Echocardiography (II of II). *N Engl J Med* 1990;323:165.

34. Kaul S, Spotnitz WD, Galsheen WP, et al. Mechanism of ischemic mitral regurgitation: an experimental evaluation. *Circulation* 1991; 84:2167.

35. Sharma SK, Seckler J, Isreael DJ, et al. Clinical, angiographic, and anatomic findings in acute severe ischemic mitral regurgitation. *Am J Cardiol* 1992;70:277.

36. Mongano DT, Browner WS, Hollenberg M, et al. Association of perioperative myocardial ischemia with cardiac morbidity and mortality in men undergoing noncardiac surgery. *N Engl J Med* 1990;323:1781.

37. Bayer AJ, Chadha J, Farag RR, et al. Changing presentation of myocardial infarction with increasing old age. *J Am Geriatr Soc* 1986;34: 263.

38. Gillum RF. Trends in acute myocardial infarction and coronary heart disease death in the United States. *J Am Coll Cardiol* 1994;23:1273.

39. Braunwald E. Myocardial reperfusion, limitation of infarct size, reduction of left ventricular dysfunction, and improved survival: Should the paradigm be expanded? *Circulation* 1989;79:441.

40. Califf RM. The diagnosis of acute myocardial infarction. *Chest* 1992; 101:106S.

41. Gibler WB, Lewis LM, Erb RE, et al. Early detection of acute myocardial infarction in patients presenting with chest pain and nondiagnostic ECGs: serial CK-MB sampling in the emergency department. *Ann Emerg Med* 1990;19:1359.

42. Sobel BE, Shell WE. Serum enzyme determinations in the diagnosis and assessment of myocardial infarction. *Circulation* 1972;45:471.

43. Roberts R, Henry PD, Witteveen SAFG, Sobel BE. Quantification of serum creatine phosphokinase (CPK) isoenzyme activity. *Am J Cardiol* 1974;33:650.

44. Puleo PR, Meyer D, Wathen C, et al. Use of rapid assay of subforms of creatine kinase MB to diagnose or rule out acute myocardial infarction. *N Engl J Med* 1994;331:561.

45. Adams JE, Bodor GS, Davila-Roman VG, et al. Cardiac Troponin I: A marker with high specificity for cardiac injury. *Circulation* 1993; 88:101.

46. Pending FDA clearance. Boehringer Mannheim Corporation.

47. Katus HA, Schefford R, Remppis A, Zehlein J. Proteins of troponin complex. *Lab Med* 1994;23:311.

48. D'Agostino AN, Chicga M. Mitochondrial mineralization in human myocardium. *Am J Clin Pathol* 1970;58:820.

49. Willerson JT. Radionuclide assessment and diagnosis of acute myocardial infarction. *Chest* 1988;93:7S.

50. Willerson JT, McGhie I, Parkey RW, Bonte FJ, Buja LM, Corbett JR. Infarct avid imaging. In: Marcus ML, Skorton DJ, Schelbert HR, Wolf GL, eds. *Cardiac imaging: a companion to Braunwald's Heart Disease.* New York: Saunders; 1991:1074.

51. Buja LM, Parkey RW, Dees JH, et al. Morphologic correlates of technetium-99m stannous pyrophosphate imaging of acute myocardial infarcts in dogs. *Circulation* 1975;52:596.

52. Beller GA. Myocardial perfusion imaging with thallium-201. In: Marcus ML, Skorton DJ, Schelbert HR, Wolf GL, eds. *Cardiac imaging: a companion to Braunwald's Heart Disease.* New York: Saunders; 1991:1047.

53. DePasquale EE,, Nody AC, Depuey EG, et al. Quantitative rotational thallium-201 tomography for identifying and localizing coronary artery disease. *Circulation* 1988;77:316.

54. Younis L, Stratmann H, Takase B, Byers S, Chaitman BR, Miller DD. Preoperative clinical assessment and dipyridamole thallium-201 scintigraphy for prediction and prevention of cardiac events in patients having major noncardiovascular surgery and known or suspected coronary artery disease. *Am J Cardiol* 1994;74:311.

55. Gruentzig AR. Transluminal dilation of coronary artery stenosis [Letter to Editor]. *Lancet* 1978;1:263.

56. Myoler RK, Stertzer SH. Coronary and peripheral angioplasty: historical perspective. In: Topol EJ, ed. *Textbook of interventional cardiology.* Philadelphia: Saunders; 1994:171.

57. Landau C, Lange RA, Hillis LD. Percutaneous transluminal coronary angioplasty. *N Engl J Med* 1994;330:981.

58. Killip T, Kimball JT. Treatment of myocardial infarction in a coronary care unit: a two year experience with 250 patients. *Am J Cardiol* 1967;20:457.

59. Hibbard MD, Holmes DR Jr, Bailey KR, et al. Percutaneous transluminal coronary angioplasty in patients with cardiogenic shock. *J Am Coll Cardiol* 1992;19:639.

60. Simari RD, Berger PB, Bell MR, Gibbons RJ, Holmes DR Jr. Coronary angioplasty in acute myocardial infarction: primary, immediate adjunctive, rescue, or deferred adjunctive approach. *Mayo Clin Proc* 1994;69:346.

61. Grines CL, Browne KF, Marco J, et al. A comparison of immediate angioplasty with thrombolytic therapy for acute myocardial infarction. *N Engl J Med* 1993;328:673.

62. Zijlstra F, de Boer MJ, Hoorntje CA, Reffer S, Reiber JHC, Suryapranata H. A comparison of immediate coronary angioplasty with intravenous streptokinase in acute myocardial infarction. *N Engl J Med* 1993;328:680.

63. Brodie BR, Grines CL, Ivanhoe R, et al. Six-month clinical and angiographic follow-up after direct angioplasty for acute myocardial infarction: final results from the primary angioplasty registry. *Circulation* 1994;25:156.

64. Kelsey SF, Miller DP, Holubkov R, et al. Results of percutaneous transluminal coronary angioplasty in patients greater than 65 years of age (from 1985 to 1986 National Heart, Lung, Blood Institute's Coronary Angioplasty Registry). *Am J Cardiol* 1990;66:1051.

65. Jackman JD, Navetta FI, Smith JE, et al. Percutaneous transluminal coronary angioplasty in octogenarians as an effective therapy for angina pectoris. *Am J Cardiol* 1991;68:116.

66. Ellis SG, Myler RF, King SB III, et al. Causes and correlates of death after unsupported coronary angioplasty: implications for use of angioplasty and advanced support techniques in high risk settings. *Am J Cardiol* 1991;68:1447.

67. Holmes DR, Holubkov R, Vlietstra RE, et al. Comparison of complications during percutaneous transluminal coronary angioplasty from 1977 to 1981 and from 1985 to 1986: the National Heart, Lung, and Blood Institute Percutaneous Transluminal Coronary Angioplasty Registry. *J Am Coll Cardiol* 1988;12:1149.

68. Stevens T, Kahn JK, McCallister BD, et al. Safety and efficacy of percutaneous transluminal coronary angioplasty in patients with left ventricular dysfunction. *Am J Cardiol* 1991;68:313.

69. Wohlgelernter D, Cleman M, Highman HA, et al. Regional myocardial dysfunction during coronary angioplasty: evaluation by two-dimension echocardiography and 12-lead electrocardiography. *J Am Coll Cardiol* 1986;7:1245.

70. Weber KT, Janicki JS. Intra-aortic balloon counterpulsation: a review of physiologic principles, clinical results, and device safety. *Ann Thorac Surg* 1974;17:602.

71. Kern MT. Intra-aortic balloon pumping post angioplasty: documentation of increased coronary blood flow. *Cardiac Assists* 1992;6:1.

72. Mooney MR, Mooney JF, Mathias DW, et al. Clinical applications of percutaneous cardiopulmonary bypass for high risk coronary angioplasty. *J Invest Cardiol* 1990;2:161.

73. Vogel RA. Initial report of the national registry of elective cardiopulmonary bypass supported coronary angioplasty. *J Am Coll Cardiol* 1990;15:23.

74. Vogel RA. Femorofemoral cardiopulmonary bypass support during high-risk coronary angioplasty. *Learning Center Highlights (Am Coll Cardiol)* 1992;8:19.

75. Tommaso CL, Vogel JHK, Vogel RA. Coronary angioplasty in high-risk patients with left main stenosis: results from the Nanal Registry of Elective Supported Angioplasty. *Cathet Cardiovasc Diagn* 1992; 15;169.

76. Serruys PW, de Jaegere P, Kiemeneij F, et al. A comparison of balloon-expandable-stent implantation with balloon angioplasty in patients with coronary artery disease. *N Engl J Med* 1994;331:489.

77. Reilly JM, Cunnion RE, Burch-Whitman C, Parker MM, Shelhammer JH, Parrillo JE. A circulating myocardial substance is associated with cardiac dysfunction and peripheral hypoperfusion (lactic acidemia) in patients with septic shock. *Chest* 1989;95:1072.

78. Michie HR, Manogue SR, Spriggs M, et al. Detection of circulating tumor necrosis factor after endotoxin administration. *N Engl J Med* 1988;318:1481.

79. Han JJ, Windsor A, Drenning DH, et al. Release of endothelin in relation to tumor necrosis factor-alpha in porcine *Pseudomonas aeruginosa*-induced septic shock. *Shock* 1994;1:343.

80. Parker MM, Shelhamer JH, Bacharach S, et al. Profound but reversible myocardial depression in patients with septic shock. *Ann Intern Med* 1984;100:483.

81. Parker MM, Suffredinid AF, Nathanason C, Ognibene FP, Shelhamer JH, Parrillo JE. Response of left ventricular function in survivors and nonsurvivors of septic shock. *J Crit Care* 1989;4:19.

82. Parker MM, McCarthy KE, Ognibene FP, Parrillo JE. Right ventricular dysfunction and dilation, similar to left ventricular changes, characterize the cardiac depression of septic shock in humans. *Chest* 1990;97:126.

83. Abel F. Myocardial function in sepsis and endotoxin shock. *Am J Physiol* 1989;257:R1265.

84. Vincent JL, Roman A, Kahn RJ. Dobutamine administration in septic shock: addition to a standard protocol. *Crit Care Med* 1990;18:689.

*The Critically Ill Cardiac Patient,*
edited by V. Kvetan and D. R. Dantzker,
Lippincott-Raven Publishers, Philadelphia © 1996.

CHAPTER 2

# The High-Risk Cardiac Patient for Noncardiac Surgery

Sumita D. Paul and Kim A. Eagle

In the United States alone, over 25 million patients undergo noncardiac surgery each year (1). With the significant strides made toward perfecting surgical and anesthetic techniques over the past several decades, the major cause of morbidity and mortality after noncardiac surgery now relates to cardiac complications (1, 2). Patients with preexistent cardiac disease are more likely to develop cardiac complications after noncardiac surgery (3–7). Although much has been written about the cardiac assessment of patients approaching noncardiac surgery (3–5, 8–11), the management strategies available for successfully taking a high-risk cardiac patient through noncardiac surgery have not been formally reviewed in most texts. In this chapter, we will address the specific problems and complications which the clinician must consider as well as the management of high-risk cardiac patients in an attempt to prevent or minimize early and late cardiac complications after surgery.

## IDENTIFICATION OF THE HIGH-RISK CARDIAC PATIENT

### Clinical Evaluation

In many critically ill patients the recognition that they are high-risk candidates for any type of noncardiac surgery is not difficult. This includes patients with symptomatic arrhythmias or hypotension and those with recent myocardial infarction, unstable angina, pulmonary edema, uncontrolled hypertension, or ongoing chest pain at rest. This "obvious" high-risk group also

S. D. Paul: Department of Medicine, Harvard University and Massachusetts General Hospital, Boston, Massachusetts 02115.

K. A. Eagle: Department of Internal Medicine, University of Michigan Medical Center, Ann Arbor, Michigan 48103.

includes patients with symptomatic left ventricular dysfunction or cardiomyopathy.

However, in the "not so obvious" case in which the patient is hemodynamically stable and awaiting elective noncardiac surgery, we would recommend the use of the stepwise strategy presented in Fig. 1. The first step is to determine whether the patient has had a prior coronary revascularization. If the answer to this question is yes and the patient has not experienced recurrent symptoms, no further work-up is necessary to assess the risk of inducible ischemia. This strategy is based on evidence provided later in Table 6 and described in the ensuing sections under "Role of Noninvasive Testing to Identify the High-Risk Patient" and under "Prophylactic Revascularization."

If the patient has not had a prior revascularization, the second step is to determine whether the patient has undergone an adequate coronary evaluation in the previous 2 years with negative results. Unless the patient has recurrent symptoms, there is no need to repeat the coronary evaluation. However, if the patient has not had an adequate study in the previous 2 years, one can often identify high-risk patients by simple clinical evaluation which forms step 3 of our stepwise strategy.

Goldman and colleagues (8, 9) have developed a clinical index (Tables 1 and 2) which can be used for preoperative assessment. Based on stepwise linear discriminant analysis, they assigned relative weights to clinical variables which were identified as independent predictors of cardiac complications after noncardiac surgery. Thus, by performing a detailed clinical evaluation, the Goldman index score can be calculated for each patient. Based on the total score, patients were divided into four prognostic classes with increasing gradient of risk for cardiac events with an increasing score. Patients with a score of at least 26 are classified in the high-risk category. In this high-risk group 22% of patients have nonfatal but life-threatening complications and 56% have cardiac death. Although the

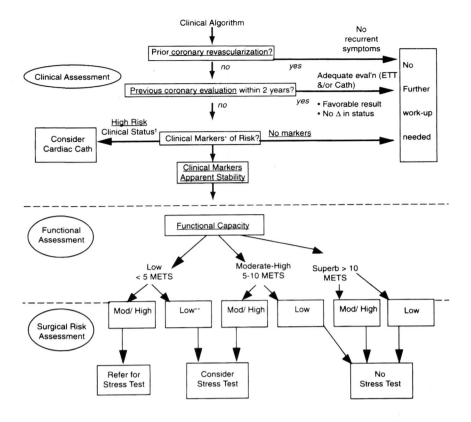

**FIG. 1.** Strategy for preoperative risk assessment for patients undergoing noncardiac surgery: (+) angina, myocardial infarction (MI) by history or electrocardiogram (ECG) (Q waves), congestive heart failure (CHF) [or ventricular tachycardia (VT)], diabetes mellitus; (†) uncontrolled angina, uncontrolled CHF, angina or CHF after recent MI; (°) moderate- or high-risk surgery—vascular, thoracic, major abdominal, orthopedic; (++) low-risk surgery—head and neck, eye, prostate, hernia, breast. Reproduced, with permission, from Paul SD, Eagle KA. *Med Clin North Am* 1995;79 (5).

Goldman index was extremely important in shaping our assessment of preoperative risk, of the 1,001 patients in the study cohort used to derive this index, only 18 were in the high-risk group. In addition, the cumbersome scoring system made this index difficult for clinicians to use routinely. Furthermore, this index surprisingly did not include variables such as angina or a history of congestive heart failure.

In an attempt to validate the Goldman index and also improve on its shortcomings, Detsky and colleagues (10, 11) modified the original index to include angina, alveolar pulmonary edema, and proximity in duration of the episode of heart failure to surgery, in addition to simplifying the scoring system by converting it into multiples of 5 (Table 3). Similar to the Goldman index, patients could be classified into risk classes with increasing likelihood ratios for developing cardiac events with increasing total score (Table 4). Thus, patients with a score greater than 30 would be classified into the high-risk group (class III) and have a likelihood ratio of developing a cardiac event of nearly 15. However, both the Goldman and the modified Goldman indices were found to have a low sensitivity for identifying high-risk patients within those classified into the intermediate-risk category, especially for elderly patients or those undergoing vascular surgery (12, 13).

More recently, Eagle and colleagues (4) have described a simple clinical index that can be used for preoperative assessment of patients undergoing vascular surgery. Fea-

tures comprising this index include age over 70 years, history of angina, myocardial infarction by history or electrocardiogram (Q waves), congestive heart failure, and diabetes mellitus. Patients who have one or two of these markers are classified in the intermediate-risk group and have been found to benefit from further risk stratification by dipyridamole stress testing with perfusion imaging. Patients classified in the intermediate clinical risk group who had reversible defects had a tenfold higher risk of cardiac complications after vascular surgery when compared to patients without such thallium defects. On the other hand, patients with more than two markers on the preoperative clinical index were classified in the high-risk category. These patients may or may not need further risk stratification by non-invasive testing to assess for ischemic risk. Some patients have such a positive clinical profile and a high likelihood of inducible ischemia that stress testing in such patients may be unnecessary. Such patients were found to have a postoperative cardiac event rate as high as 50%. The use of this index has been validated not only in patients undergoing vascular surgery but also in patients undergoing nonvascular surgery (5).

Based on data obtained by Hertzer and colleagues in a consecutive series of patients undergoing vascular surgery at the Cleveland Clinic Foundation, we have recently described a concordance of risk defined clinically (by the clinical index described by Eagle and colleagues) and angiographic coronary stenosis (14). As shown in Fig. 2,

**TABLE 1.** *The Goldman Multifactorial Cardiac Risk Index*

| Criteria | Points |
|---|---|
| **History** | |
| Age > 70 years | 5 |
| MI in previous 6 months | 10 |
| **Physical examination** | |
| $S_3$ gallop or JVD | 11 |
| Important valvular aortic stenosis | 3 |
| **Electrocardiogram** | |
| Rhythm other than sinus or PAC's on last preoperative ECG | 7 |
| > 5 PVC's/min documented at any time before operation | 7 |
| **General status** | |
| $Po_2 < 60$ or $Pco_2 > 50$ mm Hg, K < 3.0 or $HCO_3 < 20$ mEq/L, BUN > 50 or creatinine > 3.0 mg/dL, abnormal SGOT, signs of chronic liver disease, patient bed ridden from noncardiac causes | 3 |
| **Operation** | |
| Intraperitoneal, intrathoracic, or aortic operation | 3 |
| Emergency operation | 4 |
| Total | 53 |

From Goldman L, et al. *N Engl J Med* 1977;297:845, with permission.

MI, myocardial infarction; JVD, jugular vein distention; PAC's, premature atrial contractions; ECG, electrocardiogram; PVC's, premature ventricular contractions; $Po_2$, partial pressure of oxygen; $Pco_2$, partial pressure of carbon dioxide; K, potassium; $HCO_3$, bicarbonate; BUN, blood urea nitrogen; SGOT, serum glutamic oxalacetic transaminase.

there is an increasing gradient in risk for severe coronary stenosis with increasing number of clinical markers. For left main stenosis, the frequency increases from 4% to 14% depending on the presence of zero (low clinical risk) or more than two clinical predictors (high clinical risk), respectively (clinical predictors include age $\geq$ 70 years, prior angina, prior myocardial infarction, history of congestive heart failure, or diabetes mellitus).

### Role of Noninvasive Testing to Identify the High-Risk Patient

We have previously suggested that those patients who can be readily classified in the high-risk group based on clinical evaluation alone may not need stress testing. However, patients with a poor functional capacity (Table 5) may benefit from preoperative testing to determine if they have inducible ischemia even though they may only have a single clinical marker.

Those who have had a prior coronary artery bypass procedure and no recurrence of ischemic symptoms are in a group by themselves. Since they have been revascularized, they usually do not need further testing if they have a good functional capacity and no recurrence of ischemic symptoms. In a retrospective analysis of postoperative cardiac events among 567 patients undergoing vascular surgery (15), we have found that only one patient of the 68 (1.5%) who had a prior coronary bypass had a postoperative cardiac event, compared to 45 patients out of the 499 (9%) without prior coronary bypass. In addition, as shown in Fig. 3, when patients were classified based on the number of clinical markers (including a history of angina, myocardial infarction, Q waves on the electrocardiogram, or a history of congestive heart failure), an increasing gradient of risk for cardiac events was seen with increasing number of clinical markers only in the group without a prior coronary bypass (5% in those with no clinical markers vs. 27% in those with all four clinical markers, $p < 0.0003$). No such gradient of risk for cardiac events was seen with increasing number of clinical markers in the group of patients who had a prior coronary bypass.

Although prior coronary bypass appears to confer protection against postoperative cardiac events, we recommend noninvasive evaluation for patients who have recurrence of symptoms. In addition, those who had their bypass surgery more than 5 or 10 years prior to the present evaluation may need to undergo stress testing to rule out inducible ischemia.

### Exercise Stress Testing with and without Perfusion Imaging

The presence of exercise-induced ischemia and poor functional capacity as assessed by exercise testing has been found to be useful for preoperative risk stratification of patients undergoing vascular surgery (Table 6) (12, 16–24). Patients who are unable to attain a reasonable workload with achievement of 75% or 85% of predicted maximum heart rate have a higher complication rate in the postoperative period. This is especially true for patients with inducible ischemia at a low workload. Furthermore, the addition of ventricular imaging helps, not

**TABLE 2.** *The Goldman Risk Groups*

| Risk group | Number of patients | Goldman score | Life-threatening complications (non-fatal) | Cardiac death |
|---|---|---|---|---|
| I | 537 | 0–5 | 4 (0.7%) | 1 (0.2%) |
| II | 316 | 6–12 | 16 (5%) | 5 (2%) |
| III | 130 | 13–25 | 15 (11%) | 3 (2%) |
| IV | 18 | ≥26 | 4 (22%) | 10 (56%) |

Adapted, with permission, from Goldman L, et al. *N Engl J Med* 1977;297:845.

**TABLE 3.** *The modified multifactorial cardiac risk index*

| Variables | Risk points |
|---|---|
| Coronary artery disease | |
| MI within 6 months | 10 |
| History of MI > 6 months back | 5 |
| Angina (Canadian Cardiovascular Society) | |
| Class 3 | 10 |
| Class 4 | 20 |
| Unstable angina within 3 months | 10 |
| Alveolar pulmonary edema | |
| Within 1 week | 10 |
| Ever | 5 |
| Valvular disease | |
| Suspected critical aortic stenosis | 20 |
| Arrhythmias | |
| Atrial premature beats or rhythm other than sinus on last preoperative ECG | 5 |
| > 5 ventricular premature beats at any time before surgery | 5 |
| Poor general medical status[a] | 5 |
| Age > 70 years | 5 |
| Emergency operation | 10 |

Adapted, with permission, from Detsky AS, et al. *J Gen Intern Med* 1986;1:211; and Detsky AS, et al. *Arch Intern Med* 1986;146:2131.

[a]Oxygen pressure < 60 mm Hg; carbon dioxide pressure > 50 mm Hg; serum potassium < 3.0 mEq/L (<3.0 mmol/L); serum bicarbonate < 20 mEq/L (20 mmol/L); serum urea nitrogen > 50 mg/dL (>18 mmol/L); serum creatine > 3 mg/dL (>260 mmol/L); aspartate aminotransferase abnormal; signs of chronic liver disease; and/or bedridden because of noncardiac causes.

only by improving the sensitivity of the test for identifying patients who are likely to develop cardiac complications, but also by enabling the quantitation of the amount of myocardium at risk based upon the extent of the perfusion defects.

Although numerous studies have suggested that exercise testing may be a valuable noninvasive modality for preoperative risk assessment (Table 6), this may not be a feasible option for the critically ill patient or a patient with comor-

**TABLE 4.** *The risk groups for the modified multifactorial cardiac risk index*

| Risk class | Total risk points on preoperative assessment | Likelihood ratios of cardiac event |
|---|---|---|
| I | 0–15 | 0.42 |
| II | 16–30 | 3.58 |
| III | > 30 | 14.93 |

Adapted, with permission, from Detsky AS, et al. *J Gen Intern Med* 1986;1:211; and Detsky AS, et al. *Arch Intern Med* 1986;146:2131.

By using the pretest probability of cardiac complications for each major surgery, the modified Goldman index helps to determine the probability of a cardiac event for each risk score stratum, based on Bayesian analysis, by using the likelihood ratios for each stratum.

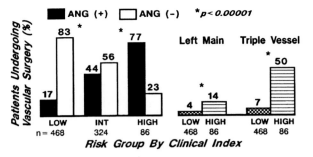

**FIG. 2.** Concordance of clinical risk with coronary angiography in patients undergoing vascular surgery. Ang (+) refers to the presence of stenoses identified by coronary angiography, defined as triple vessel (≥50% stenosis in each vessel), two vessel (≥50% stenosis in one vessel when the other is ≥70% stenosis of the left anterior descending), or left main disease (≥50% stenosis). From Paul SD, et al. *Circulation* 1994;90(1):95A. Copyright 1994 American Heart Association; with permission.

bid illnesses which preclude exercising. This has been a major factor in the development and widespread use of pharmacologic stress testing with perfusion imaging.

## Pharmacologic Stress Testing with Perfusion Imaging

Boucher and colleagues (25) were the first to define the utility of dipyridamole-thallium imaging for preoperative risk assessment. Since their original study, many studies have confirmed the value of preoperative dipyri-

**TABLE 5.** *Specific activity scale*

| Class | Patient can perform to completion |
|---|---|
| I | Activity requiring ≥ 7 METS[a]<br>Carry 24 lb up 8 steps<br>Carry objects that weigh 80 lbs<br>Outdoor work (shovel snow, spade soil)<br>Recreation (ski, basketball, squash, handball, jog/walk 5 mph) |
| II | Activity requiring ≥5 (but not ≥7) METS:<br>Have sexual intercourse without stopping<br>Walk at 4 mph on level ground<br>Outdoor work (garden, rake, weed)<br>Recreation (roller skate, dance fox trot) |
| III | Activity requiring ≥2 (but not ≥5) METS:<br>Shower/dress without stopping, strip and make bed<br>Walk at 2.5 mph on level ground<br>Outdoor work (clean windows)<br>Recreation (play golf, bowl) |
| IV | No activity requiring ≥2 METS (cannot carry out activities listed above) |

Adapted, with permission, from Goldman L, et al. *Circulation* 1981;64:1227.

[a]Metabolic equivalents.

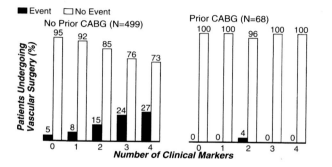

**FIG. 3.** Study of 68 patients with prior coronary artery bypass grafting (CABG) and 499 without prior CABG who underwent vascular surgery. From Paul SD, et al. *J Am Coll Cardiol* 1994;1A:484A. Reprinted with permission from the American College of Cardiology.

damole-thallium testing for predicting postoperative cardiac complications (3, 4, 26, 27). Although initial studies identified reversible defects to be associated with an increased risk of postoperative cardiac events, subsequent studies also identified fixed defects to have prognostic value, especially for long-term risk prediction (5, 28–30). In addition, semiquantitation of dipyridamole-thallium scanning has been found to be more useful since increasing numbers of regions of perfusion defects were associated with an increasing gradient of risk for cardiac complications (31, 32).

### Pharmacologic Stress Testing with Echocardiography

Another modality for preoperative assessment of cardiac risk is the stress echocardiography. More recently, dobutamine has become the most widely used pharmacologic agent for stress echocardiography. The identification

of regional wall motion abnormalities or loss of myocardial thickening after dobutamine infusion has been found be valuable for predicting both postoperative and late cardiac complications after noncardiac surgery (33–38).

The advantage of stress echocardiography when compared to perfusion imaging is its ability to assess for valvular abnormalities (including ischemic mitral regurgitation) and left ventricular dysfunction. In addition, this modality of stress testing may be preferred over dipyridamole-thallium imaging in patients with bronchospasm because of dipyridamole's potential to induce bronchospasm. Furthermore, since dipyridamole induces hypotension, it may be less desirable to use dipyridamole stress testing with thallium imaging in patients with critical carotid stenosis. In such circumstances, dobutamine stress echocardiography may be the preferred modality for determining the presence of inducible ischemia.

However, in patients who have had a previous infarct, it may be a challenge to distinguish resting wall motion abnormalities due to scar tissue from those resulting from ischemia. Other technical difficulties with echocardiographic imaging include patients with poor transducer access "windows" due to narrow intercostal space, pectus excavatum, or lung disease. Furthermore, in those with a predisposition to life-threatening arrhythmias, it may be prudent to avoid dobutamine infusion. Since institutions generally vary with regard to their experience in stress echocardiography vs. nuclear scanning, we generally recommend the use of the stress testing modality with which the institution has the most experience.

### Role of Coronary Angiography to Identify the High-Risk Patient

Patients at high clinical risk should be considered for coronary angiography on an individual basis. Depending

**TABLE 6.** *Impact of poor functional capacity on perioperative cardiac risk*

| Type of exercise test | Type of surgery | Number of patients | Exercise level achieved | Frequency of cardiac events | Reference |
|---|---|---|---|---|---|
| ETT | Peripheral vascular | 130 | >75% PMHR no ischemia | 0 of 35 | 17 |
| | | | >75% PMHR with ischemia | 6 of 23 (no deaths) | |
| | | | <75% PMHR with ischemia | 10 of 26 (5 deaths) | |
| ETT or arm ergometry | Peripheral vascular | 101 | >85% PMHR | 2 of 30 | 19 |
| | | | <85% PMHR | 17 of 70 | |
| | | | <85% PMHR with ischemia | 7 of 21 | |
| ETT or bicycle or arm ergometry | Abdominal or thoracic or vascular | 200 | >5 METS | 1 of 92 | 18 |
| | | | <5 METS | 5 of 106 | |
| Ex RNA | Abdominal or thoracic | 155 | HR > 100 and ED > 2 min | 4 of 84 | 12 |
| | | | HR < 100 and ED < 2 min | 19 of 61 | |
| Ex RNA | Peripheral vascular | 110 | >5 METS | 0 of 47 | 103 |
| | | | <5 METS | 8 of 63 (5 deaths) | |

Reprinted, with permission, from Abraham SA, et al. *Prog Cardiovasc Dis* 1991;34:205.
ETT, exercise treadmill test with electrocardiographic monitoring; PMHR, predicted maximal heart rate with vigorous exercise; Ex RNA, exercise radionuclide angiography with electrocardiographic monitoring; HR, heart rate; ED, exercise duration.

upon whether patients are good coronary revascularization candidates based on comorbid illnesses, selected patients may benefit from preoperative coronary revascularization. However, it needs to be emphasized that there are no randomized trials which prove that prophylactic coronary revascularization can reduce the subsequent risk for coronary complications for patients undergoing noncardiac surgery. This is especially true for elderly patients in whom the risk of coronary artery bypass grafting (CABG) is significant (39, 40) and one can argue that this risk may equal or exceed the risk of noncardiac surgery. Coronary artery bypass grafting may be justified in some individuals for its protective effect against long-term cardiac complications such as those with left main stenosis or three-vessel disease (41, 42). The justification for such an aggressive approach in certain selected high-risk patients is more evident in the discussions given in the ensuing sections of this chapter.

### Role of Transesophageal Echocardiography During Surgery

This has been suggested to be a useful monitoring device for the critically ill cardiac patient during noncardiac surgery (43). Since transesophageal echocardiography allows for an excellent view of the left ventricle, preliminary reports have suggested that it is very sensitive for identifying wall motion abnormalities (including hypokinesis, akinesis, or dyskinesis) suggestive of ischemia during surgery.

However, Eisenberg and colleagues (44), in their study of 332 male veterans undergoing noncardiac surgery, found that this technique is associated with a poor specificity for identifying those who are unlikely to suffer a postoperative ischemic event. Of the 321 patients who did not develop a postoperative cardiac event, 50 were found to have intraoperative "ischemia" identified by transesophageal echocardiography. With the additional consideration of the technical difficulty of performing the test as well as the added expense, the role of transesophageal echocardiography during noncardiac surgery is not entirely clear.

## PERIOPERATIVE MANAGEMENT OF THE HIGH-RISK CARDIAC PATIENT: PREOPERATIVE STRATEGIES

### General Measures

In addition to maintaining hemodynamic stability prior to noncardiac surgery, it is extremely important to address issues related to comorbid illnesses which may have an impact on increasing the likelihood of developing cardiac complications after surgery. Such factors include electrolyte imbalances predisposing to arrhythmias and renal insufficiency which may predispose to perioperative volume overload. It is helpful to maintain a reasonable hematocrit (usually ≥30) for cardiac patients undergoing noncardiac surgery, in order to minimize supply-demand imbalances.

Also, careful management of diabetes, thyroid disease, and respiratory disease is particularly important for the critically ill patient approaching noncardiac surgery. For cardiac patients who are intubated, it may be prudent to delay ventilator weaning until several days after noncardiac surgery to minimize the workload on the heart prior to and immediately after surgery.

### Medications

Cardiac medications also need to be carefully evaluated prior to noncardiac surgery. It is routine practice to discontinue aspirin 4 days prior to noncardiac surgery. Oral anticoagulants are also discontinued several days prior to surgery. Patients who are at high risk for thromboembolism with discontinuation of anticoagulants should be placed on intravenous heparin as their prothrombin times decline after discontinuation of oral anticoagulants. Intravenous heparin can be discontinued several hours prior to noncardiac surgery. If the prothrombin time remains elevated, fresh frozen plasma may be used. The use of vitamin K may result in a protracted postoperative period to reachieve adequate oral anticoagulation.

The management of patients on beta-blockers deserves a special mention. The abrupt withdrawal of beta-blockers may precipitate a sympathetic nervous system rebound with increased workload on the heart leading to myocardial ischemia and infarction. This can be particularly important in the perioperative setting since postoperative catecholamine surges are routine after major surgery (45–52). In fact, several studies have found that patients on beta-blockers have significantly fewer cardiac ischemic complications after noncardiac surgery (53–55). In addition, the use of beta-blockers was found to be safe with no significant increase in the occurrence of hypotension or bradycardia during the perioperative period. For the high-risk cardiac patient who is not already on beta-blockers, we would recommend initiating beta-blocker therapy unless otherwise contraindicated. This can be started with metoprolol at 25 mg given twice a day and continued on the morning of surgery and during the postoperative period. There are no convincing data regarding the role of prophylactic use of nitroglycerine or calcium channel blockers during the perioperative period. However, it is self-evident that if patients have required nitrates or calcium channel blockers to control ischemic symptoms in the recent past, these should be carefully maintained in the perioperative period when myocardial ischemia is especially common.

Other medications which need to be continued in the perioperative period include antihypertensive medications and digitalis (particularly if the patient has atrial fibrillation or congestive heart failure). However, Rauwolfia alkaloids should be discontinued prior to surgery since they may potentiate the effects of preoperative medications. In addition, in patients without a clear indication for digitalis, this should be discontinued prior to surgery. Furthermore, when possible, diuretics should also be discontinued at least 1 day prior to surgery since severe diuresis can predispose to hypovolemia and hypotension during anaesthesia. Furthermore, electrolyte imbalances associated with diuretic therapy may predispose patients to developing arrhythmias.

## Cardiac Arrhythmias

The management of patients with cardiac arrhythmias deserves special consideration. In addition to ensuring the aggressive management of electrolyte imbalances, it is important to ensure adequate rate control for those with tachyarrhythmias. Patients with atrial fibrillation may benefit from digitalization and, if necessary, the use of beta-blockers to ensure adequate rate control. For those who have recent-onset atrial fibrillation and underlying poor left ventricular function, an attempt to establish sinus rhythm seems reasonable since the contribution of the left atrium to the cardiac output may be significant for such patients. Either quinidine/procainamide or electric cardioversion may be attempted. Cardioversion may be preferred for those with a rapid ventricular response.

For patients with nonsustained ventricular tachycardia, there is no evidence to suggest that treating such episodes has any impact on subsequent prognosis. Sustained ventricular tachycardia, however, needs to be treated with agents such as lidocaine. Since ischemia may be an important cause for such arrhythmias, a careful evaluation including coronary angiography and/or electrophysiologic testing in selected patients is necessary before such patients proceed to noncardiac surgery.

Patients with bradyarrhythmias also deserve careful evaluation prior to noncardiac surgery. Often the bradycardia may be precipitated by atrioventricular (AV) nodal blocking agents given to the patients, and this should be the first thing to rule out in any such situation. In the presence of high-grade AV block, it may be prudent to place a prophylactic temporary wire to tide the patient over an urgent noncardiac surgery with a subsequent evaluation for the need for a permanent pacer after surgery.

## Prophylactic Revascularization

As displayed in Table 7, several studies have found that patients who have had a prior coronary bypass have a better cardiac prognosis after noncardiac surgery, by both lower rates of postoperative cardiac complications and greater event-free survival rates. However, with the absence of data from randomized trials, each case merits individual consideration based on whether the patient is otherwise a candidate for undergoing major cardiac surgery, as well as the risk of the proposed noncardiac surgery, in addition to the relative urgency of the noncardiac surgery. Among patients enrolled in the Coronary Artery Surgery Study (CASS) registry (56), patients who received medical therapy and subsequently required noncardiac surgery had a mortality rate of 2.4%, compared to a mortality of 0.9% among those who underwent CABG prior to noncardiac surgery.

The role of prophylactic coronary angioplasty prior to noncardiac surgery is still unclear. The three studies that have examined this have been retrospective and have not demonstrated significant reductions in postoperative cardiac events (57–59). Huber and colleagues (57), in their study of 55 patients with severe coronary disease undergoing coronary angioplasty prior to noncardiac surgery, found that in this small cohort 9% required emergent coronary bypass surgery after unsuccessful coronary

**TABLE 7.** *Impact of prior coronary bypass surgery on early and late death after noncardiac surgery*

| Total sample size | Prior coronary artery bypass graft | Postoperative death (%) | Late death (%) | Reference |
|---|---|---|---|---|
| 251[a] | Yes: 216 (CABG mortality 5.5%) | 2 | 12 | 7, 105 |
| | No: 35 | 12 | 26 | |
| 14,180 | Yes: 1,237 | 1.5 | 21 | 56 |
| | No: 1,337 (patients with CAD) | 6.8 | 41 | |
| | No: 1,782 (patients without evidence of CAD) | 1.3 | 20 | |
| 1093 | Yes: 255 simultaneous with vascular surgery | 4 | — | 106 |
| | Yes: 279 during same admission as vascular surgery | 4 | | |
| | Yes: 559 had preoperative CABG, then vascular surgery on separate admission | 0.2 | | |
| 42 | Yes: 20[b] (7–10 days preoperatively) | None | — | 107 |

Reproduced, with permission, from Paul SD, Eagle KA. *Med Clin North Am* 1995;79(5).
[a]Number of patients with severe, correctable CAD.
[b]Number of patients with triple-vessel disease or left main disease.
CABG, coronary artery bypass grafting; CAD, coronary artery disease.

angioplasty. Among the 50 patients who underwent successful coronary angioplasty, 3 patients suffered an acute myocardial infarction in the postoperative period and 1 patient died. In another study from the Mayo Clinic, Elmore and colleagues (58) examined 2,452 patients who underwent abdominal aortic aneurysmorrhaphy between 1980 and 1990 and identified 14 patients who had undergone preoperative coronary angioplasty and 86 who had a previous coronary bypass. Although the perioperative mortality was zero in the coronary angioplasty group and 5.8% in the coronary bypass group, late cardiac events occurred in 57% of patients in the coronary angioplasty group vs. 27% in the coronary bypass group.

In yet another study involving 110 patients who underwent coronary angioplasty prior to major vascular surgery (59), 3 patients went on to get emergent coronary bypass surgery because of an unsuccessful attempt at coronary angioplasty and 4 patients had a procedure-related non-Q-wave infarction. In addition, 3 patients went on to have a postoperative nonfatal myocardial infarction and 1 patient died after surgery. Thus, further study is needed to determine if coronary angioplasty is indeed protective against the development of postoperative or long-term cardiac events in patients with coronary artery disease.

## Prophylactic Use of Intra-aortic Balloon Pumps

Intra-aortic balloon pumps (IABPs) are often used prophylactically in critically ill patients with coronary disease (60–63) who are undergoing CABG to facilitate weaning off cardiopulmonary bypass and to improve perioperative coronary perfusion. There are case reports of similar use of the IABP prior to urgent noncardiac surgery in high-risk cardiac patients (64, 65). The potential for reducing fatal postoperative cardiac events by using the IABP needs to be weighed against the potential for serious vascular complications. Thus, further study is needed before this can be considered as the routine clinical practice for the high-risk cardiac patient approaching noncardiac surgery.

## Patients with Aortic Valvular Disease

Severe aortic stenosis has been described by Goldman and colleagues (8, 9) to be a major risk factor for developing postoperative cardiac complications in patients undergoing noncardiac surgery. In addition, Skinner and Pierce (66) have described a 25% mortality rate in a small cohort of patients with aortic stenosis who underwent intrathoracic or intra-abdominal surgery. Prophylactic correction of symptomatic aortic stenosis has been recommended prior to noncardiac surgery. However, determining whether severe aortic stenosis is in fact symptomatic is difficult in the elderly patient with severe comorbid illnesses. Furthermore, the high operative mortality rate for aortic valve replacement in this cohort must be considered.

In a retrospective study of patients with aortic stenosis undergoing noncardiac surgery at the Mayo Clinic, there were no perioperative cardiac deaths (67). In this study, O'Keefe and colleagues examined a cohort of 48 patients with moderate or severe aortic stenosis, defined as a peak instantaneous Doppler-derived aortic valve gradient of 3.5 to 4.4 and ≥4.5 m/s, respectively, or an aortic valve area of 0.76 to 0.99 and ≤0.75 cm², respectively. It is important to note that while all patients had either advanced valve gradients or significantly low valve areas, they did not have advanced symptoms.

In contrast, in a study by Roth, Palacios, and Block (68), percutaneous aortic balloon valvuloplasty was found to be useful in symptomatic patients with critical aortic stenosis prior to noncardiac surgery. Others have shown similar benefits (69, 70). We generally recommend aortic valve replacement for the young patient with symptomatic disease. Valvuloplasty may be indicated for the elderly patient with severe comorbid illnesses which preclude valve replacement. For patients with good functional capacity who have mild or asymptomatic valvular disease, we generally recommend the use of the pulmonary arterial line to carefully monitor hemodynamics during and immediately after surgery. Maintenance of adequate preload and avoidance of hypotension are especially important.

Particular vigilance is also needed for patients with aortic regurgitation since they are extremely sensitive to bradycardia and vasodilation (71). The optimal heart rate for such patients during surgery is 80 to 100, and when possible, bradycardia should be prevented. Careful use of sodium nitroprusside or angiotensin-converting enzyme inhibitors along with monitoring of the pulmonary capillary wedge pressure may be helpful in improving stroke volume and decreasing left ventricular end-diastolic volume and pressure.

## Patients with Mitral Valvular Disease

Noncardiac surgery is usually well tolerated in patients with mitral disease (66). Patients with mitral stenosis and a large left atrium have a tendency to developing atrial fibrillation and may benefit from digitalization prior to noncardiac surgery. Since these patients are also prone to develop fluid overload, they may benefit from careful hemodynamic monitoring. In addition, anaesthetic techniques which are less likely to be associated with tachycardia may be preferable for such patients (e.g., the use of scopolamine in place of atropine).

Noncardiac surgery is usually well tolerated in patients with mitral regurgitation. Patients with symptomatic disease may benefit from the use of inotropic agents and afterload reduction with vasodilators.

## Patients with Cardiomyopathy

Patients with hypertrophic obstructive cardiomyopathy benefit from the use of beta-blocking agents (72) or calcium channel blockers (73) and should be maintained on these agents prior to and following noncardiac surgery. Shorter acting agents may be preferred if major surgery is planned in order to have more flexibility in dosage adjustment with hemodynamic swings during and immediately after surgery. Two important issues to keep in mind for such patients are that, first, these patients do worse with increased contractility and, second, these patients do worse with significant declines in preload or afterload. Since Thompson and colleagues (74) have demonstrated a decrease in systemic vascular resistance after spinal anesthesia in patients with hypertrophic cardiomyopathy, it may be prudent to prefer the use of general anesthesia for such patients.

In contrast, patients with dilated cardiomyopathy benefit from the use of vasodilators and low-dose beta-blockers (75, 76). In addition, in the absence of significant coronary artery disease, a low dose of inotropic agents may be useful for such patients along with pulmonary arterial pressure monitoring, particularly if the planned surgery is likely to lead to major fluid shifts or hemodynamic changes.

## Patients with Congenital Heart Disease

Patients with cyanotic congenital heart disease have a tendency to develop polycythemia and, thus, a predisposition to thrombus formation. Patients with a hematocrit of 55% to 65% should be hydrated prior to surgery. Intravenous fluids can be started the night prior to noncardiac surgery (77). Diuretics should be held. Since an increase in blood viscosity may aggravate the postoperative prothrombotic tendency, patients with an extremely high hematocrit may benefit from plasmapheresis prior to noncardiac surgery (rather than phlebotomy, which can lead to an increase in cyanosis).

Patients with tetralogy of Fallot have certain specific management problems. The focus of perioperative management for such patients is on arrhythmias. James and colleagues (78) have reported a high incidence of premature ventricular contractions both during rest and after exercise in a small cohort of asymptomatic patients with tetralogy of Fallot followed 14 years after surgical repair. In addition, since short runs of ventricular tachycardia and/or bigeminy were seen in patients with multifocal ventricular premature beats, it has been suggested that patients with tetralogy of Fallot who are approaching noncardiac surgery should undergo exercise testing or 24-hour Holter monitoring to identify those who have a tendency to develop ventricular tachyarrhythmias for whom therapy may be prescribed. There is, however, no data that such therapy is useful in preventing postoperative cardiac complications. Other conduction abnormalities to consider in patients with tetralogy of Fallot include bifascicular block. The analysis of His bundle recordings for such patients can help to assess the risk for late onset of complete heart block (79, 80) and, when performed as part of preoperative assessment, may help to identify those patients who may benefit from prophylactic temporary pacing for the perioperative period.

Among patients with longstanding left-to-right shunts, Tikoff and colleagues (81) have found that residual hemodynamic abnormalities exist even after surgical repair. Lueker and colleagues (82) have also demonstrated decreased postoperative cardiac output in response to exercise in such patients. Aggressive management of congestive heart failure is important before such patients undergo noncardiac surgery. Patients who have a large shunt without significant increase in pulmonary artery resistance may benefit from cardiac repair prior to noncardiac surgery, although definitive data are not available for such a prophylactic strategy as yet. Elective noncardiac surgery should be avoided in those with irreversible pulmonary artery hypertension since these patients are at very high risk of perioperative death.

## Impact of Type of Anesthesia and Type of Surgery

Previous studies have suggested that the type of anesthesia used does not have any significant impact upon the development of postoperative cardiac complications (1, 83, 84). In their study involving 100 patients undergoing elective vascular surgery, Christopherson and colleagues (85) randomized patients into two different standardized anaesthetic strategies: general anesthesia followed by intravenous patient-controlled analgesia and epidural anesthesia followed by epidural analgesia. The immediate and delayed (6 months) complication rates for the two groups did not differ.

However, in a study of 1,001 patients undergoing noncardiac surgery, Goldman and colleagues (9) described a higher incidence of new or worsened congestive heart failure among those who received general anesthesia when compared to those who received spinal or epidural anesthesia. It is generally accepted that the negative inotropic action of general anesthetics makes spinal anesthesia preferable (when possible) for patients with severe left ventricular dysfunction.

The surgical risk involved for the type of procedure planned also needs to be considered before a decision is made to take a high-risk cardiac patient through noncardiac surgery. Obviously, emergency surgery is attended with a much higher risk than is elective surgery (8, 9). Among elective procedures, those undergoing vascular procedures have a higher pretest probability for postoperative cardiac events (13%), when compared to thoracic or abdominal surgery (8%) (10, 11). The lowest pretest probability for cardiac events is seen among

**TABLE 8.** *Controlled studies of pulmonary artery catheterization with clinical outcomes*

| Study | Reference | Location | N[a] | Clinical setting | Study design | Significant clinical outcomes[b] | Comments |
|---|---|---|---|---|---|---|---|
| **General surgery** | | | | | | | |
| Shoemaker et al. (1988) | 109 | Los Angeles, CA | 146 | General surgery in high-risk patients | RCT: groups = CVC, PAC normal, PAC supranormal | Postoperative mortality, mean ICU stay, ventilator use lower in PAC-supranormal group | Small size sample, poor control for confounding, uncertain case mix |
| Rao et al. (1983) | 110 | Maywood, IL | 733/364 | Noncardiac surgery in patients with prior MI | Obs-historical control; 1977–1982 cohort vs. 1973–1976 cohort | Lower perioperative reinfarction and mortality rates in study cohort | Historical controls, nonrandom selection, uncertain case mix, role of hemodynamic monitoring unclear |
| **Peripheral vascular surgery** | | | | | | | |
| Berlauk et al. (1991) | 111 | Minneapolis, MN | 89 | Vein graft arterial bypass for limb salvage | RCT; groups = PAC 12 and 3 hr before surgery, no preoperative PAC | Fewer intraoperative hemodynamic disorders and postoperative graft thromboses | Uncertain group assignment methods, discrepancies in data reporting regarding cardiac morbidity |
| **Aortic reconstruction** | | | | | | | |
| Isaacson et al. (1990) | 112 | Atlanta, GA | 102 | Abdominal aortic reconstruction | RCT; groups = CVC, PAC | No difference in morbidity, mortality, ICU or hospital stay | Possible type II error |
| Joyce et al. (1990) | 113 | Toronto, Canada | 40 | Abdominal aortic aneurysm repair | RCT; groups = CVC, PAC; comparison group of 11 high-risk patients | ICU stay longer in CVC and PAC (combined), then PAC | Small sample size, comparison of CVC and PAC ICU stay not reported |
| Headorffer et al. (1987) | 114 | Johannesburg, South Africa | 61, 87 | Abdominal aortic aneurysm repair | Obs-historical controls; 1983–1984 cohort vs. 1980–1982 cohort | Lower perioperative hypotensive episodes and mortality in study cohort than historical controls | Historical controls, nonrandom selection, does not compare PAC use, inconsistent data, uncertain attrition, statistical significance not reported |

Adapted, with permission, from *Anesthesiology* 1993;78(2):380.

[a] In observational studies with historical controls, sample size of study group and historical cohort reported.

[b] Does not include outcomes for which no significant benefit observed.

RCT, randomized controlled trial (composition of randomized groups described); Obs-historical, observational study with historical controls; PAC, patients monitored by pulmonary artery catheter; CVP = patients monitored by central venous pressure measurements; ICU, intensive care unit; CVC, central venous catheter.

patients undergoing prostate, or ophthalmologic procedures (<3%) (10, 11, 86).

## INTRAOPERATIVE AND IMMEDIATE POSTOPERATIVE STRATEGIES

### Hemodynamic Monitoring

The role of perioperative intensive hemodynamic monitoring with the use of Swan-Ganz catheters is difficult to assess objectively because of the widespread use of such monitoring for the critically ill patient undergoing noncardiac surgery. Table 8 summarizes the various studies that have evaluated the use of the Swan-Ganz catheter in the perioperative period for noncardiac surgery.

More recently, the American Society of Anesthesiologists Task Force on Pulmonary Artery Catheterization has published guidelines for pulmonary artery catheterization (87). The task force recommends the perioperative use of such invasive monitoring in surgical settings where there is a potential for increased hemodynamic risk based on three variables: patient characteristics, procedural risk, and practice setting, as shown in Fig. 4.

Thus, the use of such invasive perioperative monitoring appears justified for the high-risk cardiac patient with evidence of left ventricular dysfunction, in particular when either the left ventricular dysfunction is extremely severe and/or the operation is likely to cause large hemodynamic stresses and/or fluid shifts.

### Ischemia Monitoring

Ischemia monitoring has been evaluated as a pre-, intra-, and postoperative strategy to identify patients who may

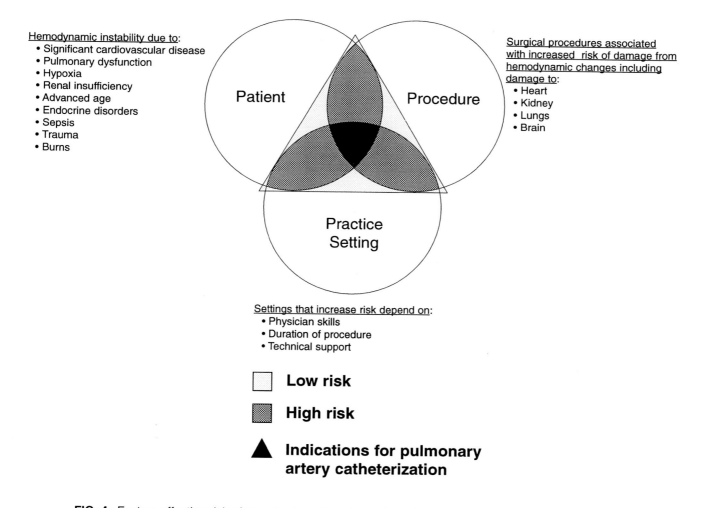

**FIG. 4.** Factors affecting risk of complications from hemodynamic changes. Adapted, with permission, from *Anesthesiology* 1993;78(2):380.

develop myocardial infarction after surgery—both immediate and late (88–90). Mangano and colleagues (88), in their study of 474 men undergoing noncardiac surgery at Veterans Administration hospitals, documented a 9.2-fold increase in the odds of an ischemic cardiac event in the postoperative period for those who had postoperative ischemia. The presence of ischemia on preoperative or intraoperative monitoring was not identified to be an independent predictor of cardiac events in their study. In another study, Raby and colleagues (89) found that the presence of postoperative ischemia was associated with a relative risk of 16 for postoperative cardiac events. Unfortunately, the positive predictive value of ischemia was only 8%. At the moment, early postoperative ischemia monitoring is a promising but experimental tool.

## Medications

The role of prophylactic beta-blockers during the perioperative period has been examined and found to be useful in several reports (Table 9). Stone and colleagues (53) randomized 128 patients to four groups: no beta-blockers, 100 mg of labetalol, 50 mg of atenolol, or 20 mg of oxprenolol (with the beta-blockers being given as a single dose 2 hours prior to the induction of anesthesia). While 28% of patients in the control group developed myocardial ischemia, only 2% had ischemia in the group who received a beta-blocker. Pasternack and colleagues (54) also demonstrated such a beneficial effect of a single

dose of beta-blocker (50 mg of metoprolol) given immediately before surgery in a study of 200 patients undergoing vascular surgery. Patients in the beta-blocker group had significantly fewer episodes of ischemia along with a lower total ischemic time.

In another study (55), the same investigators followed the initial preoperative oral dose of metoprolol with an additional dose of 10 to 15 mg given intravenously as soon as the patients were brought into the recovery room and subsequently repeated this every 12 hours for 5 days. Compared to historical controls undergoing similar surgery without receiving beta-blockers, the beta-blocker group had a lower incidence of postoperative myocardial infarction. The data on the prophylactic use other anti-ischemic agents such as intravenous nitroglycerine or calcium channel blockers is less convincing (91, 92). In another small study involving 45 patients with stable angina (Canadian Cardiovascular Society class II or III), the incidence of intraoperative myocardial ischemia was reduced in the group receiving 1 μg/kg/min of intravenous nitroglycerin (93). However, there was no difference in perioperative myocardial infarction or death. Thus, based on the existing data, we recommend the use of beta-blockers for the high-risk cardiac patients undergoing noncardiac surgery, unless otherwise contraindicated, and intravenous nitroglycerin only if the patient is hemodynamically stable and having ongoing ischemia.

Several other medications have been suggested to be beneficial based on their mechanism of action (94–98). The basis for their proposed beneficial effect is the possi-

**TABLE 9.** *Impact of anti-ischemic medications on perioperative myocardial ischemia in noncardiac surgery*

| Medication | Modality of ischemia detection | Type of surgery | Number of patients | Comment | Reference |
|---|---|---|---|---|---|
| Oral beta-blockers | Continuous lead V₅ or oscilloscope with intermittent paper recordings | Abdominal and vascular | 128 | 13 of 128 had ischemia; 2 of 89 treated patients vs. 11 of 39 untreated | 53 |
| Oral metoprolol | Holter monitor | Vascular | 200 | 48 treated patients, 152 untreated (historical controls); treatment resulted in twofold to threefold decrease in ischemic episodes and duration of ischemia | 54 |
| Oral metoprolol | Holter monitor | Abdominal aortic aneurysm | 83 | 10 of 83 had MI; 1 of 32 treated patients vs. 9 of 51 untreated (historical controls) | 55 |
| Intravenous diltiazem | Holter monitor | Vascular | 30 | 17 of 83 had ischemia; 6 of 15 treated patients vs. 11 of 15 untreated | 91 |
| Intravenous nitroglycerine | Holter monitor | Abdominal and vascular | 45 | 18 of 45 had ischemia; 14 of 22 on 0.5 μg/kg/min[a] vs. 4 of 23 on 1.0 μg/kg/min | 93 |

Reproduced, with with permission from Abraham SA, et al. *Prog Cardiovasc Dis* 1991;34:205.
[a]Micrograms per kilogram of patient body weight per minute.

ble role of postoperative catecholamine surges in the development of myocardial ischemia. One such agent is clonidine (94–96). Other agents include high-dose fentanyl, which can block afferent pain signals and thus result in a blunting of postoperative catecholamine surges (97). In addition, epidural anesthesia has been suggested to have the potential to prevent postoperative catecholamine surges by decreasing afferent pain signals in one study (98) but has not been confirmed by another study (99). Thus, although these medications may help to alter the postoperative neurohormonal milieu in a favorable direction, further studies are needed to determine the impact of these medications on clinical outcomes after noncardiac surgery before they can be recommended for widespread use.

## RISK STRATIFICATION FOR LONG-TERM PROGNOSIS

In assessing the risk for cardiac complications for a patient approaching noncardiac surgery, it is important to consider not only the immediate postoperative period but also the long-term risks. Patients who have unstable angina or other nonfatal cardiac complications in the perioperative period have a worse cardiac prognosis in the long term when compared to patients who have an uneventful postoperative period (100, 101). Such patients need aggressive management of any traditional cardiac risk factors including hypertension, diabetes mellitus, hyperlipidemia, smoking, and obesity, as well as a consideration for long-term beta-blocker therapy in addition to further work-up including coronary angiography.

## REFERENCES

1. Mangano DT. Perioperative cardiac morbidity. *Anesthesiology* 1990; 72:153.
2. Goldman L. Cardiac risk and complications of noncardiac surgery. *Ann Intern Med* 1983;98:504.
3. Eagle KA, Singer DE, Brewster DC, et al. Dipyridamole-thallium scanning in patients undergoing vascular surgery. *JAMA* 1987;257: 2185.
4. Eagle KA, Coley CM, Newell JB, et al. Combining clinical and thallium data optimizes preoperative assessment of cardiac risk before major vascular surgery. *Ann Intern Med* 1989;110:859.
5. Coley CM, Field TS, Abraham SA, et al. Usefulness of dipyridamole-thallium scanning for preoperative evaluation of cardiac risk for nonvascular surgery. *Am J Cardiol* 1992;69:1280.
6. Jamieson WRE, Janusz MT, Miyagishima RT, et al. Influence of ischemic heart disease on early and later mortality after surgery for peripheral occlusive vascular disease. *Circulation* 1982;66:92.
7. Hertzer NR, Beven EG, Young JR, et al. Coronary artery disease in peripheral vascular patients: a classification of 1000 coronary angiograms and results of surgical management. *Ann Surg* 1984;199:223.
8. Goldman L, Caldera DL, Nussbaum SR, et al. Multifactorial index of cardiac risk in noncardiac surgical procedures. *N Engl J Med* 1977; 297:845.
9. Goldman L, Caldera DL, Southwick FS, et al. Cardiac risk factors and complications in noncardiac surgery. *Medicine* 1978;57:357.
10. Detsky AS, Abrams HB, McLaughlin JR, et al. Predicting cardiac complications in patients undergoing noncardiac surgery. *J Gen Intern Med* 1986;1:211.
11. Detsky AS, Abrams HB, Forbath N, et al. Cardiac assessment for patients undergoing noncardiac surgery: a multifactorial clinical risk index. *Arch Intern Med* 1986;146:2131.
12. Gerson MC, Hurst JM, Hertzberg VS, et al. Cardiac prognosis in noncardiac geriatric surgery. *Ann Intern Med* 1985;103:832.
13. Jeffrey CC, Kunsman J, Cullen DJ, et al. A prospective evaluation of cardiac risk index. *Anesthesiology* 1983;58:462.
14. Paul SD, Eagle KA, Kuntz KM, Young JR, Hertzer NR. Concordance of a validated clinical risk index with coronary angiography prior to vascular surgery (VAS): the Cleveland Clinic (CCF) experience. *Circulation* 1994;90(4):I-95A.
15. Paul SD, L'Italien GJ, Hendel RC, et al. Influence of prior heart disease on morbidity and mortality after vascular surgery: role of coronary artery bypass grafting. *J Am Coll Cardiol* 1994;1A:484A.
16. McCabe CJ, Reidy NC, Abbott WM, Fulchino DM, Brewster DC. The value of electrocardiogram monitoring during treadmill testing for peripheral vascular disease. *Surgery* 1981;89:183.
17. Cutler BS, Wheeler HB, Paraskos JA, et al. Applicability and interpretation of electrocardiographic stress testing in patients with peripheral vascular disease. *Am J Surg* 1981;141:501.
18. Carliner NH, Fisher ML, Plotnick GD, et al. Routine preoperative exercise testing in patients undergoing major noncardiac surgery. *Am J Cardiol* 1985;56:51.
19. McPhail N, Calvin JE, Shariatmadar A, et al. The use of preoperative exercise testing to predict cardiac complications after arterial reconstruction. *J Vasc Surg* 1988;7:60.
20. Arous EJ, Baum PL, Cutler BS. The ischemic exercise test in patients with peripheral vascular disease. Implications for management. *Arch Surg* 1984;119:780.
21. Leppo J, Plaja J, Gionet M, Tumolo J, Paraskos JA, Cutler BS. Noninvasive evaluation of cardiac risk before elective vascular surgery. *J Am Coll Cardiol* 1987;9:269.
22. von Knorring J, Lepantalo M. Prediction of perioperative cardiac complications by electrocardiographic monitoring during treadmill exercise testing before peripheral vascular surgery. *Surgery* 1986;99: 610.
23. Gardine RL, McBride K, Greenberg H, Mulcare RJ. The value of cardiac monitoring during peripheral arterial stress testing in the surgical management of peripheral vascular disease. *J Cardiovasc Surg* 1985; 26:258.
24. Hanson P, Pease M, Berkoff H, Turnipseed W, Detmer D. Arm exercise testing for coronary artery disease in patients with peripheral vascular disease. *Clin Cardiol* 1988;11:70.
25. Boucher CA, Brewster DC, Darling RC, et al. Determination of cardiac risk by dipyridamole-thallium imaging before peripheral vascular surgery. *N Engl J Med* 1985;312:389.
26. Lette J, Waters D, Lapointe J, et al. Usefulness of the severity and extent of reversible perfusion defects during thallium-dipyridamole imaging for cardiac risk assessment before noncardiac surgery. *Am J Cardiol* 1989;64:276.
27. McEnroe CS, O'Donnell TF Jr, Yeager A, et al. Comparison of ejection fraction and Goldman risk factor analysis to dipyridamole-thallium 201 studies in the evaluation of cardiac morbidity after aortic aneurysm surgery. *J Vasc Surg* 1990;11:497.
28. Paul SD, L'Italien GJ, Coley CM, et al. Perioperative and late cardiac prognosis after geriatric vascular surgery: Implications for preoperative screening. *Am J Geriatric Cardiology* 1996 (in press).
29. Josephson MA, Brown BG, Hecht HS, et al. Non-invasive detection and localization of coronary stenosis in patients: comparison of resting dipyridamole and exercise thallium-201 myocardial perfusion imaging. *Am Heart J* 1982;103:1008.
30. Leppo JA. Dipyridamole-thallium imaging: the lazy man's stress test. *J Nucl Med* 1989;30:281.
31. Lane SE, Lewis SM, Pippin JJ, et al. Predictive value of quantitative dipyridamole-thallium scintigraphy in assessing cardiovascular risk after vascular surgery in diabetes mellitus. *Am J Cardiol* 1989;64: 1275.
32. Levinson JR, Boucher CA, Coley CM, et al. Usefulness of semiquantitative analysis of dipyridamole-thallium-201 redistribution for improving risk stratification before vascular surgery. *Am J Cardiol* 1990;66:406.
33. Davila-Roman VG, Waggoner AD, Sicard GA, et al. Dobutamine

stress echocardiography predicts surgical outcome in patients with an aortic aneurysm and peripheral vascular disease. *J Am Coll Cardiol* 1993;21:957.

34. Langan EM, Youkey JR, Franklin DP, Elmore JR, Costello JM, Nassef LA. Dobutamine stress echocardiography for cardiac risk assessment before aortic surgery. *J Vasc Surg* 1993;18:905.

35. Eichelberger JP, Schwarz KQ, Black ER, Green RM, Ouriel K. Predictive value of dobutamine echocardiography just before noncardiac vascular surgery. *Am J Cardiol* 1993;72:602.

36. Poldermans D, Fioretti PM, Forster T, et al. Dobutamine stress echocardiography for assessment of perioperative cardiac risk in patients undergoing major vascular surgery. *Circulation* 1993;87:1506.

37. Lalka SG, Sawada SG, Dalsing MC, et al. Dobutamine stress echocardiography as a predictor of cardiac events associated with aortic surgery. *J Vasc Surg* 1992;15:831.

38. Lane RT, Sawada SG, Armstrong WF, Feigenbaum H. Dobutamine stress echocardiography for assessment of cardiac risk before noncardiac surgery. *Am J Cardiol* 1991;68:976.

39. Gersh BJ, Kronmal RA, Frye RL. Coronary arteriography and coronary artery bypass surgery; morbidity and mortality in patients ages 65 or older. A report from the Coronary Artery Surgery Study. *Circulation* 1983;67:483.

40. Gersh BJ, Kornmal RA, Schaff HB. Comparison of coronary artery bypass surgery and medical therapy in patients 65 years of age and older. *N Engl J Med* 1985;313:217.

41. Coronary Artery Surgery Study (CASS): a randomized trial of coronary artery bypass surgery. *Circulation* 1983;68:939.

42. Varnauskas E. Twelve-year follow-up of survival in the randomized European coronary surgery study. *N Engl J Med* 1988;319:332.

43. Gewertz BL, Kremser PC, Zarins CK, et al. Transesophageal echocardiographic monitoring of myocardial ischemia during vascular surgery. *J Vasc Surg* 1987;5:607.

44. Eisenberg MJ, London MJ, Leung JM, et al. Monitoring for myocardial ischemia during noncardiac surgery: a technology assessment of transesophageal echocardiography and 12-lead electrocardiography. *JAMA* 1992;268:210.

45. Brismar B, Hedenstierna G, Lundh R, et al. Oxygen uptake, plasma catecholamines, and cardiac output during neuroleptic nitrous oxide and halothane anaesthesias. *Acta Anaesth Scand* 1982;26:541.

46. Brown FF, Owens WD, Felts JA, et al. Plasma epinephrine and norepinephrine levels during anesthesia: enflurane-N20-O2 compared with fentanyl-N20-O2. *Anesth Analg* 1982;61:366.

47. Ponten J, Biber B, Henriksson BA, et al. Longterm beta-receptor blockade—adrenergic and metabolic response to surgery and neuroleptic anaesthesia. *Acta Anaesth Scand* 1982;26:570.

48. Riles TS, Fisher FS, Schaefer S, Pasternack PF, Baumann FG. Plasma catecholamine concentrations during abdominal aortic aneurysm surgery: the link to perioperative myocardial ischemia. *Ann Vasc Surg* 1993;7:213.

49. Breslow MJ, Jordan DA, Christopherson R, et al. Epidural morphine decreases postoperative hypertension by attenuating sympathetic nervous system hyperactivity. *JAMA* 1989;261:3577.

50. Stanley TH, Berman L, Green O, et al. Plasma catecholamine and cortisol responses to fentanyl-oxygen anesthesia for coronary artery operations. *Anesthesiology* 1980;53:250.

51. Engquist A, Fog-Moller F, Christiansen C, et al. Influence of epidural analgesia on the catecholamine and cyclic AMP responses to surgery. *Acta Anaesth Scand* 1980;24:17.

52. Breslow MJ. The role of stress hormones in perioperative myocardial ischemia. *Int Anesth Clinics* 1992;30(1):81.

53. Stone JG, Foex P, Sear JW, et al. Myocardial ischemia in untreated hypertensive patients: effect of a single small oral dose of a beta-adrenergic blocking agent. *Anesthesiology* 1988;68:495.

54. Pasternack PF, Grossi EA, Baumann FG, et al. Beta blockade to decrease silent myocardial ischemia during peripheral vascular surgery. *Am J Surg* 1989;158:113.

55. Pasternack PF, Imparato AM, Baumann FG, et al. The hemodynamics of β-blockade in patients undergoing abdominal aortic aneurysm repair. *Circulation* 1987;76(Suppl 3):III-1.

56. Foster ED, Davis KB, Carpenter JA, et al. Risk of non-cardiac operation in patients with defined coronary disease: the Coronary Artery Surgery Study (CASS) Registry experience. *Ann Thorac Surg* 1986;41:42.

57. Huber KC, Evans MA, Bresnahan JF, Gibbons RJ, Holmes DR. Outcome of noncardiac operations in patients with severe coronary artery disease successfully treated preoperatively with coronary angioplasty. *Mayo Clin Proc* 1992;67:15.

58. Elmore JR, Hallett JW, Gibbons RJ, et al. Myocardial revascularization before abdominal aortic aneurysmorrhaphy: effect of coronary angioplasty. *Mayo Clin Proc* 1993;68:637.

59. Jones SE, Raymond RE, Whitlow PL, Simpfendorfer CC. Using coronary angioplasty as a bridge to major vascular surgery: is it helpful? *Circulation* 1992;86(Suppl I):11A.

60. Leinbach RC, Gold HK, Harper RW, Buckley MJ, Austen WG. Early intraaortic balloon pumping for anterior myocardial infarction without shock. *Circulation* 197;58:204.

61. Weintraub RM, Voukydis PC, Aroesty JM, et al. Treatment of preinfarction angina with intraaortic balloon counterpulsation and surgery. *Am J Cardiol* 1974;34:809.

62. Buckley MJ, Craver JM, Gold HK, Mundth ED, Daggett WM, Austen WG. Intraaortic balloon pump assist for cardiogenic shock after cardiopulmonary bypass. *Circulation* 1973;48(Suppl III):III9-4.

63. Kern MJ, Aguirre FV, Tatineni S, et al. Enhanced coronary blood flow velocity during intraaortic balloon counterpulsation in critically ill patients. *J Am Coll Cardiol* 1993;21:359.

64. Siu SC, Lowalchuk GJ, Welty FK, Benotti PN, Lewis SN. Intraaortic balloon counterpulsation support in the high-risk cardiac patient undergoing urgent noncardiac surgery. *Chest* 1991;99:1342.

65. Grotz RL, Yeston NS. Intraaortic balloon counterpulsation in high-risk patients undergoing noncardiac surgery. *Surgery* 1989;106:1.

66. Skinner JF, Pierce ML. Surgical risk in the cardiac patient. *J Chron Dis* 1964;17:57.

67. O'Keefe JH, Shub C, Rettke SR. Risk of noncardiac surgical procedures in patients with aortic stenosis. *Mayo Clin Proc* 1989;64:400.

68. Roth RB, Palacios IF, Block PC. Percutaneous aortic balloon valvuloplasty: its role in the management of patients with aortic stenosis requiring major noncardiac surgery. *J Am Coll Cardiol* 1989;13:1039.

69. Levine MJ, Berman AD, Safian RD, et al. Palliation of valvular aortic stenosis by balloon valvuloplasty as preoperative preparation for noncardiac surgery. *Am J Cardiol* 1988;62:1309.

70. Hayes SN, Holmes DR, Nishimura RA, Reeder GS. Palliative percutaneous aortic balloon valvuloplasty before noncardiac operations and invasive diagnostic procedures. *Mayo Clin Proc* 1989;64:753.

71. Bolen JL, Alderman EL. Hemodynamic consequences of afterload reduction in patients with chronic aortic regurgitation. *Circulation* 1976;53:879.

72. Bonow RO, Maron BJ, Leon MB, et al. Medical and surgical therapy of hypertrophic cardiomyopathy. *Cardiovasc Clin* 1988;19:221.

73. Chatterjee K. Calcium antagonist agents in hypertrophic cardiomyopathy. *Am J Cardiol* 1987;59:146B.

74. Thompson RC, Liberthson RR, Lowenstein E. Perioperative anesthetic risk of noncardiac surgery in hypertrophic obstructive cardiomyopathy. *JAMA* 1985;254:2419.

75. Massin EK. Current treatment of dilated cardiomyopathy. *Texas Heart Inst J* 1991;18:41.

76. Waagstein F, Caidahl K, Wallentin I, et al. Longterm beta-blockade in dilated cardiomyopathy. Effects of short- and longterm metoprolol treatment followed by withdrawal and readministration of metoprolol. *Circulation* 1989;80:551.

77. Smith RM. *Anesthesia for infants and children.* 3rd ed. St. Louis: Mosby; 1968.

78. James FW, Kaplan S, Schwartz DC, et al. Response to exercise in patients after total surgical correction of tetralogy of Fallot. *Circulation* 1976;54:671.

79. Downing JW, Kaplan S, Bove KE. Postsurgical left anterior hemiblock and right bundle branch block. *Br Heart J* 1972;34:263.

80. Godman JM, Roberts NK, Izukawa T. Late postoperative conduction disturbances after repair of ventricular septal defect and tetralogy of Fallot. Analysis of His bundle recordings. *Circulation* 1974;49:214.

81. Tikoff G, Keith TB, Nelson RM, Kuida H. Clinical and hemodynamic observations after closure of large atrial septal defects complicated by heart failure. *Am J Cardiol* 1969;23:810.

82. Lueker RD, Vogel JH, Blount SG Jr. Cardiovascular abnormalities following surgery for left to right shunts: observations in atrial septal defects, ventricular septal defects, and patent ductus arteriosus. *Circulation* 1969;40:785.

83. McGowan SW, Smith GFN. Anaesthesia for transurethral prostatec-

tomy: a comparison of spinal intradural analgesia with two methods of general anaesthesia. *Anaesthesia* 1980;35:847.

84. Mclaren AD, Stockwell MC, Reid VT. Anesthetic techniques for surgical correction of fractured neck of femur. *Anaesthesia* 1978;33: 10.

85. Christopherson R, Beattle C, Frank SM, et al. Perioperative morbidity in patients randomized to epidural or general anesthesia for lower extremity vascular surgery. *Anesthesiology* 1993;79:422.

86. Backer CL, Tinker JH, Robertson DM, et al. Myocardial reinfarction following local anesthesia for ophthalmic surgery. *Anesth Analg* 1980;59:257.

87. Practice guidelines for pulmonary artery catheterization: a report by the American Society of Anesthesiologists Task Force on pulmonary artery catheterization. *Anesthesiology* 1993;78(2):380.

88. Mangano DT, Browner WS, Hollenberg M, et al. Association of perioperative myocardial ischemia with cardiac morbidity and mortality in men undergoing noncardiac surgery. *N Engl J Med* 1990;323:1781.

89. Raby KE, Barry J, Creager MA, Cook EF, Weisberg MC, Goldman L. Detection and significance of intraoperative and postoperative myocardial ischemia in peripheral vascular surgery. *JAMA* 1992;268 (2):222.

90. Raby KE, Goldman L, Creager MA, et al. Correlation between preoperative ischemia and major cardiac events after peripheral vascular surgery. *N Engl J Med* 1989;321:1296.

91. Godet G, Coriat P, Baron JF, et al. Prevention of intraoperative myocardial ischemia during noncardiac surgery with intravenous diltiazem: a randomized trial versus placebo. *Anesthesiology* 1987;66: 241.

92. Dodds TM, Stone JG, Coromilas J, Weinberger M, Levy DG. Prophylactic nitroglycerin infusion during noncardiac surgery does not reduce perioperative ischemia. *Anesth Analg* 1993;76:705.

93. Coriat P, Dalaz M, Bousseau D, et al. Prevention of intraoperative myocardial ischemia during noncardiac surgery with intravenous nitroglycerin. *Anesthesiology* 1984;61:193.

94. Flacke JW, Bloor BC, Flacke WE, et al. Reduced narcotic requirement by clonidine with improved hemodynamic and adrenergic stability in patients undergoing coronary bypass surgery. *Anesthesiology* 1987;67:11.

95. Ghignone M, Calvillo O, Quintin L. Anesthesia and hypertension: the effect of clonidine on perioperative hemodynamics and isoflurane requirements. *Anesthesiology* 1987;67:3.

96. Helbo-Hansen S, Gletcher R, Lundberg D, et al. Clonidine and the sympatico-adrenal response to coronary artery bypass surgery. *Acta Anaesthesiol Scand* 1986;30:235.

97. Stanley TH, Berman L, Green O, et al. Plasma catecholamine and cortisol responses to fentanyl-oxygen anesthesia for coronary artery operations. *Anesthesiology* 1980;53:250.

98. Engquist A, Fog-Moller F, Christiansen C, et al. Influence of epidural analgesia on the catecholamine and cyclic AMP responses to surgery. *Acta Anaesth Scand* 1980;24:17.

99. Riles TS, Fisher FS, Schaefer S, Pasternack PF, Baumann FG. Plasma catecholamine concentrations during abdominal aortic aneurysm surgery: the link to perioperative myocardial ischemia. *Ann Vasc Surg* 1993;7:213.

100. Paul SD, Coley CM, Field TS, et al. Predicting long-term cardiac complications after vascular surgery: importance of preoperative clinical features, thallium data and perioperative complications. *Circulation* 1991;84(4):II-22.

101. Cheney PH, Bry JDL, O'Donnell TF, Mackey WC, Udelson JE. Long-term prognostic implications of perioperative myocardial infarction in patients undergoing peripheral vascular surgery. *Circulation* 1994;90(4):I-95A.

102. Goldman L, Hashimoto B, Cook EF, Loscalzo A. Comparative reproducibility and validity of systems for assessing cardiovascular functional class: advantages of a new specific activity scale. *Circulation* 1981;64:1227.

103. Kopecky SL, Gibbons RJ, Hollier LH. Preoperative supine exercise radionuclide angiogram predicts perioperative cardiovascular events in vascular surgery. *J Am Coll Cardiol* 1986;7:226A.

104. Abraham SA, Coles NA, Coley CM, et al. Coronary risk of noncardiac surgery. *Prog Cardiovasc Dis* 1991;34:205.

105. Hertzer NR, Young JR, Beven EG, et al. Late results of coronary bypass in patients with peripheral vascular disease: I. Five-year survival according to age and clinical cardiac status. *Cleve Clin Q* 1986; 53:133.

106. Reul GJ, Cooley DA, Duncan JM, et al. The effect of coronary bypass on the outcome of peripheral vascular operations in 1093 patients. *J Vasc Surg* 1986;3:788.

107. Acinapura AJ, Rose DM, Kramer MD, et al. Role of coronary angiography and coronary artery bypass surgery prior to abdominal aortic aneurysmectomy. *J Cardiovasc Surg* 1987;28:552.

108. Paul SD, Eagle KA. A stepwise strategy for coronary risk assessment for noncardiac surgery. *Med Clin North Am* 1995;79(5):1241.

109. Shoemaker WC, Appel PL, Kram HB, et al. Prospective trial of supranormal values of survivors as therapeutic goals in high-risk surgical patients. *Chest* 1988;94:1176.

110. Rao TLK, Jacobs KH, El-Etr AA. Reinfarction following anesthesia in patients with myocardial infarction. *Anesthesiology* 1983;59:499.

111. Berlauk JF, Abrams JH, Gilmour IJ, et al. Preoperative optimization of cardiovascular hemodynamics improves outcome in peripheral vascular surgery: a prospective, randomized clinical trial. *Ann Surg* 1991;214:289.

112. Isaacson IJ, Lowdon JD, Berry AJ, et al. The value of pulmonary artery and central venous monitoring in patients undergoing abdominal aortic reconstructive surgery: a comparative study of two selected, randomized groups. *J Vasc Surg* 1990;12:754.

113. Joyce WP, Provan JL, Ameli FM, et al. The role of central hemodynamic monitoring in abdominal aortic surgery: a prospective randomized study. *Eur J Vasc Surg* 1990;4:633.

114. Headorffer CS, Milne JF, Meyers AM, et al. The value of Swan-Ganz catheterization and volume loading in preventing renal failure in patients undergoing abdominal aneurysmectomy. *Clin Nephrol* 1987; 28:272.

*The Critically Ill Cardiac Patient,*
edited by V. Kvetan and D. R. Dantzker,
Lippincott - Raven Publishers, Philadelphia © 1996.

CHAPTER **3**

# Ventilatory Support in Cardiac Failure

Steven M. Scharf

Respiratory failure resulting in the need for ventilatory support is not uncommon in patients with severe cardiac dysfunction. Various forms of positive-pressure ventilatory support have been used to treat pulmonary edema since the early part of this century (1). While the salutary effects of mechanical ventilatory support on gas exchange are obviously therapeutic, it is less well appreciated that ventilatory support can be an effective, efficient way of supporting and improving the function of the failing heart above and beyond any effects on gas exchange. The degree to and the circumstances under which this is the case have been the subject of intensive investigation for the last 10 to 15 years. It is the object of this chapter to review some of the essential features of these studies. In the first section we review the basic principles of heart-lung interactions which underlie the clinical use of respiratory maneuvers to support the circulation. These include the effects of cardiac failure on respiratory function, the effects of lung volume, changes in autonomic tone, effects of ventricular interdependence, and the effects of changes in intrathoracic pressure on cardiocirculatory function. In the second section, we review the topic of ventilatory support in cardiac failure, with an eye to the ways in which ventilatory support can aid cardiac function in the failing or ischemic heart. We will discuss a number of clinical observations which can best be understood in terms of current ideas of cardiorespiratory interactions and make a few specific recommendations to physicians involved in the care of patients with heart disease. We have made no attempt to be all-inclusive in this review and acknowledge that many worthy studies are not specifically referenced. This is to be viewed as a limitation of the scope of this chapter and the room available in the current text.

## BASIC PRINCIPLES OF HEART-LUNG INTERACTIONS

### Effects of Heart Failure on Respiratory Function

The factors governing the transfer of fluid across capillary and precapillary microcirculation have been extensively reviewed in a number of different publications (2–4). As is well known from basic physiology, Starling's law of diffusion describes most of the relevant factors, which include forces tending to transfer fluid from the *vascular compartment* to *pulmonary interstitium*—the balance of hydrostatic forces—and factors tending to move fluid from the *interstitium* to the *pulmonary vasculature,* the difference in oncotic pressure between microvasculature and interstitium. The degree to which alterations in the balance of forces produces actual fluid accumulation within the lung is modulated by the *permeability* of endothelium to water and small solutes. The *reflection coefficient* of these layers represents the permeability of the endothelium to proteins and the *competency* of the pulmonary lymphatic network.

Early in the development of cardiogenic pulmonary edema interstitial fluid accumulates around arterioles and bronchioles. This leads to perivascular and peribronchial cuffing. Whether this leads to decreased luminal diameter is still controversial (5), but decreased dynamic compliance suggests that this is the case (6). Further, bronchial reactivity may increase during this stage of fluid accumulation (6). Pulmonary compliance expressed in terms of gas volume decreases with the onset of fluid accumulation (7). Pulmonary compliance abnormalities are further exacerbated by interference with the normal action of pulmonary surfactant by edema fluid and closure of terminal airway units, primarily in the bases of the lung. As a result of increased airway resistance and decreased lung compliance, the work of breathing increases dramatically as left atrial pressure increases. This in turn reduces the efficiency and increases the oxygen cost of breathing (8).

S. M. Scharf: Pulmonary and Critical Care Division, Long Island Jewish Medical Center, Long Island Campus for the Albert Einstein College of Medicine, New Hyde Park, New York 11042.

The increased workload placed on the muscles of respiration naturally increases their energy requirement and hence requirement for blood flow. This results in an increase in the proportion of total cardiac output being diverted to these muscles.

With worsening pulmonary edema arterial hypoxemia ensues, primarily as a result of poor match between ventilation and perfusion. In many patients increasing $PaCO_2$ attests to severe ventilation/perfusion mismatch and/or alveolar hypoventilation (9). Finally, metabolic acidosis (10), usually lactic acidosis (11), is not uncommonly observed in patients with severe heart failure and hypoperfusion of peripheral organs. Blood gas abnormalities and stimulation of intrapulmonary receptors by edema fluid (12) lead to increased ventilatory effort. Given the large increase in oxygen demand by respiratory muscles and the limitation of blood flow by virtue of shock and decreased cardiac output in severe heart failure, it is to be expected that fatigue of the respiratory muscles would be common with cardiac failure. In fact, in experimental cardiogenic shock, death usually occurs by virtue of respiratory muscle fatigue rather than cardiac arrest (13). Further, the primary source of lactate production in this situation is the muscles of respiration (14). These factors are reviewed more thoroughly in Chapter 3.

Thus, if for no other reason than resting the respiratory muscles until hemodynamic stability can be achieved, mechanical ventilatory support would be advantageous in many patients with cardiogenic shock. This would seem especially important in patients experiencing acute ischemia. Efforts should be made to use mechanical ventilatory support early and continue it until one is sure that respiratory muscle function is normal and fatigue is no longer a factor.

## Heart-Lung Interactions in Respiratory Failure

During normal respiration, the effects of respiratory perturbations on cardiovascular function are relatively small, and one may ignore the effects of ventilatory mechanics when assessing the cardiovascular system. However, in patients with respiratory failure, there are substantial changes in respiratory mechanics which alter cardiovascular mechanics and modify the interpretation of many of the usual hemodynamic measurements made while caring for these patients. Cardiovascular changes in respiratory failure are classified as *indirect* and *direct*. Indirect changes are the result of alteration in arterial blood gas tensions such as hypoxia and hypercapnia. Direct consequences are the result of changes in ventilatory mechanics. The former have been reviewed elsewhere (15, 16); hence we will concentrate on the latter. Suffice it to say that correction of hypoxemia and *severe* acidosis (pH < 7.25) should be one of the primary goals of ventilatory therapy in patients with respiratory failure. To understand the direct consequences of respiratory failure, one must understand the effects of changes in lung volume, factors controlling venous return, the diastolic interactions between the ventricles, and the effects of changes in intrathoracic pressure on cardiac, specifically left ventricular (LV), function.

## Changes in Lung Volume

### Changes in Pulmonary Vascular Resistance

A number of investigators have noted a biphasic relationship between lung volume and pulmonary vascular resistance and capacitance (17, 18). In the normal lung, As lung volume increases from residual volume to functional residual capacity (FRC), pulmonary vascular resistance decreases, and vascular capacitance increases. Then as lung volume increases from FRC to total lung capacity, pulmonary vascular resistance increases, and capacitance decreases. Thus, increases in lung volume above FRC lead to increased pulmonary vascular resistance and decreased capacitance. At constant pulmonary arterial pressure this leads to decreased blood flow and decreased pulmonary vascular volume. This biphasic behavior of the pulmonary vasculature has been explained by postulating at least two kinds of pulmonary vessels (19). Pulmonary microvasculatures located within interalveolar septa that are exposed to pulmonary transmural pressure and constricted when lung volume increases are called *intra-alveolar* vessels. Pulmonary vessels located in the corners where alveoli join or within peribronchial spaces that are actually exposed to expanding forces when lung volume increases are called *extra-alveolar* vessels. As lung volume increases from residual volume to FRC, the effects on extra-alveolar vessels predominate and pulmonary vascular resistance decreases. As lung volume increases above FRC, the effects on intra-alveolar vessels predominate and pulmonary vascular resistance increases. Further, lung-volume-related increases in pulmonary vascular resistance will be compounded by the presence of edema fluid around vessels, hypoxia- and acidosis-mediated pulmonary vasoconstriction, and emboli within the pulmonary vasculature, all of which may occur in respiratory failure.

Right ventricular (RV) afterload is partly related to RV wall stress, which in turn is a function of RV end-systolic volume and pressure (20). Clearly, as lung volume increases above FRC, as long as cardiac output is kept reasonably constant, RV end-systolic pressure and volume will increase. Thus, increased lung volume can impose an increase in afterload on the RV. This can be hemodynamically significant when lung volume is increased with high levels of positive end-expiratory pressure (PEEP), cardiac output is preserved, and there is concomitant pulmonary edema. In fact, in patients with adult respiratory distress syndrome (ARDS) this combination of circumstances can lead to RV failure (21). On the other hand, with increased airway pressure, preload may decrease due to decreased venous return. In this case, the hemodynamic effects on the RV are not usually dominated by increases in afterload, but rather by changes in preload (see discussion of venous return below).

### The Concept of Transmural Pressure

Critically ill patients frequently require monitoring of intravascular pressures. Various measures of preload, including central venous (right atrial) pressure and pulmonary artery wedge (left atrial) pressure, are often recorded via balloon-tipped flow-directed catheter. These measures are often said to reflect the "filling pressure" of the right and left ventricles, respectively. As an intrathoracic organ, the heart is subject to perturbations of pressure within the chest. These can be large negative swings in inspiratory pressure with respiratory distress and large increases in end-expiratory and end-inspiratory pressure with mechanical ventilation, especially with the use of PEEP. If an intrathoracic vascular pressure is measured in reference atmospheric pressure, as is usually done, then changes in this pressure will reflect not only changes in the pressure gradient across the wall of the heart, the filling pressure, but also transmitted intrathoracic pressure changes as well. In most cases the state of filling of the heart is best reflected by measuring the pressure across its wall, the transmural pressure (22). This is the difference between intracardiac and cardiac surface pressure. It is this pressure difference which comprises the end-diastolic and end-systolic stresses.

Many studies of cardiac function during respiratory failure attempt to estimate transmural RV and LV filling and end-systolic transmural pressures. Often, esophageal pressure is used as the reference pressure for intravascular pressures. While changes in body position and the weight of mediastinal contents on the esophagus can change baseline esophageal pressure (23), it is assumed that changes in cardiac surface pressure are adequately reflected by changes in esophageal pressure. Unfortunately, this assumption may not always be valid. As lung volume increases, there are mechanical interactions between the heart and lungs which are not adequately reflected by esophageal pressure. Thus, at large lung volumes, the heart may be mechanically compressed by the expanding lung (24–26). This can result in increases in cardiac surface pressure (pericardial pressure) greater than those measured in the esophagus (23). Further, the pericardium normally limits cardiac expansion even at physiologic volumes (27). Thus, as the heart enlarges or decreases in size, overlying cardiac surface (intrapericardial) pressure increases and decreases in a manner not

reflected in esophageal pressure (28). The smaller the heart, the more the principal determinant of cardiac surface pressure is cardiac fossa pressure external to the pericardium. However, as cardiac volume increases, the elastic properties of the pericardium become more important and at large enough cardiac volume become the prime determinant of cardiac surface pressure, being less subject to cardiac fossa or intrathoracic pressure (29). Finally, surface pressure over the left ventricle decreases during ventricular ejection as the left ventricle decreases in size (28). These changes are not reflected in esophageal pressure (28), and calculations of end-systolic wall stress (end-systolic transmural pressure) made on the basis of esophageal pressure can therefore be misleading. Having made these provisos, the *concept* of transmural pressure is extremely important for the critical care physician to understand, and estimates of intrathoracic pressure using esophageal pressure as the reference pressure may still often provide useful information. Changes in intrathoracic pressure during ventilatory support are often made using esophageal balloons by standard techniques (30). If one assumes that RV compliance is extremely high (31), swings in central venous pressure during respiration become fairly accurate measures of respiratory swings in pericardial pressure. Finally, during mechanical ventilation with PEEP, one can briefly discontinue PEEP. Pressure measured by the wedged pulmonary arterial catheter will drop immediately by the amount that PEEP had increased cardiac surface pressure and then will usually begin to rise again as venous return increases. Thus, with discontinuation of PEEP the *nadir* wedge pressure can be used as a measure of LV end-diastolic filling pressure, and the difference between pulmonary wedge pressure on PEEP and the nadir pressure equals the amount by which cardiac surface pressure increased with PEEP (32). Using this pressure difference allows for better estimations of changes in transmural filling pressure during PEEP positive-pressure ventilation with high airway pressure.

### Changes in Autonomic Tone

While there are many mechanical interactions between the lungs and the heart, of perhaps equal importance are changes in autonomic tone, both sympathoadrenal and vagal, with changes in respiratory status. Vasomotor and respiratory neurons both emanate from common medullary centers, thus affording ample opportunity for interaction at the level of the central nervous system (33). Large increases in lung volume can lead to vagally mediated circulatory collapse with hypotension, decreased cardiac output, and severe bradycardia (34). Increases in only a small portion of the lung to its specific total lung capacity are sufficient to induce this reflex (35). On the other hand, the role of vagal circulatory inhibition with increased lung volume produced by PEEP in the clinical range is unclear (36). There are many other reflex links between cardiac and circulatory systems which relate to changes in chest wall and/or respiratory mechanoreceptors. A good example is the cardiocirculatory response to hypoxia. Stimulation of the carotid chemoreceptors produces an increase in vagal discharge, whereas stimulation of aortic and central chemoreceptors produces a sympathetic discharge. The balance between these effects is modulated by mechanical changes in the respiratory system. When experimental animals are made hypoxic, but hyperventilation is not allowed to occur (paralyzed, constantly ventilated), severe bradycardia and circulatory collapse may occur at relatively mild levels of hypoxia (37). On the other hand, with hyperventilation, the balance falls in favor of sympathoadrenal tone and tachycardia ensues at mild to moderate levels of hypoxia (37, 38), with circulatory collapse occurring only at $PaO_2 < 20$ torr. The neural link between respiration and circulation is also illustrated in animal studies, demonstrating that when all respiratory motion ceases (apnea), hypoxia induces blood pressure waves with a periodicity of 4 to 8 per minute. These waves are synchronous with respiratory motoneuron output (39). Finally, during mechanical ventilation there are often seen inspiratory increases in arterial pressure, sometimes called *reverse pulsus paradoxus*. While there are a number of factors that contribute to this phenomenon, including changes in stroke output and transmitted changes in intrathoracic pressure (40), part of the rise in arterial pressure is mediated by sympathetic alpha-adrenergic tone which "locks into" the respiratory frequency (40, 41). Changes in lung volume and chest wall mechanoreceptors as well as respiratory-mediated changes in baroreceptor output are likely responsible for this. The clinical implications of these findings discussed above have not been well investigated, but it is possible that future studies will reveal that the effects of ventilation on the circulation are quite a bit more than the mechanical effects usually discussed in reviews of this type.

Pathologic changes in the pulmonary airways and parenchyma induce reflex alterations in respiration and circulation. A relevant example in the intensive care unit is the effect of increased lung water, whether due to raised pulmonary intravascular pressure (hemodynamic pulmonary edema) or increased endothelial permeability (ARDS). Increased pulmonary vascular congestion and lung water is associated with tachypnea, hyperventilation (unless the mechanical defects are very severe), and tachycardia. These reflex changes are unrelated to changes in arterial oxygenation and are observed even though arterial blood is fully saturated with $O_2$. The relevant afferent impulses are probably carried by unmyelinated C-fibers in the vagus nerve. The trigger may be related to stimulation of intraparenchymal receptors close to the pulmonary capillaries, called J-receptors (42, 43). This mechanism is probably responsible, at least in part, for the clinical observation that patients with pulmonary edema or ARDS "overtrigger" ventilators and hyperventilate to a mild to moderate respiratory alkalosis (44). This is usually not of concern unless accompanied by metabolic alkalosis which makes the pH dangerously high.

## Determinants of Venous Return

It has long been recognized that the heart cannot pump out more blood than it receives from the periphery, the venous return. In the early 1950s, Guyton et al. (45) elaborated the model of determination of cardiac output which is still in use today for understanding the relationship between changes in cardiac and venous function. Figure 1 illustrates a model of the circulation. This model consists of a simple reservoir of compliance C, which drains through the venous circuit into the right atrium. The right atrium serves as a "priming chamber" for the lumped heart-lung unit which pumps blood back into the chamber. The pressure head in the peripheral reservoir is equal to the product of the compliance of the chamber and the "stressed" volume of the chamber: $P_s = (C)(V_s)$. The concept of stressed volume is important. Any elastic chamber, including the peripheral circulation, will fill with a certain volume, called the "unstressed" volume, without changing the pressure, or distending the chamber. Unstressed volume is a significant part, perhaps as much as 25%, of total blood volume and constitutes a significant reservoir for internally recruiting volume into the system. The difference between the total volume in the system and its unstressed volume is the relevant volume

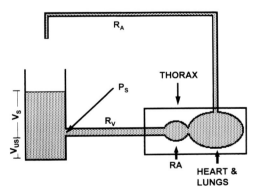

**FIG. 1.** Model of the systemic circulation illustrating venous return. The peripheral capacitance vessels are lumped as a reservoir draining through a venous resistance (RV) into the right atrium. The rest of the heart and lungs are lumped and pump blood out through an arterial resistance (RA) back into the reservoir. Reservoir volume is divided into two components, the unstressed volume (VUS) and the stressed volume (VS), the latter of which is responsible for producing the relevant upstream pressure draining the reservoir (PS). This pressure is also called mean circulatory pressure. Right atrial pressure thus constitutes the back pressure for venous return.

for causing pressure in the chamber, the stressed volume. The pressure head driving blood from the periphery to the right atrium is the difference between $P_s$ and right atrial pressure ($P_s$ - $P_{ra}$). Venous return will therefore be equal to ($P_s$ - $P_{ra}$)/$R_v$, where $R_v$ is the resistance to venous return. As $P_{ra}$, the back pressure to venous return, decreases, venous return increases and vice versa. Actually one can draw a curve describing the relationship between $P_{ra}$ and venous return, as shown in Fig. 2. As $P_{ra}$ increases, venous return decreases until $P_{ra}$ is equal to the pressure in the peripheral reservoir, called the mean circulatory pressure, at which point flow is zero. As $P_{ra}$ decreases, venous return increases, until $P_{ra}$ is a few torr below zero. At this point further decreases in $P_{ra}$ fail to elicit increases in venous return, and venous return is said to be "flow limited." Flow limitation probably occurs because of collapse of the great veins at the entrance to the thorax. Thus the ability of decreases in $P_{ra}$ to increase influx into the chest is limited. Since the right atrium is located within the chest and is normally exposed to swings of pressure within the chest, increases in intrathoracic pressure lead to decreases in venous return and vice versa (within the limits set by flow limitation).

Cardiac function is also a part of the scheme, as shown in Fig. 2. The cardiac function curve is represented by the curve plotting cardiac output as a function of right atrial

end-diastolic pressure, which thus represents the preload. Since, in the steady state, cardiac output must equal venous return, the point at which the two systems exist in equilibrium is represented by the point of intersection of the cardiac function (Frank-Starling) and venous return curves. Thus for any given set of cardiac function and venous return curves there exists only one combination of right atrial pressure and cardiac output (= venous return) at which steady-state conditions apply.

### Effect of PEEP on Venous Return

Mechanical ventilation with increased airway pressure is frequently used to ventilate patients with hypoxemic respiratory failure and pulmonary edema. The goal of increased airway pressure, usually delivered by increasing levels of PEEP, is to increase lung volume, thus maintaining terminal airway patency. As lung volume increases, there is an increase in intrathoracic pressure, which is transmitted to the right atrium. This is expected to decrease venous return in a manner demonstrated in Fig. 3. The cardiac function curve is displaced rightward by the amount by which intrathoracic pressure is increased, thus maintaining the same transmural pressure–cardiac output relations. This moves the intersection of the cardiac function and the venous return curves "downward" on the venous return curve. In effect, right atrial pressure increases, which increases the back pres-

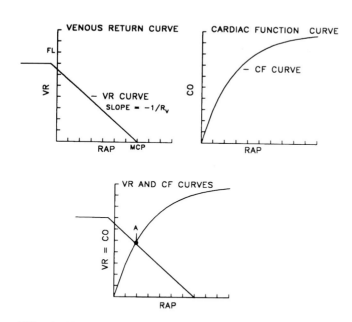

FIG. 2. Venous return (VR) and cardiac function (CF) curves. As right atrial pressure (RAP) increases, venous return decreases until RAP equals mean circulatory pressure (MCP). As RAP decreases, VR increases until the point of flow limitation (FL). The slope of the VR curve is equal to -1/RV. The CF curve is essentially a form of the Frank-Starling curve. In steady state the system exists at the point of intersection of the curves (point A). Reprinted from Scharf, SM. *J Crit Care* 1992;7:268, with permission.

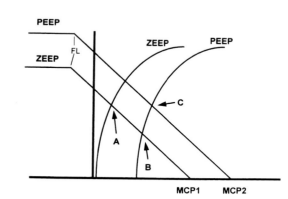

FIG. 3. Theoretic effects of positive end-expiratory pressure (PEEP) on venous return and cardiac function curves. PEEP leads to an increase in intrathoracic pressure and a shift right in the cardiac function curve. If there were no change in the venous return curve, then cardiac output and venous return would decrease, as shown in the shift from point A to point B. However, if there is a compensatory increase in mean circulatory pressure (from MCP1 to MCP2), then the system will exist in equilibrium at point C, at which the decrease in cardiac output and venous return is markedly less than if there were no changes in the venous return curve. Mean circulatory pressure can increase either by an increase in stressed volume or sympathoadrenal stimulation. ZEEP, zero end-expiratory pressure.

sure to venous return, and decreases the gradient for venous return. This simple observation was originally thought to account for the decrease in cardiac output commonly observed in patients placed on PEEP (reviewed in ref. 46). On the other hand, early observations (47) suggested that ventilation with PEEP must increase mean circulatory pressure, thus shifting the venous return curve to the right (Fig. 3). It was found that alpha-adrenergic blockade severely exacerbated the effects of PEEP on cardiac output (48). This suggested that sympathoadrenal homeostatic mechanisms played an important role in buffering the adverse effects of PEEP on cardiac output. Later work demonstrated that mean circulatory pressure increases approximately the same amount as does right atrial pressure with PEEP, and thus there was no demonstrable decrease in the gradient for venous return (49), and that this was again dependent on sympathoadrenal mechanisms. Finally, a recent study (50) confirmed earlier preliminary observations (22) that with PEEP the venous return curve changes by shifting the point of flow limitation to the right (Fig. 4). This means that mechanisms related to lung inflation cause the great veins to collapse at higher pressure than normal; i.e., there is an increase in the critical closing pressure of these vessels. The exact mechanisms of this are under investigation, but possible mechanisms include direct mechanical compression by the inflating lungs and/or mechanical compression by intra-abdominal contents, primarily the liver (seee ref. 46 for discussion).

These studies serve to illustrate the dynamic interplay between factors which govern the control of cardiac output during mechanical ventilation with increased airway pressures. Given the importance of venous return, it is not surprising that the effects of PEEP on cardiac output are exaggerated when blood volume and sympathoadrenal

tone are low. Conversely, increasing blood volume and increasing sympathoadrenal tone (infusion of sympathetic agents) can usually successfully counter the tendency of high levels of PEEP to decrease cardiac output (51).

### Effects of PEEP on RV Function

As discussed above, increased lung volume with PEEP would be expected to have different, and possibly opposing, effects on RV function. Increased intrathoracic pressure when transmitted to the right atrium, coupled with changes in the venous return curve, leads to decreased venous return, thus decreasing RV preload. On the other hand, increased lung volume with PEEP increases pulmonary vascular resistance and could lead to increases in RV afterload. Again the resultant effect depends on initial conditions. Under normovolemic blood volume conditions, increasing PEEP is associated with decreased cardiac output and decreased RV end-diastolic volume, i.e., preload (52–54). However, if cardiac output is held constant with PEEP by volume resuscitation, RV effects are easily demonstrated (55, 56). These consist of an increase in RV end-diastolic and end-systolic volumes with PEEP, especially at higher levels (≥15 cm $H_2O$). Further, when baseline RV function is compromised, the application of PEEP has been reported to lead to further deterioration of RV systolic function (53, 54, 57–59). In fact, when baseline RV function is severely compromised, in the presence of severe ARDS circulatory collapse on the basis of RV failure has been reported following the application of PEEP (60). Therefore, while preload effects are usually evident during the application of PEEP, when blood volume is high, baseline RV function in depressed, PEEP levels are high, and/or baseline pulmonary vascular resistance is already elevated, deterioration of RV function leading to RV end-systolic and end-diastolic dilation can occur.

### Diastolic Ventricular Interdependence

The right and left ventricles are connected *in series* through the pulmonary circulation. However, the two ventricles share common fiber bundles and a common septum and coexist within the same pericardial space. These features lead to the presence of *parallel* interactions between the ventricles whereby the function of one ventricle influences the function of the other. If the diastolic volume of one ventricle increases, then the diastolic compliance of the other ventricle decreases (reviewed in ref. 61). This interaction is amplified by the presence of the pericardium. For respiratory maneuvers, the most important diastolic interactions are those due to increased RV volume. This occurs during spontaneous inspiration when decreased intrathoracic pressure leads to increased venous return during the inspiratory phase and with RV

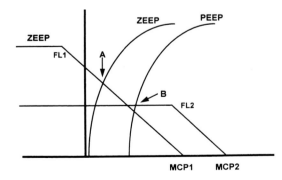

**FIG. 4.** Another more likely scheme for the changes in venous return with PEEP. If there is an increase in the pressure at which flow limitation occurs, then the ability of an increase in mean circulatory pressure to buffer PEEP-induced decreases in venous return is markedly less. FL1, flow limiting point at ZEEP; FL2, flow limiting point with PEEP. The venous return/cardiac output equilibrium point moves from A to B.

dilation as discussed above during mechanical ventilation with PEEP when venous return is preserved. Decreased LV preload has been observed as well in humans with mechanical ventilation with PEEP and exacerbations of asthma (62, 63). Pulsus paradoxus, the exaggerated inspiratory fall in arterial pressure occurring with breathing against obstructed airways, can be at least partly attributed to decreased LV preload caused by diastolic interdependence between the ventricles (64–66). As well, LV compliance has been observed to decrease with mechanical ventilation with PEEP (67, 68). These effects have been attributed to increased RV volume and interdependence. Finally, the effects of PEEP on LV compliance are exacerbated by RV ischemia, presumably because RV volumes increase more under these circumstances and interdependence effects are greater (54).

## Mechanical Heart-Lung Interactions

Earlier we alluded to mechanical compression of the heart by the lungs (23–26). Since the heart is located between the lungs, mechanical forces generated by the expanding lungs can be manifest which are not reflected in measurements of changes in intrathoracic pressure outside the cardiac fossa. This leads to limitation of diastolic filling by the expanding lungs above and beyond changes due to interdependence and the pericardium. This factor will presumably be greater with mechanical ventilation with large tidal volumes and high levels of PEEP when lung volume will be the greatest. Modes of ventilation which minimize lung volume such as apneic or high-frequency ventilation and ventilation with small tidal volumes and low levels of PEEP will minimize this factor. Mechanical compression of the heart by the lungs would be expected to have its greatest effect on the ventricular free walls since these are the cardiac surfaces exposed to forces in the cardiac fossa, thus altering cardiac configuration. While studies of RV configuration are difficult to perform with mechanical ventilation and PEEP, studies of LV configuration have revealed a decrease in the septal-lateral dimension relative to other LV dimensions with high levels of PEEP (25, 26, 35, 55). Furthermore, compressive effects by the heart appear to be greatest when the lower lobes of the lungs are inflated (23, 24). Pathologic conditions such as emphysema and asthma which lead to increased lung volume at FRC should maximize these effects, and those conditions in which lung volumes are decreased would minimize these effects. With emphysema increased lung volume in the lower lobes during exercise is a major contributor to observed increases in the pulmonary wedge pressure under this condition (24). During mechanical ventilation of patients with obstructve airways disease, increasing respiratory rate can lead to the phenomenon of gas trapping, or *auto-PEEP*. Presumably, pulmonary wedge pressure can increase under these circumstances as well, a finding which, if misinterpreted, could lead to inappropriate therapeutic measures.

One must be careful to distinguish between lung gas volume and actual lung (tissue + fluid + gas) volume. While conditions such as pulmonary edema and ARDS are associated with decreased gas volume in the lung, total lung volume is actually not altered by very much (69). This probably explains why mechanical ventilation with PEEP often demonstrates similar changes in cardiac output in experimental ARDS as with normal lungs even though lung gas volume is less (70). Total lung volume is actually unchanged and mechanical effects on venous return and cardiac compression are probably not greatly altered except by the severest of disease.

## Effects of Changes in Intrathoracic Pressure on Cardiac Function

From what has been said above it must be clear that the term *intrathoracic pressure* does not per se specify a pressure. Rather, one must ask "which intrathoracic pressure, esophageal, pleural, cardiac fossa, or cardiac surface?" However, this term is commonly used in discussing cardiocirculatory interactions and is used when discussing the use of respiratory maneuvers to support circulatory function. We will continue to use the term, but in general the meaning will be cardiac surface pressure, unless otherwise specified.

In 1850 the great physiologist Donders (71) recognized that just as decreased intrathoracic pressure would encourage the influx of blood (venous return) *into* the chest, decreased intrathoracic pressure would also hinder the efflux of blood *from* the chest. In modern parlance, decreased intrathoracic pressure acts to impede LV ejection, or as an increase in LV afterload. The converse is that increased intrathoracic pressure can act to aid LV ejection or as a decrease in LV afterload. Figure 5 illustrates one way of thinking about this. If one considers the left ventricle to be a pump raising a bolus of blood equal to stroke volume from the potential energy of the left atrium to that of the aorta, then from the left ventricle's point of view it makes little difference if the aortic pressure is raised or the left atrial pressure is decreased. The effective afterload has increased. Another way of looking at this is to consider LV wall stress as LV end-systolic transmural pressure. If, during a maneuver which decreases intrathoracic pressure, LV end-systolic pressure decreases less than LV surface pressure, then the pressure difference across the LV wall (end-systolic transmural pressure) will actually increase. Numerous studies have studied LV function during the performance of the Mueller maneuver (sustained decrease in intrathoracic pressure—the converse of the Valsalva maneuver). In most cases there have been measured increases in LV

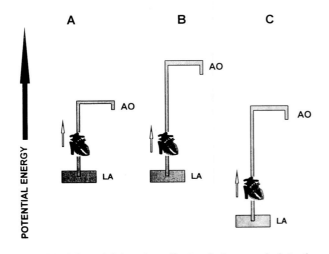

**FIG. 5.** Model explaining the effects of changes in intrathoracic pressure on cardiac function. The left ventricle is a pump which lifts blood from the potential energy of the left atrium (LA) to that of the aorta (AO). If AO pressure is increased (panel B), then cardiac work is increased. Conversely, if LA pressure is decreased at constant AO pressure (panel C), cardiac work is also increased. The former could occur with vasoconstrictors, the latter with decreases in intrathoracic pressure which are transmitted to the LA. Increased intrathoracic pressure would act in the opposite manner, aiding ventricular ejection.

end-systolic volume and/or transmural pressure (72–75). As well, in patients with ischemic heart disease regional wall akinesis has been recorded during the Mueller maneuver consistent with increased transmural pressure (76, 77). It is not clear how these findings relate to cyclical swings in intrathoracic pressure as seen with obstructed respiration or respiratory distress, a debate beyond the scope of this chapter. However, it is reasonable to assume that in patients on ventilators, decreasing mean intrathoracic pressure could increase the overall afterload against which the LV must eject and that this could be most important in patients in whom LV function is already compromised.

The converse of the above is, of course, that increased intrathoracic pressure could aid the function of the failing left ventricle. This could work in two ways. First, changes in intrathoracic pressure are transmitted to the thoracic aorta (78, 79). This would be especially important in young individuals in whom this vessel is rather compliant (80). Thus, increasing intrathoracic pressure would increase intra-aortic pressure in the thoracic portion of the aorta relative to the rest of the arterial system. This would lead to efflux of blood from the thorax, which would occur from veins as well as arteries. When pressure in the chest falls again, blood would move back into the chest via the veins, but only minimally via the arterial system because of the presence of the aortic valve. If increases in intrathoracic pressure were periodic, then the result would

be the net movement of blood from the venous to the arterial system. This notion has been called the *thoracic pump* and is one of the principal mechanisms by which "cardiac" massage aids in supporting the circulation (81, 82). Indeed, increasing intrathoracic pressure by any means would lead to support of the circulation by this mechanism. In 1976 Criley et al. (83) reported eight patients who underwent ventricular fibrillation while at cardiac catheterization and were able to support their circulation by repetitive coughing long enough for electrical defibrillation to be instituted, thereby obviating the need for external cardiac massage. Theoretically, if increases in intrathoracic pressure were timed to ventricular diastole, then blood would flow from the aorta into the extrathoracic arterial system during this phase of the cardiac cycle. At the next ventricular systole, the ventricle would be ejecting into a relatively empty aorta and its ejection could be greater than if it were ejecting into a full aorta. This may be the mechanism whereby increases in intrathoracic pressure timed to diastole can lead to increased stroke volume in the failing heart (80, 84, 85). On the other hand, with aortic emptying, aortic input impedance increases (84), a change which would tend to increase LV afterload and could limit the increase in stroke volume observed with diastolic phasic increases in intrathoracic pressure. Most current work concentrates on systolic increases in intrathoracic pressure, as will be reviewed in the section on respiratory treatment in heart failure.

### Effect of Increased Cardiac Surface Pressure on Coronary Blood Flow

FInally, when cardiac surface pressure is increased relative to aortic pressure, this increase could be transmitted to the epicardial vessels of the heart. Either increased cardiac surface pressure could act as an increase in the critical closing pressure of these vessels or right atrial pressure could act to increase the back pressure to coronary perfusion. Either way, increased LV surface pressure might be expected to impede coronary flow. In an isolated heart preparation, Fessler et al. (86) demonstrated that raising cardiac surface pressure relative to aortic (coronary perfusion) pressure led to decreases in coronary flow and corresponding worsening cardiac function. These changes were accompanied by myocardial lactate production, suggesting the onset of myocardial ischemia. While these changes were consistent with the above predictions, they were only seen when cardiac surface pressure had been increased by 60 torr. At lower levels of increased cardiac surface pressure, evidence of improved cardiac function was seen.

A number of investigators have studied the effects of mechanical ventilation with PEEP on coronary blood flow. In 1973 Tucker and Murray (87) measured decreases in coronary blood flow with PEEP, which appeared out of proportion to decreases in cardiac work (related to decreased venous return and blood pressure). They suggested that if PEEP led to decreases in coronary flow out of proportion to metabolic needs (i.e., out of proportion to autoregulatory demands), then this mode of ventilatory support could be dangerous when coronary flow reserve is limited. Venus and Jacobs (88) studied regional myocardial blood flow in dogs during the administration of PEEP. They found a decrease in LV and septal myocardial blood flow in all regions and RV endocardial blood flow with 15 and 25 cm $H_2O$ PEEP. The authors concluded that PEEP could reduce LV function above and beyond preload effects. They suggested that decreased myocardial blood flow could be an effect of reflexes triggered by lung inflation (see above). In humans, Tittley et al. (89) studied patients post–coronary arterial bypass graft on mechanical ventilation with levels of PEEP of 0 to 15 cm $H_2O$. In 17 of 33 patients, decreased lactate utilization was observed at 15 cm $H_2O$ PEEP. The authors concluded that at the greatest level of PEEP, *ischemic metabolism* was observed in one-half the patients. Finally, in anesthetized dogs, Hassapoyannes et al. (90) studied the effects of increased cardiac surface pressure (15 and 30 torr) confined to cardiac systole on myocardial blood flow and metabolism. These authors concluded that coronary blood flow decreased in proportion to decreased LV energy demands, that is, coronary flow changes were autoregulatory in nature. However, since aortic diastolic pressure decreased, a limit may exist to increasing cardiac surface pressure above which coronary blood flow may decrease out of proportion to changes in myocardial energy demands, thus posing the danger of ischemia, especially in patients with limited coronary flow reserve.

In the next section we will review experimental and clinical effects of various respiratory maneuvers, all of which increase intrathoracic pressure. As will be seen, there are a number of contradictory findings. Possibly one of the reasons for seemingly contradictory findings in the literature is that the effects of potential changes in coronary blood flow have not been accounted for. The studies just quoted impose a cautionary note on the routine clinical use of increasing intrathoracic pressure to treat patients with ischemic heart disease and suggest that more study be undertaken to determine the clinical importance of these findings.

## RESPIRATORY TREATMENT IN HEART FAILURE

In this section we review some of the experimental and clinical data relevant to the topic. One must be careful in generalizing from one study to the next. Conditions vary from study to study, and generalizations from one mode of ventilatory support to another are not often possible.

For example, experimental studies with mechanical ventilation and PEEP are usually performed on anesthetized, paralyzed animals. This means that intrathoracic pressure invariably rises on inspiration since the animals do not use their inspiratory muscles. Further, the anesthetic interferes with cardiopulmonary homeostatic reflexes. On the other hand, clinical studies with mechanical ventilation with PEEP are usually performed on unanesthetized (although possibly sedated) patients. They may be on *intermittent mandatory* mode of ventilation, where spontaneous inspiration is possible between ventilator-mandated breaths, or they may be on *assist-control* mode of ventilation, where mechanical breaths are triggered. In these cases, intrathoracic pressure may not behave as in the paralyzed control ventilation situation. Even during the assist-control mode of ventilation, patients often continue to use their inspiratory muscles throughout inspiration. Thus, intrathoracic pressure may not rise at all, or may even fall, as the force generated by the inspiratory muscles may counterbalance the increase in intrathoracic pressure due to the increase in lung volume. In the ensuing discussion we will point out some of the pitfalls along the way which the reader should be aware of when attempting to understand and place in context much of the recent literature on the topic.

### Continuous Positive Airway Pressure

Continuous positive airway pressure (CPAP) ventilatory support refers to the application of pressure to the airway of the spontaneously breathing patient throughout all phases of respiration. This mode of ventilatory support is quite old and has been used clinically at least since the beginning of this century (91). This may be done while the patient is intubated or via face or nose mask. A commonly used system today is the use of a low-resistance spring-loaded valve with a high airflow passing through the system. This allows for airway pressure to be relatively stable throughout all phases of respiration (92, 93). In 1936 Pulton and Oxon reported using a home-made CPAP device (made from a vacuum cleaner!) to treat a variety of forms of respiratory failure including left-sided heart failure and pulmonary edema (1). Subsequently, CPAP has become an accepted mode of therapy for treating respiratory distress and pulmonary edema in children and adults (93–96). Improved gas exchange and decreased work of breathing have been documented in patients receiving CPAP therapy for pulmonary edema and ARDS (96–98). However, the concept that CPAP could actually improve the functioning of the failing heart by mechanisms above and beyond improving gas exchange and ventilatory mechanics has received a fair degree of attention only relatively recently.

Continuous positive airway pressure is being used commonly in the treatment of obstructive sleep apnea

(99). As a result of its widespread nocturnal use in patients with concomitant sleep apnea and LV dysfunction, clinical observations suggested that, in addition to resolution of symptoms of sleep apnea, there was often marked improvement in LV function as well (100). In a preliminary study of five patients without obstructive sleep apnea but with severe congestive heart failure and Cheyne-Stokes respiration, the nocturnal use of nasal CPAP 12.5 cm $H_2O$ was associated with improvements in mean arterial $O_2$ saturation at night and resolution of symptoms of fragmented sleep. Most important there was a significant increase in the mean resting LV ejection fraction measured during the day (31% to 38%) and marked improvement in symptoms of congestive heart failure, including improvements in the New York State Heart Association disability classification. A recent controlled trial of the treatment of congestive heart failure by nocturnal CPAP (101) confirmed improvement of LV ejection fraction and daytime functioning. These trials demonstrate improvement in LV functioning comparable to those seen with vasodilator trials, suggesting nocturnal nasal CPAP as a viable nonpharmacologic treatment for congestive heart failure and Cheyne-Stokes respiration. On the other hand, two small uncontrolled patient trials failed to demonstrate significant daytime improvement in indices of heart failure using nocturnal CPAP (102, 103), and one (102) actually reported deterioration in three patients. While the reason for the different clinical observations is unclear, differences in baseline cardiac and autonomic function may well be responsible, and standardized large trials will need to be undertaken to assess whether nocturnal respiratory support with CPAP can improve daytime cardiac function in the failing heart.

The question of the acute effects of CPAP on cardiac function have been investigated both clinically and experimentally. In 22 patients with dilated cardiomyopathy, Bradley et al. (104) demonstrated acute improvements in cardiac output when 5 cm $H_2O$ CPAP was applied, but only in patients in whom baseline pulmonary wedge pressure was greater than > 12 cm $H_2O$. Patients with wedge pressure in the normal range demonstrated decreased cardiac output with CPAP. This mode of respiratory support has been evaluated in acutely ill patients with congestive heart failure in a few small studies. In a single patient receiving inotropic and intra-aortic balloon counterpulsation support, Pery et al. (97) demonstrated improved cardiac output, increased mixed venous $O_2$ saturation, and decreased pulmonary wedge pressure when 7 cm $H_2O$ CPAP was added. Improved gas exchange, decreased respiratory muscle work, and decreased LV afterload due to raised intrathoracic pressure were all postulated to be contributing mechanisms. Baratz et al. (105) studied 13 patients with acute decompensation of congestive heart failure with CPAP levels up to 15 cm $H_2O$. Seven of the patients responded with an increase in cardiac output of at least 400 mL/min. Since all of these patients had pul-

monary wedge pressures of more than 20 torr, the effect of baseline wedge pressure could not be determined as in the previous study done in stable patients at catheterization (104). Further, these patients were administered a variety of cardiac support medications, including vasodilators, inotropes, and antianginal medications, all of which could be confounding factors. Räsänen et al. (106) reported on the effects of increasing CPAP in 14 patients with acute respiratory failure complicating acute myocardial infarction. Overall, respiratory effort as measured by swings in pleural pressure was diminished. While there was no overall trend in cardiac output, patients with only moderate LV dysfunction (stroke volume index > 20 mL/m$^2$) demonstrated decreased output, while those with poor LV function (stroke volume index < 20 mL/m$^2$) demonstrated a nonsignificant trend to improved output.

From the above clinical data it is apparent that CPAP can be associated with improved cardiac function at least in some patients, probably those with the most severe dysfunction. The mechanisms by which CPAP aids LV ejection either acutely or over the long term are poorly understood. Mechanisms for acutely improved ejection include decreased LV afterload and improved contractility. Left ventricular afterload could decrease if cardiac surface pressure increased relative to intracavitary pressure, or if there were changes in vasomotor arterial tone (vasodilation).

Recently, using previously instrumented unanesthetized, sedated pigs, our laboratory has been investigating the mechanisms whereby CPAP could improve LV ejection in normal and abnormal hearts (107). In the first study, normal animals were studied under two conditions, normal blood volume and when made hypervolemic by infusion of hetastarch. The later condition raised LV end-diastolic pressure (LVEDP) from the baseline of approximately 12 torr to approximately 25 torr. A second study (108) was performed in animals in which congestive cardiomyopathy had been produced by 7 days of rapid ventricular pacing. Figure 6 shows changes in cardiac output from these studies. It can be seen that with normovolemia CPAP led to decreases in cardiac output. However, with both hypervolemia in normal hearts and cardiomyopathy, there were increases in cardiac output of 5 cm $H_2O$ CPAP followed by decreases towards baseline. These results could be explained by the interaction of the dual effects of CPAP on circulatory function. First, increased intrathoracic pressure acts to decrease venous return. Second, CPAP aids ventricular ejection by one of the mechanisms just discussed. Using graphic analysis, we demonstrated that when blood volume is low, i.e., low mean circulatory pressure, and cardiac function good, the major effect would be on venous return and cardiac output would fall with CPAP. On the other hand, when blood volume is elevated and/or baseline cardiac function poor, then at low levels of CPAP, the effects on ventricular ejection outweigh those on venous return and cardiac output increases. Figure 7 demonstrates a decrease in LV end-diastolic and

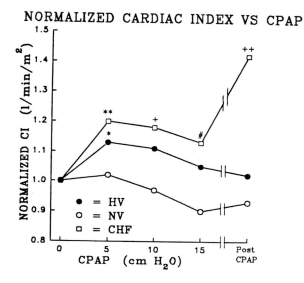

**FIG. 6.** Effects of continuous positive airway pressure (CPAP) on cardiac index (CI; normalized to baseline) in sedated pigs. NV, normovolemic conditions; HV, hypervolemic conditions; CHF, rapid ventricular pacing induced cardiomyopathy with congestive heart failure. (*) p 0.05 compared with baseline; (**) p 0.003 compared with baseline; (+) p 0.01 compared with baseline; (#) p 0.05 compared with baseline; (++) p 0.001 compared with baseline.

end-systolic volume with increasing levels of CPAP in a single animal. Note the decrease in both end-diastolic and end-systolic volume with increased CPAP. Decreased end-diastolic volume is consistent with decreased venous return and preload; decreased end-systolic volume is consistent with decreased afterload and/or improved contractility. One additional finding was demonstrated in the myopathic animals (Fig. 6). When the CPAP was removed, a sustained increase in cardiac output, considerably above baseline levels, was observed. This was not seen in animals with normal hearts. These studies indicate

that there are circulatory changes induced by CPAP which may be present even when CPAP is removed. Post-CPAP increases in cardiac output were associated with vasodilation and raise the question of CPAP-mediated changes in autonomic tone. Possibly, post-CPAP vasodilation unloaded the left ventricle enough to lead to sustained increases in cardiac output. Indeed, during this phase, substantial decreases in systemic vascular resistance were observed. Finally, we tested the hypothesis that increased cardiac output with CPAP was due to increased cardiac surface pressure (109), which subsequently led to decreased LV afterload. Figure 8 shows the results of measurements of intrapericardial pressure with increased CPAP in animals with normal hearts under normo- and hypervolemic conditions. Under normovolemic conditions, increased CPAP was associated with increased cardiac surface pressure, as expected. However, under hypervolemic conditions, while baseline cardiac surface pressure was increased (increased cardiac volume), increasing CPAP was associated with decreasing cardiac surface pressure. The difference in response between normo- and hypervolemia was not explained by differences in lung mechanics or changes in intrathoracic pressure as measured from esophageal pressure. Actually, this somewhat surprising finding was not altogether unprecedented (29, 110) and was explained by assuming, as had others (28, 29), that pericardial pressure resulted from the summation of extrapericardial and pericardial elastic forces. With CPAP, extrapericardial pressure increases because of increased intrathoracic pressure and direct mechanical heart-lung interactions. However, increased CPAP was associated with decreased cardiac volume (Fig. 7). This tends to lead to decreases in cardiac surface pressure. Under normovolemic conditions, when cardiac volume is normal, changes in extrapericardial pressure predominate and cardiac surface pressure increases with CPAP. When cardiac volume is large (hypervolemia), the decrease in LV volume predominates and cardiac surface

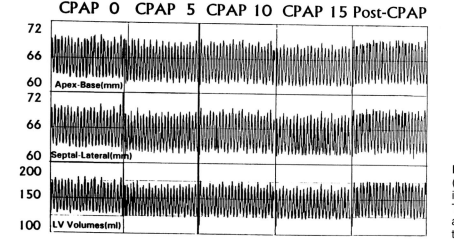

**FIG. 7.** Raw data tracing of left ventricular (LV) volume changes with increasing CPAP in a single pig with congestive heart failure. Two axes and calculated ventricular volume are shown. Note decreased diastolic and systolic volumes with CPAP.

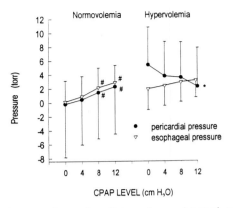

**FIG. 8.** Change in pericardial and esophageal pressures with CPAP in sedated pigs. See discussion in text.

pressure falls with increased CPAP. These findings suggest that the beneficial effects of CPAP are not related simply to increased cardiac surface pressure unloading the left ventricle. If afterload decreases, then it is by some other mechanism besides increased intrathoracic pressure, possibly arterial vasodilation. On the other hand, if there is autonomic stimulation with CPAP, then cardiac contractility might in fact increase. These possibilities are currently under investigation.

To summarize, CPAP can lead to clinical improvement in patients with congestive heart failure. This improvement lasts beyond the time in which CPAP is actually applied. Part of this improvement is related to improvement in lung mechanics (decreased work of breathing, recruitment of collapsed alveoli) and gas exchange, but there are definitely patients in whom LV ejection is improved. These patients probably constitute a subset of patients with the poorest baseline LV function. The mechanisms by which the improvement occurs are not yet clear but may relate partly to changes in peripheral vasomotor tone and autonomic mediated changes in cardiac function. However, CPAP shows great promise as an acute and chronic mode of therapy for the failing left ventricle. Further investigation should yield clinical guidelines upon which to decide to initiate and continue therapy with CPAP.

## Mechanical Ventilation in Patients with Ischemic Heart Disease

We have already alluded to changes in pulmonary and respiratory muscle function which occur with cardiorespiratory failure. Further, the changes in cardiocirculatory function related to mechanical ventilation and PEEP have been discussed. In this section we will discuss the role of mechanical ventilation as a therapeutic adjunct in patients with ischemic heart disease.

Generally, when patients are weaned off ventilators, there is a small increase in cardiac output. This is likely related to increased metabolic demands and sympathetic adjustments as well as a decrease in mean intrathoracic pressure leading to increased venous return. In 1973 Beach et al. (111) reported on the effects of discontinuing mechanical ventilation on cardiac output in 37 patients. They observed that cardiac output actually decreased in 18 of 37 patients when they were weaned from mechanical ventilation. They could not predict the hemodynamic response to weaning from any changes in arterial blood gas tensions. The patients in whom output decreased upon weaning had somewhat worse preweaning cardiac function, as demonstrated by a greater central venous pressure and lower preweaning cardiac output. Pulmonary vascular resistance was also greater in this group. The authors speculated that changes in sympathoadrenal function associated with weaning might have been responsible. An equally likely hypothesis is that cardiocirculatory changes associated with mechanical ventilation had a beneficial effect on circulatory function in the patients with the poorer baseline cardiac function.

In 1984 Räsänen et al. (112) studied the cardiopulmonary effects of ventilatory support in 12 patients with acute myocardial infarction complicated by respiratory failure. They found 5 of 12 who developed EKG evidence of ischemia upon assuming spontaneous ventilation. They also calculated an index called the *endocardial viability ratio,* defined as the ratio between arterial diastolic pressure-time integral and tension-time index and found that this fell significantly during spontaneous compared with mechanical ventilation. Lemaire et al. (113) studied a group of patients with known ischemic heart disease who could not be weaned off mechanical ventilators following an episode of respiratory failure. Although arterial blood gas tensions were well maintained and there were few indicators of cardiac ischemia (EKG, chest pain), these authors documented increases in transmural LV filling pressure (pulmonary wedge minus esophageal pressure) during weaning attempts. Several days of therapy with calcium channel blockers and nitrates was enough to make the patients weanable. At this point, increased transmural wedge pressures were not observed. The authors suggested that unsuspected LV failure in patients with ischemic heart disease be considered as a cause of failure to wean. Hurford et al. (114) then investigated the cause of failure to wean in 14 unweanable patients with coronary heart disease. These authors demonstrated LV ischemia by radiolabeled thallium perfusion studies in 7 of 14 of these patients. Thus, clinically silent ischemia may occur in a large percentage of patients with coronary heart disease which is suppressed by mechanical ventilation. Ischemia was not related to changes in arterial blood gas tensions. Again the mechanism for ischemia is unknown. Adjustments of sympathoadrenal tone associated with increased metabolic demands of spontaneous ventilation may be partly responsible. However, increased LV stroke work due to increased LV transmural pressure (decreased mean intrathoracic pressure) and/or increased stroke output may also contribute by increasing myocardial oxygen demand and unfavorably altering demand-supply ratios. Whatever the mechanisms, these considerations should be brought to bear in caring for patients with ischemic heart disease and concomitant ventilatory failure requiring mechanical ventilation. Prudence would dictate avoiding hasty weaning attempts, especially if acute ischemia is present. In the unweanable patient, consideration should be given to the diagnosis of clinically silent LV failure due to ischemia. The diagnosis will not necessarily be made by measuring the pulmonary wedge pressure in the normal way (referencing to atmospheric pressure) since intrathoracic pressures may decrease with increasing respiratory distress. Measuring wedge pressure relative to esophageal pressure may be a useful and simple clinical tool for making this assessment.

FInally, is there a role for increasing intrathoracic pressure with mechanical ventilation above and beyond the needs of ventilation? That is, can the ventilator be used as a tool for supporting the failing heart and increasing cardiac output? In 1982 Grace and Greenbaum (115) reported on the effects of PEEP on cardiac performance in patients with cardiac dysfunction. In studies reminiscent of previously quoted studies with CPAP they found that 3 to 5 cm $H_2O$ PEEP added to mechanical ventilation raised cardiac output (mean increase 500 mL/min) in patients with a baseline pulmonary wedge pressure of more than 19 torr and either had no effect on or decreased output when the wedge pressure was lower. In the same year Mathru et al. (116) studied patients post–cardiopulmonary bypass and compared controlled ventilation with intermittent mandatory ventilation (IMV) with IMV plus 5 cm $H_2O$ PEEP. In patients with severe congestive heart failure (LVEDP > 16 torr), institution of IMV led to decreased cardiac output and increased pulmonary artery wedge pressure, signs of decreasing cardiac function. Adding PEEP to IMV in turn increased cardiac output and decreased wedge pressure back to the levels of controlled ventilation. Pinsky et al. produced cardiac failure by injecting large doses of propranolol into pentobarbital-anesthetized dogs (117). The animals were mechanically ventilated using large tidal volumes (30 mL/kg), and to further increase inspiratory intrathoracic pressure swings, chest and abdominal compliances were decreased by binding. With binding, inspiratory intrathoracic pressure increased by 12.1 torr, as opposed to 1.2 torr with no binding. With the bound condition there was an upward shift in the Frank-Starling function curve compared to the unbound state. Pinsky and Summer (118) reported using inspiratory phasic increases in intrathoracic pressure in mechanically ventilated patients with cardiogenic shock. They applied binders to the chest and abdomen to a degree sufficient to increase esophageal pressure by 5 torr during inspiration but loose enough to leave expiratory esophageal pressure unchanged. This led to increased cardiac output in five of seven patients. There was no correlation between baseline wedge pressure and the response to increased intrathoracic pressure. In an accompanying editorial Robotham coined the term *ventilator-assisted myocardial performance* (VAMP) to describe the use of ventilatory maneuvers to assist circulatory function in the failing heart (119).

### Cardiac Cycle Specific Increases in Intrathoracic Pressure

One problem with using high-tidal-volume ventilation with chest wall binding is the effect of these maneuvers on venous return. One could imagine disastrous consequences from substantially increasing intrathoracic pressure if circulating blood volume was low. Further, chest and abdominal binding could decrease lung volume at end expiration, which in turn would have adverse consequences on gas exchange. Finally, large-tidal-volume ventilation could be problematic in terms of the regulation of gas exchange. To address the problem of the balance between venous return and LV function effects, a number of studies have utilized cardiac cycle specific increases in intrathoracic pressure. This approach attempts to limit increased intrathoracic pressure to that phase of the cardiac cycle in which it would do the most good, i.e., during systole.

In an early study Pinsky et al. (120) studied the effects of phasic increases in intrathoracic pressure in anesthetized dogs with propranolol-induced heart failure. Pressure pulses were produced by a jet ventilator and exaggerated by respiratory binding. They altered respiratory timing and duty cycle while maintaining constant mean intrathoracic pressure. They found that when cardiac function was normal, LV stroke volume decreased. However, when cardiac function was abnormal (LV filling pressure > 17 torr), they observed increases in stroke volume. They found that changes in intrathoracic pressure could account for all observable changes steady-state hemodynamic changes, independent of respiratory frequency, phasic respiratory swings in intrathoracic pressure, or respiratory cycle timing. However, this study did not attempt to synchronize intrathoracic pressure with cardiac cycle. This was done in a later study in anesthetized animals (84) in which the jet ventilator pulses were timed to occur in early and late systole and early and late diastole. Again abdominal binders were used to increase the swings in intrathoracic pressure while not altering lung volume. With pharmacologically induced LV failure, pulses timed to systole had the greatest effect on improving stroke volume while decreasing LV transmural filling pressure. In a clinical study in nine patients prior to cardiac transplant study Pinsky et al. (121) compared the effects of intermittent positive pressure ventilation with jet ventilation set at the heart rate, the latter unsynchronized with heart rate or timed to occur during the upstroke of the arterial pressure. As shown in Fig. 9, jet ventilation synchronous with LV ejection produced statistically significant increases in cardiac output compared to standard ventilation of asynchronous jet ventilation. These results suggested that data from the animal studies could be extrapolated to human cardiac failure and that the key was timing increased intrathoracic pressure to occur during LV ejection.

In a mathematical analysis of timed increases in intrathoracic pressure, Beyar et al. (122) concluded that maximum flow augmentation would occur when the onset of the increase in intrathoracic pressure is simultaneous with the onset of LV isovolumic contraction and has a duration of 400 msec. The magnitude of flow augmentation would be a function of the amplitude of the rise in intrathoracic pressure. These predictions were more or less borne out by experimental data in anesthetized dogs, although they found that there was little further flow augmentation when the rise in intrathoracic pressure was more that 30 to 40 torr. In this case, intrathoracic pressure was increased using a rapidly inflating/deflating external vest. This has great potential importance since this method of cardiac assist could be applied noninvasively and does not require intubation or respiratory apparatus.

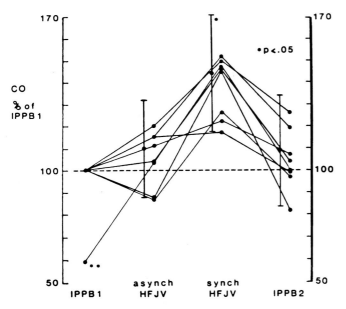

**FIG. 9.** Effects of high-frequency jet ventilation (HFJV) in humans with congestive heart failure. IPPB, standard ventilation with intermittent positive pressure breathing; asynch HFJV, HFJV at heart rate but not synchronized to any cardiac phase; synch HFJV, HFJV synchronized to cardiac systole. Cardiac output (CO) is normalized to the value with IPPB1. Reprinted from Pinsky MR, et al. *Chest* 1987;91:709, with permission.

Other experimental studies have addressed the question as to whether synchronized jet ventilation is effective in other forms of cardiac dysfunction. In a study on experimental mitral regurgitation, Stein et al. (123) found that both systolic and diastolic timed jet ventilation led to increased stroke volume but that systolic increases were greater than diastolic increases. Thus, even with normal LV contractility, when mitral regurgitation impedes forward flow, increased intrathoracic pressure could aid in LV ejection. Guimond et al. (124) studied the effects of synchronized jet ventilation during endotoxemia in anesthetized dogs. In this case there were no increases in stroke volume noted with either synchronized or unsynchronized increases in intrathoracic pressure. The authors pointed out the complex interrelationships between cardiac and peripheral circulatory function. They suggested that changes in cardiac function due to phasic increases in intrathoracic pressure were masked by the combination of arterial vasodilation and increased venous return associated with endotoxin and fluid resuscitation.

In a recent study using chronically instrumented dogs, Peters and Ihle (125) evaluated the cardiovascular effects of single and repetitive increases in intrathoracic pressure produced by external vest inflation in anesthetized dogs before and after autonomic blockade and myocardial ischemia. Although single inflations coupled to late systole led to augmented stroke volume, repetitive inflations coupled to all cardiac cycle phases led to nonspecific flow increases (40%). This was not observed after beta-adrenergic blockade either before or following coronary arterial occlusion. Thus, the effects of vest inflations appeared to be related to changes in sympathoadrenal tone rather than increased intrathoracic pressure per se. The authors noted that previous studies were done in acutely anesthetized animals where cardiac failure was induced by pharmacologic autonomic blockade. The authors felt that differences in study conditions accounted for differences in results and suggested that cyclical changes in lung volume in previous studies could have accounted for the increases in output seen in these studies. That is, direct compression of the heart with the jet ventilator could have given the cardiac assist. They concluded (123) that "there remain several unresolved issues with respect to assisting a failing heart by pleural pressure increments," a sentiment shared by the author of this chapter.

## CONCLUSIONS

From what has been said, it should be clear that numerous factors govern the cardiac and peripheral circulatory response to ventilatory maneuvers in patients with normal and failing hearts. Traditionally, the balance between venous return and cardiac function has been the model by which experimental and clinical observations have been interpreted. It is clear that other factors may, under the right circumstances, play an important role. These include central arterial compliance, changes in coronary blood flow, and changes in autonomic tone. Since at least some patients with failing hearts respond to ventilatory support, and since effective nonpharmacologic therapy for poor cardiac function offers many advantages, it behooves the critical care community to further evaluate the role of ventilatory support in caring for acutely ill cardiac patients. Future studies directed at elucidating the complex interactions between all the contributing factors can be expected to reward the clinician with another weapon in our armamentarium for treating the most critically ill patient.

## REFERENCES

1. Poulton EP, Oxon DM. Left-sided heart failure with pulmonary oedema: its treatment with the 9pulmonary plus pressure machine.9 *Lancet* 1936;1:981.
2. Smulyn H, Gilbert R, Eich RH. Pulmonary effects of heart failure. *Surg Clin North Am* 1974;54:1077.
3. Oppenheimer L, Goldberg HS. Pulmonary circulation and edema formation. In: Scharf SM, Cassidy SS, eds. *Heart-lung interactions in health and disease.* New York: Marcel Dekker; 1989:93.
4. Bates DV. *Respiratory function in disease.* 3rd ed. Philadelphia: Saunders; 1989:250.
5. Chung KF, Keyes SJ, Morgan BM, Jones PW, Snashall PD. Mechanisms of airway narrowing in acute pulmonary oedema in dogs: influence of the vagus and lung volume. *Clin Sci* 1983;65:289.
6. Kikuchi R, Sekizaea K, Sasaki H, et al. Effects of pulmonary congestion on airway reactivity to histamine aerosol in dogs. *J Appl Physiol* 1984;57:1640.
7. Sharp JT, Griffith GT, Bunnell IL, Greene DG. Ventilatory mechanics in pulmonary edema in man. *J Clin Invest* 1958;37:111.
8. Hoeschen RJ, Gold LHA, Cuddy TE, Cherniak RM. Oxygen cost and efficiency of respiratory system in hypoxia and in congestive heart failure. *Circ Res* 1962;11:825.
9. Anthonisen NR, Smith HJ. Respiratory acidosis as a consequence of pulmonary edema. *Ann Intern Med* 1965;62:991.
10. Avery WG, Samet P, Sackner MA. The acidosis of pulmonary edema. *Am J Med* 1970;48:320.
11. Fulop M, Horowitz M, Aberman A, Jaffe ER. Lactic acidosis in pulmonary edema due to left ventricular failure. *Ann Intern Med* 1973; 79:180.
12. Roberts AM, Bhattacharya, Schultz J, Coleridge HD, Coleridge JCG. Stimulation of pulmonary vagal afferent C-fibers by lung edema in dogs. *Circ Res* 1986;58:512.
13. Aubier M, Trippenbach T, Roussos C. Respiratory muscle fatigue during cardiogenic shock. *J Appl Physiol* 1981;56:499.
14. Aubier M, Viires N, Syllie G, Moses R, Roussos C. Respiratory muscle contribution to lactic acidosis in low cardiac output. *Am Rev Respir Dis* 1982;126:648.
15. Heistad DD, Abboud FM. Circulatory adjustments to hypoxia. *Circulation* 1980;61:463.
16. Richardson EW, Wasserman AJ, Patterson JL. General and regional circulatory responses to change in blood pH and carbon dioxide tension. *J Clin Invest* 1961;40:41.
17. Permutt S, Howell JBL, Proctor D, Riley R. Effects of lung inflation on static pressure-volume characteristics of pulmonary vessels. *J Appl Physiol* 1961;16:64.
18. Whittenberger JL, MacGregor M, Berglund E, Borst MC. Influence of state of inflation of the lung on pulmonary vascular resistance. *J Appl Physiol* 1960;15:878.
19. Scharf SM, Greenberg H. The normal adult pulmonary circulation. In: Baum G, Wolinsky E, eds. *Textbook of pulmonary diseases.* Boston: Little, Brown; 1993:1265.
20. Maughan WL. Right ventricular function. In: Scharf SM, Cassidy SS, eds. *Heart-Lung interactions in health and disease.* New York: Marcel Dekker; 1989:179.
21. Dhainaut JF, Schlemmer B, Monsallier JF, Fourestié V, Carli A. Behavior of the right ventricle following PEEP in patients with mild and severe ARDS. *Am Rev Respir Dis* 1984;129:A99.
22. Robotham J, Scharf SM. The effects of positive and negative pressure ventilation on cardiac performance. In: Matthey RA, Matthey MA, Dantzker D, eds. *Cardiovascular pulmonary interactions in normal and diseased lungs.* Philadelphia: WB Saunders; 1983:161.
23. Marini JJ, O'Quinn R, Culver BH, Butler J. Estimation of transmural cardiac pressures during ventilation with PEEP. *J Appl Physiol* 1982; 53:384.
24. Butler J, Schrijen F, Henriquez A, Polu J-M, Albert RK. Cause of the raised wedge pressure on exercise in chronic obstructive pulmonary disease. *Am Rev Respir Dis* 1988;138:350.
25. Wallis TW, Robotham JL, Compean R, Kindred MK. Mechanical heart-lung interaction with positive end-expiratory pressure. *J Appl Physiol* 1983;54:1039.
26. Cassidy SS, Ramanathan M. Dimensional analysis of the left ventricle during PEEP: relative septal and lateral wall displacements. *Am J Physiol* 1984;246:H792.
27. Glantz SA, Misbach WY, Moores DG, et al. The pericardium substantially affects the left ventricular diastolic pressure-volume relationship in the dog. *Circ Res* 1978;42:433.
28. Scharf SM, Brown R, Warner KG, Khuri S. Esophageal and pericardial pressures and left ventricular configuration with respiratory maneuvers. *J Appl Physiol* 1989;66:481.
29. Takata M, Mitzner W, Robotham JL. Influence of the pericardium on ventricular loading during respiration. *J Appl Physiol* 1990;68:1640.
30. Milic-Emili J, Mead J, Turner J, Glauser EM. Improved technique for estimating a pleural pressure from esophageal balloons. *J Appl Physiol* 1964;19:207.
31. Pinsky MR, Desmet J-M, Vincent J-L. Effect of positive end-expiratory pressure on right ventricular function in humans. *Am Rev Respir Dis* 1992;146:661.
32. Pinsky M, Vincent JL, DeSmet JM. Estimating left ventricular filling pressure during positive end-expiratory pressure in humans. *Am Rev Respir Dis* 1991;143:25.
33. Daly M DeB. Interactions between respiration and circulation. In: Fishman AP, Cherniack N, eds. *Handbook of physiology* (Sec 3, Vol II, Pt 2). Baltimore: Williams and Wilkins; 1986.
34. Angell James JE, Daly M DeB. Cardiovascular responses in apnoeic asphyxia: role of arterial chemoreceptors and the modification of their effects by a pulmonary vagal inflation reflex. *J Physiol (Lond)* 1969;201:87.
35. Cassidy SS. Stimulus-response curves of the lung inflation cardiodepressor reflex. *Respir Physiol* 1984;57:259.
36. Scharf SM, Caldini P, Ingram RH. Cardiovascular effects of positive airway pressure in dogs. *Am J Physiol* 1977;232:H35.
37. Levinson RD, Millman RP. Causes and consequences of blood pressure alterations in obstructive sleep apnea. *Arch Intern Med* 1991; 1512:455.
38. Kontos HA, Verovec GW, Richardson DW. Role of carotid chemoreceptors in circulatory response to hypoxia in dogs. *J Appl Physiol* 1970;28:561.
39. Shykoff BE, Naqvi SSJ, Menon AS, Slutsky AS. Respiratory sinus arrhythmia in dogs: effects of phasic afferents and chemostimulation. *J Clin Invest* 1991;87:1621.
40. Scharf SM, Ingram RH. Influence of abdominal pressure and sympathetic vasoconstriction on the cardiovascular response to PEEP. *Am Rev Respir Dis* 1977;116:661.
41. Okada H, Fox IJ. Respiratory grouping of abdominal sympathetic activity in the dog. *Am J Physiol* 1967;213:48.
42. Kaufman MP, Cassidy SS. Reflex effects of lung inflation and other stimuli on the heart and circulation. In: Scharf SM, Cassidy SS, eds. *Heart-lung interactions in health and disease.* New York: Marcel Dekker; 1989:339.
43. Paintal AS. Mechanism of stimulation of type J pulmonary receptors. *J Physiol (Lond)* 1969;203:511.
44. Hudson LD, Hurlow RS, Craig KC, Pierson DJ. Does intermittent mandatory ventilation correct respiratory alkalosis in patients receiving assisted mechanical ventilation? *Am Rev Respir Dis* 1985;132:1071.
45. Guyton AC, Jones CE, Coleman TG. *Circulatory physiology: cardiac output and its regulation.* Philadelphia: WB Saunders; 1973.

46. Scharf, SM. Cardiovascular effects of positive pressure ventilation. *J Crit Care* 1992;7:268.

47. Scharf SM, Caldini P, Ingram RH Jr. Cardiovascular effects of increasing airway pressure in the dog. *Am J Physiol* 1977;232:H35.

48. Scharf SM, Ingram RH Jr. Influence of abdominal pressure and sympathetic vasoconstriction on the cardiovascular response to positive end-expiratory pressure. *Am Rev Respir Dis* 1977;116:661.

49. Fessler HE, Brower RG, Wise RA, et al. Effects of positive end-expiratory pressure on the gradient for venous return. *Am Rev Respir Dis* 1991;143:19.

50. Fessler HE, Brower RG, Wise RA, et al. Effects of positive end-expiratory pressure on the canine venous return curve. *Am Rev Respir Dis* 1992;146:4.

51. Noble WH, Kay JC. The effect of dobutamine, nitroprusside and volume expansion on cardiac output and lung water after CPPV. *Can Anaesth Soc J* 1986;33:48.

52. Fewall JE, Abendschein DR, Carlson J, et al. Mechanisms of decreased right and left ventricular end-diastolic volumes during continuous positive pressure ventilation in dogs. *Circ Res* 1981;47:467.

53. Schulman DS, Biondi JW, Zohghi S, et al. Coronary flow limits right ventricular performance during positive end-expiratory pressure. *Am Rev Respir Dis* 1990;141:1531.

54. Schulman DS, Biondi JW, Aoghi S, et al. Left ventricular diastolic function during positive end-expiratory pressure. *Am Rev Respir Dis* 1992;145:515.

55. Scharf SM, Brown R. Influence of the right ventricle on left ventricular function with PEEP. *J Appl Physiol* 1982;52:254.

56. Sibbald WH, Calvin JE, Driedger AA. RIght and left ventricular preload and diastolic ventricular compliance: implications of therapy in critically ill patients. *Critical care: state of the art*, vol 3. Fullerton, CA: Society of Critical Care; 1982.

57. Schulman DS, Biondi J, Barash P, et al. Effect of positive end-expiratory pressure on right ventricular performance: importance of baseline right ventricular function. *Am J Med* 1988;84:57.

58. Terai C, Venishi M, Sugimoto H, et al. Transesophageal echocardiographic dimensional analysis of four cardiac chambers during positive end-expiratory pressure. *Anesthesiology* 1985;63:640.

59. Potkin R, Hudson L, Weaver J, et al. Effect of positive end-expiratory pressure on right and left ventricular function in patients with the adult respiratory distress syndrome. *Am Rev Respir Dis* 1987;134:307.

60. Dhainaut J-F, Aouate P, Brunet FP. Circulatory effects of positive end-expiratory pressure in patients with acute lung injury. In: Scharf SM, Cassidy SS, eds. *Heart-lung interactions in health and disease.* New York: Marcel Dekker; 1989:809.

61. Janicki JS, Shroff SG, Weber KT. Ventricular interdependence. In: Scharf SM, Cassidy SS, eds. *Heart-lung interactions in health and disease.* New York: Marcel Dekker; 1989:285.

62. Jardin F, Farcot J-C, Boisant L, Curien N, Margairaz A, Bourdarias JP. Influence of positive end-expiratory pressure on left ventricular performance. *N Engl J Med* 1981;304:387.

63. Jardin F, Farcot JC, Boisante L, et al. Mechanism of paradoxic pulse in bronchial asthma. *Circulation* 1982;66:887.

64. Scharf SM. Mechanical cardiopulmonary interactions in asthma. *Rev Allergy* 1985;3:487.

65. Scharf SM, Graver LM, Khilnani S, Balaban K. Respiratory phasic effects of inspiratory loading in left ventricular hemodynamics in vagotomized dogs. *J Appl Physiol* 1992;73:995.

66. Scharf SM, Brown R, Saunders NA, Green LH. Effects of normal and loaded spontaneous inspiration on cardiovascular function. *J Appl Physiol* 1979;47:582.

67. Scharf SM, Brown R, Saunders N, Green LH. Changes in canine left ventricular size and configuration with positive end-expiratory pressure. *Circ Res* 1979;44:672-678.

68. Haynes JB, Carson SD, Whitney WP, et al. Positive end-expiratory pressure shifts left ventricular diastolic pressure-area curves. *J Appl Physiol* 1980;48:670.

69. Slutsky AS, Scharf SM, Brown R, Ingram RH. The effect of oleic acid induced pulmonary edema on lung and chest wall mechanics in dogs. *Am Rev Respir Dis* 1980;121:9.

70. Scharf SM, Ingram RH. The effects of decreasing lung compliance on the cardiovascular response to PEEP. *Am J Physiol* 1977;232:H635-H641.

71. Donders FC. Contribution to the mechanism of respiration and circulation in health and disease. In: West JB, ed. *Translations in respiratory physiology.* Stroudsburg, PA: Dowden, Hutchinson and Ross; 1975:298.

72. Buda AJ, Pinsky MR, Ingels NB, et al. Effect of intrathoracic pressure on left ventricular performance. *N Engl J Med* 1979;301:453.

73. Scharf SM, Ingram RH. The effects of decreasing lung compliance on the cardiovascular response to PEEP. *Am J Physiol* 1977;232:H635.

74. Scharf SM, Brown R, Tow DE, Parisi AF. Cardiac effects of increased lung volume and decreased pleural pressure in man. *J Appl Physiol* 1979;47:257.

75. Brinker AA, Weiss JL, Lappe DL, et al. Leftward septal displacement during right ventricular loading in man. *Circulation* 1980;61:626.

76. Scharf SM, Bianco JA, Tow DE, Brown R. The effects of large negative intrathoracic pressure on left ventricular function in patients with coronary artery disease. *Circulation* 1981;63:871.

77. Scharf SM, O'Beirne Woods B, Brown R, Parisi AF, Miller MM, Tow DE. Effects of Mueller maneuver on global and regional left ventricular function in angina pectoris with or without previous myocardial infarction. *Am J Cardiol* 1987;59:1305.

78. Scharf SM, Brown R, Saunders NA, Green LH. Hemodynamic effects of positive pressure inflation. *J Appl Physiol* 1980;49:124.

79. McIntyre K, Scharf SM. The use of Valsalva's and Mueller's maneuvers as diagnostic tests for coronary artery disease. In: Scharf SM, Cassidy SS, eds. *Heart-lung interactions in health and disease.* New York: Marcel Dekker; 1989:1021.

80. Lichtenstein SV, Slutsky A, Salerno TA. Noninvasive right and left ventricular assist. *Surg Forum* 1985;36:306.

81. Rudikoff MT, Maughan WL, Elfron M, Freund P, Weisfeldt ML. Mechanisms of blood flow during cardiopulmonary resuscitation. *Circulation* 1980;61:345.

82. Hausknecht M, Brower R, Wise R, Permutt S. The contribution of left ventricular stroke volume to CPR blood flow depends upon the duty cycle. *Am J Emerg Med* 1984;2:350.

83. Criley JM, Blaufuss AH, Kissel GL. Cough-induced cardiac compression. *JAMA* 1976;236:1246.

84. Pinsky MR, Matuschak GM, Bernardi L, Klain M. Hemodynamic effects of cardiac cycle-specific increases in intrathoracic pressure. *J Appl Physiol* 1986;60:604.

85. Fessler HE, Brower RG, Wise RA, Permutt S. Mechanism of reduced LV afterload by systolic and diastolic positive pleural pressure. *J Appl Physiol* 1986;65:1244.

86. Fessler HE, Brower RG, Wise R, Permutt S. Positive pleural pressure decreases coronary perfusion. *Am J Physiol* 1990;258:H814.

87. Tucker HJ, Murray JF. Effects of end-expiratory pressure on organ blood flow in normal and diseased dogs. *J Appl Physiol* 1973;34:573.

88. Venus B, Jacobs HK. Alterations in regional myocardial blood flows during different levels of positive end-expiratory pressure. *Crit Care Med* 1984;12:96.

89. Tittley JG, Fremes SE, Weisel RD, et al. Hemodynamic and myocardial metabolic consequences of PEEP. *Chest* 1985;88:496.

90. Hassapoyannes C, Harper JF, Stuck LM, Hornung CA, Abel FL. Effects of systole-specific pericardial pressure increases on coronary flow. *J Appl Physiol* 1991;71:104.

91. Bunnell S. The use of nitrous oxide and oxygen to maintain anesthesia and positive pressure for thoracic surgery. *JAMA* 1912;58:835.

92. Duncan AW, Oh TE, Hillman DR. PEEP and CPAP. *Anaesth Intens Care* 1986;14:236.

93. Samodelov LF, Falke KJ. Total inspiratory work with modern demand valve devices compared to continuous flow CPAP. *Intens Care Med* 1988;14:632.

94. Gregory GA, Kitterman JA, Phibbs RH, Tooley WH, Hamilton WK. Treatment of idiopathic respiratory distress syndrome with continuous positive airway pressure. *N Engl J Med* 1971;284:1333.

95. Venus B, Jacobs HK, Lim L. Treatment of the adult respiratory distress syndrome with continuous positive airway pressure. *Chest* 1979;76:257.

96. Perel A, Willionson DC, Modell JH. Effectiveness of CPAP by mask for pulmonary edema associated with hypercarbia. *Intens Care Med* 1983;9:17.

97. Pery N, Payen D, Pinsky MR. Monitoring the effect of CPAP on left ventricular function using continuous mixed-blood saturation *Chest* 1991;99:512.

98. Räsänen J, Heikkilä J, Downs J, Niiki P, Väisänen I, Viitanen A. Con-

tinuous positive airway pressure by face mask in acute cardiogenic pulmonary edema. *Am J Cardiol* 1985;55:2986.

99. McNamara SG, Strohl KP, Cistulli PA, Sullivan CE. Clinical aspects of sleep apnea. In: Saunders NA, Sullivan CE, eds. *Sleep and breathing*. 2nd ed. New York: Marcel Dekker; 1994;493.

100. Malone S, Liu PP, Holloway R, Rutherford R, Xie A, Bradley TD. Obstructive sleep apnea in patients with dilated cardiomyopathy: effect of continuous positive airway pressure. *Lancet* 1991;338: 1480.

101. Naughton MT, Liu PP, Benard DC, Goldstein RS, Bradley TD. Treatment of congestive heart failure and Cheyne-Stokes respiration during sleep by continuous positive airway pressure. *Am Rev Respir Crit Care Med* 1995;151:92.

102. Davies RJO, Harrington KJ, Ormerod OJM, Stradling JR. Nasal continuous positive airway pressure in chronic heart failure with sleep-disordered breathing. *Am Rev Respir Dis* 1993;147:630.

103. Buckle P, Millar R, Kryger M. The effect of short-term CPAP on Cheyne-Stokes respiration on congestive heart failure. *Chest* 1992; 102:3.

104. Bradley TD, Holloway RM, McLaughlin PR, Ross BL, Walters J, Liu PP. Cardiac output response to continuous positive airway pressure in congestive heart failure. *Am Rev Respir Dis* 1992;145:377.

105. Baratz DM, Westbrook PR, Shah PK, Mohsenifar A. Effect of nasal continuous positive airway pressure on cardiac output and oxygen delivery in patients with congestive heart failure. *Chest* 1992;102: 1397.

106. Räsänen J, Väisänen I, Heikkilä J, Nikki P. Acute myocardial infarction complicated by left ventricular dysfunction and respiratory failure. The effects of continuous positive airway pressure. *Chest* 1985; 87:159.

107. Genovese J, Moskowitz M, Tarasiuk A, Graver LM, Scharf SM. Effects of CPAP on cardiac output in normal and hypervolemic unanesthetized pigs. *Am J Resp Crit Care Med [in press]*.

108. Genovese J, Huberfeld S, Tarasiuk A, Moskowitz M, Scharf SM. Effects of CPAP on Cardiac Output in Pigs with Pacing-Induced Congestive Heart Failure. *Am J Respir Crit Care Med* 1995;152:1847.

109. Huberfeld S, Genovese J, Tarasiuk A, Scharf SM. Effects of CPAP on pericardial pressure, transmural left ventricular pressures and respiratory mechanics in hypervolemic unanesthetized pigs. *Am J Respir Crit Care Med* 1995;152:142.

110. Cabrera MR, Nakamura GE, Montaugue DA, Cole RP. Effect of airway peressure on pericardial pressure. *Am Rev Respir Dis* 1989;140: 659.

111. Beach T, Millen E, Grenvik A. Hemodynamic response to discontinuance of mechanical ventilation. *Crit Care Med* 1973;1:85.

112. Räsänen J, Nikki P, Heikkilä J. Acute myocardial infarction complicated by respiratory failure. The effects of mechanical ventilation. *Chest* 1984;85:21.

113. Lemaire F, Teboul JC, Cinotti L, et al. Acute left ventricular dysfunction during unsuccessful weaning from mechanical ventilation. *Anesthesiology* 1988;69:171.

114. Hurford WE, Lynch KE, Strauss HW, Lowenstein E, Zapol WM. Myocardial perfusion as assessed by thallium-201 scintigraphy during the discontinuation of mechanical ventilation in ventilator-dependent patients. *Anesthesiology* 1991;74:1007.

115. Grace MP, Greenbaum DM. Cardiac performance in response to PEEP in patients with cardiac dysfunction. *Crit Care Med* 1982;10:358.

116. Mathru M, Rao T, El-Etr AA, Pifarre R. Hemodynamic response to changes in ventilatory patterns in patients with normal and poor left ventricular reserve. *Crit Care Med* 1982;10:423.

117. Pinsky MR, Summer WR, Wise RA, Permutt S, Bromberger-Barnea B. Augmentation of cardiac function by elevation of intrathoracic pressure. *J Appl Physiol* 1983;54:950.

118. Pinsky MR, Summer WR. Cardiac augmentation by phasic high intrathoracic pressure support in man. *Chest* 1983;84:370.

119. Robotham JL. Ventilatory-assisted myocardial performance (VAMP). *Chest* 1983;84:366.

120. Pinsky MR, Matuschak GM, Klain M. Determinants of cardiac augmentation by elevations in intrathoracic pressure. *J Appl Physiol* 1985;58:1189.

121. Pinsky MR, Marquez J, Martin D, Klain M. Ventricular assist by cardiac cycle-specific increases in intrathoracic pressure. *Chest* 1987;91: 709.

122. Beyar R, Halperin HR, Tsitlik J, et al. Circulatory assistance by intrathoracic pressure variations: optimization and mechanisms studied by a mathematical model in relation to experimental data. *Circ Res* 1989; 64:703.

123. Stein KL, Kramer DJ, Killian A, Pinsky MR. Hemodynamic effects of synchronous high-frequency jet ventilation in mitral regurgitation. *J Appl Physiol* 1990;69:2120.

124. Guimond J-G, Pinsky MR, Matuschak GM. Effect of synchronous increase in intrathoracic pressure on cardiac performance during acute endotoxemia. *J Appl Physiol* 1990;69:1502.

125. Peters J, Ihle P. ECG synchronized thoracic vest inflation during autonomic blockade, myocardial ischemia or cardiac arrest. *J Appl Physiol* 1992;73:2263.

*The Critically Ill Cardiac Patient,*
edited by V. Kvetan and D. R. Dantzker,
Lippincott-Raven Publishers, Philadelphia © 1996.

# CHAPTER 4

# Oxygen Transport and Utilization

David R. Dantzker

## THE METABOLIC REQUIREMENT FOR OXYGEN

Sufficient energy is required to maintain the integrity of cell membranes and allow for activities such as muscular contraction, synthetic processes, and active transport. Energy is extracted from food predominantly through oxidative phosphorylation via the tricarboxylic acid (TCA), or Krebs, cycle (1). The TCA cycle is a series of oxidation-reduction reactions during which the energy released during the metabolism, predominantly of carbohydrates and free fatty acids, is captured. This involves the reduction of nicotinamide adenine dinucleotide ($NAD^+$) to NADH, a shuttling of the electrons from NADH into mitochondria, transferring the electrons along a series of electron-carrier enzymes, the cytochrome chain, located in the inner mitochondrial membrane, and finally the capture of the energy in the easily manageable high-energy phosphate bonds of adenosine triphosphate (ATP). For the TCA cycle to function, adequate $O_2$ must also diffuse into the mitochondria, where it serves as the final electron acceptor reacting with cytochrome $aa_3$. Oxidative phosphorylation is the most efficient means of energy generation, producing 36 mol ATP/mol glucose metabolized.

When $O_2$ is insufficient to support oxidative phosphorylation, ATP is produced anaerobically, almost entirely through glycolysis, and pyruvate serves as the terminal electron receptor. This is a much less efficient means of energy production since only 2 mol ATP are produced per mole of glucose. Lactate is an end product in this reaction since it is necessary to regenerate the NAD required for continued glycolysis. An elevated lactate level is thus a marker of anaerobic ATP production.

An alternative anaerobic means of ATP production, at least in cardiac and skeletal muscle as well as in brain, is the creatine kinase reaction (2). In this reaction, a high-energy phosphate bond is transferred from the storage compound, phosphocreatine (PCr), to adenine diphosphate (ADP) to form ATP. While this constitutes a ready source of energy under conditions of $O_2$ scarcity in tissues containing PCr, its usefulness is limited by the relatively small PCr stores when compared to energy requirements.

The ATP diffuses out of the mitochondria to cellular sites requiring energy utilization and the energy is released via ATP hydrolysis:

$$ATP + H_2O \rightarrow ADP + Pi + H^+ + energy$$

Under conditions of sufficient $O_2$, the products of ATP hydrolysis are reutilized to form ATP via oxidative phosphorylation. Thus, despite the fact that as much as 150,000 mmol $H^+$ is produced each day by energy utilization, there is virtually no change in pH. The $H^+$, however, is not reutilized when ATP is produced by glycolysis and this is the source of the acidosis associated with tissue hypoxia (3). Thus anaerobic metabolism via glycolysis leads to the production of equimolar amounts of $H^+$ and lactate, i.e., lactic acidosis. The creatine kinase reaction, by contrast, utilizes $H^+$ in the production of ATP, therefore temporizing the development of metabolic acidosis that would otherwise occur.

The amount of $O_2$ required for oxidative phosphorylation is substantial. For example, it takes the $O_2$ found in 650 lters of air to metabolize 1 mol of glucose. Yet at the level of the mitochondria it requires a $Po_2$ of less than 1 mm Hg to maintain cellular respiration at maximal levels. The transport of $O_2$ from the environment to the cell is achieved by a series of diffusion and convection steps. Pulmonary gas exchange, a complex process on its own, has been well reviewed elsewhere (4) and will not be further discussed.

Convective $O_2$ transport to the tissues ($To_2$) is defined as

$$To_2 = cardiac\ output \times arterial\ O_2\ content$$

As such, it is determined by $Pao_2$, $O_2$ saturation, hemoglobin concentration, and the complex factors which reg-

D. R. Dantzker: Long Island Jewish Medical Center and Albert Einstein College of Medicine, New Hyde Park, New York 11040.

ulate cardiac output. The $To_2$ must be clearly differentiated from oxygen delivery ($Do_2$), which is a much more complex process and represents the actual amount of $O_2$ reaching the tissue mitochondria. The differences between the two should be evident, although they are often spoken of as if they were interchangeable.

Factors intrinsic to cardiac function such as contractility, valvular integrity, and coronary blood flow set limits on the cardiac output, but its moment-to-moment control is regulated by the peripheral vasculature as it alters vascular resistance and venous return (5). The distribution of the cardiac output to individual organs depends on the ability of the regional vascular bed to respond to differing stresses and metabolic demands as well as the anatomic integrity of the vessels and microvasculature (6).

Organ blood flow is primarily controlled at the level of the microvasculature which alters local vascular resistance and controls the number of open capillaries. Two mechanisms appear to be involved in maintaining the required blood flow. The first of these is myogenic control, which is responsible for keeping flow constant in the face of varying intravascular pressures through alterations in vascular smooth muscle tone (7). This type of autoregulation appears to be regulated through the release of vasoactive mediators from the endothelial cells. Dilating substances like endothelium-derived relaxing factor (EDRF) (8) and constricting substances such as endothelin (9) have been identified. Endothelium-derived relaxing factor has been shown to be nitric oxide, which explains the mechanism of action of the clinically important vasodilators, sodium nitroprusside and nitroglycerine, which also release nitric oxide. Other important vasodilators like acetylcholine stimulate the release of EDRF and are thus dependent on the presence of a functioning endothelium (10).

A second mechanism controlling regional blood flow distribution is the metabolic controller which alters local $To_2$ to accommodate for continuously varying metabolic demands (11). Local blood flow is in some way linked to local $O_2$ utilization; while increases in $Po_2$ constrict and decreases dilate the microvessels, it is probably not $Po_2$ itself which is sensed, but rather, some substance released in response to an imbalance between $O_2$ requirements and supply which acts as the signal to the metabolic controller. Possible mediators include adenosine, a potent vasodilator produced during the degradation of ATP, or inorganic phosphate, which accumulates in the setting of insufficient ATP production.

The ability of any particular microvascular bed to increase flow and recruit additional capillaries in response to increased metabolic demand differs from organ to organ. For example, skeletal muscle can increase its capillary density by as much as three times and its total flow by about sevenfold. The heart, on the other hand, is almost totally flow dependent. In response to various stresses such as hypotension, hemorrhage, or hypoxemia, local vascular beds differ significantly in their ability to main-

tain or increase overall $To_2$. For example, during hypoxemia, total blood flow increases to the brain, myocardium, adrenals, and skeletal muscle but declines to the kidney and most of the gastrointestinal (GI) tract (12).

## TISSUE OXYGEN DIFFUSION

After reaching the nutritive vessels, $O_2$ diffuses into the tissues. The factors which determine the diffusion of $O_2$ from the capillaries into the tissues can be defined as follows:

$$O_2 \text{ transfer} = D(P\text{cap}o_2 - P\text{mit}o_2)$$

where $D$ represents the factors which determine tissue $O_2$ diffusibility, such as the cross-sectional area of the microvessels, and $P\text{cap}o_2$ and $P\text{mit}o$ are the $Po_2$ in the capillary and mitochondria, respectively, i.e., the driving pressure.

The driving pressure necessary to maintain an adequate diffusion of $O_2$ is unknown, largely because of the difficulty in measuring $Po_2$ along the pathway from the capillary to the mitochondria. Experimental studies have demonstrated metabolic evidence of tissue hypoxia when the arterial $Po_2$ falls below 35 to 40 mm Hg (13). However, adequate tissue function at lower arterial $Po_2$ has been seen in normal individuals acclimated to high altitude (14). Measurements of tissue $Po_2$ are particularly difficult to accurately obtain. Gayeski et al., however, were able to make measurements of tissue $Po_2$ in working skeletal muscle and found values in the 2 to 3 mm Hg range (15). Measurements this low were seen in the muscle just adjacent to a capillary as well as deeper in the tissue. This large pressure drop between the capillary and adjacent tissue suggests a significant resistance to $O_2$ diffusion. The location of this resistance is unknown but is thought to reside either in the relatively stagnant layer of fluid which develops at the outer margins of the capillaries or in the tissue's interstitium. At the mitochondrial level, a $Po_2$ of less than 1 mm Hg is all that is necessary for normal aerobic function (16).

The factor $D$ is determined by the diffusion and solubility coefficients for oxygen, the surface area available for exchange to take place, and the distance from the capillary to the cell. The latter two are regulated by the regional vascular beds through the recruitment and decruitment of microvessels. Other factors which alter $D$, such as the presence of tissue edema or inflammation, may impair $O_2$ diffusion into the tissues and require more than the 35 to 40 mm Hg driving pressure described above to ensure adequate tissue oxygenation.

Since it is almost impossible to accurately measure the $Po_2$ along the pathway from blood to mitochondria, many of our concepts of tissue oxygenation are based on calculations derived from simple physiologic models of tissue blood flow and $O_2$ diffusion. In the most commonly utilized model, a core of tissue with a single perfusing capillary, the $Pcap_{O_2}$ is assumed to fall progressively from the arterial to venous value as it moves down the vessel (17). Using this model, Tenney suggested that the venous $P_{O_2}$ would be a good estimate of mean tissue $P_{O_2}$, as long as the $O_2$ requirements of the tissue were normal and the capillary density resulted in a normal diffusion distance between the blood and tissue (18). Unfortunately, the results of this theoretical study of a single core of tissue have been often extrapolated to conclude that the mixed venous blood could be considered representative of the mean tissue $P_{O_2}$ of the whole body. This extrapolation fails to account for the difference between a single core of tissue and a flow-weighted mean from tissues with differing flows and metabolic requirements. In addition, Tenney showed that even in this simple model of the tissues, the venous $P_{O_2}$ would be misleading as an index of tissue $P_{O_2}$ in situations in which $T_{O_2}$ or $V_{O_2}$ were abnormal or where capillary density did not match $O_2$ demands.

The simple tissue model described above also fails to take into account a number of other complexities of the microcirculation. For example, it fails to consider the time it takes for $O_2$ to be released from the red blood cells, which under certain circumstances is likely to be an important determinant of $Pcap_{O_2}$ (19). In the setting of a reduced $T_{O_2}$, increased $V_{O_2}$, or reduced capillary transit time, there may be insufficient time for $O_2$ release from the red cell to keep up with its removal from the blood. This will result in a lower $Pcap_{O_2}$ than might otherwise be predicted and a venous $P_{O_2}$ that may overestimate even the $P_{O_2}$ at the venous end of the capillary no less tissue $P_{O_2}$.

Arteries and veins run parallel to each other as they penetrate into many tissues, and under these circumstances $O_2$ may diffuse directly from the arteries to the veins in a countercurrent system, effectively creating an $O_2$ shunt (20). Similar to the effect of the time-dependent release of $O_2$ from hemoglobin, it would result in a tissue $P_{O_2}$ that is considerably lower than that predicted from the arterial and venous $P_{O_2}$. Unlike the problem raised by the time dependence of $O_2$ release from hemoglobin, a countercurrent shunt would be more of a problem during low-flow states since this would increase the time available for arterial to venous $O_2$ diffusion.

The $P_{O_2}$ in the capillary may also be affected by alterations in the capillary hematocrit. As the red cells move through the capillaries, they are oriented in the center of the stream and travel faster than the flow of the surrounding plasma which is retarded by its contact with the endothelial surface (21). This relatively stagnant layer of plasma serves to dilute the red cells, resulting in a capillary hematocrit that is usually less than 50% of that found in the arterial blood. Major alterations in the systemic hematocrit may have little effect on the volume flow of red cells in the microcirculation since there is not a fixed ratio of the systemic to capillary value. For example, in one study, a reduction of the systemic hematocrit by 50% was associated with an unchanged capillary red cell flux

because the smaller reduction in capillary hematocrit was offset by an increase in red cell velocity due to the reduction in whole blood viscosity (22). At this point in time, the factors that alter and regulate the capillary hematocrit and its relationship to systemic hematocrit are not well defined, nor is the effect of various stresses such as hypoxemia, hypotension, etc. However, if the microvascular hematocrit falls low enough, it may significantly reduce the $Pcap_{O_2}$. In addition, changes in the relatively slower moving plasma layer surrounding the inside of the capillary could alter the resistance to $O_2$ diffusion.

An additional factor contributing to the overall relationship between hematocrit and $T_{O_2}$ is the effect that changes in the systemic hematocrit have on the viscosity of the blood. Alternatives in whole blood viscosity have important, poorly quantified effects on cardiac work, microvascular vasomotion, and the regional distribution of cardiac output. Given this complexity, it is not surprising that data can be found which support the maintenance of all ranges of hematocrit in order to optimize $T_{O_2}$ from normal values to significant hemodilution. For example, the optimal hematocrit in one series of postoperative patients was found to be about 32% (23). In the normal brain, decreasing the hematocrit to 30% increases cerebral blood flow and tissue oxygenation (24). During experimentally induced hemorrhagic shock, whole body $V_{O_2}$ was maximal at a hematocrit of 45% while the heart did best at 25% (25). Clearly, any firm recommendations on optional hematocrit at this time would be foolhardy.

## REGULATION OF $O_2$ UTILIZATION

In normal subjects, the level of $V_{O_2}$ is determined by the body's demand for energy. During incremental exercise, the best studied and most easily controlled alteration in metabolic demand, $T_{O_2}$ increases simultaneously with the onset of work and in a linear relationship to the energy output (26). This increase in $T_{O_2}$ is accomplished mainly through an increase in cardiac output. While the increase in $T_{O_2}$ at maximal exercise in conditioned individuals may be as high as four to five times basal levels, it is not sufficient to supply all of the body's requirements for increased energy since $V_{O_2}$ can increase 10- to 15-fold. The additional $O_2$ is provided by an increase in $O_2$ extraction. The normal $O_2$ extraction ratio ($ER = V_{O_2}/T_{O_2} = Ca_{O_2}/Ca_{O_2} - Cv_{O_2}$) is about 0.3 but can increase during exercise to 0.8 or higher. An increase in the ER is made possible by improvements in $O_2$ diffusion primarily through an increase in capillary density.

Even an increase in ER to levels of 0.7 or greater is usually not sufficient to supply all of the increased $O_2$ requirements at high levels of metabolic demand, and the body eventually calls upon glycolysis to anaerobically produce additional ATP. The level of work at which the onset of glycolysis can be identified is called the anaerobic threshold (AT), and in sedentary individuals, this may occur as low as 40% of maximum $V_{O_2}$ (27). With improved conditioning, the AT can be increased to as high as 60% or more, presumably through a combination of better cardiac performance and more effective peripheral $O_2$ delivery and utilization. In patients with cardiovascular disease, or those who are poorly conditioned, the AT will be lower than normal. In most individuals, the ER at the AT is about 60% and continues to increase as the metabolic load increases despite an apparent increasing dependency on anaerobic sources of energy. The skeletal muscles are well designed to increase $O_2$ extraction through their ability to increase overall blood flow and to recruit additional microvessels. This ability is necessary since skeletal muscles are repeatedly required to increase their energy expenditure significantly over basal requirements. Unfortunately, many visceral organs are not as well endowed with diffusion reserve or the ability to increase blood flow and for this reason are more prone to hypoxia under conditions of increased metabolic stress.

A reduction in $T_{O_2}$ below basel levels is an unusual occurrence in normal subjects, even with environmental reductions of the $FI_{O_2}$. At extreme altitude, for example, an increase in cardiac output is normally sufficient to maintain an adequate $T_{O_2}$ (14). Even in the face of significant anemia, an increasing cardiac output is usually able to make up for the reduction in red cell mass, at least at rest (28). However, if cardiac insufficiency is severe or combined with hypoxemia or anemia, $T_{O_2}$ may no longer be able to match metabolic requirements.

Any acute reduction in $T_{O_2}$ to levels insufficient to supply resting $O_2$ requirements can initially be compensated for by an increase in ER. However, if $T_{O_2}$ continues to fall, a point is eventually reached (the critical $T_{O_2}$ or $T_{O_2}$crit) where, despite a continued increase in the ER, $T_{O_2}$ is insufficient to sustain $O_2$ needs, and $V_{O_2}$ below this point will fall (29). This fall in $V_{O_2}$ is associated with the onset of anaerobic metabolism and, ultimately, a fall in tissue energy levels. Presumably, unless this situation can be reversed, tissue ischemia and death will ensue, since energy stores are small and anaerobic means of ATP production inefficient. Values for the $T_{O_2}$crit in animal studies have varied from 6 to 10 mL/kg/min (30) and were even lower in one study in critically ill patients (31). While the effects of a controlled reduction of $T_{O_2}$ cannot be studied in normal humans, a similar biphasic relationship between $T_{O_2}$ and $V_{O_2}$ was demonstrated in a series of patients in whom cardiopulmonary support was gradually withdrawn following a decision to remove life support (31). The ER at $T_{O_2}$crit (the critical ER or ERcrit) appears to vary from about 45 to 80% depending upon the underlying method of $T_{O_2}$ reduction and the animal specimens studied.

In the setting of chronic reductions of $T_{O_2}$, as seen, for example, in congestive heart failure, some investigators have suggested the presence of an adaptive response to reduced $O_2$ availability (32). In some experimental settings, this appears to result from a modification of intra-cellular enzyme activity, while in others, there seems to be an actual downregulation of metabolic requirements (33). This downregulation has been shown to be present in both the heart and other visceral organs (34). The clinical importance of these observations remains conjectural at this time.

Some critically ill patients, especially those with the systemic inflammatory response syndrome, seem to be hypoxic as assessed by the usual clinical indicators (see below), but this apparent insufficiency of tissue oxygenation is noted in conjunction with what would appear to be normal levels of oxygen transport and a normal or even low oxygen extraction ratio (35). In some of these patients, increasing $T_{O_2}$ was associated with a concomitant increase in oxygen utilization. This so-called pathologic supply dependency, pathologic because it occurred at apparently normal levels of $T_{O_2}$ and a low ER, has been ascribed to an abnormally increased oxygen requirement and/or a decreased ability to extract or utilize oxygen. The latter has been attributed either to an abnormality in the microvascular bed or to some defect of oxygen utilization at the cellular level.

Many of the measurements suggesting pathologic supply dependency in both acute and chronically ill patients have been challenged on the basis of the fact that the measurement of oxygen consumption and oxygen transport shared the common variables of cardiac output and arterial oxygen content (36). Measurements in which oxygen consumption were obtained from expired gas analysis, in many cases, failed to reproduce the findings of supply dependency. However, whether or not true supply dependency exists, it is still incumbent upon us to explain why these patients have low oxygen extraction in the setting of apparent clinical hypoxia.

Because of the apparent finding of pathologic supply dependency, a number of clinical studies have tried to increase $T_{O_2}$ as a way of improving the survival of a wide array of seriously ill patients. The few attempts to study this question in a controlled fashion have produced disparate results, with some showing that an increased oxygen transport leads to an improved outcome (37, 38) and others showing no difference between the treatment and the control group (39, 40). In a recently reported controlled trial, the study group, in whom an increase in oxygen transport was achieved, actually had a worse outcome than the control patients (41). Unfortunately, a valid interpretation of all these data is difficult at this time because of the aforementioned inability to actually measure oxygen delivery, as opposed to transport, as well as the absence of a true index of adequate tissue oxygenation.

## MONITORING THE ADEQUACY OF TISSUE OXYGENATION

A number of indices have been commonly followed as measures of tissue oxygenation. The available indices can be divided, for convenience of discussion, into input, utilization, and output variables as well as direct measurements of tissue bioenergetics. With the exception of measurements of tissue bioenergetics, these indices treat the tissues as a "black box," a particularly risky thing to do when inside the box is as complicated a process as cellular respiration. Each of these parameters differs in the ease of measurement and its ability to actually quantitate tissue oxygenation.

The input variables are the easiest to obtain and the ones most commonly measured. The $Pa_{O_2}$ and $O_2$ saturation are accurate indices of lung function but have no necessary relationship to the level of oxygenation of the peripheral tissues. Patients are rarely exposed to the levels of hypoxemia that have been shown experimentally to lead to tissue hypoxia in normal animals, and the critical $Pa_{O_2}$ in humans in unknown. In fact, the critical $Pa_{O_2}$ is likely to differ from person to person and organ to organ depending on the underlying disorder and the integrity of the $O_2$ transport pathway. The $T_{O_2}$ is more useful since it monitors the bulk delivery of $O_2$. However, as discussed above, $T_{O_2}$ has a complex and unclear relationship to oxygen delivery, and the $T_{O_2}crit$, like the critical $P_{O_2}$, is likely to vary from situation to situation, making any individual number difficult to interpret.

The major utilization variable is $V_{O_2}$, a good measurement of overall aerobic metabolism. It is most easily measured using the principle of conservation of mass:

$$V_{O_2} = VI \times FI_{O_2} - VE \times FE_{O_2}$$
$$= Q (Ca_{O_2} - Cv_{O_2})$$

where VI and VE are the inspired and expired minute ventilations, $FI_{O_2}$ and $FE_{O_2}$ are the inspired and expired fractional concentrations of oxygen, Q is the cardiac output, and $Ca_{O_2}$ an $Cv_{O_2}$ are the arterial and mixed venous $O_2$ contents. Whether measured by analysis of expired gas or calculated from the product of cardiac output and the arteriovenus $O_2$ content difference, an accurate measurement requires the patient to be in steady state such that metabolic demands VE and Q are all constant. The accuracy of the specific method chosen in any particular clinical situation is conditioned by the ability to accurately measure each of the individual variables. However, under ideal conditions each technique should provide the same results.

Measurement from the gas side is noninvasive but depends on the ability to accurately measure the $FI_{O_2}$ and $FE_{O_2}$. In a patient breathing room air, this measurement is easy and accurate. However, in patients breathing an increased $FI_{O_2}$, especially those on mechanical ventilation, the accuracy is limited by the consistency of the $O_2$ delivery system. Quantitation of $V_{O_2}$ from the blood side, although invasive, requiring measurement of cardiac output as well as the sampling of mixed venous and arterial blood, bypasses the problem of consistency of inspired $O_2$ and thus is the method used most commonly in critically ill patients. Its major disadvantage is the large number of variables (partial pressures and saturations of arterial and mixed venous blood, hemoglobin concentration, and cardiac output) that must be measured, each of which is subject to error. In the setting of lung inflammation, it has been suggested that measurement from the blood side might underestimate true $V_{O_2}$ by as much as 15%, missing the increased contribution from the diseased lung (42).

While $V_{O_2}$ is a good measurement of overall aerobic metabolism, by itself it is an unreliable measure of tissue oxygenation. The appropriate level of $V_{O_2}$ for any individual patient depends on metabolic demands, which may vary widely both from patient to patient and from moment to moment. It has been suggested that monitoring the relationship between $T_{O_2}$ and $V_{O_2}$ might increase the usefulness of both measurements. However, as opposed to laboratory experiments, patients undergo spontaneous variations of both $T_{O_2}$ and $V_{O_2}$. A primary change in $V_{O_2}$ would be expected to result in a concomitant change in $T_{O_2}$, as we see, for example, in normal subjects during exercise. Conversely, a primary change in $T_{O_2}$ would likewise cause an alteration in $V_{O_2}$ if supply dependency is present. In the clinical setting, it may be quite difficult to tell which is the dependent and which is the independent variable without a controlled attempt to perturb one or the other value. In other words, by simply following serial measurements of $T_{O_2}$ and $V_{O_2}$, it may be impossible to know if the system is behaving in a physiologic or pathologic fashion.

If we were to assume that the finding of supply dependency is an index of inadequate tissue oxygenation, then increasing $T_{O_2}$ until $V_{O_2}$ reaches a plateau, indicating the supply-independent region, might seem reasonable. Unfortunately, while many investigators have demonstrated that $V_{O_2}$ can be increased by increasing $T_{O_2}$, none have yet demonstrated an ability to achieve a plateau (43). Other problems with monitoring this relationship as well as the conflicting results of increasing $T_{O_2}$ have already been pointed out. The extraction ratio is merely a derivative of the $T_{O_2}$-$V_{O_2}$ relationship and adds no additional information.

The output variables have been the traditional measures of adequate tissue oxygenation. The $Pv_{O_2}$, or mixed venous saturation, has been commonly assumed to represent the mean tissue $P_{O_2}$. We have already discussed why the $Pv_{O_2}$ is not necessarily a good approximation of the end-capillary $P_{O_2}$ in the tissue, no less a helpful measure of mean tissue $P_{O_2}$. The $Pv_{O_2}$ has the added disadvantage of being a blood-flow-weighted mean of the venous effluent from each of the tissue beds and not necessarily equal to any of them. Thus, the $Pv_{O_2}$ is influenced by the relative contributions from tissues with differing metabolic rates, and changes in the $Pv_{O_2}$ may reflect only an alteration in blood flow distribution. For example, in sepsis, a high $Pv_{O_2}$ probably indicates inadequate tissue $V_{O_2}$ or severe maldistribution of peripheral flow, and a fall in the PvO2 may actually be a good sign, indicating the return of local microvascular control. Clinical studies have suggested that values of PvO2 below 28 mm Hg are associated with a poor prognosis (44), and yet values of PvO2 considerably lower are found in situations in which apparently normal tissue function is present, such as during very high levels of exercise or at high altitude. It seems likely that the prognostic information inherent in a low PvO2 is most likely to stem more from its association with other physiologic abnormalities such as low cardiac output or severe anemia than from its ability to predict tissue PO2.

When there is insufficient O2 to sustain oxidative phosphorylation, glycolysis is utilized to maintain tissue ATP levels, and lactate is produced. Some tissues, such as the red blood cell, the renal medulla, and portions of the eye, routinely depend on glycolysis for energy production. Their overall contribution of lactate is small, about 40 g/day. Under normal circumstances, skeletal muscle, brain, intestine, and skin may also produce small amounts of lactate; the muscle contribution can increase dramatically during exercise, especially in unconditioned individuals. The lactate may undergo further oxidation through the TCA cycle or serve as a substrate for gluconeogenesis. Both of these processes require adequate amounts of oxygen. When glycolysis is carried out under conditions of insufficient O2, lactate accumulates. The normal lactate level is about 1 mEq/L; increased levels are often considered as de facto evidence of inadequate tissue oxygenation.

Unfortunately, factors other than tissue hypoxia can result in increased lactate production. Lactate will be elevated by factors that increase the rate of glycolysis in excess of the ability of pyruvate to be utilized in the TCA cycle (45). These would include alkalosis, excess insulin, or catecholamine release, as well as factors that reduce the levels of acetyl coenzyme A, such as starvation and diabetes. During sepsis lactate accumulates even in the absence of clearly defined tissue hypoxia. It has been suggested that, under these circumstances, a metabolic block may prevent substrate from entering the TCA cycle, leading to pyruvate accumulation and increased lactate production. Finally, drugs and chemicals such as ethanol, methanol, ethylene glycol, salicylates, and phenformin can elevate lactate levels by interfering with gluconeogenesis.

There are also factors that may limit the production of lactic acid and thus decrease the lactate level present in the setting of significant tissue hypoxia. In malnourished patients, for example, glycogen deposits may be inadequate to supply sufficient substrate for glycolysis. More importantly, as tissue pH falls, glycolytic flux is inhibited, providing a sort of feedback control on the level of blood lactate.

On the other side of the balance sheet, lactate is removed from the circulation predominantly by the liver.

In fact, it is generally thought that the ability of the liver to remove lactate is severalfold greater than the ability of the peripheral tissues to produce it. Thus, any compromise in liver function can have a dramatic effect on the level of lactate present for any given rate of accelerated glycolysis (46). In addition, lactate produced by one organ can be used as substrate by another, in particular the heart and skeletal muscle. Both of these means of lactate clearance further reduce the sensitivity of lactate as an index of inadequate tissue oxygenation unless the defect is global in nature.

Directly monitoring the onset of organ hypoxia by looking for the presence of tissue acidosis may become a useful way of detecting inadequate tissue oxygenation. As already mentioned, protons are produced during the hydrolysis of ATP and are reutilized during aerobic production of ATP. When energy is derived from glycolysis, protons accumulate, leading to acidosis. It has been demonstrated that the onset of tissue acidosis in the gastrointestinal tract can be detected accurately by a tonometric technique (47). As the pH in the wall of the GI tract falls, the hydrogen ions are buffered by bicarbonate producing carbon dioxide which freely diffuses into the lumen of the stomach or intestine. This rise in $CO_2$ can be detected and has been shown in experimental studies to correlate with the onset of anaerobiosis. The gastrointestinal tract, as an organ to monitor, has some seeming advantages. Because of the pattern of countercurrent blood supply to the micropapillae, it is particularly sensitive to the onset of reductions in oxygen transport. Thus it may serve as an early warning sign of impending tissue hypoxia in other organs. The GI tract is also felt to play a significant role in the development of multiple organ failure syndrome, perhaps because it serves as a reservoir for endotoxin- and exotoxin-producing bacteria (48).

A number of studies have now demonstrated that a fall in the interstitial pH of the GI tract can be used as a prognostic indicator of increased morbidity and mortality (49, 50), and one recent study suggested it can provide guidance to the adequacy of overall oxygen transport (51). However, more and better control studies will be necessary before the clinical usefulness of this technique can be fully evaluated.

Other, more direct measurements of tissue bioenergetics are available and have proven useful in the experimental laboratory. Magnetic resonance spectroscopy (MRS) is a noninvasive means of measuring the key biologic molecules involved in the energy balance sheet. When tissue is placed in a strong magnetic field and subjected to radio frequency waves, certain isotopic species will absorb and then admit some of the energy in the form of a radio frequency signal that can be characterized and quantitated. Phosphorus-31 is a stable isotope that forms a part of the key molecules involved in the storage and transfer of energy in the cell: ATP, ADP, PCr, and Pi. The PCr/Pi ratio is the equivalent of the cellular phosphate potential and is easily measured in those tissues that contain PCr, namely skeletal muscle, heart, and brain (52). The MRS measurements can be made in intact tissue and, when combined with tomographic imaging, could become quite useful in patients, providing access to a magnetic resonance device could be made more easily. Another technique for direct quantitation of cellular bioenergetics is the optical monitoring of the reduction-oxidation status of the mitochondrial energy chain by near-infrared spectroscopic measurements of cytochrome $aa_3$ (53). Unfortunately, at the moment, it is difficult to calibrate optical techniques, and they may be useful in the near future only as a way of following trends, and not as a measure of any absolute level of tissue oxygenation.

## SUMMARY

The evolution from single cell to complex organism in an aerobic environment requires the development of an intricate delivery system to guarantee that an adequate amount of oxygen would be available to support the requirements for energy generation. Our understanding of that transport system is still somewhat rudimentary, and our ability to monitor the end result, the adequacy of tissue oxygenation, is also modest. Multicenter clinical trials are now planned or underway which will test the number of hypotheses regarding an approach to optimizing oxygen transport, but, as yet, the answers are unclear and should preclude the development of dogmatic approaches to patient care.

## REFERENCES

1. Newsholme EA, Leech AR. *Biochemistry for the medical sciences.* New York: Wiley; 1983.
2. Chance B, Leigh JS, Clark BJ, et al. Control of oxidative metabolism and oxygen delivery in human skeletal muscle: a steady state analysis of work/energy cost transfer acidosis function. *Proc Natl Acad Sci USA* 1985;82:8384.
3. Zilva J. The origin of the acidosis in hyperlactatemia. *Ann Clin Biochem* 1978;15:40.
4. Dantzker DR. *Pulmonary gas exchange in pulmonary and critical care medicine.* Chicago, IL: Mosby; 1992.
5. Guyton AC, Jones CE, Coleman TG. *Circulatory physiology: cardiac output and its regulation.* Philadelphia: WB Saunders; 1973.
6. Heistad PD, Abboud FM. Circulatory adjustments to hypoxia. *Circulation* 1980;61:463.
7. Johnson P. Autoregulation of blood flow. *Circ Res* 1986;59:483.
8. Ignarro LJ, Buga GM, Wood KS, et al. Endothelium derived relaxing factor produced and released from artery and vein is nitric oxide. *Proc Natl Acad Sci USA* 1987;84:9265.
9. Yanagisawa M, Inoue A, Ishikawa T, et al. Primary structure, synthesis and biological activity of rat endothelium-derived vasoconstrictor peptide. *Proc Natl Acad Sci USA* 1988;85:6964.
10. Furchott RF, Zawadzki JV. The obligatory role of endothelial cells in the relaxation of arterial smooth muscle by acetylcholine. *Nature* 1980;288:373.
11. Sparks HV. Effect of local metabolic factors on vascular smooth muscle. In: Bohr DR, Somlyo AP, Sparks HV, eds. *The cardiovascular system: vascular smooth muscle.* Bethesda, MD: American Physiological Society; 1980:475.
12. Johnson P. Autoregulation of blood flow. *Circ Res* 1986;59:483.
13. Maker HS, Niclas WJ. In: Robin E, ed. *Biochemical responses of body organs to hypoxia and ischemia in extrapulmonary manifestations of respiratory disease.* New York: Marcel Dekker; 1978:107.
14. Wagner PD, Sutton JR, Reeves JT, Cymerman A, Groves BM, Malconian MK. Operation Everest II. Pulmonary gas exchange throughout a simulated ascent of Mt. Everest. *J Appl Physiol* 1987;63:2348.
15. Gayeski TEJ, Honig CR. $O_2$ gradients from sorcolemma to cell interior in red muscle at maximal $V_{O_2}$. *Am J Physiol* 1986;251:H789.
16. Araki R, Tamura M, Yamazaki I. The effect of intracellular oxygen concentration on lactate release, pyridine nucleotide reduction and respiratory rate in rat cardiac tissue. *Circ Res* 1983;53:448.
17. Krogh A. The number and distribution of capillaries in muscles with calculations of the oxygen pressure head necessary for supplying the tissue. *J Physiol (Lond)* 1919;52:409.
18. Tenney SM. A theoretical analysis of the relationship between venous blood and mean tissue oxygen pressures. *Respir Physiol* 1974;20:283.
19. Gutierrez G. The rate of oxygen release and its effect on capillary $O_2$ tension: a mathematical analysis. *Respir Physiol* 1985;63:69.
20. Piper J, Meyer M, Scheid. Dual role of diffusion in tissue gas exchange: blood-tissue equilibrium and diffusion shunt. *Respir Physiol* 1984;56:131.
21. Desjardins C, Duling BR. Micro vessel hematocrit: measurement and implications for capillary oxygen transport. *Am J Physiol* 1987;252:H494.
22. Arfors KF. Increase in capillary blood flow and relative hematocrit in rabbit skeletal muscle following normovolemic anemia. *Acta Physiol Scand* 1988;134:503.
23. Czer LSC, Shoemaker WC. Optical hematocrit value of critically ill post operative patients. *Surg Gynecol Obstet* 1978;147:363.
24. Brown MM, Marshall J. Regulation of cerebral blood flow in response to changes in blood viscosity. *Lancet* 1985;1:604.
25. Jan K, Heldman J, Chen S. Coronary hemodynamics and oxygen utilization after hematocrit variations in hemorrhage. *Am J Physiol* 1980;239:H326.
26. Astrand P, Cuddy TE, Saltin B, Steaberg J. Cardiac output during submaximal and maximal work. *J Appl Physiol* 1964;19:268.
27. Wasserman K, Whipp BJ, Koyal SN, Beauer WL. Anaerobic threshold and respiratory gas exchange during exercise. *J Appl Physiol* 1973;35:236.
28. Woodson RD, Wills RE, Lenfant C. Effect of acute and established anemia on $O_2$ transport at rest, submaximal and maximal work. *J Appl Physiol: Respir Environ Exercise Physiol* 1978;44:36.
29. Stainsby WN, Otis AB. Blood flow, oxygen tension, oxygen uptake and oxygen transport in skeletal muscle. *Am J Physiol* 1964;206:858.
30. Cain SM. Oxygen delivery in dogs during anemic and hypoxic hypoxia. *J Appl Physiol* 1977;43:228.
31. Ronco JJ, Fenwick JC, Tweeddale MG, et al. Identification of the critical oxygen delivery for anaerobic metabolism in critically ill septic and nonseptic humans. *JAMA* 1993;270:1724–1730.
32. Rady MY, Sayeed J, Rives EP, Alexander M. Characterization of systemic oxygen transport in end stage chronic congestive heart failure. *Am Heart J* 1994;128:744.
33. Meldrum DR, Mitchell MB, Banerjee A, Harleen AH. Cardiac preconditioning: induction of tolerance to ischemia-reperfusion injury. *Arch Surg* 1993;128:1208.
34. Bristow JD, Arai AE, Anselone CG, Pantely GA. Response to myocardial ischemia as a regulated process. *Circulation* 1991;84:2580.
35. Danek SJ, Lynch JP, Weg JG, Dantzker DR. The dependence of oxygen uptake on oxygen delivery in the adult respiratory distress syndrome. *Am Rev Respir Dis* 1980;122:387.
36. Phang PT, Cunningham KF, Ronco JJ, Wiggs BR, Russell JA. Mathematical coupling explains dependence of oxygen consumption or oxygen delivery in ARDS. *Am J Respir Crit Med* 1994;150:318.
37. Shoemaker WC, Appel PL, Kram HB, Waxman K, Lee TS. Prospective trial of supra normal values of survivors as therapeutic goals in high risk patients. *Chest* 1988;94:1176.
38. Shoemaker WC, Appel PL, Kram HB. Role of oxygen debt in the development of organ failure, sepsis and death in high-risk surgical patients. *Chest* 1992;102:208.
39. Bone RC, Slotman G, Maunder R, et al. Randomized double-blind multicenter study of prostaglandin E in patients with adult respiratory distress syndrome. *Chest* 1989;96:114.
40. Yu M, Levy MM, Smith P, Takiguchi SA, Miyasaki A, Myers SA. Effect of maximizing oxygen delivery on morbidity and mortality rates in critically ill patients; a prospective randomized controlled study. *Crit Care Med* 1993;21:830.

41. Hayes MA, Timmins AC, Yau EHS, Palazzo M, Hinds CJ, Watson D. Elevation of systemic oxygen delivery in the treatment of critically ill patients. *N Engl J Med* 1994;330:1717.

42. Light B. Intra pulmonary oxygen consumption in experimental pneumococcal pneumonia. *J Appl Physiol* 1988;64:2490.

43. Dantzker DR, Gutierrez G, Foresman B. Oxygen supply and utilization relationships; a re-evaluation. *Am Rev Respir Dis* 1991;143:675.

44. Kasnitz P, Druger DL, Yorra, et al. Mixed venous oxygen tension and hyperlactatemia. *JAMA* 1976;236:570.

45. Hochachka PW. Defense strategies against hypoxia and hypothermia. *Science* 1986;231:234.

46. Kreisberg PA. Lactate homeostasis and lactic acidosis. *Ann Intern Med* 1980;92:227.

47. Grum CM, Fiddian-Green RG, Pittenger GL, Grant BJ, Rothman ED, Dantzker DR. Adequacy of tissue oxygenation in infant dog intestine. *J Appl Physiol* 1984;56:1065.

48. Meakins JL, Marshall JC. The gut as the motor of multiple system organ failure. In: Marston A, Bulkley GB, Fiddian-Green RG, Haglund UH, eds. *Splanchnic ischemia and multiple organ failure.* London: Edward Arnold; 1989:339.

49. Doglio GR, Pusajo JF, Egurrola MA, et al. Gastric mucosal pH as a prognostic index of mortality in critically ill patients. *Crit Care Med* 1991;19:1037.

50. Maynard N, Bihari D, Beale R, et al. Assessment of splanchnic oxygenation by gastric tonometry in patients with acute circulatory failure. *JAMA* 1993;270:1203.

51. Gutierrez G, Palizas F, Doglio G, et al. Gastric intra mucosal pH as a therapeutic index of tissue oxygenation in critically ill patients. *Lancet* 1992;339:195.

52. Kadda GK. The use of NMR spectroscopy for the understanding of disease. *Science* 1986;233:640.

53. Hampson NB, Piotadosi CA. Near infrared monitoring of human skeletal muscle oxygenation during forearm ischemia. *J Appl Physiol* 1988;64:2449.

*The Critically Ill Cardiac Patient,*
edited by V. Kvetan and D. R. Dantzker,
Lippincott-Raven Publishers, Philadelphia © 1996.

# CHAPTER 5

# Regional Circulation in Critical Illness

Ronald J. Lis and Stephen McCarthy Pastores

Monitoring of regional blood flow is one of the greatest difficulties and challenges for those caring for critically ill patients. It is well recognized that despite what appears to be adequate or supranormal central hemodynamics, as assessed by a pulmonary artery catheter, inadequate regional blood flow can occur (1–5). Inadequate blood flow may, along with the various mediators of critical illness, result in multisystem organ dysfunction. As more organ systems fail, the prognosis for survival of the critically ill patient worsens.

In this chapter, we will review the regulation and perturbations in blood flow associated with critical illness to several regional organ beds, including the brain, heart, kidneys, diaphragm, liver, and intestine. Pulmonary circulation, which can partially be assessed by the use of pulmonary artery catheter, will not be reviewed. The normal distribution of blood flow and oxygen extraction among the different regional organs are shown in Table 1. Currently available techniques for assessment of regional blood flow in critically ill patients are shown in Table 2. It is important to recognize that it is not possible to measure total regional organ blood flow in humans with reliable accuracy. Because of inherent difficulties in measuring regional blood flow in humans, most of the available scientific evidence is based on studies done in nonhuman species. However, caution must be used when attempting to apply the results of animal studies to humans. Some animal models of critical illness may not accurately mimic the physiologic changes seen in humans. For example, intravenous bolus administration of bacterial lipopolysaccharide (LPS) in dogs without volume resuscitation may not result in the vasodilated, high-cardiac-output state typical of volume resuscitated human septic shock. Similarly, although acute surgical cardiac tamponade results in a low cardiac output, results from this model may not be applicable to chronic

congestive heart failure (CHF) with its chronic alterations in the neurohumoral axis and vascular remodeling. Anesthetic agents can alter and often exaggerate the response to hemodynamic insults (e.g., hemorrhage), decrease oxygen extraction, and change the point of critical oxygen delivery via their peripheral vasodilator effects (6). In addition, anesthetic agents can alter vascular smooth muscle response to vasoconstrictors and attenuate endothelium-derived relaxing factor (ERDF) production (7, 8).

Vascular smooth muscle tone is regulated through endothelium-dependent and endothelium-independent mechanisms (9, 10). The principal site for the regulation of regional blood flow occurs in vessels less than 200 to 150 μm in diameter. It is at this level that the vasculature tone is significantly influenced by local metabolic factors. As the need of a tissue for a substrate increases, the extraction of the substrate from the bed can increase and/or the delivery of the substrate can be increased via increased blood flow. Products of metabolism with vasodilator properties such as adenosine can act locally to increase blood flow. Inadequate tissue oxygen levels directly or via mediators can lead to local vasodilation. The coupling of local vascular resistance to metabolic needs is referred to as metabolic regulation. It is important to recognize that, for tissues with a high baseline level of substrate extraction, increasing extraction will provide only a limited reserve for meeting metabolic demands. In these tissues significant increases in substrate utilization will need to be met by increases in flow (11–13). During critical illness regional redistribution of blood flow can occur. Under these conditions changes in the neurohumoral axis, endothelial cell physiology, and vascular smooth muscle physiology may result in the redistribution of blood flow toward vital regional beds at the expense of other regional beds (13).

Blood vessels have the ability to maintain constant flow over a wide range of perfusion pressures. Vessels contract in response to increases in transmural pressure

---

R. J. Lis and S. M. Pastores: Albert Einstein College of Medicine/Montefiore Medical Center, Bronx, New York 10467.

**TABLE 1.** *Regional blood flow and oxygen extraction.*

| | Blood flow (mL/min/100 g) | Oxygen extraction ratio (%) |
|---|---|---|
| Cerebral | 50 | 35 |
| Renal | 400 | 10 |
| Cardiac | 80 | 65 |
| Diaphragm | 2–10 | 25 |
| Liver | 100 | 20 |
| Intestine | 50–70 | 15–20 |

and relax in response to decreases in transmural pressure. This is known as the myogenic response and is mediated by mechanoreceptors (14, 15). Extrinsic regulation of blood vessels occurs via both neuronal and humoral mechanisms (11, 12).

During critical illness alterations in endothelium and vascular smooth muscle occur. The etiology of these changes are multifactorial. In heart failure remodeling of the cardiovascular system (16), endothelial changes (17), and changes in myocardial and vascular receptor function (18) have been reported. The peripheral vasodilatation which characterizes septic shock can result from the administration of bacterial LPS (19), interleukin-1 (IL-1) (20), and tumor necrosis factor (TNF) (21). Nitric oxide, produced by the inducible form of nitric oxide synthase, is felt to have a significant role in the vasodilatation seen during sepsis (22–24). The eicosanoids prostaglandin $I_2$ and prostaglandin $E_2$ (25) can also contribute to the vasodilatation seen with sepsis. Similarly, elevated levels of the vasoconstrictor endothelin are found in sepsis (26). Thus, local imbalances between vasodilators and vasoconstrictors may contribute to redistribution of regional blood flow (27, 28).

## CEREBRAL CIRCULATION

The brain supplies arterial blood via two pairs of vessels. Internal carotid arteries originate from the common carotid arteries. The cerebral portion of the internal

**TABLE 2.** *Techniques for assessment of regional flow in the critically ill patient.*

*Central nervous system:* infrared spectroscopy, transcranial Doppler, jugular venous bulb oximetry, radiolabeled scans
*Renal:* clearance studies, renal vein thermodilution catheter, Doppler, radiolabeled scans
*Respiratory muscles:* infrared spectroscopy
*Splanchnic organs:* indocyanine green, galactose clearance; duplex Doppler, computed tomography, magnetic resonance imaging, abdominal angiogram; gastric or intestinal tonometry

carotid arteries give off the ophthalmic arteries and then branch into the anterior and middle cerebral arteries. The vertebral arteries originate from the subclavian arteries and travel vertically through the transvere foramina of the cervical vertebrae. At the level of the pons the vertebral arteries unite to form the basilar artery. Extracranial-to-intracranial anastomosis, such as between the maxillary and internal carotid, exists. The circle of Willis is an important anastomosis between the vertebral and internal carotid arteries. The circle of Willis is formed by the internal carotid, anterior cerebral, anterior communicating, posterior communicating, and posterior cerebral arteries. Originating off the main cerebral vessels and the circle of Willis are two types of vessels. Cortical vessels supply superficial areas. Central arteries penetrate into the brain and supply deep structures (29, 30).

Although accounting for only 2% of total body weight, the brain receives approximately 20% of cardiac output and accounts for 20% of whole body oxygen consumption. Normally, cerebral blood flow is approximately 50 mL/100 g/min. The normal rate of cerebral oxygen consumption ($CMRO_2$) is 3.4 mL/100 g/min. Venous blood obtained from the internal jugular vein has been used to reflect mixed venous cerebral blood flow. Normal jugular bulb mixed venous oxygen saturation is 62%. Utilizing internal jugular vein saturation, the arterial-venous difference and oxygen extraction ratio across the cerebral circulation has been calculated to average 6.7 volume percent and 35%, respectively (31–33).

Maintaining ionic homeostasis and neurotransmitter synthesis accounts for the majority of the brain's metabolic activity. Of the total energy requirements, 45% is required to maintain cellular integrity and 55% is utilized for neurotransmission. Because the brain lacks reserves of oxygen as well as significant reserves of glucose and high-energy phosphate compounds, it is particularly subject to the dangers of disturbances in blood flow (34). Decreasing cerebral blood flow to 50% baseline value results in altered sensorium and electroencephalographic disturbances (32). Decreasing cerebral blood flow to 18 to 20 mL/100 g/min is accompanied by the loss of EEG activity. Cerebral blood flow rates less than 10 to 12 mL/100 g/min are accompanied by ion pump failure (35, 36). Within several minutes of ion pump failure cytotoxic cell edema and cell death can be expected to occur (37, 38). It is important for clinicians to realize that cerebral blood flow may decrease up to 50% before clinically apparent changes can be detected. It is also obvious that measures of global cerebral blood and metabolism do not necessarily reflect what is occurring regionally within the brain.

### Cerebral Autoregulation

The brain has the ability to regulate cerebral blood flow (CBF) over a wide range of perfusion pressures.

When intracranial pressure (ICP) is greater than central venous pressure (CVP), cerebral perfusion pressure (CPP) is defined by the difference between mean arterial pressure (MAP) and ICP. Normally CBF is maintained over a range of CPPs varying between 50 and 150 mm Hg (31). The brain must not only be able to regulate global CBF over a wide range of CPP, it must also be able to regulate regional cerebral blood flow (rCBF) to meet regional changes in metabolism. Regional increases in neuronal activity are felt to result in similar changes in regional metabolism (39).

Paired measurements of $CMRO_2$ and CBF obtained at rest have documented regional coupling of $CMRO_2$ and rCBF (40). Increased neuronal activity caused by processes such as thinking (41), stereognostic testing, and visual stimulation have been found to increase rCBF (42). Positron emission tomography studies during periods of somatosensory stimulation have shown that stimulus-induced augmentation of rCBF may exceed the local increase in $rCMRO_2$ (43, 44). This finding suggests that regulation of rCBF may be mediated by a mechanism dependent on neuronal firing but to a certain extent independent of $rCMRO_2$. Multiple mechanisms and sites of regulation allow the brain to accomplish this complex process of autoregulation of both global and regional cerebral blood flow. The exact relationship between these mechanisms and autoregulation of CBF are incompletely understood (33). Micropuncture studies in different species suggest that the large cerebral arteries are important resistance vessels for the cerebral circulation. Vessels greater than 200 μm in diameter have been found to account for up to 45% of total cerebral vascular resistance (45–48). The behaviors of large and small vessels do not necessarily parallel each other (48). In anesthetized cats the intravenous infusion of vasopression decreased resistance of arteries greater than 200 μm in diameter, resulting in an increase in pressure in smaller vessels. Small-vessel resistance increased in response to the elevation of pressure, and there was no change in CBF (49). When pharmacologic agents or physiologic stimuli result in parallel changes of large- and small-vessel resistance, the degree of change in each group of vessels may vary. In rabbits seizures produce a preferential reduction in the resistance of vessels less than 100 μm in diameter. In studies of anesthetized rabbits and cats, sympathetic stimulation increased resistance in large arteries while resistance in small vessels did not change (50). In the same model, systemic arterial hypertension was associated with an increase in small-vessel resistance which exceed the increase in large-vessel resistance. Clearly the site and value of change of the resistance generated in response to different stimuli can vary. There are multiple possible mechanisms which can be responsible for these changes in vascular resistance. Neuronal regulation of cerebral blood flow can occur through several possible mechanisms. Cerebral blood vessels are richly innervated with sympathetic neurons arising primarily from cervical ganglion (51, 52). Cerebral blood vessels are also innervated by noradrenergic neurons (53).

Nitric oxide synthase has been detected in up to 2% of parenchymal brain neurons (54). Excitatory amino acids such as glutamate, aspartate and N-methyl-D-aspartate (NMDA) produce dilation of cerebral arterioles. The NMDA-mediated vasodilatation of pial arterioles is blocked by the NMDA receptor antagonist as well as by the nitric oxide synthase inhibitor and $N^G$-nitro-L-arginine (L-NAME). This implies that nitric oxide is both neuronally derived and requires neuronal activation for release (55, 56). Evidence suggests that large cerebral arteries and pial arterioles are innervated by nitric oxide synthase containing neurons. Numerous studies have investigated the effect of various nitric oxide synthase inhibitors on CBF (57–59). In different animal species nitric oxide synthase inhibitors appear to attenuate the vasodilator response normally seen with hypercapnia (59). The exact role of nitric oxide in controlling CBF during periods of normal and abnormal physiology has yet to be defined.

Properties intrinsic to the vascular smooth muscle and endothelium may play an important role in the autoregulation of cerebral blood flow (60). The myogenic response, the contraction of vascular smooth muscle which follows the stretch of a blood vessel, has been demonstrated in cerebral blood vessels. Flow-induced changes in resistance have been demonstrated in both arteries and veins. Rabbit pial arteries in vitro demonstrate flow-induced changes in resistance. Flow-induced changes in vascular resistance are not entirely dependent on the presence of an intact endothelium (61). By-products of metabolism, such as extracellular potassium, calcium, hydrogen ion, and adenosine, may play a role in coupling rCBF to regional cerebral metabolism (33).

## Measurement of Cerebral Blood Flow

Assessment of CBF in the critically ill patient is essential in order to ensure that CBF is adequate for the patient's cerebral metabolic rate. Indirectly, physicians can assess the adequacy of CBF by their physical examination and electrophysiologic testing. At CBF rates approximately 50% of normal, alterations in level of consciousness and EEG can be expected. Further decreases in CBF are associated with dense neurologic deficits and flattening of the EEG. Cerebral blood flow rates on the order of 12 to 17 mL/100 g/min are associated with loss of evoked potentials (34, 35). Unfortunately, physical examination and electrophysiologic testing are not sensitive to early changes in CBF. By the time changes on physical exam or EEG are detected, a significant reduction in CBF has already occurred. In addition alterations in mental status in the critically ill patient can be secondary to a wide array of toxic-metabolic disturbances or medications.

Cerebral perfusion pressure can provide an indirect assessment of the adequacy of CBF. If one were to assume abnormal cerebral metabolic rate and cerebral vascular resistance with intact autoregulatory mechanisms, then a normal CPP, or a CPP above the lower limit of autoregulation, should be associated with adequate CBF. Unfortunately both the cerebral metabolic rate and autoregulatory mechanisms are often abnormal in the head-injured and critically ill patient; therefore, a normal CPP cannot be assumed to reliably predict adequate CBF (62).

Transcranial Doppler studies utilize ultrasound technology to measure blood flow velocity in the large cerebral arteries in the base of the brain. A low-frequency ultrasonic signal is emitted and reflected off flowing red blood cells. The resulting Doppler shift is measured and used to calculate the velocity of blood flow. Transcranial Doppler studies report only velocity in centimeters per second. Transcranial Doppler studies do not report flow rate nor tissue perfusion (milliliters per 100 g of tissue per minute). Maximal flow velocity, mean flow velocity, flow direction, and the pulsatile index [(systolic velocity − diastolic velocity)/mean velocity] can be reported. Vessel diameter, absolute flow, along with several other physiologic factors can influence velocity. Only when vessel diameter remains constant can changes in velocity be taken to represent changes in flow. When vessel diameter remains constant, increased flow velocity will be associated with increased flow rates. Under conditions of constant flow, velocity will increase if vessel diameter is decreased (63–65). The consistency of large cerebral artery diameter at the base of the brain during systemic physiologic disturbances has been subject to controversy (66, 67). Direct observations of human cranial arteries subject to moderate changes in systemic blood pressure and $PaCO_2$ revealed less than a 4% change in the diameter of internal carotid, middle cerebral, and vertebral arteries. Smaller blood vessels such as the anterior cerebral artery and more distal segments of the middle cerebral artery exhibited changes in diameter of up to 20% (68). Direct measurements of hemispheric cerebral blood flow correlate poorly with middle cerebral artery flow velocities (69). Although transcranial Doppler studies cannot be used to quantify cerebral blood flow, transcranial Doppler studies can be used to detect and assess relative changes in blood flow (70). Besides changes in vessel diameter and flow, a number of other physiologic changes commonly encountered in the critically ill patient can alter flow velocity. Decreasing $PaO_2$ and hematocrit are associated with increased flow velocities. Decreasing cerebral metabolism is associated with decreased flow velocities (65, 71). Three-dimensional transcranial Doppler studies not only provide information about blood flow, but also may provide imaging of the vessel (72).

A small hand-held probe is used to perform most transcranial Doppler studies. Three transcranial "windows" are most commonly used. The transtemporal window can be used to evaluate the middle cerebral artery. The ipsilateral ophthalmic artery and segments of the ipsilateral internal carotid siphon can be evaluated via the transopthalmic window. The suboccipital window directs signals through the foramen magnum and is used for the evaluation of the basilar and vertebral arteries. The noninvasive nature of the test is one of the advantages of transcranial Doppler studies. The ability to perform repetitive testing and the portable equipment which allows testing to be done at the bedside are other advantages associated with transcranial Doppler studies. Potential pitfalls of transcranial Doppler monitoring include failure to recognize that absolute velocity is influence by patient age, hematocrit, $PaCO_2$, and the angle of isonation (73).

Transcranial Doppler studies have found their greatest use in the neurosurgical arena, where they have been employed for the detection of vasospasm following subarachnoid hemorrhage or trauma, evaluating collateral circulation in patients with stenosis and flow in arteriovenous malformations. By assessing changes in flow velocity in response to alterations in CPP or $PaCO_2$ it is possible to evaluate for the presence or absence of intact autoregulatory mechanisms in the critically ill patient (74, 75). Transcranial Doppler studies can be used for the evaluation of cerebral circulatory arrest and may have a role in future brain death protocols (76–78). Detection of air emboli in patients with patent foramen ovale or undergoing surgical procedures and the detection of particulate emboli in patients with prosthetic heart valves or undergoing carotid endarterectomy are other uses of transcranial Doppler studies which have been reported but still require continued investigation (79–81). Continuous bilateral transcranial Doppler monitoring of the middle cerebral blood flow may prove to be of benefit in patients undergoing carotid endarterectomy, cardiopulmonary bypass (82, 83). Continuous bilateral monitoring of CBF may eventually serve as a research and possibly a management tool in the care of critically ill patiens with hemodynamic instability (84).

In 1945, Kety and Schmidt described a technique to measure CBF based on the Fick principle using inhaled nitrous oxide. In this technique patients inhale a low dose of nitrous oxide. Over 10 minutes, serial samples of arterial and jugular venous blood are obtained. The decay curve of the venous concentration of nitrous oxide combined with the arterial-venous nitrous oxide difference and a known partition coefficient of the brain for nitrous oxide allows for the calculation of global CBF (85). Limitations of this technique include its invasive nature and need for instrumentation which measures blood nitrous oxide concentration. Also differences of up to 15% between the right and left internal jugular bulb oxygen saturations have been recorded in normals (86). These differences result from naturally occurring variability in cerebral venous drainage and/or inadequate mixing of venous blood in the jugular venous bulb.

The $^{133}$Xenon clearance technique is commonly used to measure CBF in the critically ill ICU patient. Xenon-133 is a gamma emitter with cerebral uptake and clearance that can be detected by extracranial scintillation counters. Xenon-133 can be dissolved in liquid and administered intravenously or can be administered as a gas. Arterial concentrations of the radioisotope (estimated from end tidal gas concentrations), dynamic changes in cerebral $^{133}$Xe concentrations, and a mathematical model which assumes a normal blood-brain partition coefficient for $^{133}$Xe are required to calculate CBF. For the patient in the intensive care unit (ICU) typically eight scintillation counters are utilized for each hemisphere. Advantages of the $^{133}$Xe clearance technique include its portable and noninvasive nature. Xenon-133 has a short half-life, allowing for repeated measurements over a short period of time. That only relatively superficial CBF is measured and the lack of sensitivity for detecting focal areas of markedly decreased CBF are potential disadvantages of the technique (87, 88).

Continuous or intermittent monitoring of jugular bulb venous oxygen saturation (SjvO$_2$) has been used to assess the adequacy of CBF for CMRO$_2$ (86). By the Fick equation CMRO$_2$ = AVDO$_2$ × CBF, where AVDO$_2$ equals arterial oxygen content (CaO$_2$) minus mixed jugular vein oxygen content. The Fick equation can be rearranged such that AVDO$_2$ = CMRO$_2$/CBF. The normal arterial-jugular oxygen difference is 6.7 volume percent. The normal cerebral oxygen extraction ratio is approximately 32% (89). If CBF and CMRO$_2$ remain coupled, then changes in CMRO$_2$ are met by parallel changes in CBF and the AVDO$_2$ would be expected to remain relatively constant. Under pathologic conditions CBF may not be tightly coupled to CMRO$_2$ (90). Under these conditions, AVDO$_2$ changes may reflect the adequacy of CBF. A decrease in AVDO$_2$ would suggest that CBF may be excessive for CMRO$_2$. An increased AVDO$_2$ would imply that CBF may be inadequate for CMRO$_2$. Lactate can also be measured in blood obtained from the jugular venous bulb. This value subtracted from the arterial lactate concentration can be used to calculate the cerebral arterial-venous lactate difference (AVDL). Normally the AVDL is .02 μmol/g/min. The lactate oxygen index (LOI) is defined by AVDL/AVDO$_2$. The addition of AVDL and LOI to jugular bulb saturation monitoring assists in assessing the adequacy of CBF. Robertson used the Kety-Schmidt technique to measure CBF and determined AVDO$_2$ and LOI in comatose head-injured patients (91). Utilizing AVDO$_2$ and LOI, it was possible to classify CBF into nonischemic and ischemic/infarcted patterns.

Retrograde cannulation of the internal jugular vein with a fiberoptic catheter makes continuous monitoring of SjVO$_2$ possible. Potential complications and limitations of this technique include its invasive nature. Carotid artery puncture has been reported to occur in up to 3% of attempts. Adequate catheter position is required in order to assure the adequacy of the measurement (86, 92). In some studies, up to 50% of SjVO$_2$ desaturations were found to be incorrect (93). Artifactual changes in SjVO$_2$ may be secondary to inaccurate placement of the catheter or changes in catheter position following movement of the head or neck. Differences between right and left SjVO$_2$ are another potential limitation of SjVO$_2$ monitoring. In trauma patients the catheter is usually placed on the side with computed tomography (CT) abnormality. In the absence of unilateral roetengenographic abnormality the catheter is placed on the side of dominant venous drainage, which is usually the right. Another potential limitation of SjVO$_2$ monitoring is the influence of extracranial blood flow on SjvO$_2$ under pathologic conditions (86). Normally extracranial blood flow is only a small percentage of jugular venous flow. However, it is unclear to what extent extracranial flow contributes to jugular venous flow under pathologic conditions.

Jugular venous saturation monitoring has been utilized extensively in the monitoring of the head-injured patient. Jugular venous saturation monitoring is frequently employed with other techniques such as ICP monitoring (94), transcranial Doppler (95), and direct measurements of direct CBF to assess the adequacy of CBF, the adequacy of cerebral hemodynamic reserve, and the "intactness" of autoregulatory mechanisms (96).

Thermal diffusion flow probes have been used to measure rCBF. In this technique, two small probes are placed in contact with the surface of the brain. The probes are several millimeters apart from each other. One plate is heated, while the second plate monitors tissue temperature. Blood flow is inversely proportional to the temperature gradient between the two plates (97, 98). Cerebral blood flow measured by the thermodilution technique has been correlated with CBF measured with $^{133}$Xenon and hydrogen clearance (99). The technique has been utilized for intraoperative and postoperative monitoring (100). Continuous monitoring of rCBF is one of the potential advantages of this technique. Thus, the potential for detection of significant changes in CBF prior to clinical deterioration and at a time when intervention may change outcome exists. Potential complications include cerebrospinal fluid (CSF) leaks and infection. Potential disadvantages include the fact that only rCBF is monitored and its invasive nature. Loss of contact with the brain and placement over a large vessel will interfere with the reliability of the technique. Further investigation of the clinical utility, reliability, and potential impact on patient outcome is required.

Cerebral near-infrared spectroscopy (NIRS) utilizes near-infrared light (wavelength 700 to 1000 nm) as a noninvasive method to detect changes in the concentrations of oxyhemoglobin, deoxyhemoglobin, and oxidized cytochrome $a,a_3$. Cytochrome $a,a_3$ is located on the inner mitochondrial membrane and catalyzes the last step of oxidative phosphorlyation of adenosine diphosphate (ADP) in the electron transport chain. If adequate oxygen is available, the enzyme exists in its oxidized state. Light with the wavelengths utilized can penetrate through the scalp, skull, and several centimeters of cerebral contents. Spectrophotometers typically utilize four to six wavelengths. Light is conducted by an optical fiber to the head. The iron-porphyrin complexes of oxyhemoglobin, deoxyhemoglobin, and the oxidized copper atom of cytochrome $a,a_3$ absorb light (101). Light entering tissue is either transmitted through the skull in small infants or scattered in tissues with portions being returned though the surface. One or more sensors capture returning light. The attenuation of transmitted or scattered light is attributed to absorption by the light-absorbing molecules and is proportional to their concentrations. Use of multiple sensors and placement of a sensor near the light source allows for subtraction of attenuation secondary to the scalp and skull. By inducing changes in systemic arterial oxygen saturation, it is possible to use the Fick principle to calculate both cerebral blood flow and volume (101–103).

Cerebral near-infrared spectroscopy has been most studied in newborn infants (104, 105). In adults, because of large head size and the scattering of light, different transmission lengths are more problematic. Large clinical trials on the value of NIRS in adults are lacking. In adult volunteers, NIRS has been used to study the effects of hypocapnia and normocapnic hypoxemia on cerebral oxyhemoglobin, oxidized cytochrome $a,a_3$ concentrations, and cerebral blood volume (106). Cerebral blood volume increased in both groups, with normocapnic subjects having a significantly greater increase in blood volume than hypocapnic subjects. While both groups had significantly decreased concentrations of oxyhemoglobin, hypocapnic patients had significantly greater decreases than normocapnic subjects. Changes in brain oxyhemoglobin preceded changes in heart rate, blood pressure, or ventilation. Changes in oxyhemoglobin concentrations preceded changes in oxidized cytochrome $a,a_3$ concentrations.

For the adult patient, NIRS would appear to be a potentially valuable tool. Allowing physicians to noninvasively and continuously monitor the effect of alterations in physiology or therapeutics on cerebral blood volume and oxyhemoglobin contents may allow them to recognize a "brain at risk" before neurologic changes are manifest. Potential problems with long-term NIRS monitoring exist. Changes in plasma volume will not be detected; therefore estimates of cerebral volume may not be reliable if hematocrit changes.

Changes in CBF and $CMRO_2$ may affect CBV measurements (101, 104).

### Cerebral Blood Flow During Sepsis and Septic Shock

Animal studies employing different species and different models of sepsis have found no difference or decreased CBF during sepsis and septic shock. The clinical relevance and applicability of these studies to human sepsis is ques-

tionable. Dogs treated with LPS generally demonstrate decreased CBF with an increased $CMRO_2$. Canine studies suggest that the increase $CMRO_2$ may be mediated by circulating catecholamines (107). Animal studies demonstrate the LPS can damage the blood-brain barrier (108). Disruption of the blood-brain barrier allows circulating catecholamines access to the CNS (109, 110). Pretreatment of dogs with propranolol prior to LPS administration blocks the increase in $CMRO_2$ (111). Studies in humans demonstrate that intracarotid or intravenous administration of epinephrine, norepinephrine, and angiotensin do not significantly change rCBF (112). Canine studies also have shown that although rCBF may be uniformly decreased, changes in rCVR may vary (113).

Rat models of sepsis have generally demonstrated no alterations in CBF (3). In rats the peripheral administration of LPS results in the production of mRNA for TNF-$\alpha$, IL-1, and IL-6 (114). Prostaglandin $E_2$ immunoreactivity in the choroid plexus and microvasculature of the rat brain is increased by the peripheral administration of LPS (115). This experimental evidence might suggest that the local production of arachadonic metabolites or cytokines may influence cerebral function in sepsis (116). The possibility and role of local cerebral production of these metabolites in human sepsis have yet to be investigated.

Swine-made hypotensives by LPS administration develop intracranial hypertension, reduced cerebral oxygen extraction, and increased blood volume. An equivalent decrease in systemic blood pressure secondary to hemorrhage did not result in elevated intracranial pressures. The increased cerebral blood volume was felt to at least partially account for the elevated intracranial pressure.

Two studies have investigated the effect of sepsis on CBF in humans. Small numbers of patients were present in both studies. Bowton used [133]Xenon clearance to study cerebral blood flow in nine patients with sepsis and multiorgan system failure (117). For septic patients, the mean CBF was of $29.6 \pm 15.8$ (SD) mL/100 g/min, vs. $44.9 \pm 6.2$ mL/100 g/min in age-matched historical controls. There was no correlation between CBF and MAP. Mackeawa measured CBF and $CMRO_2$ in six patients with sepsis and multisystem organ failure (118). All of these patients were receiving mechanical ventilation. The average total bilirubin was $13.4 \pm 5.2$ mg/dL. The Glasgow Coma Scale varied between 4 and 10. Five of these six patients eventually died from their illness. Cerebral perfusion pressure was calculated as the difference between MAP and jugular bulb pressure and was $79 \pm$ mm Hg. Cerebral blood flow varied over a wide range but was significantly less in the septic vs. nonseptic control patients (17 to 37 mL/100 g/min, $28 \pm 3$ vs. $46 \pm 2$ mL/100 g/min).

### Cerebral Blood Flow in Congestive Heart Failure

Paulson has used [133]Xenon to measure cerebral blood flow in patients with New York Heart Association class

III and IV CHF (119, 120). Mean cerebral blood flow was reduced in patients compared to controls. Cerebral blood flow was unchanged after the administration of captopril, even in those patients who had a significant reduction in systemic blood pressure.

## CORONARY BLOOD FLOW

Under resting conditions human coronary blood flow is estimated to be 60 to 100 mL/min/100 g tissue. Myocardial oxygen consumption has been estimated to 6 to 8 mL $O_2$/min. Myocardial oxygen extraction is approximately 65%, resulting in a coronary sinus hemoglobin oxygen saturation of 35% (121). During exercise the myocardial oxygen extraction ratio may increase to 80% (122). Because of the baseline high extraction of oxygen, increases in myocardial oxygen extraction provide only a limited reserve to meet increasing myocardial oxygen requirements; therefore increases in myocardial oxygen consumption must be accompanied by increases in flow (123). Smith investigated the different components of myocardial oxygen consumption. Beating canine hearts were found to have a myocardial oxygen consumption of 10.3 mL/100 g/min (124). During asystole and ventricular fibrillation oxygen consumption fell to 2.0 and 3.8 mL/min. Coarse ventricular fibrillation was associated with greater oxygen consumption than fine ventricular fibrillation. Therefore the majority of oxygen consumption is related to myocardial mechanical activity. Approximately 20% of total myocardial oxygen consumption represents basal cellular metabolism. Electrical activity without mechanical activity adds little to myocardial oxygen consumption. On a per-weight basis subendocardial oxygen consumption and blood flow are 20% greater than those of the subepicardial myocardium. Increased cell shortening and greater wall stress lead to the increased subendocardial oxygen requirements (121, 122). The primary determinants of myocardial oxygen consumption are systolic wall tension (125–127), contractility (128–131), and heart rate (132, 133). During stable inotropic states, the left ventricular systolic pressure volume area has been found to be a reliable marker of myocardial oxygen consumption (134–137).

Coronary blood flow is regulated by anatomic, physiologic, metabolic, myogenic, and neurologic factors. Coronary blood flow is autoregulated over a wide range of perfusion pressures ranging from 60 to 130 mm Hg. Coronary perfusion pressure can be defined as the difference between aortic root pressure and right atrial or left ventricular diastolic pressure. Clinically diastolic pressure is often used to approximate aortic root pressure (138).

In addition to perfusion pressure gradients, it is also necessary to consider the fact that intramyocardial vessels are subject to compressive forces during the various phases of the cardiac cycle (139). Intramyocardial wall tension will increase with increases in loading condition and contractility. Intramyocardial pressure is greatest during systole; therefore most of left ventricular blood flow occurs diastole. As intermyocardial pressure is less for the right ventricle, the right ventricular coronary flow occurs during both systole and diastole. Subendocardial vessels are exposed to greater compressive forces than subepicardial vessels (122, 138). Decreases in perfusion pressure are accompanied by relatively greater decreases in subendocardial than subepicardial myocardial blood flow (140). This contributes to the susceptibility of the subendocardium to ischemia (141, 142). As tachycardia is associated with decreased time spent in diastole, tachycardia will result in reduced blood flow (122, 138).

Coronary vessels are innervated with alpha-1, alpha-2, beta-1, and beta-2-adrenergic and parasympathetic neurons. Alpha-1- and alpha-2-receptors mediate vasoconstriction while the beta receptors mediate vasodilitation. Some beta-receptor vasodilatation may be mediated via increased metabolic demands secondary to stimulation of myocardial beta-receptors (133).

### Myocardial Blood Flow in Sepsis and Septic Shock

The typical hemodynamic profile of volume-resuscitated septic shock is characterized by an increased cardiac output, low systemic vascular resistance, and normal oxygen extraction ratio (143–145). Because vasodilatation and third spacing of fluids typically are part of the inflammatory response to sepsis, fluid loading to achieve an adequate preload is often required for a typical hemodynamic profile (146). Clinical and laboratory studies show that gram-positive and gram-negative organisms result in a similar cardiovascular response (147, 148). Despite the elevated cardiac output, right and left ventricular dysfunction has been found during sepsis and septic shock. Both right and left ventricular stroke work indices are reduced early in sepsis (149, 150). Serial radionucleotide and hemodynamic measurements have found a dynamic process to occur. Biventricular dilatation occurs within the first several days of septic shock. Stroke volume is maintained, while end-systolic and end-diastolic volumes increase. Ejection fraction is reduced. These changes resolve over a period of 10 to 14 days (151). The ratio of peak systolic pressure to end-systolic pressure is also reduced in patients with septic shock compared to nonseptic critically ill patients (152). Survivors of septic shock have lower initial peak systolic pressure/end-systolic pressure ratio than nonsurvivors. The peak systolic pressure/end-systolic pressure ratio increased with time in survivors and did not change in nonsurvivors. In one study with a small number of patients, those patients who did not survive their episode of septic shock tended not to have cardiac dilatation. Persistent tachycardia and failure for the hyperdynamic state to resolve have also been found to be markers of a poor prognosis (153). In addition to systolic dysfunction, animal models of sepsis and human studies have found evidence of diastolic dysfunction during sepsis and septic shock (154, 155) .

Myocardial ischemia, alterations in serum constituents, and the presence of circulating myocardial depressant factors have all been postulated to account for the alterations in cardiac function observed during sepsis and septic shock. Animal studies have yielded conflicting results concerning the contribution of ischemia to the myocardial dysfunction observed during sepsis. Various animal models have suggested that a limitation of global coronary blood flow or a redistribution of myocardial blood flow may account for the cardiac dysfunction observed during sepsis (156–158). Flow redistribution involved a decrease in subendocardial-to-epicardial blood flow ratios (159, 160). Limitations of these studies include the fact that models were often not hyperdynamic, relied on endotoxin boluses, were not volume resuscitated, were of short duration, or involved isolated heart. Two studies have compared coronary blood flow and myocardial metabolism in septic patients without known coronary artery disease to that of control patients (161, 162). Increased coronary blood flow, especially at high heart rates, and a reduction in coronary artery resistance have been found in septic patients. Coronary sinus hemoglobin saturation is increased and myocardial oxygen extraction ratio is reduced compared to controls. Myocardial oxygen consumption was not significantly different from that of control patients. Metabolic studies revealed elevated lactic acid uptake and reduced uptake of free fatty acid, glucose, and ketone bodies during sepsis and septic shock. There was no correlation between serum lactate levels and lactate uptake in septic patiens. Nonsurvivors had lower myocardial free fatty acid and glucose uptake than survivors. Only 6 of 40 patients who underwent these metabolic studies had zero or negative lactic acid clearance. These 6 patients had reduced cardiac indices, coronary perfusion pressures, and coronary sinus blood flow. There was no difference in myocardial oxygen extraction ratios (162). If this is considered a marker of myocardial ischemia, then only a minority of patients with septic shock had metabolic evidence of myocardial ischemia. Positive lactate clearance can occur during periods of regional ischemia; therefore a positive lactate clearance does not with 100% certainty exclude the possibility of regional ischemia (163). Thus it seems that in the majority of patients inadequate coronary blood flow does not account for the observed changes in cardiac function.

Studies have investigated the effect of coronary artery disease on cardiac performance during sepsis and septic shock in humans. Limitations of these studies include the use of history, ECG changes, or wall motion abnormalities as markers of coronary artery diseases. Patients with coronary artery disease tend to be older than the patients without coronary artery disease. Ellrodt performed hemo-dynamic and radionucleotide studies in 35 patients with septic shock (164). Fifteen patients had heart disease. Eleven of the 15 had coronary artery disease. Segmental wall motion abnormalities were detected in 22 patients and was more frequently detected in patients with cardiac disease than those without (87% vs. 45%). No differences in coronary perfusion pressure were found between those patients with segmental wall motion abnormalities and those without. Raper compared hemodynamic and gated radionucleotide studies in patients with nonhypotensive sepsis (165). Twenty patients had coronary artery disease, as evidenced by a history of angina, ECG evidence of infarction or ischemia, and the presence of focal wall motion abnormalities on gated cardiac scintigraphy. Compared to patients without coronary artery disease, patients with coronary artery disease were older, had reduced left ventricular end-diastolic volume, left ventricular end-systolic volume, left ventricular systolic work, and cardiac and stroke volume indexes. The differences in left ventricular end-diastolic indexes occurred despite pulmonary artery occlusion pressures being equal between the two groups, suggesting reductions in ventricular compliance in the patients with coronary artery disease. It therefore appears that preexisting heart disease can alter the cardiac response to volume-resuscitated sepsis and septic shock. The role of coronary artery disease and possible limitations of coronary blood flow in determining the cardiac response to sepsis in these patients is unknown.

In the absence of inadequate coronary blood flow a "circulating myocardial depressant factor" was felt to account for the changes in cardiac function observed during sepsis. Serum obtained from septic shock patients results in a decreased velocity and extent of shortening of newborn rat myocardial myocytes (166, 167). Cytokine-mediated expression of inducible nitric oxide synthase appears to account for the myocardial depression. Nitric oxide has been shown to attenuate cardiac myocyte contraction (168). Rat ventricular myocytes exposed to the medium of activated macrophages exhibit a depressed response to beta-adrenergic agonists. Increased content of cyclic guanosine monophosphate, nitrite concentrations, and the fact that effect is blocked by the addition of nitric oxide synthase inhibitors implicate nitric oxide as a cause of the decreased myocardial function (169).

The cytokines IL-1, beta-interferon, and gamma-interferon have been demonstrated to induce the expression of inducible nitric oxide synthase in rat myocytes (170, 171). Tumor necrosis factor alpha may also result in myocardial depression via induction of calcium-independent nitric oxide synthase activity (172, 173).

## Myocardial Blood Flow During Hemorrhagic Shock

Various animal models have been used to investigate the effect of hemorrhagic shock on myocardial blood flow and metabolism. Interspecies variation, differences in the depth and duration of hypotension, the influence of anesthetic agents, and the use of heparin to prevent the clotting of extracorporeal circuits need to be considered when attempting to apply these studies to humans. The majority of studies have shown that hemorrhagic shock is accompanied by reductions in coronary blood flow, coronary artery resistance, and myocardial oxygen delivery. Myocardial oxygen consumption is reduced while oxygen extraction and arterial venous oxygen differences are increased (174–176). Depending upon the degree and duration of hypotension evidence of anaerobic metabolism may be found. Endocardial blood flow is reduced to a greater amount than epicardial blood flow (177, 178). Pathologically, subendocardial injury predominates. Subendocardial hemorrhage and necrosis have been found in experimental hemorrhagic shock. Disruption in myocardial cell membrane integrity and impaired volume regulation have been found in hemorrhagic shock (179, 180). These alterations predominate in the subendocardial region. Experimentally myocardial edema is manifested by a decrease in the dry-to-wet-weight ratio.

Experimentally hemorrhagic shock is accompanied by impaired left ventricular contractility. The degree of dysfunction appears to be related to the depth and duration of hypotension (181–183). After a prolonged period reinfusion of blood will not reverse or prevent a progressive decline in left ventricular function.

The restoration of coronary arterial pressure during hemorrhagic shock would appear to clinically make intuitive sense and experimental evidence supports this. Restoring aortic pressure or intermittently increasing coronary artery pressure has been found to maintain or restore myocardial contractility. Iguidbashian used an ovine model of hemorrhagic shock to investigate the effect of different resuscitation protocols on survival, myocardial blood flow, and contractility (184). Resuscitation protocols included volume alone, volume with an infusion of epinephrine to maintain a mean arterial pressure of 50 to 60 mm Hg, and cardiopulmonary bypass to maintain a mean arterial pressure of 50 mm Hg. All of the sheep receiving cardiopulmonary bypass survived, all of the sheep who received volume alone died, while sheep who received the epinephrine infusion in addition to volume resuscitation had intermittent survival rates. All animals had an increase in myocardial weight, suggesting that myocardial edema had occurred. Sheep in the epinephrine infusion protocol had a 60% reduction in end-systolic length relationships ($E_{ES}$). Sheep in the cardiopulmonary support protocol had only a 20% reduction in $E_{ES}$. During shock all groups had a reduction in subendocardial blood flow. After resuscitation from shock subendocardial blood flow was normal in the cardiopulmonary support animals while subendocardial blood flow was increased in the epinephrine infusion group.

Although there are no studies evaluating the effect of coronary artery disease on hemorrhagic shock, it would seem that preexisting coronary artery disease would lead to further compromise of myocardial blood flow and greater disturbances of myocardial metabolism and function. Experimental evidence also suggests that the development of subendocardial ischemia is a significant problem during hemorrhagic shock. Experimental studies also show the importance of adequate restoration of blood pressure as soon as possible before a period of inevitable deterioration occurs.

## RENAL BLOOD FLOW

In a 70-kg man the kidney receives approximately 1,000 to 1,200 mL of blood per minute, or roughly 20% of the cardiac output. Both kidneys normally weigh approximately 300 g; therefore renal blood flow is approximately 400 mL/100 g tissue/min. Within the kidney there is a heterogeneous distribution of blood flow. Eighty percent of flow is directed to the cortex and 20% to the inner and outer medulla. The inner medulla receives only 1% to 3% of the total renal blood flow (185–187). Low medullary blood flow helps prevent washout of solutes necessary for the maintenance of concentrating gradients within the kidney. The length of the vasa recta, an increased plasma protein content in medullary blood vessels, and crenation of red blood cells in a hypertonic environment possibly account for the decreased medullary blood flow (188).

Renal oxygen consumption averages 18 to –20 mL/min. Because of a high renal blood flow, renal oxygen delivery which is normally 240 mL/min is generally in excess of renal demands. Normally the kidney extracts only 8% to 10% of available oxygen, resulting in an arteriovenous oxygen difference of 1 to 2 mL/dL and a renal vein $PaO_2$ of 70 mm Hg (185). Although overall oxygen delivery would appear to be in excess of tissue requirements, significant gradients for oxygen availability exist within the kidney. Microelectrode studies have documented medullary tissue $PO_2$ in the range of 10 mm Hg under normal conditions (189). Thus medullarly tissue $PO_2$ may be lower than renal vein $PvO_2$. Organization of blood vessels with the medulla contributes to the corticomedullary $PO_2$ gradient. Blood vessels forming the vasa recta loop down into the medulla as the accompany tubules (190). As a result of this arrangement, oxygen can diffuse from the arterial to the venous system in a countercurrent manner. This results in a lower oxygen supply to deeper portions of the kidney.

Axial streaming resulting from branching of afferent arterioles at angles of 90 degrees from parent arteries may result in regional differences in hematocrit within the kidney. Axial streaming refers to the fact that formed elements of the blood tend to travel in the center of the vessel, resulting in a plasma-rich relative acellular layer forming at the vessel wall. Arteries branching off the parent artery will therefore receive blood relatively rich in plasma with a decreased hematocrit. Studies in rats have found medullary hematocrit which are approximately one-half the systemic hematocrit (190, 191).

Tubule cells of the thick medullarly limb (mTAL) are located in this area. These metabolically active cells are involved in the active transport of Na and Cl. Because these cells operate in an area of borderline oxygenation, they may be particularly prone to effects of limited oxygen flow to the kidney. Studies have shown that, during ischemic insults, some of the earliest morphologic changes occur in the cells of the mTAL. Decreasing the oxygen requirements of the cells by inhibiting the active reabsorption of solutes by the cells offers some degree of protection from ischemic insults (192).

Normally over 99% of filtered solutes are reabsorbed by the kidney. Reabsorption is an energy-consuming active process. The majority of renal oxygen consumption is utilized to support these active transport mechanisms (193). Renal blood flow is in fact regulated primarily to maintain glomerular filtration rate (GFR), not to meet the metabolic needs of the kidney (194). As GFR can vary with renal blood flow (RBF), it can appear that renal oxygen consumption is flow dependent (195). The parallel decreases in renal oxygen consumption with decreases in renal blood flow represent a decreased need for oxygen consumption as the need for the active reabsorption of solutes decreases. In anesthetized dogs subjected to hemorrhage renal $V_{O_2}$ must decrease to 63% of the baseline value before the oxygen extraction ratio increases and lactate clearance decreases (193).

## Regulation of Renal Blood Flow

The kidney has the ability to regulate blood flow over a wide range of perfusion pressures. The afferent and efferent arterioles are the major sites of renal vascular resistance. Autoregulation is primarily dominated by the need to maintain GFR. An autoregulatory mechanism can originate intrinsically or extrinsically to the kidney. Rapidly occurring mechanisms tend to be functional while more chronic mechanisms may involve structural changes (194). Several hypotheses concerning the autoregulation of RBF exist. In addition to the myogenic and metabolic hypothesis of blood flow regulation, the tubuloglomerular feedback mechanism needs to be considered. In the tubuloglomerular feedback hypothesis each nephron regulates its blood flow to maintain that nephron's GFR. Tubuloglomerular feedback involves sensing of distal NaCl delivery in the distal tubule by the macula densa. The macula densa then regulates GFR in the same nephron by altering pre- and postglomerular vessel resistance and the glomerular ultrafiltration coefficient. If an excess amount of solute is detected in the distal tubule, the afferent arteriole resistance would be increased so as to decrease blood flow to that nephron and thereby reduce that individual nephron's GFR (196).

Multiple potential mediators to regulate RBF have been identified. The kidney is richly innervated by adrenergic nerve fibers. Studies in various species utilizing different microscopic techniques have detected nerve fibers not only innervating vascular segments but also surrounding tubule cells and in the region of the juxtaglomerular apparatus. In humans stimulation of the adrenergic nervous alpha-1-receptors appear to predominate. Serotonin, dopamine 1, dopamine 2, alpha-2, beta-2, neuropeptide Y, and vasoactive intestinal peptide receptors have also been found in various species (197–200). Under normal resting conditions renal nerve activity is felt to have little influence on the renal circulation. Animal studies utilizing different species have found that large increases in renal nerve activity are required before renal blood flow is altered (201). By comparing renal vein with renal artery neurotransmitter concentrations, it is possible to assess the degree of renal nerve activity. The "spillover," or excess amount, of neurotransmitter found in the venous blood can serve as a marker for renal nerve activity. Graded exercise and mental stress have been found to increase renal nerve activity (202, 203). Dynamic and physical activity appear to be potent stimulants of renal nerve activity and are associated with increases in renal vascular resistance and diminished renal blood flow (203). Renal nerve activity directly or indirectly through the renin-angiotensin system may account for these observations (204).

In addition to renal nerve activity, it is necessary to consider the multiple biologically active substances that can be produced within or outside the kidney and influence renal blood flow. The effects of atrial natriuretic factor, angiotensin, bradykinin, endothelin, nitric oxide, vasopressin, vasoactive intestinal peptide, adenosine, prostaglandins, and various catecholamines have been investigated (204, 205). Because of the complex nature and often multiple interactions of these substances, it is often impossible to have one clear direct causal effect of an individual substance. Also, the alterations in systemic hemodynamics and changes in endothelial cell function, receptor activity, regional cytokine production, and regional prostaglandin production in critically ill patients make it even more difficult to clearly identify the effect of an individual agent on renal blood flow during a critical illness.

## Measurement of Renal Blood Flow

The clearance of $p$-aminohippurate (PAH) is commonly used to determine renal blood flow. The PAH is filtered by the glomerulus and secreted by tubule cells. Clearance of PAH can be calculated by the following formula:

$$c_{PAH} = U_{PAH}V/P_{PAH}$$

Here, $U_{PAH}$ is the concentration of PAH in the urine, V is the urine flow rate, and $P_{PAH}$ is the plasma concentration of PAH. If 100% of PAH is cleared during passage through the kidney, then the clearance of PAH ($c_{PAH}$) will be equal to renal plasma flow (RPF). Normal renal plasma flow is approximately 650 mL/min. Knowing RPF it is possible to calculate RBF by the following formula:

$$RBF = RPF/ 1 - Hct$$

Under normal conditions the kidney actually extracts approximately 90% of PAH ($E_{PAH}$); therefore RBF calculated from RPF may underestimate actual RBF. The extraction of PAH is defined by the following equation:

$$A_{PAH} - V_{PAH}/A_{PAH}$$

Here, $A_{PAH}$ is the concentration of PAH in arterial blood and $V_{PAH}$ is the venous concentration of PAH. Animal studies as well as human studies have found that $E_{PAH}$ can be reduced in sepsis, chronic renal failure, hypotensive hemorrhagic shock, and oliguric renal failure and during fluid loading. Decreases in $E_{PAH}$ may result in erroneous RBF measurements when $C_{PAH}$ is used to calculate RBF in critically ill patients. Renal vein blood can be sampled and PAH concentration determined so that a corrected $C_{PAH}$ can be calculated. The corrected $C_{PAH}$ can then be used to calculated RBF (206, 207).

Thermodilution catheters have been used to measure RBF. In this technique, the renal vein is cannulated with an indwelling catheter. Like PA catheters, these catheters have a thermositer probe and utilize changes in temperature to calculate blood flow. Both instantaneous bolus and continuous measurements are possible. For thermodilution-determined RBF measurements to be accurate, there must be only one renal vein on the side studied and there must be equal blood flow to each kidney. There must also be minimal flow from other vessels which drain into the renal vein. The invasive indwelling nature of the catheter as well as the fact that the relatively short renal veins make catheter displacement relatively easy are potential disadvantages of this methodology.

Several studies have correlated RBF determined by the thermodilution technique with RBF measured by corrected clearance methods. The correlation between the two methods has been disappointing in humans. In a small number of patients with sepsis and septic shock, some of whom were receiving catecholamine therapy, bolus thermodilution RBF measurements correlated with RBF determined by corrected $c_{PAH}$ with an $r$ value of 0.62. In vitro and in vivo validation studies utilizing a continuous thermodilution catheter to measure porcine RBF have shown good correlations with actual RBF ($r^2 = 0.98$ and $r^2 = 0.85$, respectively) (208). The catheter was also studied in 16 patients who were undergoing cardiac catheterization for the evaluation of angina pectoris (209). Thirty minutes after the catheterization RBF was determined by thermodilution and the corrected clearance of $^{131}I$ orthoiodohippurate. Correlation of the two methods in humans was less than in the animal studies($r^2 = 0.64$).

Other methods used clinically to measure RBF include renal artery ultrasound with Doppler (210), inert gas washout techniques, and magnetic resonance imaging (MRI) angiography. Inert gas washout techniques allow for the measurement of distribution of intrarenal blood flow. Research methods to measure RBF include microsphere techniques and magnetic flow probes applied to the renal arteries (211).

### Renal Blood Flow in Sepsis and Septic Shock

Animal studies investigating the effect of sepsis and septic shock on renal blood flow have resulted in variable and sometimes conflicting results. Disturbances in systemic hemodynamics as well as biologically active mediator release need to be considered when one evaluates the effect of sepsis on renal blood flow. Differences in species, degree of hypotension, adequacy of volume resuscitation, anesthetic agents, and methods used to measure renal blood flow account for some of this variability. Utilization of different models of sepsis and the agent used to initiate the "septic response" also contribute to these variable results. Studies utilizing boluses of LPS versus continuous infusions of LPS, cecal ligation with perforation, the intraperitoneal instillation of bacteria, or the intravenous administration of live bacteria may result in different inflammatory, biochemical, and hemodynamic responses and therefore may have different effects on renal blood flow. In general, with few exceptions, acute bolus models, especially when accompanied by a decrease in both blood pressure and cardiac output, are associated with a decrease in renal blood flow (212). More chronic models such as cecal ligation and perforation and continuous infusion of low-dose endotoxin, particularly associated with preservation or increase in cardiac output, are accompanied by preservation or increased RBF compared to control animals (213, 214). These may be better models of volume-resuscitated hyperdynamic sepsis.

Disturbances in renal blood flow can occur locally within the kidney and can occur without major disturbances in systemic hemodynamics. In a hydronephrotic rat model, videomicroscopy has been used to assess the response of video microscopy and Doppler studies have been used to assess the effect of live *Escherichia coli* infusion on interlobular artery, afferent arteriole, and efferent arteriole diameter. Interlobular artery blood flow was quantified by Doppler velocimetry. The tubuloglomerular feedback mechanism is not functional in this model. In this study, there were no significant changes in blood pressure, and cardiac output tended to increase. Bacteremic rats had decreased intralobular diameter (–22%) and afferent arteriole diameter (–20%). Interlobular blood flow decreased by 56% (215). Topical application of the nitric oxide synthase inhibitor, L-

NAME, resulted in further decreases in afferent and efferent arteriole diameter and also led to a decrease in efferent arteriole diameter (–30%). Topical L-NAME resulted in a 75% decrease in interlobular flow. Topical administration of L-arginine ameliorated the observed changes in bacteremic rats. This experiment shows the importance of nitric oxide in maintaining preglomerular vascular tone. This model suggests that different pre- and postglomerular nitric oxide mediated mechanisms for controlling vasculature tone exist between basal and bacteremic animals. Elevated endothelin levels have been detected during and experimental and human sepsis (216). Endothelin 1 is known to be a potent constrictor of the renal vasculature. Elevated endothelin levels are detected in rats bolused with intravenous endotoxin. Administration of anti-endothelin 1 antibodies to endotoxin-treated rats is associated with improvement in indices of renal function. This suggests that endothelin may play a role in the regulation of renal function and the disturbance in renal blood flow associated with sepsis and septic shock (217).

There have been several studies of renal blood flow in human sepsis. Tristani utilized an indicator dilution technique via catheterization of the renal artery and renal vein to measure renal blood flow in 17 patiens with shock and 7 control volunteers (218). Systemic hemodynamics as well as the effect of various interventions were also reported. No pulmonary artery occlusion pressure measurements were available. Eleven of the 17 patients were felt to have sepsis as the major etiology of their shock. One patient had sepsis complicated by myocardial infarction, 2 patients had myocardial infractions, and 1 patient had pancreatitis. Compared to control subjects, patients had decreased RBF [225 ± 25 SEM (standard error of the mean) vs. 399 ± 38 mL/min/kidney]. The small number of patients with low cardiac output made intragroup comparisons impossible. Eight patients with low central venous pressures received 500 mL of dextran for volume expansion. After the volume infusion cardiac output, mean arterial pressure, and renal blood flow improved. This suggests that some of these patients may have been volume depleted. Lucas evaluated renal function in 40 patients with sepsis (219). *Para*-aminohippurate clearance was used to measure renal plasma flow. Renal vein catheters were place in 11 of these patients so that corrected $c_{PAH}$ could be calculated. The extraction ratio of PAH in these patients was 46%. True renal plasma flow averaged 1116 mL/min ± 582 (SD) versus a reported normal value of 725 ± 150 mL/min/175 m². Renal blood flow averaged to be 19.2 ± 4.6% of cardiac output in these patients. Brenner measured renal blood flow by corrected $c_{PAH}$ in eight septic patients, some of whom were receiving catecholamine therapy (220). The corrected extraction rate of PAH in this study was 53.6%. Renal blood flow ranged from 112 to 1,767 mL/min with a mean of 690 ± 179 mL/min. Renal blood flow did not correlate with any systemic hemodynamic parameter or catecholamine dose. Renal blood flow as a percentage of cardiac output was reduced. Repeat studies performed later in the patients' clinical course as their sepsis resolved revealed that total RBF and RBF as a percentage of cardiac index increased as systemic vascular resistance increased, the implication being that the profound systemic vasodilatation seen during the early septic hemodynamic response was not matched by an equal degree of vasodilatation in the renal circulation. The unequal vasodilatation between systemic and renal vascular beds may contribute to the early decrease in percentage of cardiac output going to the kidneys. As systemic vascular resistance increases later in the patients' course, an increase in percentage of cardiac output could return to the kidneys.

Quite often critically ill patients with sepsis and septic shock have inadequate urine outputs despite adequate systemic hemodynamics. These patients may be on catecholamine for its alpha-1 effect to maintain systemic blood pressures. Quite often, in an attempt to restore urine output and improve renal blood flow, *renal dose dopamine* is infused at a rate of 0.5 to 2 µg/kg/min. Unfortunately there are few clinical studies which physicians can use to decide if this is a valid conclusion (221). In animal studies norepinphrine infusions can lead to the development of renal failure (222). In human volunteers, norepinephrine infusions can lead to increases in renal vascular resistance and decreased renal plasma flow. This effect is mediated by constriction of afferent and arteriole vessels (223, 224). Unfortunately there are no large studies of renal blood flow in patients with septic shock who are receiving intravenous catecholamines for their alpha-1 effect. Human studies would suggest that reestablishment of a systemic perfusion pressure is the most important factor in reestablishing renal blood flow (225–227).

The kidney is innervated with DA1 and DA2 receptors. Postsynaptic DA1 receptors lead to vasodilatation. Presynaptic DA2 receptors lead to decreased release of the vasoconstrictor norepineprhine (228). This has led to the widespread use of renal dose dopamine in patients with vasodilated shock. Dopamine has a direct effect on tubule cells, leading to inhibition of the reabsorption of sodium chloride. In subjects with normal renal function as well as patients with CHF, the intravenous administration of dopamine can lead to increases in plasma flow and increased sodium excretion (229, 230). Because changes in systemic hemodynamics are often recorded, it is difficult to ascribe these effects solely to the effect of dopaminergic receptors on the kidney. Animal studies have yielded conflicting results as to the benefit of renal dose dopamine in maintaining renal blood flow during septic shock in animals receiving norepinephrine (231–234).

In summary, studies of RBF in a large number of patients with sepsis and septic shock are lacking. From animal studies and the available human studies it seems clear that disturbances in systemic hemodynamics and perfusion pressures alone cannot account for all of the alterations in RBF observed during sepsis and septic shock. Alterations in various hemodynamically mediated mediators can apparently effect total as well as intrarenal distribution of blood flow.

## Renal Blood Flow in CHF and Cardiogenic Shock

Alterations in renal perfusion pressure, cardiac output, endothelial function (235), and perhaps more importantly the neurohumoral axis can affect renal blood flow in patients with CHF and cardiogenic shock. Activation of the renin-angiotensin system and elevated atrial natriuretic factor, norepinephrine, arginine vasopressin, angiotesin, and aldosterone levels are frequently detected in CHF (236–239). Norepinephrine spillover studies indicate activation of the cardiac and renal sympathetic nervous system in patients with CHF (240, 241). Complicating the interpretation of these studies is the fact that administration of diuretics can, through the production of relative volume depletion, lead to activation of the renin-angiotensin system. Evidence of activation of the renin-angiotension system can also be demonstrated in patients who have recently sustained an acute myocardial infarction not accompanied by clinical evidence of CHF (236).

Experimental studies utilizing rats indicate the importance of the renin-angiotensin system in determining renal blood flow after myocardial infarction and in the setting of CHF. In rats with myocardial infarction following ligation of the left coronary artery, significant intrarenal vasoconstriction can be demonstrated. The intrarenal vasoconstriction occurs without detectable differences in cardiac output or mean arterial blood pressure. Angiotensin-converting enzyme inhibition (ACEI) and renin inhibitors reverse the intrarenal vasoconstriction (242). Other investigators utilizing rats with myocardial infarction secondary to ligation of the left coronary artery and accompanied by decreases in mean arterial pressure and elevation of left ventricular end-diastolic pressure have found reduced glomerular plasma flow and a lesser decline in GFR (243). Elevation of efferent arteriole tone secondary to angiotensin II is felt to account for the majority of these changes (243, 244). The ACEI led to reversal of these changes.

Studies of patients with CHF have demonstrated that although some variability exists, renal blood flow is often reduced in CHF. Renal blood flow as a percent of cardiac output is generally reduced as well (245, 246). The reduction in renal blood flow occurs in patients with mean arterial pressures above that commonly expected to maintain renal blood flow autoregulation. Studies investigating the effects of ACEI in CHF patients have generally demonstrated decreased renal vascular resistance, increased absolute renal blood flow, and increased renal blood flow

as a percentage of cardiac output (247–249). If ACEI is accompanied by a significant decrease in systemic blood pressure to a level close to that of the minimal requirement for renal autoregulation, then renal blood flow may not increase after the initiation of ACEI (250). As ACEI is often accompanied by decreases in both serum catecholamine and angiotensin II levels, as well as increased cardiac output, it is difficult to clearly identify one specific mechanism that accounts for increased renal blood flow after ACEI. One also needs to consider the fact that improvements in cardiac output may perhaps decrease activation of the sympathetic nervous and renin-angiotensin systems which accompanies heart failure. Studies in which cardiac output increased after the administration of hydralazine (251, 252) and catecholamines (253) in patients with CHF have demonstrated increases in renal blood flow. Studies of the neurohumoral axis are not available. However, studies which demonstrate improvements in renal blood flow prior to or without changes in indices of cardiac function suggest that alterations in neurohumoral axis and not pump function per se may account for a majority of the decline in renal blood flow which accompanies CHF.

## Renal Blood Flow During Hemorrhage

Multiple experimental models have been used to investigate the effect of hemorrhage on renal blood flow. The use of different species, experimental models, and anesthetic techniques has provided some variable results as to the effect of hemorrhage on renal blood flow. This is particularly true at low volumes of hemorrhage. The importance of anesthetic agents is illustrated by the fact that pentobarbital has been shown to decrease the volume of hemorrhage necessary to obtain a set decrease in blood pressure (254). Pentobarbital has also been shown to increase the minimal systemic pressure necessary to maintain intact autoregulation of renal blood flow during hemorrhage (255).

Alterations in cardiac output, systemic perfusion pressure, and neurohumoral, cytokine, and endothelin activity can all influence renal blood flow during hemorrhage. Elevations in renal nerve activity, endothelin (256), renin-angiotensin, arginine vasopressin, and catecholamine levels can all increase during hemmorhage. The fact that alterations in renal blood flow during hemorrhage are not simply or directly mediated by central hemodynamic changes can be illustrated by the following experimental data. For a given decrease in blood pressure plasma renin activity increases to a greater extent after hemorrhage than sodium nitroprusside infusion (257). Total renal blood flow and the intrarenal distribution of blood flow undergo greater changes during hemorrhagic hypotension than afer an equivalent degree of hypotension from a low cardiac output state induced by inflating a balloon in the left atrium (258).

During graded experimental hemorrhage total renal blood flow decreases while renal vascular resistance increases. In some studies the alterations in renal blood flow are greater than those changes in systemic hemodyamics (259). Generally the intrarenal distribution of blood flow is also changed, with outer cortical blood flow sustaining a greater decrease in blood flow than the inner cortex and medulla (260, 261). Cortical and medullarly $PO_2$ levels decrease during progressive hemorrhage. Decreases in cortical $PO_2$ are more rapid than the decrease in medullary $PO_2$ (262). During early hemorrhage in anesthetized dogs renal lactate clearance remains relatively stable. Lactate production was detected only after a 40% blood loss. At this time a 94% reduction in renal blood flow had occurred and cortical $PO_2$ was severely reduced (262). The relative late increase in lactate production occurring only at the time when cortical $PO_2$ was greatly decreased and increases in real vascular resistance which accompany hemorrhage are consistent with the theory that the kidney regulates blood flow primarily to maintain GFR and blood volume, not metabolic needs.

## DIAPHRAGM BLOOD FLOW

Due to its location and associated difficulties in measurement, the vast majority of diaphragm blood flow studies have been conducted in animals. Arterial blood flow for the superior aspect of the diaphragm includes the superior phrenic arteries and two branches of the internal thoracic artery, the musculophrenic and pericardiophrenic arteries. The inferior phrenic arteries also supply the diaphragm (263, 264). A topographic gravity-independent distribution of blood flow has been observed in the canine diaphragm (265). Diaphragm blood flow will vary with the amount of work the diaphragm is performing. This fact combined with different animal models leads to a wide variation in reported blood flow. Diaphragm blood flow rates between 0.1 and 8 mL/100 g/min have been reported in the literature. Arterial-venous oxygen differences are in the range of 5 to 8 volume percent (266–268).

The increased oxygen and substrate requirements associated with elevated work rates are met by both an increased arterial blood flow and increased oxygen extraction (269). Increases in diaphragm blood flow and oxygen extraction have been documented to occur during the increased work of breathing associated with inspiratory and expiratory loading (266, 270), hyperventilation (271), hypoxemia (267, 272), oleic acid lung injury (273), and endotoxin infusion (274) and during cardiac tamponade (275). Canine studies document that phrenic artery blood flow is autoregulated over a wide range of perfusion pressures (276, 277). Because diaphragm blood flow must be maintained with increasing work, it is unclear what the lower pressure limit of autoregulation is. In a canine study evaluating the effect of hemorrhagic shock the lower limit of autoregulation was felt to be a mean arterial pressure of approximately 50 mm Hg (268). The importance of maintaining adequate diaphragm blood flow for the amount of work being performed by the diaphragm is the fact that an imbalance between substrate delivery and the needs of the diaphragm is felt to play a role in the development of diaphragmatic fatigue. Biopsies analyzed from fatigued diaphragms during times of limited perfusion contain decreased concentrations of adenosine triphosphate (ATP), creatinine phosphate, and glycogen. Lactate levels are increased (278). Mechanical hyperperfusion has been found to partially reverse fatigue in diaphragm strips (279). In eight mechanically ventilated patients with chronic obstructive pulmonary disease the intravenous infusion of dopamine was found to increase diaphragm strength. Dopamine resulted in increased cardiac output, heart rate, and blood pressure. In three patients phrenic artery blood flow was also measured and was found to increase significantly during the dopamine infusion. The hemodynamic and increased transdiaphragmatic force generation associated with dopamine resolved 15 minutes after the infusion was stopped (280). The implications being that increased perfusion of the diaphragm accounted for the improved diaphragmatic performance.

Besides increasing the delivery of substrates such as oxygen, increased perfusion may improve diaphragm performance by other mechanisms. More homogenous distribution of blood flow, recruitment of new capillary beds during higher perfusion pressures, a direct catecholamine effect, and changes in the extracellular milieu may contribute to the improved diaphragm performance associated with hyperperfusion (281, 282).

Although diaphragm blood flow has been documented to increase during times of increasing work load, several studies have found that diaphragm blood flow can be limited during elevated work rates. For limb muscles blood flow can become limited at 10% to 30% of maximum tension generation (283, 284). The limitation of diaphragm blood flow during contraction appears to be best related to the duty cycle (the time of the respiratory cycle spent in inspiration) and the amount generated by diaphragm tension (285, 286). Twisting and shearing of blood vessels during contraction, as well as the rise in intramuscular pressure associated with contraction, may limit diaphragm blood flow during periods of excessive work. At low tensions vascular dilatation may overcome the effects of increases in intramuscular pressure and vascular shearing. Further increase in intramuscular pressure secondary to increased tension generation may decrease blood flow during contraction. Blood flow during relaxation may increase to compensate for the decreased contraction phase flow. Increased relaxation phase blood flow may prevent a decrease in total diaphragmatic blood flow (287). As the time spent in inspiration increases (Increased duty cycle), the time for relaxation phase blood flow decreases. During less than maximal diaphragm tension generation a higher duty cycle is required before a limitation of diaphragm blood flow occurs (288, 289). At times of maximal transdiaphragmatic tension generation, limitation of diaphragmatic blood flow can occur at a lower duty cycle.

## Diaphragmatic Blood Flow During Sepsis and Septic Shock

Canine models utilizing endotoxin boluses have frequently been used as a model to study the effects of sepsis on respiratory muscle function and blood flow. A limitation of this model is that the hypotension is accompanied by a low cardiac output and therefore does not completely mimic the high cardiac output—hyperdynamic state typically found in volume-resuscitated septic shock. Minute ventilation and indices of work performed by the diaphragm typically increase after endotoxin infusion. Absolute diaphragm blood flow has been found to increase by a factor of 6 to 7 while the percent of cardiac output going to the respiratory muscles increases from 1.9% to 8.8%. Diaphragmatic oxygen consumption has been found to increase approximately by a factor of 10. Phrenic vein oxygen content decreases while phrenic vein lactate levels increase (274, 290, 291). Diaphragm glycogen concentration is decreased and lactate concentration is increased (292). In spontaneously breathing dogs with endotoxin shock electrical activity of the phrenic nerve and diaphragm increase over time while the pressure-generating ability of the diaphragm decreases (290). A decrease in the pressure-generating ability of the diaphragm, while electrical activity of the phrenic nerve and diaphragm increase suggest the development of respiratory muscle fatigue. This finding, along with the results of diaphragm biopsies, suggests that inadequate blood flow for the needs of a muscle subjected to increase metabolic demands may contribute to the respiratory muscle dysfunction seen with sepsis.

A regional redistribution of blood flow has been observed in dogs with endotoxin shock. Endotoxin shock is accompanied by increased blood flow to the respiratory muscles while blood flow to the gut, spleen, kidney, and brain are reduced. Intubation with mechanical ventilation and paralysis not only prevents the increase in blood flow to the respiratory muscles following endotoxin shock, but also decreases respiratory muscle blood flow compared to preendotoxin values. Mechanical ventilation with paralysis attenuated the decrease in blood flow to the gut and brain (274).

Intraperitoneal administration of a fecal inoculum in the rat has been used as a model of chronic sepsis. There was no difference in absolute blood flow in milliliters per minute per gram of diaphragm between control and experimental animals during the first 2 days postinoculation. During the final 2 days of the study diaphragm blood flow was significantly less in experimental compared to control animals; however, there was no consistent change in diaphragmatic blood flow in experimental animals during the course of the study. The fractional distribution of cardiac output to the diaphragm did not change during the study.

The effects of intravenous endotoxin infusion of rat diaphragm microvasculature has been studied with videomicroscopy. Rats were mechanically ventilated and received both pentobarbital and pancuronium bromide. Both endotoxin and hemorrhage to an equal degree of hypotension as induced by endotoxin were found to result in constriction of second-generation but not in third- or fourth-generation arterioles. Increased sympathetic tone in response to hypotension may account for the observed vasoconstrtiction. This vasoconstriction may explain the decreases in respiratory muscle blood flow observed in mechanically ventilated paralyzed dogs with endotoxic shock. Endotoxin, but not hemorrhagic shock, increased the number of nonperfused capillaries by a factor of four. Capillary obstruction by granulocytes may account for this observation (293). The decrease in functional capillaries may contribute to the development of fatigue despite the fact the diaphragmatic blood flow is markedly increased during endotoxic shock.

Animal studies have generally found that skeletal muscle blood flow decreases during sepsis (294). Alterations in skeletal muscle function independent of changes in blood flow have been reported (295). It is unlikely that the respiratory muscle dysfunction seen during critical illness is purely a result of an imbalance between substrate delivery and utilization by the respiratory muscles. Changes in plasma and intracellular acid-base status (296), the development of neuropathies, and a direct or indirect effect of the mediators of the systemic inflammatory response on skeletal muscle may also contribute to the respiratory muscle dysfunction (295a).

## Diaphragm Blood Flow During Congestive Heart Failure and Cardiogenic Shock

Dyspnea and fatigue are major complaints of patients with CHF. Extensive studies of diaphragm blood flow in humans with CHF and cardiogenic shock are lacking. Peripheral muscle function and blood flow autoregulation have been more extensively studied than that of the diaphragm. It is unclear if the effects of chronic CHF on peripheral skeletal muscle are also found in the diaphragm. The increased fatigability of peripheral skeletal muscle in patients with chronic CHF is most likely multifactorial (302, 303). The expected normal skeletal muscle arteriole vasodilator response and increase in skeletal muscle blood flow to exercise are reduced. Studies of forearm and leg muscles have demonstrated reduced blood flow and increased vascular resistance compared to normals during exercise. These changes in blood flow are accompanied by reductions in maximal oxygen consumption, increased oxygen extraction, and early onset of lactate production from the muscle groups (304–306). Although acute dobutamine infusions can increase cardiac output in CHF patients, exercise capacity is not increased (307, 308). Administration of diuretics to remove excess fluids (309), which may lead to vascular compression, the use of alpha-adrenergic blocking agents, and sympathetic nervous system blockade, does not normalize the vasodilator response to exercise (310). The short-term administration of ACEIs, while improving systemic hemodynamics, does not restore to normal the vasodilator response and maximal oxygen uptake in regional skeletal muscle beds at maximal exercise (311). Long-term administration of ACEIs can be associated with improvements in maximal skeletal muscle blood flow and oxygen consumption (312, 313). It is unclear if this is a pharmacologic effect on the vasculature or if the long-term use of an ACEI allowed for increased exercise training.

In addition to abnormalities in blood flow, changes in skeletal muscle biochemistry, metabolism, and histology have been demonstrated in patients with CHF (314). Atrophy and deconditiong of muscles occurs (315). Decreased oxidative enzyme concentrations, 3-hydroxy-acyl-CoA-dehydrogenase (involved in the beta oxidation of fatty acids) levels, and decreased glycogen content are found in the skeletal muscle of patients with CHF (316). Nuclear magnetic resonance studies have found an early onset of glycolysis in the skeletal muscle of patients with CHF (317). Reduced percentages of slow-twitch type I muscle fibers and an increased percentage of type IIB fast fibers have been found (316).

Abnormalities in the central drive and the neuromuscular junction do not appear to account for the enchanced fatigue seen in patients with CHF (318). Exercise training has been found to increase maximal exercise capacity and delay the anaerobic threshold and has been linked to increased oxidative enzyme concentrations in the skeletal muscle of patients with chronic CHF (319). This implies that deconditioning plays some role in the observed peripheral skeletal muscle abnormalities. It remains unclear if deconditiong is the only or major cause of the abnormalities in skeletal muscle fatigue, histology, and biochemistry. Other possible contributing factors include underperfusion, malnutrition, elevated levels of tumor necrosis factor, and catecholamines (303, 320).

It is difficult to know to what extent, if any, the changes found in peripheral skeletal muscle structure, biochemistry, and blood flow autoregulation may occur in the diaphragm. One would expect the diaphragm not to be subject to disuse atrophy. In a small number of patients histologic abnormalities have been found in the diaphragm in some patients with ischemic myopathy and idiopathic dilated cardiomyopathy in whom diaphragm biopsies were obtained at the time of cardiac transplantation (321). No significant differences in fiber size or type were found between transplant patients and patients who were undergoing coronary artery bypass grafting. Histologic abnormalities were most marked in patients with idiopathic dilated cardiomyopathy, suggesting the possibility of a generalized skeletal and cardiac myopathic process in these patients. In another study coastal diaphragmatic biopsies were obtained from normal subjects and patients undergoing cardiac transplantation (322). Biopsy specimens were analyzed for myosin isoforms and enzyme markers of oxidative and glycolytic metabolism. Biopsies obtained from heart failure patients had an increased percentage of slow myosin isoforms, decreased glycolytic capacity, and increased oxidative capacity. These biochemical and histologic changes are the opposite of those found in peripheral skeletal muscle and are similar to those found with endurance training. The hyperventilation which occurs at rest and during exercise in patients with CHF may account for these findings.

Respiratory muscle weakness, as evidenced by reductions in maximal inspiratory and expiratory pressure generation, has been reported in patients with chronic CHF (323, 324). Inspiratory muscle weakness has been correlated with the patients' sense of exertional dyspnea (325). Compared to controls, CHF patients have an abnormal ventilatory response but maintain a normal arterial blood gas response to exercise. Increased minute ventilation and an increased amount of work performed by the diaphragm for a given level of exercise has been documented. Early onset of the anaerobic threshold may account for some of the observed elevations in minute ventilation. The pulmonary ratio of dead space to tidal volume increases during exercise in CHF patients, while this ratio remains unchanged in normals and may account for some of the excess minute ventilation (326–328). Activation of pulmonary J receptors by chronic pulmonary interstitial changes may lead to the development of rapid shallow breathing and thereby an increased dead-space-to-tidal-volume ratio. Inadequate pulmonary perfusion may also lead to increased dead space during exercise. From the exercise studies it seems that patients with chronic CHF have an increased work of breathing and might be expected to have increased diaphragm blood flow or increased oxygen extraction during exercise.

Studies assessing diaphragm blood flow in humans with CHF are lacking. Near-infrared spectroscopy has detected early accessory respiratory muscle deoxygenation during submaximal exercise in patients with chronic CHF (329, 330). This suggests that inadequate blood flow, at least to the accessory muscles of respiration, may occur during submanximal exercise in these patients. Various animal models have been used to study the effect of cardiogenic shock and CHF on diaphragm blood flow.

In a canine model of CHF induced by rapid ventricular pacing, isometric force generation due to phrenic nerve stimulation was reduced. Phrenic artery blood flow tended to be greater in experimental than in control animals, but this was not statistically significant. The phrenic artery blood flow response to transient occlusion of the phrenic artery was altered in CHF dogs. In experimental animals, postocclusive phrenic artery flow was characterized by reductions in peak postocclusion flow and hyperemic volume over the first minute after release of the occlusion. However, the duration of the postocclusive hyperemic response was longer in experimental animals. This longer duration of the postocclusion hyperemic response resulted in no difference in the total hyperemic volume in experimental and control animals. During fatigue blood flow was reduced in the experimental animals. This reduction in blood flow was not simply a reflection of reduced force generation in experimental animals (331).

Rats with heart failure secondary to surgical ligation of the left coronary artery have attenuated blood flow to hind limb muscles during submaximal exercise compared to rats who had undergone a sham operation (332). In the same model of left ventricular failure, diaphragm blood flow increased to the diaphragm in experimental animals and was significantly related to the development of pulmonary edema. The authors estimated that at submaximal exercise the percentage of cardiac output directed to the diaphragm in experimental animals was twice that of control animals. An increased work of breathing secondary to the pulmonary congestion resulting in increased energy requirements may account for the increased diaphragm blood flow in experimental animals (333).

Cardiac tamponade has been used as a model to study the effect of cardiogenic shock on diaphragm blood flow, work, function, and regional blood flow. This model has also been used to investigate the effect of paralysis and mechanical ventilation during cardiogenic shock. Animals were randomized to spontaneous breathing or paralysis with mechanical ventilation (334). For spontaneously breathing animals there was an early increase in minute ventilation and transdiaphragmatic pressure generation. Blood flow to respiratory muscles increased by 361% (275). Toward the latter stages of the experiment minute ventilation and transdiaphragmatic pressure generation began to decrease. Electrical activity of both the phrenic nerve and diaphragm increased throughout the experiment, resulting in an increased ratio of electrical activity to pressure generation. This increased ratio implies that the respiratory failure was secondary not to neurotransmission, but rather to respiratory muscle failure. Spontaneously breathing dogs died earlier than mechanically ventilated dogs. Respiratory arrest preceded cardiac arrest. Paralysis and mechanical ventilation decreased blood flow to the respiratory muscles during tamponade. For mechanically ventilated animals only 3%, compared to 21%, of the cardiac output in spontaneously breathing dogs was directed to the diaphragm. Mechanical ventilation attenuated decreases in blood flow to the liver, brain, and quadriceps muscle resulting from tamponade (275).

### Diaphragm Blood Flow in Hemorrhagic Shock

Canine studies have investigated the effect of hemorrhage on diaphragmatic blood flow. During hemorrhagic hypotension diaphragmatic blood flow decreases. In response to metabolic stress such as inspiratory loading or pharmacologic stimulation with catecholamines diaphragmatic blood flow can increase during hemorrhagic hypotension. Oxygen extraction also increases (335). Diaphragm oxygen consumption may become compromised at a greater systemic oxygen delivery than that of other tissues (336).

To summarize, studies of diaphragm blood flow in humans with chronic CHF and cardiogenic shock are lacking. Respiratory muscle weakness, an abnormal ventilatory response to exercise and early desaturation of accessory muscle blood flow to accessory muscles of respiration, has been documented in humans with CHF.

It is clear that inadequate muscle blood flow is associated with the occurrence of muscle fatigue. Animal studies suggest that the development of shock associated with an increased work of breathing increases diaphragmatic blood flow while blood flow to other organ beds decreases. Paralysis with mechanical ventilation attenuates the redistribution of blood flow, delays the onset of respiratory muscle failure, and at least in short term-studies is associated with prolonged survival time. These findings illustrate the importance and some of the potential benefits of ventilatory support in patients with hemodynamic compromise from various etiologies.

### SPLANCHNIC CIRCULATION

### Anatomy and Physiology of Splanchnic Circulation

The splanchnic circulation is composed of the gastric, small intestinal, colonic, pancreatic, hepatic, and splenic circulations, arranged in parallel with one another (339). The splanchnic circulation is the largest regional circulation, containing 20% to 25% of systemic blood volume. Under normal, resting conditions, the splanchnic circulation in adult humans receives 1,500 mL/min, or approximately 25% of the cardiac output (340). Of this amount, the liver receives approximately 100 mL/100 g liver/min while the mesenteric circulation receives 50 to 70 mL/min/100 g tissue (341). Total splanchnic oxygen consumption at rest is 50 to 60 mL/min; thus, only 15% to 20% percent of the oxygen the splanchnic region receives each minute is extracted.

There are three primary vessels that supply blood to the splanchnic bed: the *celiac artery*, which supplies the foregut, liver, and spleen; the *superior mesenteric artery* (SMA), which supplies the intestine from the duodenal-ejunal junction to the midtransverse colon; and the *inferior mesenteric artery* (IMA), which supplies the midtransverse colon to the rectum (342). In addition, there are several, extensive, but highly variable collaterals that are present, particularly in the mesenteric circulation. Because of this collateral network, at least two of the three major splanchnic vessels must be occluded before chronic ischemic symptoms develop. Blood from all splanchnic organs drains into the inferior vena cava via several hepatic veins. The intestinal tract is also drained by an elaborate lymphatic system that serves as a major route for absorption of nutrients.

The liver receives its blood supply from two sources, the hepatic artery and the portal vein (343). Hepatic arterial and portal venous blood mix in the hepatic sinusoids, which are drained by several hepatic veins into the inferior vena cava. Approximately 25% of total hepatic blood flow is supplied by the hepatic artery and the remainder by the portal vein. The portal vein is most commonly formed by the union of the superior mesenteric and splenic veins just posterior to the head of the pancreas. At the porta hepatis it usually divides into two branches that terminate in the right and left lobes of the liver.

Although the portal vein supplies a greater amount of blood flow to the liver, the hepatic artery and portal vein supply approximately 50% each of the total hepatic oxygen delivery (344). The pressure in the hepatic artery is the same as systemic arterial blood pressure. The normal pressure in the portal vein is 5 to 10 mm Hg and is higher than the pressure in the inferior vena cava (345). The control of hepatic blood flow takes place in four areas: the hepatic arterioles, the portal venules, the hepatic venules, and indirectly the arterioles of the intestinal, splenic, and pancreatic vascular beds. The hepatic arterial system is governed by nervous, hormonal, metabolic, and local influences, similar to those that affect the intestinal circulation, as discussed below. On the other hand, control of portal venous blood is undertaken primarily outside the liver, by the prehepatic vasculature in the gastrointestinal tract and spleen. Unlike the hepatic artery, the portal venous system does not have the capacity for autoregulation and cannot maintain flow when pressure falls. Although oxygen supply to the liver may be at risk if portal venous blood flow is reduced, this effect is minimized by an increase in hepatic arterial blood flow (346). This decrease in hepatic arterial resistance resulting from reduced portal venous blood flow has physiologic importance, in that it tends to increase total hepatic blood flow and oxygen delivery in pathologic states, such as hemorrhagic shock (345). Thus, intrahepatic interaction between the arterial and portal circulations supply a local means of hepatic arterial blood flow control through the hepatic arterial "buffer" response to maintain homeostasis.

## Microscopic and Functional Anatomy of Intestinal Circulation

Most of the cardiac output that the gastrointestinal circulation receives (approximately 15% to 20%) is distributed to the small intestine (347). The small intestine is composed of three main tissue layers: the mucosa, submucosa, and muscularis propria. Each of the major functions of the small intestine (absorption, secretion, motility) is localized in one of these three layers (348). Absorption of nutrients takes place in the mucosa with its numerous villi and attending microvilli. The secretory function is subserved by the submucosa and basal region of the mucosa, where several glands are located at the base of the villi and lining the crypts, and in the submucosa proper. Lastly, intestinal motility is dependent on the contraction and relaxation of the longitudinal and circular smooth muscle fibers located in the muscularis propria. Because of the higher metabolic demands for absorption and secretion, the mucosal and submucosal layers of the small intestine receive a major portion of the resting blood flow; in humans, this is approximately 50 mL/min/100 g tissue, or 70%, of the total intestinal blood flow (349). The intramural vascular architecture is similar in the small intestine and the large intestine in many respects (350). The vasa recta penetrate the bowel wall and course obliquely through the muscularis propria to enter the submucosa. In the submucosa, large tortuous vessels surround the whole circumference of the bowel wall. These vessels anastomose freely with each other and give origin to smaller vessels which pass to the mucosa and muscularis propria. In addition, the muscularis propria also receives tributaries arising from the serosal plexus. This dual blood supply to the muscularis layer, from both the submucosal and serosal regions, may provide an anatomic explanation for the resistance of the muscularis propria to ischemia (350).

On the other hand, the mucosal vascular pattern differs between the large and small intestines. In the colon, branches of the submucosal plexus extend toward the base of the mucosa and then branch extensively, forming a basal mucosal plexus (350). Capillary channels arise from this basal plexus and pass toward the mucosal surface. The small intestine also has a rich basal mucosal plexus from which a central nutrient arteriole passes upward through the middle of the villus to reach its tip. At this point, the nutrient vessel branches into a dense subepithelial network of capillaries and is drained by an arbor of venules surrounding the inflow vessel (351). Generally, one or two veins drain from each villus and eventually join the veins located at the submucosa, the muscularis, and the serosal layers. The venous drainage from the small intestine merges with the veins of the large intestine, which then subsequently join with the splenic vein to form the portal vein. The venous drainage of the large intestine is similar to that of the small intestine and reaches the portal vein via either the superior or inferior mesenteric veins.

The vascular arrangement of the intestinal villus represents a countercurrent exchange system where the main direction of blood flow in the subepithelial capillary network and venules is opposite to that of the central nutrient vessel (352). This unique microvascular architecture makes the gut more susceptible to ischemic damage. The tips of the intestinal villi tend to be relatively hypoxic even under normal conditions, because oxygen is consumed by epithelial cells lining the villi from the base to the tip. In this system, the base-to-tip oxygen tension ($P_{O_2}$) gradient induced by oxygen consumption can be exagerrated by diffusional arteriovenous shunting present during low-flow states (347, 351, 353). Although Lundgren originally proposed that the base-to-tip $P_{O_2}$ gradient would be exaggerated under conditions of low flow, recent studies suggest that shunting actually decreases when flow is reduced (352). In experimental animals and in humans with hemorrhagic shock, tissue $P_{O_2}$ at the villus tip falls dramatically, resulting in mucosal ulceration and tissue necrosis (354).

The rate of blood flow through the splanchnic circulation is governed primarily by the arterial-to-venous pressure gradient and the mechanical resistance to the flow of blood in the splanchnic vasculature (339). In the intestine, the greatest portion of vascular resistance occurs in the small arteries and precapillary arterioles, often referred to as *resistance vessels,* while most of the transport of oxygen and other nutrients occur across capillaries, or the *exchange vessels* (341). The amount of exhange depends predominantly on the surface area or density of the villous capillaries. The small veins draining the capillaries in the intestinal wall contain about 80% of the intestinal blood volume—hence, their designation as *capacitance vessels.* These veins contribute little to blood flow regulation and serve to mobilize pooled blood central in response to systemic need (e.g., during exercise) (339). Various intrinsic and extrinsic factors control intestinal blood flow, including neural, humoral, and local mechanisms.

### Neural Control of Intestinal Blood Flow

The principal neural input to the intestinal tract is via the sympathetic nervous system (347, 348). Within the intestinal wall, sympathetic nerve fibers are located around the vessels in the muscularis propria, the submucosa, and the deeper portions of the mucosa. In the villi, few sympathetic fibers are found and there the vessels also lack smooth muscles. Although parasympathetic fibers arising from the vagi supply the small intestine, these fibers have little, if any, direct effect on intestinal blood flow but are important in the regulation of secretion and motility. Changes in secretion and motility result, however, in metabolic and mechanical alterations that may affect blood flow (339).

Mesenteric blood flow during activation of the sympathetic nervous system has been most thoroughly investigated in the cat (355, 356). Stimulation of the sympathetic nerves causes vasoconstriction and decreases blood flow to splanchnic organs. Mucosal blood flow is primarily affected, while no redistribution of flow occurs between the mucosa, submucosa, and muscularis. Mean flow in the mucosa-submucosa and in the muscularis is reduced to approximately the same extent as is total intestinal blood flow. However, blood flow to the mucosal villi is generally preserved, suggesting that the vasoconstriction occurs in the crypts of the mucosa (347). However, it appears that qualitative differences exist between species, since studies in humans have demonstrated that blood flow is diverted away from the muscularis to the mucosa-submucosa during sympathetic nerve stimulation (357). In addition, sympathetic stimulation contracts venous smooth muscle, which results in the expulsion of pooled blood from the splanchnic venous bed into the systemic circulation (339).

The intestinal and hepatic circulations respond to sustained sympathetic stimulation with a transient decrease in blood flow followed by a gradual return to near-normal levels upon release of the vasoconstrictive influence, a phenomenon termed *autoregulatory escape.* It has been suggested that this autoregulatory escape is secondary to either adaptation of the alpha-adrenergic receptors on the vascular smooth muscle of the intestinal tract or the concomitant activation of alpha-receptors, which cause vasoconstriction, and beta-receptors, which induce vasodilatation (358).

### Humoral Control of Intestinal Blood Flow

Various substances have been demonstrated to alter intestinal blood flow, including circulating catecholamines (norepinephrine, epinephrine), vasopressin, angiotensin II, and gastrointestinal hormones such as glucagon, vasoactive inhibitory peptide, cholecystokinin, gastrin, and secretin (339, 348, 353). However, none of these hormones produced in the gastrointestinal tract have, as yet, been convincingly shown to participate in the physiologic control of intestinal blood flow.

Recent evidence suggests that nitric oxide (NO) in concert with other vasoactive mediators plays an essential role in the regulation of vasomotor tone and perfusion of the gut (359). The NO is synthesized from the amino acid L-arginine by the enzyme nitric oxide synthase (NOS). Potential sources of NO in the gut include intrinsic intestinal tissue (mast cells, epithelium, smooth muscle, neural plexus), resident and/or infiltrating leukocytes (neutrophils, monocytes), and NO produced by bacterial denitrification. Under normal conditons, mucosal perfusion is regulated by NO derived from the vascular endothelium of the mesenteric bed. The NO stimulates guanylyl cyclase in vascular smooth muscle, resulting in an increase in gut mucosal blood flow. Experimental studies have shown that inhibition of basal production of NO by NOS inhibitors results in significant reduction in blood flow to the gut (360). On the other hand, excessive production of NO in response to a variety of inflammatory stimuli leads to inhibition of smooth muscle activity and consequent gut mucosal hyperemia (361).

## Local Control Mechanisms

Intrinsic control mechanisms are reflected in the ability of the intestine to locally regulate blood flow and metabolism independent of neural input and circulating vasoactive substances. These local mechanisms are often characterized as either metabolic or myogenic in nature (339, 348). Metabolic control is initiated when metabolic demand exceeds oxygen delivery. Vasodilatory substances such as hydrogen ion, potassium ion, adenosine, histamine, prostaglandins, and lactic acid are released locally and cause relaxation of arteriolar and/or precapillary sphincter smooth muscle to maintain oxygen delivery (339, 348, 362). Myogenic control arises from a tendency of vascular smooth muscle to maintain a constant wall tension despite variations in perfusion pressure (348). As transmural pressure is increased, the smooth muscle is stretched. Since wall tension is the product of transmural pressure and vessel diameter, the myogenic mechanism predicts that increased transmural pressure results in arteriolar vasoconstriction and increased vascular resistance. As the contraction proceeds and radius is reduced, wall tension falls and the stimulus for contraction dissipates (339). These adjustments serve to maintain, or "autoregulate," blood flow at near-normal levels regardless of arterial pressure (pressure-flow autoregulation). In addition to the autoregulation of total organ blood flow, the splanchnic organs respond to decreases in perfusion pressure by redistributing blood flow within the individual organs (363). This redistribution is effected by changes in the relative resistance of the arterioles and precapillary sphincters gating the intestinal microvasculature. In general, the metabolic mechanism is directed toward maintaining adequate blood flow and oxygen delivery, whereas the myogenic mechanism is directed more toward keeping intestinal capillary pressure and transcapillary fluid exchange constant (339).

## Techniques for Measuring Splanchnic Blood Flow

There are several methods that have been used to measure splanchnic blood flow, including techniques that measure total organ blood flow and techniques that measure fractionated blood flow. Among the techniques for measuring total organ blood flow in experimental and clinical studies, the indocyanine green clearance technique to estimate liver blood flow is the most commonly utilized method (364). The technique employs an intravenous bolus injection of indocyanine green and obtains serial measurements of indocyanine extraction via a hepatic vein catheter. Assuming indocyanine green is cleared exclusively and completely by the liver, systemic clearance is equal to liver plasma flow. Among the methods used to measure fractionated blood flow, the radioactive microsphere technique has been the most extensively studied but is only applicable in animal studies. This method is based on the assumption that the number of spheres trapped within an organ is proportional to blood flow. In general, these techniques have limited clinical application and are used mainly for investigative studies.

More recently, noninvasive and invasive imaging of splanchnic vasculature have been in widespread use (365–367). These include duplex Doppler ultrasound, computed tomography, magnetic resonance imaging (MRI), and abdominal angiography. In various studies, duplex ultrasound has been used to examine blood flow characteristics in the major arteries of the abdomen, splanchnic vascular responses to oral food intake, changes in mesenteric blood flow during infusion of gastrointestinal hormones, and small-volume hemorrhage as well as for the diagnosis of splanchnic arterial occlusive disease (368). It is important to recognize, however, that the anatomy of splanchnic vessels is marked by great variability. In addition, other factors can decrease the sensitivity and reproducibility of splanchnic ultrasound measurements in clinical practice, including operator-to-operator variability, presence of surgically altered anatomy, difficulties in optimally positioning the patient, and the frequency of distended gas-filled bowel loops (368).

Because of the limitations of available techniques to measure splanchnic blood flow, particularly in the critically ill, recent studies have focused on obtaining indirect measurements of splanchnic oxygenation. In particular, the monitoring of mucosal pH using gastric (or intestinal) tonometry has been intensely investigated (369–384). The technique is based on the principle that the fluid in a hollow viscus (e.g., GI tract, gallbladder, or urinary bladder) can be used to estimate the partial pressures of oxygen ($pO_2$) and carbon dioxide ($pCO_2$) of the surrounding tissues (374, 385). The tonometer is a modified nasogastric tube with a saline-filled silicone balloon that is placed in the lumen of the stomach or intestine. Simultaneous measurements of the saline $CO_2$ tension and arterial bicarbonate ($HCO_3$) allow for the calculation of the intramucosal pH (pHi) in a modified Henderson-Hasselbach equation:

$$pHi = 6.1 + \log HCO_3/pCO_2 \times 0.03$$

where 0.03 is the solubility constant of $CO_2$ in plasma and 6.1 the pK (ionization constant of carbonic acid) (386).

The technique is based on two assumptions: first, that luminal $pCO_2$ reflects the $pCO_2$ of the gastric mucosa and, second, that arterial $HCO_3$ is identical in the blood and in the gastric mucosa (387, 388). Tonometry has been validated in animal studies and in humans, where gastric pHi measurements correlate well with changes in gut blood flow (369, 370, 389, 390). Decreases in gastric pHi or mucosal acidosis indicates ongoing splanchnic hypoperfusion and has been used to predict the development of organ failure or death in critically ill patients, as well as complications after cardiac and aortic surgery (371–374, 377–380, 383, 384). However, the clinical utility of gastric tonometry in the routine monitoring of high-risk and critically ill patients remains to be conclusively proven.

## Splanchnic Blood Flow in Hemorrhagic Shock

During hypovolemic shock, generalized vasoconstriction in regional organ beds occur, especially in the GI tract and the kidneys (391). In animal models of hemorrhagic shock, cardiac ouput directed toward the splanchnic bed decreases early and is redistributed to the vital organs (brain and heart) to maintain systemic perfusion (392, 393). In addition, it has been demonstrated in animal studies that $O_2$ delivery to the gut decreases earlier than $O_2$ delivery to other regions during progressive hemorrhage and $O_2$ consumption becomes supply dependent in the gut at levels of $O_2$ delivery that continue to maintain supply independence in other organ beds (394).

The vasoconstrictor response of the splanchnic circulation observed during hypovolemic shock or low-flow states has been attributed to sympathetic stimulation, release of angiotensin II, and several mediators such as leukotrienes, thromboxane $A_2$, endothelin, and endothelium-derived contracting factor (EDCF) (363, 393, 395–399). In animal studies, the administration of ACEI as well as leukotriene and thromboxane antagonists has been shown to reduce splanchnic vasoconstriction during shock and prevent loss of the protective intestinal barrier (363, 399). Depending on the severity and duration of shock, splanchnic vasoconstriction and the resulting ischemia may lead to injury of the stomach, small intestine, large intestine, liver, gallbladder, and pancreas (347, 354, 363). In particular, ischemia of the intestinal mucosa occurs, especially at the tips of the villi of the small intestine. In the early stages, there is patchy necrosis of the superficial layer of the intestinal epithelium (347, 354, 397). With more severe degrees of injury, extensive epithelial loss ensues along with involvement of deeper layers of the intestinal wall. If the ischemia is prolonged, transmural infarction occurs and the bowel becomes nonviable.

Various mechanisms have been implicated in the gut mucosal injury during hemorrhagic shock, including ischemia and reperfusion injury and derangements in mucosal function induced by cytokines, NO, eicosanoids, and other secondary mediators (348, 353, 396, 400). Mesenteric ischemia not only leads to mucosal intracellular hypoxia, but it also causes activation of various mediators and enzyme systems (e.g., xanthine oxidase) within endothelial cells and polymorphonuclear neutrophils (PMNs), resulting in the generation of $O_2$ free radicals which can augment or accelerate tissue injury during reperfusion (396). Several experimental studies have demonstrated that blockade of toxic $O_2$ free radicals significantly ameliorates postischemic reperfusion injury (401, 402). However, the use of antioxidant therapies in critically ill patients with ischemia/reperfusion injury (e.g., myocardial infarction, pulmonary embolism, stroke, cardiopulmonary bypass, and organ transplant) remains investigational (403).

Recent evidence implicates PMN-endothelial cell adhesion and an altered metabolism of NO in the microvascular dysfunction associated with ischemia-reperfusion injury (359, 397). The PMN attachment to endothelial cells is facilitated by several adhesion molecules located on PMNs and endothelial cells. The interaction of PMNs and endothelial cells causes the elaboration of proteases, $O_2$ free radicals, and cytokines that promote tissue injury. In experimental models of ischemia-reperfusion injury manifested by significant leukocyte adherence and emigration, as well as albumin extravasation, infusion of NO donors (sodium nitroprusside, spermine-NO, S1N1) into the mesenteric microcirculation significantly attenuated the reperfusion-induced increase in venular albumin leakage via an inhibitory effect on leukocyte-endothelial cell adhesion (404).

## Splanchnic Blood Flow in Sepsis and Septic Shock

In addition to its important role in the digestion and absorption of nutrients, the gut mucosa functions as an immune organ and as an important barrier that prevents the systemic absorption of intraluminal microbes and their toxic products (e.g., endotoxin). Experimental studies have suggested that splanchnic ischemia during shock, trauma, or sepsis can lead to loss of gut barrier function (405). The latter can predispose to the phenomenon of *translocation* (movement across grossly intact epithelium) of bacteria and endotoxins from gut lumen to mesenteric lymph nodes and portal blood (405, 406). Excessive activation of the reticuloendothelial system (mainly Kupffer cells) of the liver initiates the release of cytokines and other mediators, which in concert with activated neutrophils and endothelial cells may lead to septic shock and multiple organ dysfunction syndrome (MODS), depending on the status of the host defense mechanisms (407). This has formed the basis for gut mucosal injury to be considered as the "motor" of MODS in critically ill patients (408). However, despite compelling animal data that bacterial translocation occurs, human evidence remains lacking.

Endothelial injury and unregulated mediator release play important pathophysiologic roles in sepsis-induced splanchnic organ injury (11). Endotoxin has direct pathogenic effects on splanchnic organs, including increases in epithelial and endothelial permeability, decreases and/or redistribution of splanchnic blood flow, and alterations in hepatocellular function (409). In addition, endotoxin initiates the release of vasoconstricting mediators from activated macrophages, including various cytokines, leukotriene $D_4$, and thromboxane $A_2$, as well as functional alterations in the capacity of resistance vessels in the mesenteric bed to respond approppriately to vasodilatory agonists (409–411). Interestingly, studies of total hepatosplanchnic perfusion using indocyanine green or galactose clearance techniques have demonstrated that hepatosplanchnic blood flow and $O_2$ consumption increase significantly in patients with sepsis (412–415). Because it is difficult to obtain reliable data about splanchnic perfusion in sepsis and septic shock in humans, most of the available information is derived primarily from studies of animal models of sepsis. There is, however, great variability among experimental studies, depending on the species employed, type of septic insult, and the hemodynamic patterns observed following the septic insult (405, 416, 417). In a porcine endotoxic shock model, it has been reported that mesenteric hypoperfusion occurs following infusion of LPS and is accompanied by ileal mucosal acidosis and increased permeability to various hydrophilic solutes (418). Furthermore, the degree of ileal mucosal hyperpermeability was directly proportional to the extent of the mucosal acidosis. In this model, administration of cyclooxygenase inhibitors (ibuprofen, meclofenamate) has been shown to improve mesenteric $O_2$ delivery and prevent the development of gut mucosal acidosis (419). However, in hyperdynamic endotoxemic rabbits, mesenteric perfusion is increased while hepatic and pancreatic blood flows are reduced (420).

Similarly, the hemodynamic effects of endotoxemic shock on the portal venous (PV) and hepatic arterial (HA) vascular beds contribute to the reduction in preload, increase in splanchnic blood pooling and edema formation, and hepatic dysfunction seen in experimentally induced sepsis (421). In this model, endotoxic shock leads to a time-dependent impairment of PV flow with increased PV resistance. The HA vascular bed is dilated early in shock with an absent HA buffer response. Histologic studies demonstrate focal necrosis and hemorrhage without evidence of vasoconstriction or thrombosis. Similar morphologic changes caused by endotoxemia can be demonstrated in other splanchnic organs such as the spleen and pancreas (398).

In humans with hyperdynamic septic shock, increased splanchnic blood flow and $O_2$ consumption have been demonstrated during hypotension and during vasopressor therapy with dopamine or norepinephrine (1). It was the-orized that the marked splanchnic hypermetabolism during the acute hypotensive phase of septic shock may contribute to a regional mismatch between $O_2$ demand and $O_2$ supply. Furthermore, preliminary investigations in patients with septic shock have shown that although dopamine and norepinephrine have similar systemic hemodynamic effects, dopamine may have deleterious effects on splanchnic tissue oxygenation because it causes uncompensated increases in splanchnic $O_2$ requirements (422). Further prospective studies are needed to determine whether alterations in splanchnic perfusion and oxygenation induced by vasoactive agents affect outcome in critically ill patients.

## Splanchnic Circulation in Congestive Heart Failure and Cardiogenic Shock

The majority of experimental models of cardiogenic shock have utilized pericardial tamponade to produce reductions in cardiac output and arterial pressure. In contrast to experimental models of hemorrhage or sepsis, the cardiac tamponade model produces a shock state that is fully and rapidly reversible with release of tamponade, which allows for repeat experiments in the same preparation after perturbation of the neurohumoral milieu (423). In this model, cardiogenic shock produces a profound reduction in blood flow to the liver and the entire mesenteric circulation (423–425). The primary cause of splanchnic hypoperfusion in low cardiac output or cardiogenic shock is disproportionate vasospasm of the splanchnic resistance vessels mediated primarily by the renin-angiotensin system and vasopressin (358, 363, 397). In addition, sympathetic stimulation causes sustained increases in the tone of the postcapillary venous capacitance vessels, which allows pooled splanchnic blood volume to be returned to the heart to maintain cardiac output (363). In animal models of cardiogenic shock, ACEI, not blockade of the sympathetic nervous system, abolishes the selective vasospasm of the splanchnic circulation (423–425).

Similarly, patients with low-output CHF and patients undergoing coronary artery bypass surgery have derangements in splanchnic hemodynamics and oxygen metabolism releated to the reduction in blood flow to the various organs and the effects of humoral substances (angiotensin II, vasopressin, thromboxane, catecholamines) (363, 426). In addition, alterations in baroreceptor regulation of splanchnic blood flow and endothelial dysfunction play significant roles (17, 426, 427). Although the exact mechanisms, signficance, and etiologic importance of this endothelial defect remains incompletely understood, several mechanisms may be involved, including alterations in endothelial cell surface receptors or abnormalities of postreceptor signal transduction, abnormalities of EDRF production or release; rapid inactivation of EDRF, and an increase in EDCF production and activity (17).

With respect to splanchnic blood flow, major differenceas exist between cardiovascular drug groups (e.g., vasodilators, vasoconstrictors, ACEIs, inotropic agents), between drugs within a group (e.g., the arterial dilators, parenterally administered inotropes), and between different doses of the same drug (e.g., prasozin, dopexamine) (428). For example, augmentation of hepatic-splanchnic blood flow occurs after first-dose $a_1$-adrenoceptor blockade (prazosin), suggesting that alpha-adrenergic agonism plays an important role in modifying hepatic-splanchnic blood flow and the regional distribution of cardiac output in CHF. In contrast, hepatic-splanchnic blood flow remains either unchanged or decreases slightly after administration of parenteral nitrates (nitroglycerin) and ACEIs (captopril, enalapril). However, nitroprusside infusion into patients with severe CHF has been shown to increase intestinal and hepatic blood volume (429). It was suggested that nitroprusside caused active relaxation and reduced smooth muscle tone of the capacitance vessels in these regions and that hepatic blood volume was probably reduced due to passive expulsion of blood secondary to the reduced distending pressure. Similarly, beta-agonists such as dobutamine, epinephrine, and dopexamine and phosphodiesterase inhibitors (milrinone, amrinone) have vasodilatory effects on splanchnic vasculature, in addition to their inotropic properties. On the other hand, digitalis glycosides and alpha-adrenergic agents (phenyleprine, norepinephrine) can cause splanchnic vasoconstriction (430).

## CONCLUSION

In conclusion, critical illnesses such as septic, hemorrhagic, and cardiogenic shock can be associated with disturbances in regional blood flow. Table 3 summarizes these changes. Disturbances in central hemodynamics, neuronal input, and mediators with autocrine, paracrine, and endocrine activities all contribute to these changes. It is important for clinicians to realize that these disturbances may play a role in the development of multisystem organ dysfunction and are not detectable clinically or by central hemodynamic monitoring as assessed by a pulmonary artery catheter. By greater awareness of these disturbances, along with increased use of technologies for monitoring regional blood flow, hopefully, clinicians will be able to improve patient outcome.

**TABLE 3.** *Effect of critical illness on regional blood flow.*

|  | Septic shock | Hemorrhagic shock | Cardiogenic shock |
|---|---|---|---|
| Cerebral | -/↓ | -/↓ | -/? |
| Renal | -/↓ | ↓ | ↓ |
| Myocardial | ↑/- | -/↓ | ↓ |
| Respiratory muscle | ↑/ | -/↓ | ↑ |
| Splanchnic | ↑ | ↓ | ↓ |

## REFERENCES

### Introduction

1. Ruokonen E, Takala J, Kara A, et al. Regional blood flow and oxygen transport in septic shock. *Crit Care Med* 1993;21:1296.
2. Ruokonen E, Takala J, Uusaro A. Effect of vasoactive treatment on the relationship between mixed venous and regional oxygen saturation. *Crit Care Med* 1991;19:1365.
3. Lang CH, Bagby GJ, Ferguson JL, Spitzer JJ. Cardiac output and redistribution organ blood flow in hypermetabolic sepsis. *Am J Physiol* 1984;246:R331.
4. Bersten AD, Gnideck AA, Rutledge FS, Sibbald WJ. Hyperdynamic sepsis modifies a PEEP-mediated redistribution in organ blood flows. *Am Rev Respir Dis* 1990;141:1198.
5. Schlictig R, Kramer DJ, Pinsky MR. Flow redistribution during progressive hemorrhage is a determinant of critical $O_2$ delivery. *J Appl Physiol* 1991;70(1):169.
6. van der Linden P, Gilbart E, Engleman E, Schmartz D, Vincent J-L. Effects of anesthetic agents on systemic critical $O_2$ delivery. *J Appl Physiol* 1991;71(1):83.
7. Uggeri MJ, Proctor GJ, Johns RA. Halothane, Enflurane, and Isoflurane attenuate both receptor- and non-receptor-mediated EDRF production in rat thoracic aorta. *Anesthesiology* 1992;76:1012.
8. Kon Park W, Lynch C, Johns RA. Effects of Propofol and Thiopental in isolated rat aorta and pulmonary artery. *Anesthesiology* 1992;77:956.
9. Davies MG, Hagen P-O. The vascular endothelium. A new horizon. *Ann Surg* 1993;218(5):593.
10. Brenner BM, Troy JL, Ballermann BJ. Endothelium-dependent vascular responses. *J Clin Invest* 1989;84:1373.
11. Hollenberg SM, Cunion RE. Endothelial and vascular smooth muscle function in sepsis. *J Crit Care* 1994;94(4):262.
12. Johnson PC. Autoregulation of blood flow. *Circ Res* 1986;59(5):483.
13. Sibbald WJ, Fox G, Martin C. Abnormalities of vascular reactivity in the sepsis syndrome. *Chest* 1991;100(3):155S.
14. Meininger GA, Davis MJ. Cellular mechanisms involved in the vascular myogenic response. *Am J Physiol* 1992;263:H647.
15. Berridge MJ. Inositol triphosphate and diacylglycerol as second messengers. *Biochem J* 1984;330:345.
16. Weber KT, Anversa P, Armstrong PW, et al. Remodeling and reparation of the cardiovascular system. *J Am Coll Cardiol* 1992;20:3.
17. Treasure CB, Alexander RW. The dysfunctional endothelium in heart failure. *J Am Coll Cardiol* 1993;22:129A.
18. Bristow MR. Changes in myocardial vascular receptors in heart failure. *J Am Coll Cardiol* 1993;22:61A.
19. Suffredini AF, Fromm RE, Parker MM, et al. The cardiovascular response of normal humans to the administration of endotoxin. *N Engl J Med* 1989;32:1280.
20. Okusawa S, Gelfand JA, Ikejima T, Connolly RJ, Dinarello CA. Interleukin 1 induces a shock-like state in rabbits. *J Clin Invest* 1988;81:1162.
21. Natanson C, Eichenholz PW, Danner RL, et al. Endotoxin and tumor necrosis factor challenges in dogs simulate the cardiovascular profile of human septic shock. *J Exp Med* 1989;169:823.
22. Moncada S, Higgs A. The L-arginine nitric oxide pathway. *N Engl J Med* 1993;329:2002.
23. Vallence P, Moncada S. Role of endogenous nitric oxide in septic shock. *New Horizons* 1993;1(1):77.
24. Lowenstein CJ, Dinerman JL, Snyder SH. Nitric oxide: a physiologic messenger. *Ann Intern Med* 1994;20:227.
25. Rossi V, Breviario F, Ghezzi P, Dejana E, Mantovani A. Prostacyclin synthesis induced in vascular cells by interleukin-1. *Science* 1985;229:174.
26. Weitzberg E, Lundberg JM, Rudehill A. Elevated plasma levels of endothelium in patients with sepsis syndrome. *Circ Shock* 1991;33:222.
27. Marsden PA, Brenner BM. Nitric oxide and endothelins: novel auto-

crine/paracrine regulators of the circulation. *Semin Nephrol* 1991;11 (2):169.

28. De Nucci G, Thomas R, D'Orleans-Juste P, et al. Pressor effects of circulating endothelin are limited by its removal in the pulmonary circulation and by the release of prostacyclin and endothelium-derived relaxing factor. *Proc Natl Acad Sci* 1988;85:9797.

## Cerebral Blood Flow

29. Moore KL. The head. In: Moore KL, ed. *Clinically oriented anatomy*. Baltimore: Williams and Wilkins; 1992:637.

30. Osborn AG. Normal vascular anatomy In: Patterson AS, ed. *Diagnostic neuroradiology*. St. Louis: Mosby; 1994.

31. Kelly BJ, Luce JM. Current concepts in cerebral protection. *Chest* 1993;103:1246.

32. Siesjo BK. Pathophysiology and treatment of focal cerebral ischemia. *J Neurosurg* 1992;77:169.

33. Chehrazi BB, Youmans JR. Cerebral blood flow in clinical neurosurgery. In: Edvinsson L, ed. *Cerebral blood flow and metabolism*. New York: Raven; 1993:696.

34. Bickler PE. Energetics of cerebral metabolism and ion transport. *Anesthesiol Clin North Am* 1992;10:563.

35. Branston NM, Symon L, Crockard HA, Pasztor E. Relationship between the cortical evoked potential and local cortical blood flow following acute middle cerebral artery occlusion in the baboon. *Exper Neurol* 1974;45:192.

36. Jones TH, Morawetz RB, Crowell RM, et al. Thresholds of focal cerebral ischemia in awake monkeys. *J Neurosurg* 1981;54:773.

37. Astrup J. Energy-requiring cell functions in the ischemic brain. Their critical supply and possible inhibition in protective therapy. *J Neurosurg* 1982;56:482.

38. Lou HC, Edvinsson L, MacKenzie ET. The concept of coupling blood flow to brain function: revision required? *Ann Neurol* 1987;22:289.

39. Raichle ME, Grubb RL, Gado MK, Eichling JO, Ter-Pogossian MM. Correlation between regional cerebral blood flow and oxidative metabolism. *Arch Neurol* 1976;33:523.

40. Roland PE, Friberg I. Localization of cortical areas activated by thinking. *J Neurophysiol* 1985;53:1219.

41. Roland PE, Larsen B. Focal increase of cerebral blood flow during stereognostic testing in man. *Arch Neurol* 1976;33:551.

42. Fox PT, Raichle ME. Focal physiological uncoupling of cerebral blood flow and oxidative metabolism during somatosensory stimulation in human subjects. *Neurobiology* 1986;83:1140.

43. Fox PT, Raichle ME, Mintun MA, Dence C. Nonoxidative glucose consumption during focal physiologic neural activity. *Science* 1988; 241:462.

44. Faraci FM, Heistad DD. Regulation of large cerebral arteries and cerebral microvascular pressure. *Circ Res* 1990;66:8.

45. Stromberg DD, Fox JR. Pressures in the pial arterial microcirculation of the cat during changes in systemic arterial blood pressure. *Circ Res* 1972;23:229.

46. Tamaki K, Mayhan W, Heistad D. Effects of vasodilator stimuli on resistance of large and small cerebral vessels. *Am J Physiol* 1986;251: H1176.

47. Shapiro HM, Stromberg DD, Lee DR, Wiederhielm CA. Dynamic pressures in the pial arterial microcirculation. *Am J Physiol* 1971;221: 279.

48. Kontos HA, Wei EP, Navari RM, et al. Responses of cerebral arteries and arterioles to acute hypotension and hypertension. *Am J Physiol* 1978;234(4):H371.

49. Faraci FM, Mayhan WG, Scmid PG, Heistad DD. Effects of arginine vasopressin on cerebral microvascular pressure. *Am J Physiol* 1988; 255:H70.

50. Baumbach GL, Heistad DD. Effects of sympathetic stimulation and changes in arterial pressure on segmental resistance of cerebral vessels in rabbits and cats. *Circ Res* 1983;52:527.

51. Chrorobski J, Penfield W. Cerebral vasodilator nerves and their pathway from the medulla oblongata. *Arch Neurol Psychiatry* 1932;28: 1257.

52. McCalden TA. Sympathetic control of the cerebral circulation. *J Auton Pharmacol* 1981;1:421.

53. Bevan JA, Brayden JE. Nonadrenergic neural vasodilator mechanisms. *Circ Res* 1987;60(3):309.

54. Faraci FM, Heistad DD. Regulation of cerebral blood vessels by humoral and endothelium-dependent mechanisms. Update on humoral regulation of vascular tone. *Hypertension* 1991;17:917.

55. Iadecola C, Zhang F, Xu Xiaohong. Role of nitric oxide synthase-containing vascular nerves in cerebrovasodilation elicited from cerebellum. *Am J Physiol* 1993;264:R738.

56. Marshall JJ, Wei EP, Kontos HA. Independent blockade of cerebral vasodilation from acetylcholine and nitric oxide. *Am J Physiol* 1988; 255:H847.

57. Prado R, Watson B, Wester P. Effects of nitric oxide synthase inhibition on cerebral blood flow following bilateral carotid artery occlusion and recirculation in the rat. *J Cereb Blood Flow Metab* 1993;13: 720.

58. Muhonen MG, Heistad DD, Faraci FM, Loftus CM. Augmentation of blood flow through cerebral collaterals by inhibition of nitric oxide synthase. *J Cereb Blood Flow Metab* 1994;14:704.

59. Sandor P, Komjati K, Reivich M, Nyary I. Major role of nitric oxide in the mediation of regional $CO_2$ responsiveness of the cerebral and spinal cord vessels of the cat. *J Cereb Blood Flow Metab* 1994;14:49.

60. Garcia-Roldan J-L, Bevan JA. Flow-induced constriction and dilation of cerebral resistance arteries. *Circ Res* 1990;66:1445.

61. Bevan JA, Joyce EH, Wellman GC. Flow-dependent dilation in a resistance artery still occurs after endothelium removal. *Circ Res* 1988;63:980.

62. Lang E, Chestnut R. Intracranial pressure monitoring and management. *Neurosurg Clin North Am* 1994;5(4):573.

63. Aaslid R. Cerebral hemodynamics. In: Newell DW, Aaslid R, eds. *Transcranial Doppler*. New York: Raven; 1992:49.

64. Sorteberg W. Cerebral artery blood velocity and cerebral blood flow. In: Newell DW, Aaslid R, eds. *Transcranial Doppler*. New York: Raven; 1992:57.

65. Lindegaard K-F. Indices of pulsatility. In: Newell DW, Aaslid R, eds. *Transcranial Doppler*. New York: Raven; 1992:67.

66. Kontos HA. Validity of cerebral arterial blood flow calculations from velocity measurements. *Stroke* 1989;20(1):1.

67. Newell DW, Aaslid R, Lam A, Mayberg TS, Winn HR. Comparison of flow and velocity during dynamic autoregulation testing in humans. *Stroke* 1994;25:793.

68. Giller CA, Bowman G, Dyer H, Mootz L, Krippner W. Cerebral arterial diameters during changes in blood pressure and carbon dioxide during craniotomy. *Neurosurgery* 1993;32:737.

69. Bishop CCR, Powell S, Rutt D, Browse NL. Transcranial doppler measurement of middle cerebral artery blood flow velocity. A validation study. *Stroke* 1986;17(5):913.

70. Ringelstein EB, Otis SM. Physiological testing of vasomotor reserve. In: Newell DW, Aaslid R, eds. *Transcranial Doppler*. New York: Raven; 1992:83.

71. Bereczki D, Wei L, Otsuka T, et al. Hypoxia increases velocity of blood flow through parenchymal microvascular systems in rat brain. *J Cereb Blood Flow Metab* 1993;13:475.

72. Thomsen LI, Iversen HK. Experimental and biological variation of three-dimensional transcranial Doppler measurements. *J Appl Physiol* 1993;75:2805.

73. Petty GW, Wiebers DO, Meissner I. Subspecialty Clinics: Neurology. *Mayo Clin Proc* 1990;65:1350.

74. Steiger H-J, Aaslid R, Stooss R, Seiler RW. Transcranial doppler monitoring in head injury: relations between type of injury, flow velocities, vasoreactivity, and outcome. *J Neurosurg* 1994;34:79.

75. Martin NA, Doberstein C, Zane C, et al. Posttraumatic cerebral arterial spasm: transcranial Doppler ultrasound, cerebral blood flow, and angiographic findings. *J Neurosurg* 1992;77:575.

76. Newell DW, Grady MS, Sirotta P, Winn HR. Evaluation of brain death using transcranial doppler. *J Neurosurg* 1989;24(4):509.

77. Hassler W, Steinmetz H, Pirschel J. Transcranial Doppler study of intracranial circulatory arrest. *J Neurosurg* 1989;71:195.

78. Feri M, Ralli L, Felici M, VFanni D, Capria V. Transcranial Doppler and brain death diagnosis. *Crit Care Med* 1994;22(7):1120.

79. Jauss M, Kaps M, Keberle M, Haberbosch W, Dorndorf W. A comparison of transesophageal echocardiography and Transcranial Doppler sonography with contrast medium for detection of patent foramen ovale. *Stroke* 1994;25:1265.

80. Bunegin L, Wahl D, Albin MS. Detection and volume estimation of embolic air in the middle cerebral artery using Transcranial Doppler sonography. *Stroke* 1994;25:593.

81. Georgiadis D, Grosset DG, Kelman A, Faichney A, Lees KR. Prevalence and characteristics of intracranial microemboli signals in patients with different types of prosthetic cardiac valves. *Stroke* 1994; 25:587.

82. Burrows FA. Transcranial Doppler monitoring of cerebral perfusion during cardiopulmonary bypass. *Ann Thorac Surg* 1993;56:1482.

83. Babikian V, Wechsler L. Recent developments in Transcranial Doppler sonography. *J Neuroimaging* 1994;4(3):159.

84. Lundar T, Lindegaard K-F, Nornes H. Continuous recording of middle cerebral artery blood velocity in clinical neurosurgery. *Acta Neurochir* 1990;102:85.

85. Kety SS, Schmidt CF. The determination of cerebral blood flow in man by the use of nitrous oxide in low concentrations. *Am J Physiol* 1945;145:53.

86. Cruz J, Raps EC, Hoffstad OJ, Jaggi JL, Gennarelli TA. Cerebral oxygenation monitoring. *Crit Care Med* 1993;21:1242.

87. Obrist WD, Wilkinson WE. Regional cerebral blood flow measurement in humans by Xenon-133 clearance. *Cerebrovasc Brain Metab Rev* 1990;2:283.

88. Obrist WD, Thompson HK, King CH, Wang HS. Determination of regional cerebral blood flow by inhalation of 133-Xenon. *Circ Res* 1967;20:124.

89. Gibbs EL, Lennox G, Nims LF, Gibbs FA. Arterial and cerebral venous blood. Arterial-venous differences in man. *J Biol Chem* 1942; 144:32.

90. Obrist WD, Langfitt TW, Jaggi JL, Cruz J, Gennarelli TA. Cerebral blood flow and metabolism in comatose patients with acute head injury. *J Neurosurg* 1984;61:241.

91. Robertson CS, Narayan RK, Gokaslan ZL, Pahwa R, Grossman RG, et al. Cerebral arteriovenous oxygen difference as an estimate of cerebral blood flow in comatose patients. *J Neurosurg* 1989;70:222.

92. Goetting MG, Preston G. Jugular bulb catheterization: experience with 123 patients. *Crit Care Med* 1990;18:1220.

93. Sheinberg M, Kanter MJ, Robertson CS, et al. Continuous monitoring of jugular venous oxygen saturation in head-injured patients. *J Neurosurg* 1992;76:212.

94. Obrist WD, Langfitt TW, Jaggi J, Cruz J, Gennarelli TA. Cerebral blood flow and metabolism in comatose patients with acute head injury: relationship to intracranial hypertension. *J Neurosurg* 1984; 61:241.

95. Chan K-H, Miller JD, Dearden NM, Andrews PJD, Midgley S. The effect of changes in cerebral perfusion pressure upon middle cerebral artery blood flow velocity and jugular bulb venous oxygen saturation after severe brain injury. *J Neurosurg* 1992;77:55.

96. Cruz J, Miner ME, Allen SJ, Alves WM, Gennarelli TA. Continuous monitoring of cerebral oxygenation in acute brain injury: assessment of cerebral hemodynamic reserve. *J Neurosurg* 1991;29:743.

97. Kuwayama N, Takaku A, Harada J, Fukuda O, Endo S, Saito T. Modified thermal diffusion flow probe for the continuous monitoring of cortical blood flow. *J Neurosurg* 1991;29(4):583.

98. Carter LP, Graham T, Bailes JE, Bichard W, Spetzler RF. Continuous postoperative monitoring of cortical blood flow and intracranial pressure. *Surg Neurol* 1991;35:36.

99. Wei D, Shea M, Saidel GM, Jones SC. Validation of continous thermal measurement of cerebral blood flow by arterial pressure change. *Cereb Blood Flow Metab* 1993;13:693.

100. Dickman CA, Carter LP, Baldwin HZ, Harrington T, Tallman D. Continuoys regional cerebral blood flow monitoring in acute craniocerebral trauma. *J Neurosurg* 1991;28(3):467.

101. Elwell CE, Cope M, Edwards AD, Wyatt JS, Reynolds EOR, Depy DT. Measurement of cerebral blood flow in adult humans using near infrared spectroscopy—methodology and possible errors. In: Erdmann W, Bruley DF, eds. *Oxygen transport to tissue,* vol XIV. New York: 1992.

102. McCormick PW, Stewart M, Goetting MG, Dujovny M, Lewis G, Ausman JI. Noninvasive cerebral optical spectroscopy for monitoring cerebral oxygen delivery hemodynamics. *Crit Care Med* 1991;19(1): 89.

103. Wyatt JS, Cope M, Delpy DT, Richardson CE, Edwards AD, Wray S, Reynolds OR. Quantitation of cerebral blood volume in human infants by near-infrared spectroscopy. *J Appl Physiol* 1990;68(3): 1086.

104. von Siebenthal K, Bernert G, Casaer P. Near-infrared spectroscopy in newborn infants. *Brain Dev* 1992;14:135.

105. Villringer A, Planck J, Hock C, Schleinkofer L, Dirnagl U. Near infrared spectroscopy (NIRS): a new tool to study hemodynamic changes during activation of brain function in human adults. *Neurosci Lett* 1993;134:101.

106. Hampson NB, Camporesi EM, Stolp BW, et al. Cerebral oxygen availability by NIR spectroscopy during transient hypoxia in humans. *J Appl Physiol* 1990;69(3):907.

107. Ekstrom-Jodal B, Haggendal J, Larsson LE, Westerlund A. Cerebral hemodynamics, oxygen uptake and cerebral arteriovenous differences of catecholamines following *E. coli* endotoxin in dogs. *Acta Anaesth Scand* 1982;26:446.

108. Ekstrom-Jodal B, Haggendal E, Larsson LE. Cerebral blood flow and oxygen uptake in endotoxic shock. An experimental study in dogs. *Acta Anaesth Scand* 1982;26:163.

109. MacKenzie ET, McCulloch J, O'Keane M, Pickard JD, Harper AM. Cerebral circulation and norepinehrine: relevance of the blood-brain barrier. *Am J Physiol* 1976;231(2):483.

110. MacKenzie ET, McCulloch J, Harper AM. Influence of endogenous norepinephrine on cerebral blood flow and metabolism. *Am J Physiol* 1976;231(2):489.

111. Westerlind A, Larsson LE, Haggendal J, Ekstrom-Jodal B. Prevention of endotoxin-induced increase of cerebral oxygen consumption in dogs by propranolol pretreatment. *Acta Anaesthesiol Scand* 1991;35: 745.

112. Olesen J. The effect of intracarotid epinephrine, norepinephrine, and angiotensin on the regional cerebral blood flow in man. *Neurology* 1972;22:978.

113. Bryan WJ, Emerson TE. Blood flow in seven regions of the brain during endotoxin shock in the dog. *Proc Soc Eper Biol and Med* 1977; 156:205.

114. Gatti S, Bartfai T. Induction of tumor necrosis factor-alpha mRNA in the brain after peripheral endotoxin treatment: comparison with interleukin-1 family and interleukine-6. *Research* 1993;624:291.

115. Van Dam A-M, Brouns M, Man-A-Hing W, Berkenbosch F. Immunocytochemical detection of prostaglandin E$_2$ in microvasculature and in neurons of rat brain after administration of bacterial endotoxin. *Brain Res* 1993;613:331.

116. Anderson P-B, Perry VH, Gordon S. The acute inflammatory response to lipopolysaccharide in CNS parenchyma differs from that in other body tissues. *Neuroscience* 1992;48:169.

117. Bowton DL, Bertels NH, Prough DJ, et al. Cerebral blood flow is reduced in patients with sepsis syndrome. *Crit Care Med* 1989;17: 399.

118. Maekawa T, Fugii Y, Sadamitsu D, et al. Cerebral circulation and metabolism in patients with septic encephalopathy. *Am J Med* 1991;9: 139.

119. Paulson OB, Jarden JO, Godtfredsen J, Vostrup S. Cerebral blood flow in patients with congestive heart failure treated with captopril. *Am J Med* 1984;76(5B)91.

120. Paulson O-B, Jarden JO, Vorstrup S, Holm S, Godtfredsen J. Effect of captopril on the cerebral circulation in chronic heart failure. *Eur J Clin Invest* 1986;16:124.

## Myocardial

121. Schremmer B, Dhainaut JF. Regulation of myocardial oxygen delivery. *Intens Care Med* 1990;16:S157.

122. Hoffman JIE. Transmural myocardial perfusion. *Prog Cardiovasc Dis* 1987;6:429.

123. Wally KR, Becker CJ, Hogan RA, et al. Progressive hypoxemia limits left ventricular oxygen consumption and contractility. *Circ Res* 1988;63:849.

124. McKeever WP, Gregg DE, Canney PC. Oxygen uptake of the nonworking left ventricle. *Circ Res* 1958;6:612.

125. Sarnoff SJ, Braunwald E, Welch GH, et al. Hemodynamic determinants of oxygen consumption of the heart with special reference to the tension-time index. *Am J Physiol* 1958;192:148.

126. Braunwald E, Sarnoff SJ, Case RB, et al. Hemodynamic determinants of coronary flow: effect of changes in aortic pressure and cardiac output on the relationship between myocardial oxygen consumption and coronary flow. *Am J Physiol* 1958;157.

127. Rodbard S, Williams C, Rodbard D, Berglund E. Myocardial tension and oxygen uptake. *Circ Res* 1964;14:139.

128. Schipke JD, Burkhoff D, Kass DA, Alexander J, Schaefer J, Sagawa K. Hemodynamic dependence of myocardial oxygen consumption indexes. *Am J Physiol* 1990;H258, H1281.

129. Sonnenblick E, Ross J, Covell JW, Kaiser GA, Braunwald E. Velocity of contraction as a determinant of myocardial oxygen consumption. *Am J Physiol* 1965;209:919.

130. Suga H, Hisano R, Goto Y, Yamada O, Igarashi Y. Effect of positive inotropic agents on the relation between oxygen consumption and systolic pressure volume area in canine left ventricle. *Circ Res* 1983; 53:306.

131. Rooke GA, Feigl EO. Work as a correlate of canine left ventricular oxygen consumption, and the problem of catecholamine oxygen wasting. *Circ Res* 1982;50:273.

132. Boerth RC, Covell JW, Pool PE, Ross J. Increased myocardial oxygen consumption and contractile state associated with increased heart rate in dogs. *Circ Res* 1969;24:715.

133. Ardehali A, Ports TA. Myocardial oxygen supply and demand. *Chest* 1990;98:699.

134. Suga H, Katabatake A, Sagawa K. Endsystolic pressure determines stroke volume from fixed enddiastolic volume in isolated canine left ventricle under a constant contractile state. *Circ Res* 1979;44:238.

135. Suga H. Total mechanical energy of a ventricle model and cardiac oxygen consumption. *Am J Physiol* 1981;H498:240.

136. Suga H, Hayashi T, Shirahata M. Ventricular systolic pressure-volume area as predictor of cardiac oxygen consumption. *Am J Physiol* 1981;H39.

137. Khalafbeigui F, Suga H, Sagawa K. Left ventricular systolic pressure-volume area correlates with oxygen consumption. *Am J Physiol* 1985; H566:248.

138. Dole WP. Autoregulation of the coronary circulation. *Prog Cardiovasc Dis* 1987;29:298.

139. Chilian WM, Marcus M. Effects of coronary and extravascular pressure on intramyocardial and epicardial blood velocity. *Am J Physiol* 1985;H170.

140. Rouleau J, Boerboom L, Surjadhana A, Hoffman JIE. The role of autoregulation and tissue diastolic pressures in the transmural distribution of left ventricular blood flow in anesthetized dogs. *Circ Res* 1979;45:804.

141. Brazier J, Cooper N, Buckberg G. The adequacy of subendocardial oxygen delivery. The interaction of determinants of flow, arterial oxygen content and myocardial oxygen need. *Circulation* 1974;49: 968.

142. Bell JR, Fox AC. Pathogenesis of subendocardial ischemia. *Am J Med Sci* 1974;268:2.

143. Winslow EJ, Loeb HS, Rahimtoola SH, Kamath S, Gunnar R. Hemodynamic studies and results of therapy in 50 patients with bacteremic shock. *Am J Med* 1973;54:421.

144. Siegel JH, Greenspan M, Del Guercio LRM. Abnormal vascular tone, defective oxygen transport and myocardial failure in human septic shock. *Ann Surg* 1967;504:165.

145. Wilson RF, Thal AP, Kindling PH, Grifka T, Ackerman E. Hemodynamic measurements in septic shock. *Arch Surg* 1965;91:121.

146. Carroll G, Snyder JV. Hyperdynamic severe intravascular sepsis depends on fluid administration in cynomolgus monkey. *Am J Physiol* 1982;R131:243.

147. Natanson C, Dann RL, Elin RJ, et al. Role of endotoxemia in cardiovascular dysfunction and mortality. *Escherichia coli* and *Staphylococcus aureus* challenges in a canine model of human septic shock. *J Clin Invest* 1989;R131:243.

148. Ahmed A, Kruse J, Haupt M, et al. Hemodynamic response to gram positive vs. gram negative sepsis in critically ill patients with and without circulatory shock. *Crit Care Med* 1991;19:1520.

149. Parker MM, McCarthy K, Ognibene FP, Parrillo JE. Right ventricular dysfunction and dilatation, similar to left ventricular changes, characterize the cardiac depression of septic shock in humans. *Chest* 1990; 97:126.

150. Ognibene FP, Parker MM, Natanson C, Shelhamer JH, Parrillo JE. Depressed left ventricular performance. Response to volume infusion in patients with sepsis and septic shock. *Chest* 1988;93:903.

151. Parker MM, Shelmer J, Bacharach S, et al. Profound reversible myocardial depression in patients with septic shock. *Ann Intern Med* 1984;100:483.

152. Parker MM, Ognibene FP, Parrillo JE. Peak systolic pressure/endsystolic volume ratio, a load-independent measure of ventricular function, is reversibly decreased in human septic shock. *Crit Care Med* 1994;22:1955.

153. Parker MM, Shelhamer JH, Natanson C, Alling DW, Parrillo JE. Serial cardiovascular variables in survivors and nonsurvivors of human septic shock: heart rate as an early predictor of prognosis. *Crit Care Med* 1987;15:923.

154. Natanson C, Fink MP, Ballantyne HK, MacVittie JT, Conklin JJ, Parrillow JE. Gram-negative bacteremia produces both severe systolic and diastolic cardiac dysfunction in a canine model that stimulates human septic shock. *J Clin Invest* 1986;78:259.

155. Jafri SM, Lavine S, Field BE, Bahorozian MT, Carlson RW. Left ventricular diastolic function in sepsis. *Crit Care Med* 1990;18:709.

156. Elkins RC, McCurdy JR, Brown PP, Greenfield LJ. Effects of coronary perfusion pressure on myocardial performance during endotoxin shock. *Surg Gynecol Obstet* 1973;137:991.

157. Peyton MD, Hinshaw LB, Greenfield LJ, Elkins RC. The effects of coronary vasodilatation on cardiac performance during endotoxin shock. *Surg Gynecol Obstet* 1976;143:533.

158. Hinshaw LB, Archer LT, Spitzer JJ, Black MR, Peyton MD, Greenfield LJ. Effects of coronary hypotension and endotoxin on myocardial performance. *Am J Physiol* 1974;227:1051.

159. Groeneveld ABJ, van Lambalgen AA, van den Bos GC, Brosveld W, Nauta JJP, Thijs LG. Maldistribution of heterogeneous coronary blood flow during canine endotoxin shock. *Cardiovasc Res* 1991;25: 80.

160. Kleinman WM, Krause SM, Hess ML. Differential subendocardial perfusion and injury during the course of gram-negative endotoxemia. *Adv Shock Res* 1980;4:139.

161. Cunnion RE, Schaer GL, Parker MM, Natanson C, Parrillo J. The coronary circulation in human septic shock. *Circulation* 1986;73:637.

162. Dhainaut JF, Huyghebaert MF, Monsallier FJ, Lefevre G. Coronary hemodynamics and myocardial metabolism of lactate, free fatty acids, glucose and ketones in patients with septic shock. *Circulation* 1987; 75:533.

163. Gertz EW, Wisneski JA, Neese R, Bistow JD, Searle GL, Hanlon JT. Myocardial lactate metabolism: evidence for lactate release during net chemical extraction in man. *Circulation* 1981;63:1273.

164. Ellrodt AG, Riedinger MS, Kimchi A, Berman DS, Maddahi J, Swan HJC, Murata G. Left ventricular performance in septic shock: reversible segmental and global abnormalities. *Am Heart J* 1985;110: 402.

165. Raper R, Sibbald WJ. The effects of coronary artery disease on cardiac function in nonhypotensive sepsis. *Chest* 1988;94:507.

166. Reilly JM, Cunnion RE, Burch-Whitman C, Parker MM, Shelhamer JH, Parrillo JE. A circulating myocardial depressant substance is associated with cardiac dysfunction and peripheral hypoperfusion (lactic acidemia) in patients with septic shock. *Chest* 1989;95:1072.

167. Parrillo JE, Burch C, Shelhamer JH, Parker MM, Natanson C, Schuette W. A circulating myocardial depressant substance in humans with septic shock. Septic shock patients with a reduced ejection fraction have a circulating factor that depresses in vitro myocardial cell performance. *J Clin Invest* 1985;76:1539.

168. Brady AJB, Warren JB, Poole-Wilson PA, Williams TJ, Harding SE. Nitric oxide attenuates cardiac myocyte contraction. *Am J Physiol* 1993;H176:265.

169. Balligand JL, Ungureanu D, Kelly RA, et al. Abnormal contractile function due to induction of nitric oxide synthesis in rat cardiac myocytes follows exposure to activated macrophage-conditioned medium. *J Clin Invest* 1993;91:2314.

170. Balligand JL, Ungureanu-Longrois D, Simmons WW, et al. Cytokine-inducible nitric oxide synthase (iNOS) expression in cardiac myocytes. *J Biol Chem* 1994;269:275.

171. Evans HG, Lewis MJ, Shah AM. Interleukin-1B modulates myocardial contraction via dexamethasone sensitive production of nitric oxide. *Cardiovasc Res* 1993;27:1486.

172. Schultz R, Panas DL, Catena R, Moncada S, Olley PM, Lopaschuk GD. The role of nitric oxide in cardiac depression induced by interleukin-1B and tumour necrosis factor-alpha. *Br J of Pharmacology* 1995;114:27.

173. Eichenholz PW, Eichacker PQ, Hoffman WD, et al. Tumor necrosis factor changes in canines: patterns of cardiovascular dysfunction. *Am J Physiol* 1992;H668:263.

174. Lundsgaard-Hansen P. Oxygen supply and anaerobic metabolism of the heart in experimental hemorrhagic shock. *Ann Surg* 1966;163:10.

175. Ratliff NB, Hackel D, Mikat E. Myocardial oxygen metabolism and myocardial blood flow in dogs in hemorrhagic shock. *Circ Res* 1969; 24:901.

176. Hackel DB, Goodale WT. Effects of hemorrhagic shock on the heart and circulation of intact dogs. *Circulation* 1955;11:628.

177. Horton JW, Poehimann DS. Regional coronary blood flow in canine hemorrhagic shock. *Circulatory Shock* 1987;23:271.

178. Carlson EL, Selinger SL, Utley J, Hoffman JIE. Intramyocardial distribution of blood flow in hemorrhagic shock in anesthetized dogs. *Am J Physiol* 1976;230:41.

179. Horton JW. Hemorrhagic shock impairs myocardial cell volume regulation and membrane integrity in dogs. *Am J Physiol* 1987;H1203:252.

180. Horton JW. Calcium-channel blockade in canine hemorrhagic shock. *Am J Physiol* 1989;257:R1012.

181. Crowell JW, Guyton AC. Further evidence favoring a cardiac mechanism in irreversible hemorrhagic shock. *Am J Physiol* 1962;248.

182. Siegel HW, Downing SE. Reduction of left ventricular contractility during acute hemorrhagic shock. *Am J Physiol* 1970;218:772.

183. Granata L, Huvos A, Pasque A, Gregg D. Left coronary hemodynamics during hemorrhagic hypotension and shock. *Am J Physiol* 1969; 216:1583.

184. Iguidbashian JP, Follette DM, Contino JP, Chao CT, Berkoff HA. Improved myocardial function using cardiopulmonary support in resuscitation for hemorrhagic shock. *Arch Surg* 1994;129:1013.

## Renal Circulation

185. Duke GJ, Bersten D. Dopamine and renal salvage in the critically ill patient. *Anaesth Intens Care* 1992;20:277.

186. Steinhausen M, Endlich K, Wiegman, D. Editorial Review. Glomerular blood flow. *Kidney Int* 1990;38:769.

187. Stein JH. Regulation of the renal circulation. *Kidney Int* 1990;38:571.

188. Zimmerhackl B, Dussel R, Steinhausen M. Erythrocyte flow and dynamic hematocrit in the renal papilla of the rat. *Am J Physiol* 1985; 249:F898.

189. Leichtweiss HP, Lubbers DW, Weiss C, Baumgartl H, Reschke W. The oxygen supply of the rat kidney: measurements of intrarenal p02. *Pflugers Arch* 1969;309:328.

190. Beeuwkes R. The vascular organization of the kidney. *Ann Rev Physiol* 1980;42:531.

191. Rasmussen K. Red cell and plasma volume flows to the inner medulla of the rat kidney. *Pflugers Arch* 1978;373:153.

192. Brezis M, Rosen SN, Epstein FH. The pathophysiological implications of medullary hypoxia. *Am J Kidney Dis* 1989;13(3):253.

193. Dies F, Valdez JM, Vilet R, Garza R. Lactate oxidation and sodium reabsorption by dog kidney in vivo. *Am J Physiol* 1981;240:F343.

194. Arendshorst WJ, Navar LG. Renal circulation and glomerular hemodynamics. In: Schrier RW, Gottschalk CW, eds. *Diseases of the kidney,* vol 1. Boston: Little, Brown; 1988.

195. Schlichtig R, Kramer DJ, Boston JR, Pinsky MR. Renal 0₂ consumption during progressive hemorrhage. *Am J Physiol* 1991;70(5):1957.

196. Blantz RC, Thomson SC, Peterson OW, Gabbai FB. Physiologic adaptations of tubuloglomerular feedback system. *Kidney Int* 1990;38:577.

197. Barajas L. Innervation of the renal cortex. *Fed Proc* 1978;37:1192.

198. Thames MD. Contribution of cardiopulmonary baroreceptors to the control of the kidney. *Fed Proc* 1978;37:1209.

199. Tidgren B, Hjemdahl P. Reflex activation of renal nerves in humans: differential effects on noradrenaline, dopamine and renin overflow to renal venous plasma. *Acta Physiol Scand* 1988;134:23.

200. DiBona GF. Neural control of renal tubular sodium reabsorption in the dog. *Fed Proc* 1978;37:1214.

201. Vatner SF. Effects of exercise and excitement on mesenteric and renal dynamics in conscious, unrestrained baboons. *Am J Physiol* 1978;234 (2):H210.

202. Tidgren B, Hjemdahl P. Renal responses to mental stress and epinephrine in humans. *Am J Physiol* 1989;26:F682.

203. Tidgren B, Hjemdahl P, Theodorsson E, Nussberger J. Renal neurohormonal and vascular responses to dynamic exercise in humans. *J Appl Physiol* 1991;70(5):2279.

204. Baer PG. Hormonal systems and renal hemodynamics. *Ann Rev Physiol* 1980;42:589.

205. Cody RJ, Atlas SA, Laragh JH, et al. Atrial natriuretic factor in normal subjects and heart failure patients. *J Clin Invest* 1986;7:1362.

206. Battilana C, Zhang H, Olshen RA, Wexler L, Myers BD. PAH extraction and estimation of plasma flow in diseased human kidneys. *Am J Physiol* 1991;30:F726.

207. Sykes BJ, Hoie J, Schenk WG. An experimental study into the validity of clearance methods of measuring renal blood flow. *Surg Gynecol Obstet* 1972;135:877.

208. Magrini F, Guo-Quing L. A critical improvement of the local thermodilution method for measuring renal blood flow in man. *Cardiovasc Res* 1982;16:350.

209. Haywood A, Stewart JT, Counihan PJ, Sneddon JF, Tighe D. Validation of bedside measurements of absolute human renal blood flow by a continuous thermodilution technique. *Crit Care Med* 1992;20:659.

210. Grunnert D, Schoning M, Rosendahl W. Renal blood flow and flow velocity in children and adolescents: Duplex Doppler evaluation. *Eur J Pediatr* 1990;149:287.

211. Aukland K. Methods for measuring renal blood flow: total flow and regional distribution. *Ann Rev Physiol* 1980;42:543.

212. Selmyer JP, Reynolds DG, Swan KG. Renal blood flow during endotoxin shock in the subhuman primate. *Surgery* 1973;137(1):3.

213. Bersten AD, Hersch M, Cheung H, Rutledge FS, Sibbald WJ. The effect of various sympathomimetics on the regional circulations in hyperdynamic sepsis. *Surgery* 1992;112:549.

214. Fish RE, Lang CH, Spitzer JA. Regional blood flow during continuous low-dose endotoxin infusion. *Circ Shock* 1986;18:267.

215. Cryer HG, Bloom ITM, Unger LS, Garrison RN. Factors affecting renal microvascular blood flow in rat hyperdynamic bacteremia. *Am J Physiol* 1993;264:H1988.

216. Spain DA, Wilson MA, Bloom ITM, Garrison RN. Renal microvascular responses to sepsis are dependent on nitric oxide. *J Surg Res* 1994;56:524.

217. Bloom IT, Bentley FR, Wilson MA, Garrison. In vivo effects of entohelin on the renal microcirculation. *J Surg Res* 1993;54(4):274.

218. Tristani FE, Cohn JN. Studies in clinical shock and hypotension. *Circulation* 1970;42:839.

219. Lucas CE, Rector FE, Werner M, Rosenber IK. Altered renal homeostasis with acute sepsis. *Arch Surg* 1973;106:444.

220. Brenner M, Schaer GL, Mallory DL, Suffredini AF, Parrillo JE. Detection of renal blood flow abnormalities in septic and critically ill patients using a newly designed indwelling thermodilution renal vein catheter. *Chest* 1990;98:170.

221. Szerlie H. Renal-dose dopamine: fact and fiction. *Ann Intern Med* 1991;115(2):153.

222. Cronin RE, De Torrente A, Miller PD, Bulger RE, Burke TJ, Schrier RW. Pathogenic mechanisms in early norepinephrine-induced acute renal failure: functional and histologic correlates of protection. *Kidney Int* 1978;14:115.

223. Gombos EA, Hulet WH, Bopp P, Goldring W, Baldwin DS, Chasis H. Reactivity of renal and systemic circulations to vasoconstrictor agents in normotensive and hypertensive subjects. *J Clin Invest* 1962; 41(2):203.

224. Pullman TN, McClure WW. The response of the renal circulation in man to constant-speed infusions of *l*-norepinephrine. *Circulation* 1954;9:600.

225. Martin C, Eon B, Saux P, Aknin P, Gouin F. Renal effects of norepinephrine used to treat septic shock patients. *Crit Care Med* 1990;18: 3,282.

226. Meadows D, Edwards JD, Wilkins RG, Nightingale P. Reversal of intractable septic shock with norepinephrine therapy. *Crit Care Med* 1988;16(2):663.

227. De La Cal MA, Miravalles E, Pascual T, Esteban A, Ruiz-Santana S. Dose-related hemodynamic and renal effects of dopamine in septic shock. *Crit Care Med* 1984;12(1):22.

228. Horn PT, Murphy MB. Therapeutic applications of drugs acting on peripheral dopamine receptors. *J Clin Pharmacol* 1990;30:674.

229. Goldberg LI, McDonald RH, Zimmerman AM. Sodium diuresis produced by dopamine in patients with congestive heart failure. *N Engl J Med* 1963;269(20):1060.

230. McDonald RH, Goldberg LI, McNay JL, Tuttle EP. Effects of dopamine. In: Goldberg LI, McDonald RH, Zimmerman AM: Sodium diuresis produced by dopamine in patients with congestive heart failure. *N Engl J Med* 1964;269(20):1060.

231. Winso O, Biber B, Martner J. Does dopamine suppress stress-induced intestinal and renal vasoconstriction? *Acta Anaesthesiol Scand* 1985; 29:508.

232. Strigle TR, Petrinec D. The effect of renal range dopamine and norepinephrine infusions on the renal vasculature. *Am Surg* 1990;56:494.

233. Rao PS, Cavanaugh D. Endotoxic shock in the primate: some effect of dopamine administration. *Am J Obstet Gynecol* 1982;144:61.

234. Schaer GL, Fink MP, Parrillo JE. Norepinephrne alone versus norepinephrine plus low-dose dopamine: enhanced renal blood flow with combination pressor therapy. *Crit Care Med* 1985;13(6):492.

235. Drexler H, Hayoz D, Munzel T, et al. Endothelia function in congestive heart failure. *Am Heart J* 1993;126:761.

236. McAlpine HM, Morton JJ, Leckie B, Rumley A, Gillen G. Neuroendocrine activation after acute myocardial infarction. *Br Heart J* 1988; 60:117.

237. Francis GS, Benedict C, Johnstone DE, et al. Comparison of neuroendocrine activation in patients with left ventricular dysfunction with and without congestive heart failure. *Circulation* 1990;82:1723.

238. Broqvist M, Dahlstrom U, Karlberg BE, Karlsson E, Marklund T. Neuroendocrine response in acute heart failure and the influence of treatment. *Eur Heart J* 1989;10:1075.

239. Packer M. The neurohormonal hypothesis: a theory to explain the mechanism of disease progression in heart failure. *J Am Coll Cardiol* 1990;20:248.

240. Kaye DM, Lambert GW, Lefkovits J, et al. Neurochemical evidence of cardiac sympathetic activation and increased central nervous system norepinephrine turnover in congestive heart failure. *J Am Coll Cardiol* 1994;23:570.

241. Hasking GJ, Esler MD, Jennings GL, Burton D, Korner PL. Norepinephrine spillover to plasma in patients with congestive heart failure: evidence of increased overalll and cardiorenal sympathetic nervous activity. *Circulation* 1986;73(4):615.

242. Mento PF, Maita ME, Murphy WR, Holt WF, Wilkes BM. Comparison of angiotensin converting enzyme and renin inhibition in rats following myocardial infarction. *J Cardiovasc Pharmacol* 1993;21:791.

243. Ichikawa I, Pfeffer JM, Pfeffer MA, Hostetter TH, Brenner BM. Role of angiotensin II in the altered renal function of congestive heart failure. *Circ Res* 1984;55:669.

244. Steinhausen M, Ballantyne D, Fretschner M, Hoffend J, Parekh N. Different responses of cortical and juxtamedullary arterioles to norepinephrine and angiotensin II. *Kidney Int* 1990;38:S55.

245. Creager MA, Halpern JL, Bernard DB, et al. Acute regional circulatory and renal hemodynamic effects of converting-enzyme inhibition in patients with congestive heart failure. *Circulation* 1981;64(3):483.

246. Zellis R, Sinoway LI, Musch TI, Davis D, Just H. Regional blood flow in congestive heart failure: concept of compensatory mechanisms with short and long time constants. *Am J Cardiol* 1988;62:2E.

247. Levine TB, Olivari MT, Garberg V, Sharkey SW, Cohn JN. Hemodynamic and clinical response to enalapril, a long-acting converting-enzyme inhibitor, in patients with congestive heart failure. *Circulation* 1984;69(3):548.

248. Cleland JG, Shah D, Krikler S, et al. Effects of lisinopril on cardiorespiratory, neuroendocrine, and renal function in patients with asymptomatic left ventricular dysfunction. *Br Heart J* 1993;69:512.

249. Motwani JG, Fenwick MK, McAlpine HM, Kennedy N, Struthers AD. Effectiveness of captopril in reversing renal vasoconstriction after Q-wave acute myocardial infarction. *Am J Cardiol* 1993;71:281.

250. Powers ER, Bannerman KS, Stone J, et al. The effect of captopril on renal, coronary, and systemic hemodynamics in patients with severe congestive heart failure. *Am Heart J* 1982;104:1203.

251. Leier CV, Magorien RD, Desch CE, Thompson MJ, Unverferth DV. Hydralazine and isosorbide dinitrate: comparative central and renal hemodynamic effects when administered alone or in combination. *Circulation* 1981;63(1):102.

252. Cogan JJ, Humphreys MH, Carlson CJ, Rapaport E. Renal effects of nitroprusside and hydralazine in patients with congestive heart failure. *Circulation* 1980;61:316.

253. Sandler H, Dodge HT, Murdaugh HV. Effects of isoproterenol on cardiac output and renal function in congestive heart failure. *Am Heart J* 1961;62:643.

254. Vatner SF. Effects of hemorrhage on regional blood flow distribution in dogs and primates. *J Clin Invest* 1974;54:225.

255. Kremser PC, Gewertz BL. Effect of pentobarbital and hemorrhage on renal autoregulation. *Am J Physiol* 1985;249:F356.

256. Chang H, Wu GJ, Wang S-M, Hung C-R. Plasma endothelin level changes during hemorrhagic shock. *J Trauma* 1993;35(6):825.

257. Simchon S, Fan F-C, Chen RYZ, et al. Effects of experimental hypo-

258. Passmore JC, Stremel RW, Hock CE, Allen RL, Bradford JB. Distribution of intrarenal blood flow consequent to left atrial balloon inflation. *Circ Shock* 1985;15:37.

259. Carriere S, Thornburn GD, O'Morchoe CCC, Barger AC. Intrarenal distribution of blood flow in dogs during hemorrhagic hypotension. *Circ Res* 1966;19:167.

260. Shirley DG, MacRae KD, Walker J. The renal vascular response to mild and severe haemorrhage in the anaesthetized rat. *J Physiol* 1991; 432:373.

261. Neiberger RE, Passmore JC. Effects of dopamine on canine intrarenal blood flow distribution during hemorrhage. *Kidney Int* 1979;15:219.

262. Nelimarkka O, Halkola L, Niinikoski J. Renal hypoxia and lactate metabolism in hemorrhagic shock in dogs. *Crit Care Med* 1984;12: 656.

## Diaphragm

263. Comtois A, Gorczyca W, Grassino A. Anatomy of diaphragmatic circulation. *J Appl Physiol* 1987;62(1):238.

264. Keith L. *Clinically oriented anatomy.* Baltimore: Williams & Wilkins; 1992:227.

265. Brancatisano A, Amis TC, Tully A, Kelly WT, Engel LA. Regional distribution of blood flow within the diaphragm. *J Appl Physiol* 1991; 71(2):583.

266. Magder S, Lockhat D, Luo BJ, Roussos C. Respiratory muscle and organ blood flow with inspiratory elastic loading and shock. *J Appl Physiol* 1985;58(4):1148.

267. Bark H, Supinski G, Bundy R, Kelsen S. Effect of hypoxia on diaphragm blood flow, oxygen uptake, and contractility. *Am Rev Respir Dis* 1988;138:1535.

268. Hussain SNA, Roussos C, Magder S. Autoregulation of diaphragmatic blood flow in dogs. *J Appl Physiol* 1988;64(1):329.

269. Robertson CH, Foster GH, Johnson RL. The relationship of respiratory failure to the oxygen consumption of, lactate production by and distribution of blood flow among respiratory muscles during increasing inspiratory resistance. *J Clin Invest* 1977;59:31.

270. Pang ML, Kim Y-L, Bazzy AR. Blood flow to respiratory muscles and major organs during inspiratory flow resistive loads. *J Appl Physiol* 1993;74(1):428.

271. Rochester DF, Bettini G. Diaphragmatic blood flow and energy expenditure in the dog. *J Clin Invest* 1976;57:661.

272. Adachi H, Strauss W, Ochi H, Wagner HN. The effect of hypoxia on the regional distribution of cardiac output in the dog. *Circ Res* 1976; 39:314.

273. Magder S, Erian R, Roussos C. Respiratory muscle blood flow in oleic acid-induced pulmonary edema. *J Appl Physiol* 1986;60(6): 1849.

274. Hussain SNA, Roussos C. Distribution of respiratory muscle and organ blood flow during endotoxic shock in dogs. *J Appl Physiol* 1985;59(6):1802.

275. Viires N, Sillye G, Aubier M, Rassidakis A, Roussos CH. Regional blood flow distribution during induced hypotension and low cardiac output. *J Clin Invest* 1983;72:935.

276. Reid MB, Johnson RL. Efficiency, maximal blood flow, and aerobic work capacity of canine diaphragm. *J Appl Physiol* 1983;54(3):763.

277. Scharf S, Bark H. Function of canine diaphragm with hypovolemic shock and beta-adrenergic blockade. *J Appl Physiol* 1984;56(3):648.

278. Ockhat D, Roussos C, Ianuzzo CD. Metabolite changes in the loaded hypoperfused and failing diaphragm. *J Appl Physiol* 1988;65(4): 1563.

279. Supinski G, Dimarco A, Ketai L, Hussein F, Altose M. Reversibility of diaphragm fatigue by mechanical hyperperfusion. *Am Rev Respir Dis* 1988;138:604.

280. Aubier M, Murciano D, Menu Y, et al. Dopamine effects on diaphragmatic strength during acute respiratory failure in chronic obstructive pulmonary disease. *Ann Intern Med* 1989;110:17.

281. Ward M, Magder SA, Hussain SNA. Oxygen delivery-independent effect of blood flow on diaphragm fatigue. *Am Rev Respir Dis* 1992; 145:1058.

282. Yanos J, Wood LDH, Davis K, Keamy M. The effect of respiratory

and lactic acidosis on diaphragm function. *Am Rev Respir Dis* 1993; 147:616.

283. Bancroft H, Dornhurst AC. Blood flow through the human calf during rhythmic exercise. *J Physiol Lond* 1949;109:402.

284. Humphrey PW, Lind AR. The blood flow through the active and inactive muscles of the forearm during sustained handgrop contractions. *J Physiol Lond* 1948;107:518.

285. Hussain SNA, Roussos C, Magder S. Effects of tension, duty cycle, and arterial pressure on diaphragmatic blood flow in dogs. *J Appl Physiol* 1989;66(2):968.

286. Bellmare F, Wight D, Lavigne CM, Grassino A. Effect of tension and timing of contraction on the blood flow of the diaphragm. *J Appl Physiol* 1983;54(6):1597.

287. Buchler B, Magder S, Roussos C. Effects of contraction frequency and duty cycle on diaphragmatic blood flow. *J Appl Physiol* 1985;58 (1):265.

288. Hussain SNA, Magder S. Diaphragmatic intramuscular pressure in relation to tension, shortening, and blood flow. *J Appl Physiol* 1991; 71(1):159.

289. Supinski GS, Dimarco AF, Altose MD. Effect of diaphragmatic contraction on intramuscular pressure and vascular impedance. *J Appl Physiol* 1990;68(4):1486.

290. Hussain SNA, Simkus G, Roussos C. Respiratory muscle fatigue: a cause of ventilatory failure in septic shock. *J Appl Physiol* 1985;58 (6):2033.

291. Hussain SNA, Rutledge F, Graham R, Magder S, Roussos C. Effects of norepinephrine and fluid administration on diaphragmatic O$_2$ consumption in septic shock. *J Appl Physiol* 1987;62(4):1368.

292. Hussain SNA, Graham R, Rutledge F, Roussos C. Respiratory muscle energetics during endotoxic shock in dogs. *J Appl Physiol* 1986;60 (2):486.

293. Boczkowski J, Vicaut E, Aubier M. In vivo effects of *Escherichia coli* endotoxemia on diaphragmatic microcirculation in rats. *J Appl Physiol* 1992;72(6):2219.

294. Jepson MM, Cox M, Bates PC, et al. Regional blood flow and skeletal muscle energy status in endotoxemic rats. *Am J Physiol* 1987; E581.

295. Gutierrez G, Hurtado FJ, Fernandez E. Inhibitory effect of *Escherichia coli* endotoxin on skeletal muscle contractility. *Crit Care Med* 1995;23:308.

295a. Boczkowski J, Dureuil B, Branger C, et al. Effects of sepsis on diaphragmatic function in rats. *Am Rev Respir Dis* 1988;138:260.

296. DeBoisblanc BP, Meszaros K, Burns A, et al. Effect of dichloroacetate on mechanical performance and metabolism of compromised diaphragm muscle. *J Appl Physiol* 1992;72(3):1149.

297. Leon A, Boczkowski J, Dureuil B, Desmonts J-M, Aubier M. Effects of endotoxic shock on diaphragmatic function in mechanically ventilated rats. *J Appl Physiol* 1992;72(4):1466.

298. Wilcox P, Osborne S, Bressler B. Monocyte inflammatory mediators impair in vitro hamster diaphragm contractility. *Am Rev Respir Dis* 1992;146:462.

299. Nashawati E, Dimarco A, Supinski C. Effects prodiced by infusion of a free radical generating solution into the diaphragm. *Am Res Respir Dis* 1993;147:60.

300. van Surell C, Boczkowski J, Pasquier C, et al. Effects of N-acetylcysteine on diaphragmatic function and malondialdehyde content in *Escherichia coli* endotoxemic rats. *Am Rev Respir Dis* 1992;148:730.

301. Pickeny M, Balon T, Nadler J. Nitric oxide is present from incubated skeletal muscle preparations. *J Appl Physiol* 1994;77:2519.

302. Myes J, Froeliche VF. Hemodynamic determinants of exercise capacity in chronic heart fatigue. *Ann Intern Med* 1991;115:377.

303. Wilson J, Mancini D. Factors contributing to the exercise limitation of heart failure. *J Am Coll Cardiol* 1993;22(A):93A.

304. Zelis R, Longhurst J, Capone RJ, Mason D. A comparison of regional blood flow and oxygen utilization during dynamic forearm exercise in normal subjects and patients with congestive heart failure. *Circulation* 1974;50:137.

305. LeJemtel T, Maskin CS, Lucido D, Chadwick BJ. Failiure to augment maximal limb blood flow in response to one-leg versus two-leg exercise in patients with severe heart failure. *Circulation* 1986;74(2):245.

306. Drexler H, Faude F, Hoing S, Just H. Blood flow distribution within skeletal muscle during exercise in the presence of chronic heart dailure: effect of milrinone. *Circulation* 1987;76(6):1344.

307. Maskin CS, Forman R, Sonneblick EH, Frishman WH, LeJemtel T.

308. Wilson JR, Martin JL, Ferraro N. Impaired skeletal muscle nutritive flow during exercise in patients with congestive heart failure: role of cardiac pump dysfunction as determined by the effect of dobutamine. *Am J Cardiol* 1984;53:1308.

309. Sinowitz L, Minotti J, Musch T, et al. Enhanced metabolic vasodilation secondary to diuretic therapy in decompensated congestive heart failure secondary to coronary artery disease. *Am J Cardiol* 1987;60: 107.

310. Wilson JR, Ferraro N, Wiener DH. Effect of the sympathetic nervous system on limb circulation and metabolism during exercise in patients with heart failure. *Circulation* 1985;72(1):72.

311. Wilson JR, Ferraro N. Effect of the renin-angiotensin system on limb circulation and metabolism during exercise in patients with heart failure. *J Am Coll Cardiol* 1985;6:556.

312. Drexler H, Banhardt U, Meinertz T, et al. Contrasting peripheral short-term and long-term effects of converting enzyme inhibition in patients with congestive heart failure. *Circulation* 1989;79:491.

313. Mancini D, Davis L, Wexler JP, Chadwick B, LeJemtel T. Dependence of enhanced maximal exercise performance on increased peak skeletal muscle perfusion during long-term captopril therapy in heart failure. *J Am Coll Cardiol* 1987;10:845.

314. Drexler H. Skeletal muscle failure in heart failure. *Circulation* 1992; 85:1621.

315. Mancini DM, Walter G, Reichek N, et al. Contribution of skeletal muscle atrophy to exercise intolerance and altered muscle metabolism in heart failure. *Circulation* 1992;85:1364.

316. Sullivan MJ, Green HJ, Cobb FR. Skeletal muscle biochemistry and histology in ambulatory patients with long-term heart failure. *Circulation* 1990;81:518.

317. Massie BM, Conway M, Rajagopalan B, et al. Skeletal muscle metabolism during exercise under ischemic conditions in congestive heart failure. *Circulation* 1988;78:320.

318. Minotti JR, Pillary P, Chang L, Wells L, Massie BM. Neurophysiological assessment of skeletal muscle fatigue in patients with congestive heart failure. *Circulation* 1992;86:903.

319. Hambrecht R, Niebauer J, Fiehn E, et al. Physical training in patients with stable chronic heart failure: effects on cardiorespiratory fitness and ultrastructural abnormalities of leg muscles. *J Am Coll Cardiol* 1995;25:1239.

320. Levine B, Kalman J, Mayer L, Fillit H, Packer M. Elevated circulation levels of tumor necrosis factor in severe chronic heart failure. *N Engl J Med* 1990;323:236.

321. Lindsay D, Lovegrove C, Dunn M, et al. Histological abnormalities of diaphragmatic muscle may contribute to dyspnea in congestive heart failure. *Circulation* 1992;86:515.

322. Tikonov B, Levine S, Mancini D. Chronic congestive heart failure elicits adaptations of endurance exercise to diaphragmatic muscle. Supplement to *Circulation* 1995;92(8):I541.

323. McParland C, Resch E, Krishnan B, et al. Inspiratory muscle weakness in chronic heart failure: role of nutrition and electrolyte status and systemic myopathy. *Am J Respir Crit Care Med* 1995;151:1101.

324. Hammond MD, Bauer KA, Sharp JT, Rocha RD. Respiratory muscle strength in congestive heart failure. *Chest* 1990;98:1091.

325. McParland C, Krishnan B, Wang Y, Gallagher CG. Respiratory muscle weakness and dyspnea in chronic heart failure. *Am Rev Respir Dis* 1992;146:467.

326. Sullivan MJ, Higginbotham MB, Cobb FR. Increased exercise ventilation in patients with chronic heart failure: intact ventilatory control despite hemodynamic and pulmonary abnormalities. *Circulation* 1988;77(3):552.

327. Mancini DM, Henson D, LaManca J, Levine S. Respiratory muscle function and dyspnea in patients with chronic congestive heart failure. *Circulation* 1992;86:909.

328. Jennings G, Esler MD. Circulation regulation at rest and exercise and the functional assessment of patients with congestive heart failure. *Circulation* 1990;81:II-1.

329. Mancini DM, Ferraro N, Nazzaro D, Chance B, Wilson JR. Respiratory muscle deoxygenation during exercise in patients with heart failure demonstrated with near-infrared spectroscopy. *J Am Coll Cardiol* 1991;18:492.

330. Wilson JR, Mancini DM, McCully K, et al. Noninvasive detection of

skeletal muscle underperfusion with near-infrared spectroscopy in patients with heart failure. *Circulation* 1989;80:1668.

331. Supinski G, DiMarco A, Dunlap-Dibner M. Alterations in diaphragm strength and fatiguability in congestive heart failure. *J Appl Physiol* 1994;76(6):2707.

332. Musch T, Terrell JA. Skeletal muscle blood flow abnormalities in rats with a chronic myocardial infarction: rest and exercise. *Am J Physiol* 1992;262:H411.

333. Musch TI. Elevated diaphragmatic blood flow during submaximal exercise in rats with chronic heart failure. *Am J Physiol* 1993;265: H1721.

334. Aubier M, Trippenbach TM, Roussos C. Respiratory muscle fatigue during cardiogenic shock. *J Appl Physiol* 1981;51(2):499.

335. Scharf S, Bark H, Einhorn S, Tarasiuk A. Blood flow to the canine diaphragm during hemorrhagic shock. *Am Rev Respir Dis* 1988;133: 205.

336. Ward ME, Chang H, Erice F, Hussein SN. Systemic and diaphragmatic oxygen delivery consumption relationships during hemorrhage. *J Appl Physiol* 1994;77(2):653.

## Splanchnic Circulation

339. Parks DA, Jacobson ED. Physiology of the splanchnic circulation. *Arch Intern Med* 1985;145:1278.

340. Rowell LB. Control of individual vascular beds: splanchnic and renal circulations. In: Rowell LB, ed. *Human circulation: regulation during physical stress.* New York: Oxford University Press; 1986:78.

341. Folkow B, Neil E. Gastrointestinal and liver circulations. In: Folkow B, Neil E, eds. *Circulation* New York: Oxford University Press; 1971:466.

342. Marston A, Pegington J. Macroscopic anatomy. In: Marston A, Bulkley GB, Fiddian-Green RG, Haglund UH, eds. *Splanchnic ischemia and multiple organ failure.* St. Louis: Mosby; 1989:3.

343. Lautt WW, Greenway C. Conceptual review of the hepatic vascular bed. *Hepatology* 1987;7:952.

344. Gurll NJ. Ischemia of the liver and pancreas. In: Marston A, Bulkley GB, Fiddian-Green RG, Haglund UH, eds. *Splanchnic ischemia and multiple organ failure.* St. Louis: Mosby; 1989:107.

345. Hawker F. The liver—anatomy, physiology and biochemistry. In: Hawker F, ed. The liver. London: WB Saunders; 1993:1.

346. Koch NG, Hahnloer P, Roding B, Schenk WG Jr. Interaction between portal venous and hepatic arterial blood flow: an experimental study in the dog. *Surgery* 1972;72:414.

347. Lundgren O. Microcirculation of the gastrointestinal tract and pancreas. In: Renkin EM, Michel CC, eds. *Handbook of physiology*, section 2, vol IV. Bethesda, MD: American Physiological Society; 1984: 799.

348. Granger DN, Richardson PDI, Kvietys PR, Mortillaro NA. Intestinal blood flow. *Gastroenterology* 1980;78:837.

349. Hulten L, Jodal M, Lindhagen J, et al. Blood flow in the small intestine of cat and man as analyzed by an inert gas washout technique. *Gastroenterology* 1976;70:45.

350. Carr ND. Microscopic anatomy. In: Marston A, Bulkley GB, Fiddian-Green RG, Haglund UH, eds. *Splanchnic ischemia and multiple organ failure.* St. Louis: Mosby; 1989:17.

351. Lundgren O. Studies on blood flow distribution and countercurrent exchange in the small intestine. *Acta Physiol Scand* 1967;303(Suppl): 1.

352. Shepherd AP, Kiel JW. A model of countercurrent shunting of oxygen in the intestinal villus. *Am J Physiol* 1992;262:H1136.

353. Granger DN, Kvietys PR, Korthuis RJ, Premen AJ. Microcirculation of the intestinal mucosa. In: *Handbook of physiology. The gastrointestinal system. Motility and circulation.* Bethesda, MD: American Physiological Society; 1989:1405.

354. Haglund U, Jodal M, Lundgren O. The small bowel in arterial hypotension and shock. In: Shepherd AP, Granger DN, eds. *Physiology of the intestinal circulation.* New York: Raven; 1984:305.

355. Silva DG, Ross G, Osborne LW. Adrenergic innervation of the ileum of the cat. *Am J Physiol* 1971;220:347.

356. Sjovall H, Redfors S, Hallback DA, et al. The effect of splanchnic nerve stimulation on blood flow distribution, villous tissue osmolality and fluid and electrolyte transport in the small intestine of the cat. *Acta Physiol Scand* 1983;117:359.

357. Hulten L, Lindhagen J, Lundgren O, et al. Regional intestinal blood flow in ulcerative colitis and Crohn's disease. *Gastroenterology* 1977;72:388.

358. Lundgren O. Physiology of the intestinal circulation. In: Marston A, Bulkley GB, Fiddian-Green RG, Haglund UH, eds. *Splanchnic ischemia and multiple organ failure.* St. Louis: Mosby; 1989:29.

359. Salzman AL. Nitric oxide in the gut. *New Horizons* 1995;3(2):352-364.

360. Kubes P, Granger DN. Nitric oxide modulates microvascular permeability. *Am J Physiol* 1992;262:H611.

361. Stark ME, Szurszewski JH. Role of nitric oxide in gastrointestinal and hepatic function and disease. *Gastroenterology* 1992;103:1928.

362. Jacobson ED, Pawlik WW. Adenosine regulation of mesenteric vasodilation. *Gastroenterology* 1994;107:1168.

363. Reilly PM, Bulkley GB. Vasoactive mediators and splanchnic perfusion. *Crit Care Med* 1993;21:S55.

364. Campra JL, Reynolds TB. The hepatic circulation. In: Arias IM, Jakoby WB, Popper H, Schacter D, Shafritz DA. eds. *The liver: Biology and pathobiology.* New York: Raven; 1988:911.

365. Koslin DB, Mulligan SA, Berland LL. Duplex assessment of the splanchnic vasculature. *Semin Ultrasound CT MRI* 1992;13:34

366. Flinn WR, Rizzo RJ, Park JS, Sandager GP. Duplex scanning for assessment of mesenteric ischemia. *Surg Clin North Am* 1990;70:99.

367. Moore JR, Finn JP, Edelman RR. Measurement of visceral blood flow with magnetic resonance imaging. *Invest Radiol* 1992;27 (Suppl):S103.

368. Dalton JM, Gore DC, Makhoul RG, Fisher MR, DeMaria EJ. Decreased splanchnic perfusion measured by duplex ultrasound in humans undergoing small volume hemorrhage. *Crit Care Med* 1995; 23:491.

369. Grum CM, Fiddian-Green RG, Pittenger GL, et al. Adequacy of tissue oxygenation in intact dog intestine. *J Appl Physiol* 1984;56:1065.

370. Montgomery A, Hartmann M, Jonsson K, Haglund U. Intramucosal pH measurement with tonometers for detecting gastrointestinal ischemia in porcine hemorrhagic shock. *Circ Shock* 1989;29:319.

371. Fiddian-Green RG. Studies in splanchnic ischemia and multiple organ failure. In: Marston A, Bulkley GB, Fiddian- Green RG, Haglung U, eds. *Splanchnic ischemia and multiple organ failure.* St. Louis: Mosby; 1989:73.

372. Fiddian-Green RG, Baker S. Predictive value of the stomach wall pH for complications after cardiac operations: comparison with other monitoring. *Crit Care Med* 1987;15:153.

373. Gys T, Hubens A, Neels H, et al. Prognostic value of gastric intramural pH in surgical intensive care patients. *Crit Care Med* 1988;16:1222.

374. Maynard N, Bihari D, Beale R, et al. Assessment of splanchnic oxygenation by gastric tonometry in patients with acute circulatory failure. *JAMA* 1993;270:1203.

375. Boyd O, Mackay CJ, Lamb G, et al. Comparison of clinical information gained from routine blood-gas analysis and from gastric tonometry for intramural pH. *Lancet* 1993;341:142.

376. Silverman HJ, Tuma P. Gastric tonometry in patients with sepsis: effects of dobutamine infusions and packed red blood cell transfusions. *Chest* 1992;102:184.

377. Landow L, Phillips DA, Heard SO, et al. Gastric tonometry and venous oximetry in cardiac surgery patients. *Crit Care Med* 1993;19: 1226.

378. Gutierrez G, Bismar H, Dantzker DR, Silva N. Comparison of gastric intramucosal pH with measures of oxygen transport and consumption in critically ill patients. *Crit Care Med* 1992;20:451.

379. Roumen RM, Vreugde JP, Goris RJ. Gastric tonometry in multiple trauma patients. *J Trauma* 1994;36:313.

380. Bjorck M, Hedberg B. Early detection of major complications after abdominal aortic surgery: predictive value of sigmoid colon and gastric intramucosal pH monitoring. *Br J Surg* 1994;81:25.

381. Krafte-Jacobs B, Carver J, Wilkinson JD. Comparison of gastric intramucosal pH and standard perfusional measurements in pediatric septic shock. *Chest* 1995;108:220.

382. Friedman G, Berlot G, Kahn RJ, Vincent JL. Combined measurements of blood lactate concentrations and gastric intramucosal pH in patients with severe sepsis. *Crit Care Med* 1995;23:1184.

383. Doglio GR, Pusajo JF, Egurrola MA, et al. Gastric mucosal pH as a prognostic index of mortality in critically ill patients. *Crit Care Med* 1991;19:1037.

384. Marik PE. Gastric intramucosal pH: a better predictor of multiorgan

dysfunction syndrome and death than oxygen-derived variables in patients with sepsis. *Chest* 1993;104:225.

385. Bergofsky EH. Determination of tissue $O_2$ tensions by hollow visceral tonometers: effect of breathing enriched $O_2$ mixtures. *J Clin Invest* 1964;43:193.

386. Fiddian-Green RG, Pittenger G, Whitehouse WM. Back-diffusion of $CO_2$ and its influence on the intramural pH in gastric mucosa. *J Surg Res* 1982;33:39.

387. Groeneveld AB, Kolkman JJ. Splanchnic tonometry: a review of physiology, methodology, and clinical applications. *J Crit Care* 1994;9:198.

388. Gutierrez G, Brown SD. Gastric tonometry: a new monitoring modality in the intensive care unit. *J Intens Care Med* 1995;10:34.

389. Antonnson JB, Boyle CC, Kruithoff KL, et al. Validity of tonometric measures of gut intramural pH during endotoxemia and mesenteric occlusion in pigs. *Am J Physiol* 1990;259:G519.

390. Poole JW, Sammartano RJ, Boley SJ. The use of tonometry in the early diagnosis of mesenteric ischemia. *Curr Surg* 1987;44:21.

391. Bryan-Brown CW. Blood flow to organs: parameters for function and survival in critical illness. *Crit Care Med* 1988;16:170.

392. Roding B, Schenk WG. Mesenteric blood flow after hemorrhage in anesthetized and unanesthetized dogs. *Surgery* 1970;68:857.

393. McNeil JR, Stark RD, Greenway CV. Intestinal vasoconstriction after hemorrhage: roles of vasopressin and angiotensin. *Am J Physiol* 1970;219:1342.

394. Nelson DP, King CE, Dodd SL, et al. Systemic and intestinal limits of $O_2$ extraction in the dog. *J Appl Physiol* 1987;63:387.

395. Feigen LP. Differential effects of leukotrienes $C_4$, $D_4$, and $E_4$ in the canine, renal, and mesenteric vascular beds. *J Pharmacol Exp Ther* 1983;225:682.

396. Haglund U. Systemic mediators released from the gut in critical illness. *Crit Care Med* 1993;21:S15.

397. Porter JM, Sussman MS, Bulkley GB. Splanchnic vasospasm in circulatory shock. In: Marston A, Bulkley GB, Fiddian-Green RG, Haglund U, eds. *Splanchnic ischemia and multiple organ failure.* St. Louis: Mosby; 1989:73.

398. Schlag G, Redl H, Hallstrom S. The cell in shock: the origin of multiple organ failure. *Resuscitation* 1991;21:137.

399. Myers SI, Hernandez R. Leukotriene $C_4$ regulation of splanchnic blood flow during ischemia. *Am J Surg* 1994;167:566.

400. Grum CM. Tissue oxygenation in low flow states and during hypoxemia. *Crit Care Med* 1993;21:S44.

401. Greenwald RA. Superoxide dismutase and catalase as therapeutic agents for human diseases: a critical review. *Free Radic Biol Med* 1990;8:201.

402. Haglund U, Gerdin B. Oxygen free-radicals and circulatory shock. *Circ Shock* 1991;34:405.

403. Tanswell AK, Freeman BA. Antioxidant therapy in critical care medicine. *New Horizons* 1995;3:330.

404. Kurose I, Wolf R, Grisham MB, Granger DN. Modulation of ischemia/reperfusion-induced microvascular dysfunction by nitric oxide. *Circ Res* 1994;74:376.

405. Fink MP. Gastrointestinal mucosal injury in experimental models of shock, trauma, and sepsis. *Crit Care Med* 1991;19:627.

406. Mainous MR, Deitch EA. Bacterial translocation and its potential role in the pathogenesis of multiple organ failure. *J Intens Care Med* 1992;7:101.

407. Pinsky JR, Matuschak GM. Multiple systems organ failure: failure of host defense homeostasis. *Crit Care Clin* 1989;5:199.

408. Meakins JL, Marshall SC. The gastrointestinal tract: the 9motor9 of MOF. *Arch Surg* 1986;121:197.

409. Ghosh S, Latimer RD, Gray BM, et al. Endotoxin-induced organ injury. *Crit Care Med* 1993;21:S19.

410. Zivot JB, Hoffman WD. Pathogenic effects of endotoxin. *New Horizons* 1995;3:267.

411. Manthous CA, Hall JB, Samsel RW. Endotoxin in human disease. Part 2: Biologic effects and clinical evaluations of anti-endotoxin therapies. *Chest* 1993;104:1872.

412. Gump FE, Price JB, Kinney KM. Whole body and splanchnic blood flow and oxygen consumption measurements in patients with intraperitoneal infection. *Ann Surg* 1970;171:321.

413. Wilmore DW, Goodwin CW, Aulick LH, et al. Effect of injury and infection on visceral metabolism and circulation. *Ann Surg* 1980;192:491.

414. Dahn MS, Lange P, Lobdel K, et al. Splanchnic and total body oxygen consumption differences in septic and injured patients. *Surgery* 1987;101:69.

415. Dahn MS, Lange MP, Wilson RF, et al. Hepatic blood flow and splanchnic oxygen consumption measurements in clinical sepsis. *Surgery* 1990;107:295.

416. Fink MP. Adequacy of gut oxygenation in endotoxemia and sepsis. *Crit Care Med* 1993;21:S4.

417. Whitworth PW, Cryer HM, Garrison RN, et al. Hypoperfusion of the intestinal microcirculation without decreased cardiac output during live *Escherichia coli* sepsis in rats. *Circ Shock* 1989;27:111.

418. Fink MP, Cohn SM, Lee PC, et al. Effect of lipopolysaccharide on intestinal intramucosal hydrogen ion concentration in pigs: evidence of gut ischemia in a normodynamic model of septic shock. *Crit Care Med* 1989;17:641.

419. Fink MP, Rothschild HR, Deniz YF, et al. Systemic and mesenteric $O_2$ metabolism in endotoxemic pigs: effect of ibuprofen and meclofenamate. *J Appl Physiol* 1989;67:1950.

420. Fink MP, Morrissey PE, Stein KL, et al. Systemic and regional hemodynamic effects of cyclooxygenase and thromboxane inhibition in normal and hyperdynamic endotoxemic rabbits. *Circ Shock* 1988;26:41.

421. Ayuse T, Brienza N, Revelly JP, et al. Alterations in liver hemodynamics in an intact porcine model of endotoxin shock. *Am J Physiol* 1995;268:H1106.

422. Marik PE, Mohedin M. The contrasting effects of dopamine and norepinephrine on systemic and splanchnic oxygen utilization in hyperdynamic sepsis. *JAMA* 1994;272:1354.

423. Bulkley GB, Oshima A, Bailey RW. Pathophysiology of hepatic ischemia in cardiogenic shock. *Am J Surg* 1986;151:87.

424. Bailey RW, Bulkley GB, Levy KI, et al. Pathogenesis of nonocclusive mesenteric ischemia: studies in a porcine model induced by pericardial tamponade. *Surg Forum* 1982;33:194.

425. Bulkley GB, Oshima A, Bailey RW, Horn SD. Control of gastric vascular resistance in cardiogenic shock. *Surgery* 1985;98:213.

426. Niinikoski J, Kuttila K. Adequacy of tissue oxygenation in cardiac surgery: regional measurements. *Crit Care Med* 1993;21:S77.

427. Creager MA, Hirsch AT, Dzau VJ, et al. Baroreflex regulation of regional blood flow in congestive heart failure. *Am J Physiol* 1990;258:H1409.

428. Leier CV. Regional blood flow responses to vasodilators and inotropes in congestive heart failure. *Am J Cardiol* 1988;62:86E.

429. Risoe C, Simonsen S, Rootwelt K, et al. Nitroprusside and regional vascular capacitance in patients with severe congestive heart failure. *Circulation* 1992;85:997.

430. Bynum TE, Hanley HG. Effect of digitalis on estimated splanchnic blood flow. *J Lab Clin Med* 1982;99:84.

*The Critically Ill Cardiac Patient,*
edited by V. Kvetan and D. R. Dantzker,
Lippincott-Raven Publishers, Philadelphia © 1996.

CHAPTER **6**

# Cardiac Metabolism and Nutrition Support

David P. Katz, Stefan Wiese, and William A. Gay, Jr.

Enormous technical and pharmacologic progress has been achieved in improving and restoring both coronary blood flow and contractile performance in patients with coronary artery disease (CAD) during the past decade. Frequently patients that undergo cardiac surgery are older and have a greater operative risk, have lengthy hospitalizations for diagnostic and therapeutic interventions, and are acutely or chronically malnourished. It is evident that severe cardiac dysfunction results in a worsening nutrition state. Therefore a greater understanding of the interaction between cardiac metabolism and nutritional support is of great value in intelligently treating the acutely ill cardiac patient.

Our knowledge of the underlying alterations in cardiac metabolism has grown, suggesting that a complex interrelationship exists between coronary reperfusion, contractile function, and fuel utilization. Efforts of investigators have produced considerable progress in our understanding of (a) the mechanism responsible for the limitation of glucose and fatty acid oxidation during states of ischemia and reperfusion, (b) the value of available high-energy phosphates [i.e., adenosine triphospahte (ATP) and phosphocreatine] as a determinant of the contractile state of myocardial cells, and (c) the importance of the functional integrity and substrate utilization of coronary artery endothelial cells for cardiac performance.

The essential link between compromised cardiac function and appropriate nutritional support, especially during states of limited oxygen and nutrient supply to the heart (i.e., ischemia) or preexisting myocardial cell damage (i.e., myocardial infarction), has been only superficially explored. Clearly, in the absence of $O_2$ supply, intracellu-

lar modifications may develop which may limit damage or promote cardiac function. An improved understanding of the altered regulation of glucose and fatty acid metabolism during these states has recently led to an enhanced body of knowledge of the potential for modified metabolic intervention. Theoretically, specific nutritional support regimens can be designed to provide substrates (e.g., Krebs cycle intermediates) for fuel utilization and energy generation in altered myocardial states and may also exert therapeutic effects by improving the intracellular conditions for utilization of the major cardiac fuels. Properties in the latter category may include such changes as a reduction of lactate and ammonia accumulation and pH normalization during severe hypoxia, ischemia, and reperfusion.

It is increasingly evident that the coronary artery endothelium plays a central role in the evolution of ischemic damage and reperfusion injury in the heart. Dysfunction of the endothelium due to ischemia and reperfusion injury may limit the recovery of the whole heart on reperfusion. Notable progress has been made in our understanding of the differences in both energy and oxygen demands between cardiomyocytes and the coronary endothelium, revealing that hypoxia and ischemia/reperfusion may have variable effects on fuel utilization and energy generation of these tissues. By providing specific nutrients that may match more precisely the substrate demands of the endothelium, nutritional therapy may have major affect not only on the functional integrity of coronary endothelial cells but also on the performance of the whole heart. The metabolic consequences of hypoxia, ischemia, and reperfusion injury suggest that provision of specific nutrients may have a major influence on supporting the cardiac patient.

## GENERAL CONSIDERATIONS

The heart has often been considered to be protected from chronic protein-energy starvation. Undernutrition,

D. P. Katz: Department of Anesthesiology, Montefiore Medical Center and the Albert Einstein College of Medicine, Bronx, New York 10467.

S. Wiese and W. Gay: Department of Anesthesiology, Montefiore Medical Center and the Albert Einstein College of Medicine, Bronx, New York 10467.

however, also affects the myocardium, and nutritional support can prevent or partially reverse the heart disease associated with undernutrition. The undernourished state characteristic of severe heart disease is usually called cardiac cachexia (1). There are two types of cardiac cachexia; the *classic* type, which occurs in patients suffering from severe heart failure, and the *nosocomial* type, which develops in the postoperative state when complications develop, preventing a resumption of normal eating after surgery. One-third of patients with class III or IV heart disease have been found to suffer from cardiac cachexia (2). A study has estimated that 6% to 7% of patients in the surgical intensive care unit suffer from nosocomial cardiac cachexia (3). Approximately one-half of hospitalized patients suffering from both types of cardiac cachexia of the cardiac patients have been found to have some degree of undernutrition diagnosed by serum albumin and anthropometric measurements (4).

Patients with classic cardiac cachexia frequently complain of poor appetite, which is compounded by the prescription of unappealing diets. There may be drug-induced vitamin and mineral losses and often some degree of malabsorption. The body weight is frequently normal, but physical and biochemical examinations indicate chronic undernutrition. In nosocomial cardiac cachexia the preoperative nutritional status usually is adequate. The cachexia develops in days or weeks postoperatively because of complications; the intake is sharply reduced and nutrient losses are excessive. The cachexia often is clinically deceptive since many patients will appear to be normally nourished according to standard assessment techniques, despite severe depletion of lean body mass (LBM). If large amounts of carbohydrates but little or none of the other essential nutrients are infused, the glucose-induced insulin response prevents breakdown of adipose tissue without completely stopping lean tissue breakdown. Nutritional support is indicated when the underlying surgical complication cannot be corrected in 3 to 5 days.

It is clear that malnutrition results in a loss of cardiac mass and that nutritional repletion can restore cardiac tissue. However, the clinical implications and appropriate use of nutritional support in the pre- and postoperative patient have been poorly studied. A profound difference in mortality and morbidity has been found between patients with cardiac disease who suffered from preoperative malnutrition compared to patients of good nutritional status (5). It has been suggested that preoperative nutritional supplementation could reduce myocardial complications following surgery (6) and result in improved myocardial function (7).

Although some studies conclude that the undernutrition of cardiac cachexia can be at least partially corrected, the available reports about the beneficial effects of nutritional support on cardiac performance are incomplete, and further controlled studies are needed to resolve these questions. There are now specifically formulated enteral and parenteral feeding solutions available for treating cardiac cachexia. Minimal recommended therapy in the classic form of cardiac cachexia is vitamin and mineral replacement; some patients may benefit from complete nutritional supplements. Postoperative complications often lead to rapid depletion of LBM, and therefore, nutritional therapy using nutrient solutions enterally or parenterally is indicated in some instances.

## WHOLE-BODY EFFECTS OF SUBSTRATE ADMINISTRATION: IMPLICATIONS FOR THE CARDIOVASCULAR SYSTEM

Nutrient intake causes characteristic changes in the cardiorespiratory pattern that varies with diet composition, route of administration, caloric amount, and underlying disease. Following oral intake or parenteral administration of a macronutrient, typical changes in the respiratory profile include an increase in $VO_2$, $VCO_2$ and minute ventilation ($V_E$). The pulmonary adaptations are primarily due to an increase of both whole-body and myocardial oxygen consumption, associated with the cardiac effects, which follow nutrient intake (8). The postprandial elevation in whole-body oxygen consumption is accompanied by a series of cardiovascular alterations, such as an increase in the circulating blood flow in organs and peripheral tissues. It has been suggested that these cardiovascular changes primarily originate from hemodynamic alterations in the splanchnic organs, which require increased mesenteric blood flow (9). Hemodynamic changes in mesenteric blood flow have been found to be partly due to, and/or enhanced by, a group of hormones, such as vasoactive intestinal peptide (VIP), histamine, and some smaller extent prostaglandin (10). Pulmonary and whole-body hemodynamic alterations following oral nutrient intake require adaptations in cardiac performance. These include an increase in both heart rate and cardiac output associated with the increase in cardiac oxygen demand (8, 11).

Diet-induced thermogenesis [formally termed specific dynamic action (SDA)] peaks at 30 to 60 minutes after food intake and continues over a period of 3 to 8 hours (11). The mechanism for the effect is unknown; however, circulatory fuel transport, transmembrane transport of substrates, fuel storage, and enzymatic induction probably all contribute. There is evidence demonstrating that thermogenesis follows administration of all three macronutrients (fat, protein, carbohydrate) with the primary effect occurring with amino acid administration. Nonprotein caloric loads (particularly glucose) that exceed energy expenditure enhance the response (12), presumably related to the need for storage. Moreover, measurements of the plasma concentration of catecholamines have shown that increased activity of the sympathetic nervous system accompanies excess caloric ingestion, and this may also play a role as a mediator of the response (13, 14).

The principal alterations in cardiac performance due to the pulmonary and hemodynamic adaptations following ingestion of substrates are comparable in healthy subjects and patients with varying degrees of heart failure (15). However, an abnormal cardiovascular response to feeding might occur, when a small noncompliant ventricle (i.e., in hypertrophic cardiomyopathy) fails to dilate with increased preload, and is unable to enhance an already supranormal ejection fraction (16).

To the extent substrate provision occurs via continuous enteral or parenteral substrate supply, rather than intermittent bolus administration, the patients may be subjected to fewer hemodynamic perturbations.. Furthermore, the cardiovascular effects of food intake in cardiac patients should be considered when interpreting hemodynamic data (17).

## FUEL UTILIZATION IN ALTERED MYOCARDIAL STATES

### Aerobic Versus Anaerobic Metabolism

In the well-oxygenated heart, free fatty acids (FFAs), lactate, and glucose are the preferred fuels that are converted to the energy required to maintain transmembrane potential as well as contractile function (i.e., energy-dependent ion pumps). Long-chain FFAs are usually the major cardiac fuel, activated to acyl CoA and then to acyl carnitine, which enters the pathway of beta oxidation. Under conditions of elevated blood lactate concentration, i.e., due to acute exercise, lactate becomes the major myocardial source of energy, whereas following a large ingestion of carbohydrates, glucose is the major fuel. Under aerobic conditions, the rate of the individual oxidative fuel utilization via the Krebs cycle is partly related to the arterial substrate concentration.

Under ischemic conditions, the amount of available oxygen is limited to support fuel utilization in the citric acid (Krebs) cycle and energy generation (i.e., ATP). The lack of oxygen is known to cause a reduction in fatty acid oxidation, and a greater proportion of ATP production is derived from anaerobic glucose utilization (18, 19). Pulse-labeling experiments have indicated that during oxygen deficiency, fatty acids are diverted from beta oxidation to deposition as tissue triglycerides (20). In CAD patients at rest, myocardial uptake of fatty acids was found to be 50% lower than in control subjects, with an additional decrease of fatty acid uptake during pacing (21), whereas glucose uptake was twice as high, reflecting the severalfold increase in anaerobic glycolysis.

In the isolated rat heart, it has been demonstrated that altering the rate of glycolytic flux from glucose may

delay or even prevent ischemic contracture (22). Only a minimal amount of glycolytic ATP from glucose is required to maintain internal calcium homeostasis through $Ca^{2+}$ uptake into the sarcoplasmic reticulum (23) or $Ca^{2+}$ extrusion by several ion pumps (24). However, it is worth keeping in mind that glucose utilization may be dependent on the availability of calcium. This suggestion is supported by data demonstrating that an increase in glucose and lactate utilization by 50% and 30%, respectively, has occurred when $Ca^{2+}$ was added to a physiologic medium containing isolated noncontracting adult rat heart myocytes, without any changes in palmitate oxidation (25). Similarly, the addition of magnesium to a cardioplegic solution improved myocardial preservation (26) and clinical outcome in both experimental animals and clinical studies (27).

By measuring high-energy phosphates (i.e., ATP, creatine phosphate), oxygen consumption, as well as ventricular performance in hearts under conditions of coronary low-flow ischemia, cardiac efficiency (the ratio between ventricular work and oxygen consumption) appeared to be greater when substrate utilization was switched from fatty acids to glucose (28). Quantitative analysis of the contribution of glucose and fatty acid utilization to overall oxidative metabolism in ischemic myocardium indicates that glucose constituted up to 70% of the substrate oxidized (29) (Fig. 1). The required glucose can be

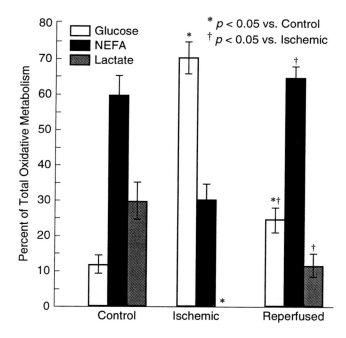

**FIG. 1.** In open-chest, anesthetized dogs, the contribution of nonesterified fatty acid (NEFA), glucose, and lactate to total oxidative metabolism is calculated. Glucose utilization is increased in the reperfused myocardium, but its contribution to total energy production is less than 30%. From Goerge G, et al. *Circ Res* 1991;68:1681, with permission.

derived from cellular uptake as well as from the breakdown of glycogen. Glycogen contributes to the flow of glucose through glycolysis, mainly during the acute onset of ischemia and/or hypoxemia, or during cyclic adenosine monophosphate (cAMP) mediated intense myocardial work (30).

However, even global ischemia appears to be a nonhomogeneous phenomenon (31), and some intercapillary areas may be more vulnerable to oxygen deficiency than others (32). Therefore, fatty acids and glucose may have variable effects in different cardiac areas during states of oxygen deficiency, particularly when one considers that the myocardium may be able to downregulate regional energy requirements as a function of the severity of ischemia (33).

## Metabolic Difference Between Hypoxia and Ischemia

A number of profound differences exist between hypoxia and ischemia. Hypoxia or anoxia are defined as states of low or respectively no oxygen tension with maintained coronary blood flow. Whereas oxygen deficiency due to ischemia is most commonly caused by a reduction or absence of coronary blood flow. Hence, ischemia, but not hypoxemia, may be accompanied by a collapse of the coronary vasculature with a loss of the contractile property. In severe ischemia, the concentration of lactic acid increases and the intracellular pH falls rapidly due to the accumulation of the acidic by-products of anaerobic glycolysis (34, 35). In contrast, under hypoxic and anoxic conditions, the maintained coronary blood flow may result in a washout of acid products of anaerobic glycolysis, thereby retarding the development of intracellular acidosis. Lowering the intracellular pH is accompanied by an inhibition of the glycolytic flux partly due to the depressed activity of phosphofructokinase, a key enzyme in the glycolytic chain, and further to the decreased phosphorylation of glucose through accumulation of glucose-6-phosphate. Thus, the glycolytic rate in the ischemic heart is about one-fourth that of the anoxic heart in a steady state, thereby providing less energy to the ischemic than to the anoxic heart.

An increase in the concentration of the intracellular calcium ion ($[Ca^{2+}]_i$) has been proposed as an explanation for the pathologic alterations that occur during ischemia/reperfusion (36). During hypoxia in the isolated heart, the intracellular ionized calcium content paralleled the increase in left ventricular (LV) diastolic pressure, while the decrease in LV systolic pressure approximated that of the control, whereas during ischemia there is a rapid fall in both LV systolic and diastolic pressure accompanied by a substantial increase in $[Ca^{2+}]_i$, indicating a desensitization of the contractile apparatus to intracellular ionized calcium (37, 38).

## Alterations During Postischemic Reperfusion

Postischemic reperfusion injury presents a complex cardiac syndrome that may include arrhythmias and contractile dysfunction as well as structural and functional changes in coronary endothelial cells resulting in a progressive decrease in microcirculatory flow (coronary *no-reflow* phenomenon). Factors determining the extent of injuries are related to both the duration and severity of ischemia as well as to the method of reperfusion (39). Glucose-loaded isolated rat hearts maintain a normal cAMP level during global ischemia and, when reperfused with a similar solution high in glucose, demonstrate a low lactate dehydrogenase (LDH) release, few arrhythmias, and a high rate of ATP regeneration (40) (Fig. 2). On the other hand, perfusion of hearts with palmitate or acetate led to a marked fall in the ATP synthesis and an acceleration of cAMP at the end of ischemia, with greatest release of LDH and most severe ventricular arrhythmias during reperfusion. An elevated content of cAMP has been linked to arrhythmogenesis through stimulation of endogenous lipolysis (41) and to high levels of intracellular cal-

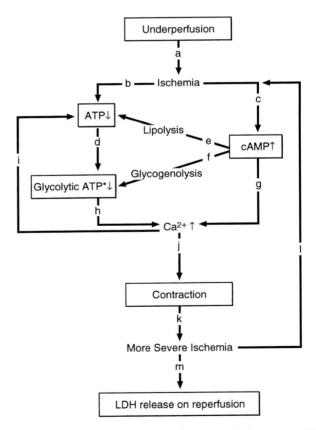

**FIG. 2.** A hypothetical scheme of events which may explain the release of enzymes during reperfusion. From Barlow CH, et al. *Science* 1976;193:909. With permission.

cium (42) that may uncouple electrical continuity with subsequent ventricular fibrillation (43). Fatty acids as the sole substrate during ischemia and reperfusion may worsen contractility and increase oxygen consumption/ unit work during reperfusion compared with glucose alone (44) (Fig. 3). On the other hand, in a study where both glucose and fatty acids were available in a perfusion buffer, the postischemic reperfused myocardium used fatty acids preferentially as substrate that provided over 90% of the ATP produced from exogenous substrates (45). Measuring $^{14}CO_2$ from both labeled glucose and fatty acids metabolized during ischemia and reperfusion has supported the concept of a competitive inhibition of glucose and/or its intermediates by the preferred utilization of fatty acids during reperfusion (46, 47). The experimental data provide evidence suggesting that the normal substrate pattern for oxidative metabolism may be restored within 30 minutes of myocardial reperfusion (45–47). Thus, during ischemia and early reperfusion, glycolysis seems to be enhanced (48) whereas fatty acid utilization is transiently depressed. When one considers the syndrome of reversibly "stunned" myocardium and hearts with signs of irreversible injury, there seems to be a pronounced dissociation of both oxidative glucose and fatty acid metabolism and contractile function in the reperfused myocardium (20).

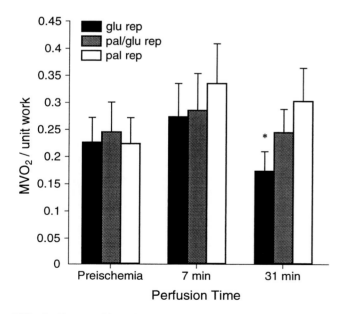

**FIG. 3.** Fatty acid and glucose metabolism in the isolated reperfused rabbit heart after 20 minutes of ischemia. Myocardial oxygen consumption (MVO2) is calculated per unit of cardiac work (micromoles oxygen per minute per rate/pressure product) for glucose (glu) and palmitate (pal). *$p < 0.05$ compared with palmitate. From Rovetto MJ, et al. *Circ Res* 1973;32:699, with permission.

## BRANCHED-CHAIN AMINO ACIDS

### Cardiac Metabolism

Several studies have demonstrated the unique character of the branched-chain amino acids (BCAAs) leucine, isoleucine, and valine on human metabolism (49–52). The BCAAs are conditionally essential amino acids that have multiple metabolic effects, which includes the regulation of protein turnover in muscle (53, 54), insulin secretion (55), release of alanine and glutamine by muscle, and gluconeogenesis (56). Their branched structure may confer special properties to proteins, altering the hydrophobic character of the molecule. The BCAAs make up about 40% of the essential amino acid carbon requirements in mammals and about 35% of the essential amino acid content of muscle protein.

Uptake of BCAAs by the myocardium is thought to be energy independent and carrier mediated, corresponding to the L-system transporter (57). The rapid entry of BCAAs yields nearly identical concentrations in muscle cytosol with that in the plasma or experimentally in the perfusate (58). Initially, the BCAAs are reversibly transaminated by the enzyme branched-chain oxo-acid transaminase, followed by an irreversible oxidative decarboxylation catalyzed by the enzyme branched-chain 2-oxo-acid dehydrogenase (BCOAD). The activity of BCOAD, localized to the inner mitochondrial membrane and considered to be the rate-limiting step in the oxidation of BCAAs, appears to be regulated by a reversible phosphorylation (59). The phosphorylation state of BCOAD is not only influenced by a specific kinase and phosphatas (60, 61) but also may be affected by the concentration of the branched-chain ketoacids (BCKAs) themselves. Thus, an increased availability of BCKAs can stimulate its utilization by the heart (62).

### Protective Impact of BCAAs on the Ischemic/Reperfused Myocardium

There are a number of studies demonstrating the beneficial biochemical and hemodynamic effects of BCAAs on myocardial ischemia/reperfusion injury. Perfusion with a 3.5-mM BCAA-enriched buffer markedly delayed the initiation of ischemic contracture and improved postischemic hemodynamic recovery of isolated reperfused rat hearts (63) (Fig. 4). The mechanism of BCAA-enhanced cardiac recovery has been hypothesized to be due to a smaller depletion of ATP during ischemia and a more rapid normalization of intracellular pH on reperfusion (Fig. 5).

The most striking effects of BCAAs have been demonstrated when these amino acids have been added to a glucose-containing oxygenated crystalloid cardioplegic solution, which significantly improved myocardial protection during global ischemia in energy-depleted rat hearts (64). The more rapid recovery of oxygen con-

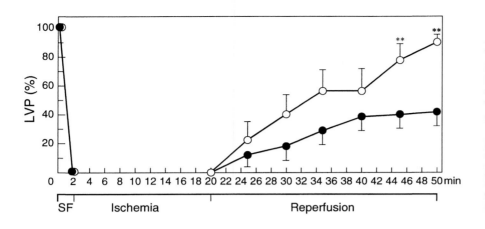

**FIG. 4.** Effects of branched-chain amino acids (BCAAs) in isolated perfused rat hearts. After 15 minutes of preischemic perfusion, left ventricular peak systolic pressure (LVP) is measured during 2 minutes of substrate free perfusion (SF), 18 minutes of global ischemia, and 30 minutes of reperfusion. Results are expressed as percentage of preischemic pressure (mean ± SD). (●-●) Krebs-Henseleit perfusion with 11.1 mM glucose; (○-○) Krebs-Henseleit perfusion + 11.1 mM glucose + 3.5 mM BCAA. **$p < 0.01$. From Buse MG, et al. *J Clin Invest* 1975;56:1250, with permission.

sumption in the BCAA hearts on reperfusion has been assumed to reflect an accelerated regeneration of high-energy phosphates (e.g., ATP and creatine phosphate) and an improved sarcolemmal integrity in the cardiac myocytes. Moreover, the BCAA-enriched oxygenated cardioplegic solution may offer an increase in tissue levels of amino acids and citric acid cycle intermediates that can become depressed during oxygen deficiency (65).

## Anabolic Effects of BCAA on Heart Muscle Protein Turnover

The importance of BCAAs on cardiac protein metabolism has been demonstrated by their ability to stimulate

protein synthesis, partly, in a dose-related fashion. Under conditions of negative protein balance in both animal and human hearts, there is an accelerated uptake of both BCAAs and their ketoacid conjugates in relation to their circulating concentration, as compared to the uptake of other essential amino acids (66, 67). (Fig. 6). In the postabsorptive state, most of the BCAAs removed by the heart are incorporated into muscle protein. The balance, as well as up to 30% of exogenously administered BCAAs, especially leucine, is directed toward oxidation and generation of ketoacid derivatives (68). However,

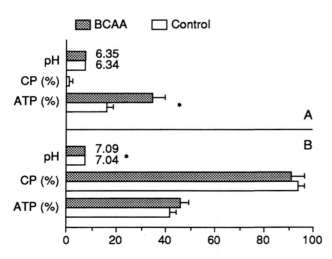

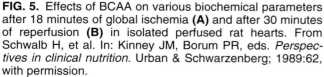

**FIG. 5.** Effects of BCAA on various biochemical parameters after 18 minutes of global ischemia **(A)** and after 30 minutes of reperfusion **(B)** in isolated perfused rat hearts. From Schwalb H, et al. In: Kinney JM, Borum PR, eds. *Perspectives in clinical nutrition.* Urban & Schwarzenberg; 1989:62, with permission.

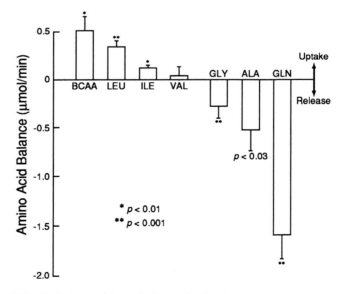

**FIG. 6.** Amino acid net balance in the basal state of dogs. Degrees of significance reflect differences in the arterial/coronary sinus concentrations of the amino acid: BCAA, branched-chain amino acid; LEU, leucine; ILE, isoleucine; VAL, valine; GLY, glycine; ALA, alanine; GLN, glutamine. From Goldberg AL, et al. *Fed Proc* 1978;37:2301, with permission.

measurements of the utilization of amino acids in normal hearts have demonstrated that amino acid oxidation accounts for only about 5% of the myocardial oxygen consumption (69, 70).

The BCAAs are thought to stimulate protein synthesis by enhancing peptide-chain initiation and elongation while inhibiting protein degradation (71). Generally, the anabolic effect of BCAAs on myocardial protein turnover, in vivo, seems to be dependent on conditions of its severalfold elevated plasma concentrations (e.g., about 5 times) which was shown in both fed and fasted rodents (62, 72). In states of enhanced energy requirements (e.g., in the working heart preparation) or during administration of competing substrates, even elevated leucine concentrations may only exert a minor effect on positive nitrogen balance (62). To date, there is considerable evidence confirming that plasma insulin may act supplementary with BCAAs to stimulate muscle protein synthesis (73, 74).

## GLUTAMATE AND ASPARTATE

### Cardioprotective Effects During Ischemia and Reperfusion

In both animal and human studies, supply of the nonessential amino acids glutamate and aspartate has been shown to exert cardioprotective effects during ischemia and following reperfusion (Fig. 7). Experimentally, when isolated hearts were subjected to cardioplegic ischemic arrest for 8 hours, provision of glutamate to the cold crystalloid potassium cardioplegic solution was found to improve cardiac performance on reperfusion, as indicated by an increase in global cardiac oxygen consumption, decreased lactate production, and less myocardial edema as compared to controls (75).

The cardioprotective properties of glutamate during ischemia and reperfusion may be enhanced by the addition of aspartate. When both amino acids were added to a blood cardioplegic solution in a setting of prolonged aortic cross-clamping in animal hearts, the functional recovery of oxygen uptake and cardiac function was almost complete (76). Additional evidence suggesting the utility of glutamate and aspartate supplementation for postischemic reperfusion injury (including coronary thrombolysis or angioplasty and cardiopulmonary bypass surgery) has been provided by a study which demonstrated that the supply of both amino acids reduced the myocardial infarct size from 60% to 37% experimentally in pigs by determining the area at risk (77).

Human studies have indicated that myocardial uptake of glutamate is accelerated in patients with (CAD) (21). In patients with stable angina, intravenous supplementation of glutamate (between 1.2 and 2.5 mg/kg body weight) was accompanied by an objectively improved stress test

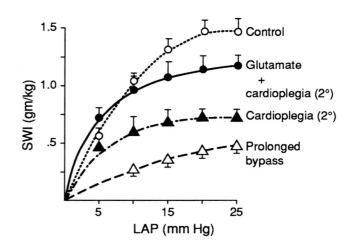

**FIG. 7.** Recovery of left ventricular performance after 45 minutes of normothermic arrest (clamping of the aorta) in dogs. Controls (no ischemia). L-Glutamate-enriched blood cardioplegia contained 0.026 M L-glutamate. During prolonged bypass in one group of dogs, the hearts were kept in the beating empty state. SWI, stroke work index; LAP, left atrial pressure. From Lazar HL, et al. *J Thorac Cardiovasc Surg* 1980;80:350, with permission.

(78). Moreover, inotropic properties were demonstrated during administration of intravenous glutamate (0.014 to 0.025 mmol/min/kg body weight) to patients with low cardiac output syndrome following open-heart surgery. After 15 minutes of glutamate infusion, an increase in both cardiac and stroke indices and a decrease in systemic vascular resistance were observed (79).

### Mechanism of Action of Glutamate and Aspartate

To date, the mechanism of action of both glutamate and aspartate remains to be defined. Glutamic acid seems to be involved in the binding of free ammonia, which can accumulate during ischemia, further inhibiting the activity of the citric acid cycle (79). In addition, glutamate taken up by the myocardium may diminish lactate accumulation during anaerobic glycolysis. The biochemical rationale suggests that less lactate may be generated from pyruvate when pyruvate is converted to alanine by transamination via glutamate (21). Moreover, glutamate may contribute to the anaerobic generation of ATP via substrate-level phosphorylation, which is independent of glycolysis. It must be considered that 1 mol ATP can be gained by the deamination of glutamate to the citric acid cycle intermediate $\alpha$-ketoglutarate and its subsequent anaerobic oxidation to succinate (80). Furthermore, glutamate and aspartate participate in the malate-aspartate shuttle that appears to affect cytosolic and mitochondrial energy metabolism, by regulating the mitochondrial redox potential (NAD/NADH ratio). Finally, during the metabolism of aspartate to malate, NADH is oxidized to nicotinamide-adenine dinucleotide (NAD) that may enter into the cytoplasm, promoting anaerobic ATP generation via glycolysis. The numerous possible mechanisms of action of both glutamate and aspartate may offer considerable evidence of their benefit, primarily by improving the altered glucose and fatty acid metabolism in the ischemic and reperfused heart.

## ADENOSINE

### Metabolic Link Between Oxygen Supply and Demand

The growing knowledge of hemodynamic and metabolic effects of adenosine, endogenously generated from the hydrolysis of homocysteine or the breakdown of cellular ATP, has suggested the potential importance of this component for maintaining energy metabolism. In the isolated working rat heart, the impact of supplied adenosine on myocardial substrate use was confirmed by an enhanced efficiency of energy generation. Glucose oxidation was found to be increased, while the reduction in glucose flux probably decreased lactate and hydrogen accumulation without affecting fatty acid oxidation (81). As a metabolic link between oxygen supply and demand, supplementation of adenosine may cause vasodilation in most vascular beds (e.g., skeletal muscle, heart, skin, brain, intestine, etc.). Under physiologic condition in humans, central venous administration of adenosine in amounts of 40 to 80 μg/min/kg body weight was found to cause a dose-related drop in systemic vascular resistance (to less than 50% of baseline), accompanied by a stimulation of the sympathetic nervous system activity (noradrenaline by 62%, adrenaline by 42%) (82). The enhanced cardiac output as well as the gradual increase of both the systolic and pulse pressure amplitude appeared to keep the mean arterial pressure almost stabilized. Generally, the duration of the vasodilative properties of adenosine is brief (5 to 30 seconds) and is found to occur in a dose-response fashion (Fig. 8) (83).

### Impact of Adenosine on Cardiac Performance During States of Oxygen Deficiency

In dogs, it has been demonstrated that intracoronary adenosine and adenosine deaminase attenuate ventricular arrhythmias caused by intracoronary norepinephrine (84). This outcome may indicate that intracoronary administration of norepinephrine, known to be accompanied by a myocardial oxygen demand exceeding oxygen supply, activates the endogenous adenosine cascade (85). During experimental regional ischemia, an accelerated concentration of adenosine can be shown in the cardiac interstitial fluid (86). It has been suggested that interstitial adenosine is linked to both cytosolic metabolism and the regulation of coronary vascular resistance (87) and, thus, may aid in

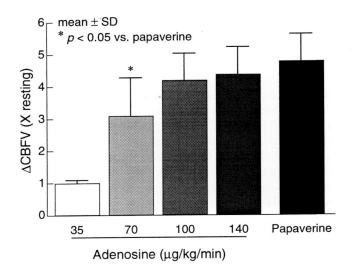

**FIG. 8.** The bar graph demonstrates changes in coronary blood flow velocity during intravenous adenosine infusion and after intracoronary papaverine in humans. From Frexes-Steed M, et al. *Am J Physiol* 1990;258:E907, with permission.

the metabolic recovery of the ischemic/reperfused myocardium (88). Therefore, it was hypothesized that exogenous supply of adenosine might be beneficial in reducing postischemic reperfusion injury, e.g., after thrombolytic therapy, myocardial infarction, cardiopulmonary bypass surgery, or coronary angioplasty (89, 90).

Preexisting coronary atherosclerosis has been postulated to limit the endothelium-dependent vasodilation of adenosine. In patients with CAD, adenosine intracoronary supplied in amounts up to 2.2 mg/min failed to demonstrate a marked vasodilation, despite an accelerated coronary blood flow (91). Supplying adenosine intracoronary in amounts greater than those responsible for maximal coronary vasodilation may provoke angina-like chest pain. The fact that the chest pain has occurred without evidence of ischemia in the electrocardiogram supported the speculation that it is probably mediated by affecting the adenosine $P_1$-receptor (92). However, the available data concerning the circulatory properties as well as the metabolic effects (e.g., antilipolytic, glycolytic) of adenosine seem to be variable, at least with respect to dose, mode, and the experimental population (93).

## OMEGA-3 FATTY ACIDS

### Anti-inflammatory and Cardiovascular Effects of *n*-3 Fatty Acids

Since the original epidemiologic observations of the health effects of *n*-3 fatty acids in Greenland Eskimos

(94), there has been progress in our understanding of their possible health benefits. It appears that the long-chain polyunsaturated n-3 fatty acids (n-3 PUFA) found in fatty fish and fish oil have beneficial effects on the cardiovascular system, in part due to their anti-inflammatory properties (95, 96). Supplement of n-3 PUFAs, at high levels of dietary intake, may affect not only plasma levels of lipids and lipoproteins that are tightly associated with the rate and severity of atherosclerosis but also thrombosis and myocardial ischemia and infarction (97, 98). The additional cardiovascular effects of "fish oils" may include the following:

1. An increase of the deformability of red blood cells, thereby improving the oxygen supply to myocardial tissue nourished by narrowed coronary vessels (99);
2. An elevation in tissue plasminogen activator and reduction in levels of inhibitors of plasminogen activator, thereby modulating the endogenous fibrinolytic activity (100);
3. A depression of the vasospastic response to catecholamines and probably to angiotensin (101); and
4. Lowering arterial blood pressure in normotensive subjects and patients with mild hypertension (102).

The interaction of platelets and the coronary endothelial vessel wall is consistent with the modern concept of the pathogenesis of atherosclerosis and acute coronary ischemic syndromes, such as unstable angina pectoris, myocardial infarction, and sudden cardiac death (103, 104). The regulation of platelet–vessel wall interaction is influenced by homeostasis between the arachidonic acid (AA) metabolites thromboxane $A_2$ (TXA$_2$), which has platelet proaggregatory and vasoconstrictory properties (105), and prostacyclin (PGI$_2$), formed primarily by the endothelium, having vasodilative effects and inhibiting platelet aggregation (106).

The rate of formation of TXA$_2$ (half-life 30 seconds) and its counteracting PGI$_2$ (half-life 3 minutes) from n-6 polyunsaturated fatty acids (n-6 PUFAs) may be altered by dietary supplementation with n-3 PUFAs. Convincing evidence from dietary studies have demonstrated that the inclusion of n-3 PUFA from seafood (fish oils) may progressively reduce the AA content in platelets. This effectively dilutes the TXA$_2$ precursor pool and may increase the content of the n-3 PUFA metabolites eicosapentaenoic acid (EPA) and docosahexaenoic acid (DHA) in the phospholipid pools of the endothelium (107, 108). Furthermore, PGI$_3$ generated from EPA has antiaggregatory properties, without affecting significantly the PGI$_2$ production from AA (109), whereas the form of thromboxane, derived from n-3 PUFA, thromboxane A$_3$ (TXA$_3$) only exerts very weak aggregatory effects but also decreases the aggregatory effects of TXA$_2$ by competitively binding to TXA$_2$ receptors on platelets.

Additionally, n-3 and n-6 PUFAs are utilized by the 5-lipoxygenase pathway, which leads to the production of leukotriene B$_4$ (LTB$_4$) and leukotriene B$_5$ (LTB$_5$) (110). The LTB$_5$, derived from n-3 PUFAs, is only one-tenth as potent as leukotriene B$_4$, generated from n-6 PUFAs, as assessed by effects on chemotaxis, adherence and aggregation of platelets, monocytes, and macrophages, and attenuating certain inflammatory responses. Additionally, DHA is considered to be a poor substrate for the lipoxygenase pathway and may inhibit the conversion of AA to LTB$_4$, thereby downregulating leukotriene synthesis (111). Thus, administration of dietary fish oils may be accompanied by a reduction of TXA$_2$ and LTB$_4$ synthesis, while prostacyclin formation (PGI$_2$ and PGI$_3$) will be enhanced (112). Considering the rheologic and antihypertensive properties of n-3 PUFAs, the favorable shift in the prostacyclin/thromboxane balance through supplementation of fish oils in endothelial cells and platelets may play a significant role in reducing myocardial ischemia and infarction (95, 113).

## Impact of n-3 Fatty Acids on Myocardial Ischemic Syndromes

The potential role of n-3 fatty acids in cardiovascular disease may be viewed in influencing coronary vascular tone, platelet activation, and atherogenesis (114). The assumption is consistent with current evidence suggesting that the pathophysiology of acute myocardial ischemic syndromes, including unstable angina and myocardial infarction, consists of reduced coronary blood flow, damaged endothelium, and platelet recruitment and thrombosis (110). Dietary fish oil supplementation may have clinical benefit in terms of secondary prevention of coronary heart disease (115). Experimentally in animals, supplementation of dietary fish oil has been demonstrated to exert direct effects on the integrity of endothelial cells, most likely by affecting patterns of eicosanoid generation (116). When animals fed with cod-liver or fish oils were subjected to ischemic stress, an improved integrity of the endothelium has been suggested by an enhanced release of endothelium-derived relaxing factors (EDRFs) over controls, thereby facilitating vasodilation in arteries and in resistance vessels (117). Furthermore, animals fed fish oils produce less platelet-derived growth factor (PDGF)-like protein in endothelial cells (118). It is well established that release of PDGF is followed by stimulation, migration, and proliferation of smooth muscle cells, fibroblasts, and macrophages in the arterial wall.

Ischemia and subsequent reperfusion are known to trigger a sequence of metabolic and biochemical changes in myocytes which may be modulated through dietary administration of n-3 fatty acids (119). In an experimental setting of coronary artery occlusion and subsequent reperfusion, feeding rats a diet supplemented with tuna fish oil, which causes an increased concentration of n-3 fatty acids in phospholipids of cardiac tissue, reduced the incidence and severity of reperfusion arrhythmias (120). This finding is supported by data demonstrating that an increment of *n*-3/*n*-6 fatty acids in the phospholipid fraction of cardiac sarcoplasmic reticulum may be cardioprotective (121), partly by modulating the $Ca^{2+}$-$Mg^{2+}$ATPase activity and by improving intracellular calcium homeostasis (122). Furthermore, in studies with adult monkeys fed dietary fish oil for several months the susceptability of the hearts to generate arrhythmias has been found to be lowered when subjected to ischemic conditions (123). Similarly, in animal experiments using ligation of a coronary artery, the amount of myocardial necrosis was significantly lowered in the group fed fish oil over controls (124). However, the large quantities of fish oils often used in animal studies are unlikely to be consumed by humans (119).

## SUBSTRATE METABOLISM IN CORONARY ARTERY ENDOTHELIAL CELLS

### Function of the Coronary Endothelium

The endothelial cells of coronary arteries perform a series of specific physiologic functions including the regulation of the vascular tone, transport of substrates, and acting as a selective permeability barrier (125). The considerable importance of the endothelium in states of oxygen deficiency is demonstrated by its potential to affect coronary blood flow by modulating the vascular tone of coronary resistance arteries (126). Endothelial cells are a source of the physiologically important EDRF nitric oxid (127) that is synthesized from the amino acid L-arginine (128). Stimulated release of nitric oxide through serotonin or the alpha-adrenergic agonist clonidine has been shown to cause endothelium-dependent relaxation in the coronary arterie (129, 130). However, modulation of coronary blood flow may be impaired by an abnormality of the endothelial function. This consideration was taken into account when normal coronary angiograms were found in patients with symptoms of angina pectoris (131). Thus, one can conclude that the nature of myocardial ischemia may be viewed as an interplay between local reactivity of coronary arteries, acute plaque disruption, as well as a disproportion of supply and demand, mainly of both oxygen and fuels (132).

### Energy and Oxygen Demand of the Coronary Endothelial Cells

In various studies there is disagreement regarding the tolerance of the coronary endothelium to oxygen deficiency, which may in part be due to the different metabolic consequences of hypoxemia and ischemia. In general, both oxygen and energy demands of coronary artery endothelial cells have been estimated to be low compared with the beating myocardium. For example, energy turnover in the myocardium at a low to moderate work load may be up to 10 times greater, i.e., 200 to 400 nmol ATP/min/mg protein, than in the coronary endothelial cells (133). In the presence of glucose, the energetic state of cultured coronary endothelial cells from rats has been shown to remain stable when the oxygen pressure was decreased from 100 to less than 0.1 torr (116). Both aerobic and anaerobic glycolysis appear to play a major role in energy generation during hypoxia. Only the presence of glucose prevented a marked degradation of myocardial ATP and a release of adenosine from endothelial cells during 3 hours of hypoxia (2 to 12 mm Hg (134). Whereas at $PO_2$ levels less than 3 torr the presence of palmitate and glutamine did not prevent a rapid decline in the adenine nucleotide content (133).

### Effect of Hypoxia and Ischemia/Reperfusion on the Coronary Endothelium

There is experimental evidence suggesting that endothelial cells are less susceptible to hypoxic damage than the myocardium. For example, anoxic perfusion of pig hearts followed by normoxic reperfusion has been shown to cause a less severe injury in coronary endothelium than in cardiomyocytes, independent of the presence of glucose (135). In contrast to conditions of hypoxemia, there are several findings that suggest that the vascular endothelial cells are the primary site of ischemia/reperfusion injury in the heart (136). Brief periods of coronary no flow could induce postischemic microvascular dysfunction reflected by a prolonged increase in the resting vascular resistance and by an impairment in the vasodilator responsiveness (137). Morphologic ultrastructural evidence of microvascular damage appears to lag behind myocardial cell injury (138). Severe ischemia in the endothelium is known to result in a rapid shift from aerobic to anaerobic metabolism, followed within minutes by a depletion of high-energy phosphates (e.g., ATP, creatine phosphate) and the accumulation of lactate, protons, ADP, and inorganic phosphates (139). The cascade of intracellular acidosis, inactivation of ion pumps, calcium overload, and stimulation of endogenous phospholipase is proposed to contribute to membrane disruption (140, 141). In addition, the generation of xanthine oxidase in animals during ischemia may lead to the generation of superoxide free radicals, presumed to act as a neutrophil chemoreactant (142, 143).

As is the case during hypoxemia, glycolysis appears to be beneficial to coronary arteries during both moderate ischemia caused by prolonged underperfusion in isolated rabbit hearts and subsequent reperfusion. Supplementation of increased glycolytic substrates (e.g., glucose and insulin) has been demonstrated to be accompanied by a decrease in coronary resistance and an enhanced coronary blood flow (144). The mechanism of action responsible for the improved cardiac performance observed has been hypothesized to be due to the combined effects of (a) increased ATP synthesis, (b) esterification of intracellular FFAs, (c) replenishment of potassium ions in the endothelium (145), and (d) a mechanism of scavenging free radicals (146). However, several findings support the view that postischemic myocardial dysfunction is not exclusively based on a limited ATP availability. Obviously, alterations of the intracellular environment, such as accumulation of inorganic phosphate and variations in pH levels (147), may all contribute to a less efficient energy utilization in all cardiac cells (148).

## An Approach for Nutritional Therapy on Endothelial Cells

Presently, there are only limited data illustrating the substrate utilization and the energy generation in coronary endothelial cells during pathophysiologic conditions. However, few investigations have demonstrated the possible benefits of nutritional therapy on the endothelium. Arginine, as previously discussed, is known to be a source of the EDRF nitric oxide (128). The cardioprotective effects of dietary supplementation of arginine were studied in isolated perfused rat hearts. Four weeks of a 5% arginine-enriched enteral diet caused a beneficial impact on both the coronary endothelium, by preserving the EDRF levels, and the myocardium, by reducing the loss of creatine kinase activity in the ischemic and reperfused heart (149).

Furthermore, the endothelium is considered to belong morphologically to the cell population of dividing cells. Especially in dividing and activated cells with an extremely high metabolic requirement, several in vitro and in vivo studies have pointed out a beneficial impact of specific nutrients, such as ribose or glutamine (150–153). The five-carbon sugar ribose may provide precursor substances for the nucleotide synthesis via the hexosemonophosphate shunt that is known to be activated in cells involved in tissue repair (152). However, it still remains to be determined if these experimental findings have a clinical impact.

## SUMMARY

Investigations of the mechanisms that modulate energy generation during states of altered cardiac metabolism reach a point where there is both need and demand for novel approaches. The evidence discussed herein strongly suggests that both energy generation and utilization in these states may be effectively strengthened by nutritional manipulation. Compared with standard treatments for ischemia/reperfusion injury or cardiac failure, nutritional therapy may present an important and less toxic approach,

by affecting the mechanisms of energy utilization during compromised cardiac states. The use of traditional energy substrates, in conjunction with those that may be conditionally important during compromised cardiac states, potentially offers a useful therapeutic modality in the treatment of the critically ill cardiac patient.

## REFERENCES

1. Pittman JG, Cohen P. The pathogenesis of cardiac cachexia. *N Engl J Med* 1964;271:403.
2. Heymsfield SB, Blieier J, Wenger N. Detection of protein calorie undernutrition in advanced heart disease. *Circulation* 1977;56(Suppl III):102.
3. Abel RM. Parenteral nutrition for patients with severe cardiac illness. In: Greep JM, Soeters PB, Wesddorp RIC, et al., eds. *Current Concepts in Parenteral Nutrition.* The Hague: Martinus Hijnoff Medical Division; 1977:147.
4. Blackburn GL, Gibbons GW, Bothe A, et al. Nutrition support in cardiac cachexia. *J Thorac Cardiovasc Surg* 1977;73:480.
5. Abel RM, Fischer JE, Buckley MJ, et al. Malnutrition in cardiac surgical patients: results of a prospective randomized evaluation of early total parenteral nutrition (TPN). *Arch Surg* 1976;111:45.
6. Lolley DM, Myers WO, Roy JR, et al. Clinical experience with preoperative myocardial nutrition management. *J Cardiovasc Surg* 1985;26:236.
7. Heymsfield SB, Bether RA, Ansley JD, et al. Cardiac abnormalities in cachectic patients before and during nutritional repletion. *Am Heart J* 1978;95:584.
8. Bagatell CJ, Heymsfield SB. Effect of meal size on myocardial oxygen requirements: implications for post-myocardial infarction diet. *Am J Clin Nutr* 1984;39:421.
9. Kelbaek H, Munck O, Christensen NJ, Godfredsen J. Central hemodynamic changes after a meal. *Br Heart J* 1989;61:506.
10. Stebbins CL, Theodossy SJ, Longhurst JC. Cardiovascular reflexes evoked by histamine stimulation of the stomach. *Am J Physiol* 1991;260:H1098.
11. Fogan TC, Sawyer PR, Gourley LA, Lee JT, Gaffney TE. Postprandial alterations in hemodynamics and blood pressure in normal subjects. *Am J Cardiol* 1986;58:636.
12. Gil K, Gump FE, Starker PM, Askanazi J, Elwyn DH, Kinney JM. Splanchnic substrate balance in malnourished patients during parenteral nutrition. *Am J Physiol* 1985;248:E409.
13. Welle S, Lilavivathana U, Campbell RG. Increased plasma norepinephrine concentrations and metabolic rates following glucose ingestion in man. *Metabolism* 1980;29:806.
14. Heymsfield SB, Hill JO, Evert M, Casper K, DiGirolamo M. Energy expenditure during continuous intragastric infusion of fuel. *Am J Clin Nutr* 1987;45:526.
15. Herrlin B, Sylven C, Nyquist O, Edhag O. Short term hemodynamic effects of converting enzyme inhibition before and after eating in patients with moderate heart failure caused by dilated cardiomyopathy: a double blind study. *Br Heart J* 1990;63:26.
16. Gilligan DM, Chan WL, Oakley CM. Effects of a meal on hemodynamic function at rest and during exercise in patients with hypertrophic cardiomyopathy. *J Am Coll Cardiol* 1991;18:429.
17. Jarvis RC, Green JA, Nara AR, Pospisil R, Kasmer RJ. Effects of food ingestion on hemodynamics in chronic congestive heart failure. *Crit Care Med* 1988;16:491.
18. Opie LH, Owen P, Riemersma RA. Relative rates of oxidation of glucose and fatty acids by ischemic and non-ischemic myocardium after coronary artery ligation. *Eur J Clin Invest* 1973;3:419.
19. Neely JR, Morgan HE. Relationship between carbohydrate and lipid metabolism and the energy balance of heart muscle. *Annu Rev Physiol* 1974;36:413.
20. Goerge G, Chatelain P, Schaper J, Lerch R. Effect of increasing degrees of ischemic injury on myocardial oxidative metabolism early after reperfusion in isolated rat hearts. *Circ Res* 1991;68:1681.
21. Thomassen A, Bagger JP, Nielsen TT, Henningsen P. Altered global myocardial substrate preference at rest and during pacing in coronary artery disease with stable angina pectoris. *Am J Cardiol* 1988;62:686.

22. Owen P, Dennis S, Opie LH. Glucose flux regulates the onset of ischemic contracture in globally underperfused rat hearts. *Circ Res* 1990;66:344.

23. Mc Donald TF, Hunter EG, MacLeod DP. ATP partition in cardiac muscle with respect to transmembrane electrical activity. *Pfluegers Arch* 1971;322:95.

24. Fossel ET, Solomon AK. Membrane mediated link between ion transport and metabolism in human red cells. *Biochim Biophys Acta* 1977; 464:82.

25. Montini J, Bagby GJ, Burns AH, Spitzer JJ. Exogenous substrate utilization in $Ca^{2+}$-tolerant myocytes from adult rat hearts. *Am J Physiol* 1981;240:H659.

26. Geffin GA, Love TR, Hendren WG, et al. The effects of calcium and magnesium in hyperkalemic cardioplegic solutions on myocardial preservation. *J Thorac Cardiovasc Surg* 1989;98:239.

27. England MR, Gordon G, Salem M, Chernow B. Magnesium administration and dysrhythmias after cardiac sugery. A placebo-controlled, double-blind, randomized trial. *JAMA* 1992;268:2395.

28. Burkhoff D, Weiss RG, Schulman SP, Kalil-Filho R, Wannenburg T, Gerstenblith G. Influence of metabolic substrate on rat heart function and metabolism at different coronary flows. *Am J Physiol* 1991;261: H741.

29. Myears DW, Sobel BE, Bergmann SR. Substrate use in ischemic and reperfused canine myocardium: quantitative considerations. *Am J Physiol* 1987;253:H107.

30. Simonsen S, Kjekshus JK. The effects of free fatty acids on myocardial oxygen consumption during arterial pacing and catecholamine infusion in man. *Circulation* 1978;58:484.

31. Barlow CH, Chance B. Ischemic areas in perfused rat hearts: measurements by NADH fluorescence photography. *Science* 1976;193: 909.

32. Chance B. Pyridine nucleotide as an indicator of the oxygen requirements for energy-linked functions of mitochondria. *Circ Res* 1976;38: 31.

33. Arai AE, Pantely GA, Anselone CG, Bristow J, Bristow JD. Active downregulation of myocardial energy requirements during prolonged moderate ischemia in swine. *Circ Res* 1991;69:1458.

34. Neely JR, Grotyohann LV. Role of glycolytic products in damage to ischemic myocardium: dissociation of adenosine triphosphate levels and recovery of perfused ischemic hearts. *Circ Res* 1984;55:816.

35. Rovetto MJ, Whitmer JT, Neely JR. Comparison of the effects of anoxia and whole heart isolated working rat hearts. *Circ Res* 1973;32: 699.

36. Nayler WG, Poole-Wilson PA, Williams A. Hypoxia and calcium. *J Mol Cell Cardiol* 1979;11:683.

37. Kihara Y, Grossman W, Morgan JP. Direct measurement of changes in intracellular calcium transients during hypoxia, ischemia, and reperfusion of the intact mammalian heart. *Circ Res* 1989;65:1029.

38. Wexler LF, Weinberg EO, Ingwall JS, Apstein CS. Acute alterations in diastolic left ventricular chamber distensibility: mechanistic differences between hypoxemia and ischemia in isolated perfused rabbit and rat hearts. *Circ Res* 1986;59:515.

39. Camacho AS, Parmley WW, James TL, et al. Substrate regulation of the nucleotide pool during regional ischemia and reperfusion in an isolated rat heart preparation: a phosphorus-31 magnetic resonance spectroscopy analysis. *Cardiovasc Res* 1988;22:193.

40. Bricknell OL, Opie LH. Effects of substrates on tissue metabolic changes in the isolated rat heart during underperfusion and on release of lactate dehydrogenase and arrhythmias during reperfusion. *Circ Res* 1978;43:102.

41. Kurien VA, Oliver MF. A metabolic cause for arrhythmias during acute myocardial hypoxia. *Lancet* 1970;1:813.

42. Greengard P. Possible role for cyclic nucleotides and phosphorylated membrane proteins in postsynaptic actions of neurotransmitters. *Nature* 1976;260:101.

43. Ashraf M. Effect of ischemia on myocardial cell gap functions. *J Mol Cell Cardiol* 1977;9(Suppl):13.

44. Johnston DL, Lewandowski ED. Fatty acid metabolism and contractile function in the reperfused myocardium: multinuclear NMR studies of isolated rabbit hearts. *Circ Res* 1991;68:714.

45. Lopaschuk GD, Spafford MA, Davies NJ, Wall SR. Glucose and palmitate oxidation in isolated working rat hearts reperfused after a period of transient global ischemia. *Circ Res* 1990;66:546.

46. Liedtke AJ, DeMaison L, Eggleston AM, Cohen LM, Nellis SH. Changes in substrate metabolism and effects of excess fatty acids in reperfused myocardium. *Circ Res* 1988;62:535.

47. Renstrom B, Nellis SH, Liedtke AJ. Metabolic oxidation of glucose during early myocardial reperfusion. *Circ Res* 1989;65:1094.

48. Boehmer JP, Becker LC. Glycolysis is important for ATP production during early reflow in globally stunned rabbit hearts. *Circulation* 1991;84(Suppl II):II-658.

49. Cerra FB, Blackburn GL, Hirsch J, Mullen K, Luther W. The effect of stress level amino acid formula and nitrogen dose on nitrogen retention in traumatic and septic stress. *Ann Surg* 1987;205:282.

50. Bower RH, Muggia-Sullam M, Vallgren S, et al. Branched chain amino enriched solutions in the septic patient. A randomized protective trial. *Ann Surg* 1986;203:13.

51. Erikson L, Conn H. Branched-chain amino acids in the management of hepatic encephalopathy: an analysis of variants. *Hepatology* 1989; 10:228.

52. Manner T, Wiese S, Katz DP, Skeie B, Askanazi J. Branched-chain amino acids and respiration. *Nutrition* 1992;8:311.

53. Tischler MF, Desautels M, Goldberg AL. Does leucine, leucyl t-RNA or some metabolite of leucine regulate protein synthesis and degradation in skeletal and cardiac muscle? *J Biol Chem* 1982;257:1613.

54. Buse MG, Reid SS. Leucine: a possible regulator of protein turnover in muscle. *J Clin Invest* 1975;56:1250.

55. Milner RDG. The stimulation of insulin release by essential amino acids from rabbit pancreas in vitro. *J Endocrinol* 1970;47:347.

56. Odessey R, Khanallah EA, Goldberg AL. Origin and possible significance of alanine production in skeletal muscle. *J Biol Chem* 1974; 249:7623.

57. Christensen HN. Interorgan amino acid nutrition. *Physiol Rev* 1982; 62:1193.

58. Morgan HE, Earl DCN, Broadus A, Wolpert EB, Giger KE, Jefferson LS. Regulation of protein synthesis in heart muscle. I. Effect of amino acid levels on protein synthesis. *J Biol Chem* 1971;246:2152.

59. Goldberg AL, Chang TE. Regulation and significance of amino acid metabolism in skeletal muscle. *Fed Proc* 1978;37:2301.

60. Kasperek GJ. Regulation of branched chain 2-oxo acid dehydrogenase activity during exercise. *Am J Physiol* 1989;256:E186.

61. Boyer B, Odessey R. Quantitative control analysis of branched-chain 2-oxo acid dehydrogenase complex activity by feedback inhibition. *Biochem J* 1990;271:523.

62. Chua BHL, Siehl DL, Morgan HE. A role for leucine in regulation of protein turnover in working rat hearts. *Am J Physiol* 1980;239:E510.

63. Schwalb H, Kushnir T, Navon G, Yaroslavsky E, Borman JB, Uretzky G. The protective effect of enriched branched chain amino acid formulation in the ischemic heart: a phosphorus-31 nuclear magnetic resonance study. *J Mol Cell Cardiol* 1987;19:991.

64. Schalb H, Izhar U, Yaroslavsky E, et al. The effect of amino acids on the ischemic heart. *J Thorac Cardiovasc Surg* 1989;98:551.

65. Buckberg GD. Studies of controlled reperfusion after ischemia. I. When is cardiac muscle damaged irreversibly? *J Thorac Cardiovasc Surg* 1986;92:483.

66. Young LH, McNulty PH, Morgan C, Deckelbaum LI, Zaret BL, Barrett EJ. Myocardial protein turnover in patients with coronary artery disease. *J Clin Invest* 1991;87:554.

67. Revkin JH, Young LH, Stirewalt WS, et al. In vivo measurement of myocardial protein turnover using an indicator dilution technique. *Circ Res* 1990;57:902.

68. Schwartz RG, Barrett EJ, Francis CK, Jakob R, Zaret BL. Regulation of myocardial amino acid balance in the conscious dog. *J Clin Invest* 1985;75:1204.

69. Opie LH. Metabolism of the heart in health and disease. *Am Heart J* 1968;76:685.

70. Bing RJ. Cardiac metabolism. *Physiol Rev* 1965;10:171.

71. Young LH, McNulty PH, Deckelbaum LS, Barrett EJ. Branch chain amino acids regulate cardiac amino acid and protein metabolism in man. *Circulation* 1989;80(Suppl II):II-498.

72. Curfman GD, O'Hara DS, Hopkins BE, Smith TW. Suppression of myocardial protein degradation in the rat during fasting. *Circ Res* 1980;46:581.

73. Dahl DM, Barrett EJ, Young LH. The anabolic effect of insulin and amino acids on canine heart. *Clin Res* 1990;38(2):271A.

74. Frexes-Steed M, Warner ML, Bulus N, Flakoll P, Abumrad NN. Role of insulin and branched chain amino acids in regulating protein metabolism during fasting. *Am J Physiol* 1990;258:E907.

75. Gharagozloo F, Melendez FJ, Hein RA, et al. The effect of amino acid L-glutamate on the extended preservation ex vivo of the heart for transplantatiom. *Circulation* 1987;76(Suppl V):V-65.

76. Rosenkranz ER, Okamoto F, Buckberg GD, Robertson JM, Vinten-Johansen J, Bugyi HI. Safety of prolonged aortic clamping with blood cardioplegia. *J Thorac Cardiovasc Surg* 1986;91:428.

77. Engelman RM, Rousou JA, Flack JE, Iyengar J, Kimura Y, Das DK. Reduction of infarct size by systemic amino acid supplementation during reperfusion. *J Thorac Cardiovasc Surg* 1991;101:855.

78. Thomassen A, Nielsen TT, Bagger JP, Pedersen AK, Henningsen P. Antiischemic and metabolic effects of glutamate during pacing in patients with stable angina pectoris secondary to either coronary artery disease or syndrome X. *Am J Cardiol* 1991;68:291.

79. Pisarenko OI, Lepilin MG, Ivanov VE. Cardiac metabolism and performance during L-glutamic acid infusion in postoperative cardiac failure. *Clin Sci* 1986;70:7.

80. Zimmermann R, Tillmanns H, Knapp WH, et al. Regional myocardial nitrogen-13 glutamate uptake in patients with coronary artery disease: inverse post-stress relation to thallium-201 uptake in ischemia. *J Am Coll Cardiol* 1988;11:549.

81. Finegan BA, Coulson CS, Lopaschuk GD, Clanachan AS. Effects of adenosine on myocardial substrate use in isolated perfused working rat hearts. *Circulation* 1991;84(Suppl II):II-276.

82. Edlund A, Sollevi A, Linde B. Hemodynamic and metabolic effects of infused adenosine in man. *Clin Sci* 1990;79:131.

83. Wilson RF, Wyche K, Christensen BV, Zimmer S, Laxson DD. Effects of adenosine on human coronary arterial circulation. *Circulation* 1990;82:1595.

84. Friedrichs GS, Merrill GF. Adenosine deaminase and adenosine attenuate ventricular arrhythmias caused by norepinephrine. *Am J Physiol* 1991;260:H979.

85. Belardinelli L, Linden J, Berne RM. The cardiac effects of adenosine. *Prog Cardiovasc Dis* 1989;32:73.

86. Van Wylen DGL, Willis J, Sodhi J, Weiss RJ, Lasley RD, Mentzer RM. Cardiac microdialysis to estimate interstitial adenosine and coronary blood flow. *Am J Physiol* 1990;258:H1642.

87. Headrick JP, Matherne GP, Berr SS, Han DC, Berne RM. Metabolic correlates of adenosine formation in stimulated guinea pig heart. *Am J Physiol* 1991;260:H165.

88. Angello DA, Headrick JP, Coddington NM, Berne RM. Adenosine antagonism decreases metabolic but not functional recovery from ischemia. *Am J Physiol* 1991;260:H193.

89. McDonald KM, Zhang J, Yoshiyama M, Francis GS, Ugurbil K, Cohn JN. Improvement of abnormal myocardial bioenergetics with adenosine in a canine model of left ventricular dysfunction. *Circulation* 1991;84(Suppl II):II-277.

90. Dorheim TA, Hoffman A, Van Wylen DGL, Mentzer RM. Enhanced interstitial fluid adenosine attenuates myocardial stunning. *Surgery* 1991;110:136.

91. Cox DA, Vita JA, Treasure CB, et al. Atherosclerosis impairs flow-mediated dilation of coronary arteries in humans. *Circulation* 1989;80:458.

92. Crea F, Pupita G, Galassi AR, et al. Role of adenosine in pathogenesis of angina pain. *Circulation* 1990;81:164.

93. Dale WE, Hale CC, Kim HD, Rovetto MJ. Myocardial glucose utilization. Failure of adenosine to alter it and inhibition by the adenosine analogue $N^6$-(L-2-phenylisopropyl)adenosine. *Circ Res* 1991;69:791.

94. Dyerberg J, Bang HO, Hjorne N. Fatty acid composition of the plasma lipids in Greenland Eskimos. *Am J Clin Nutr* 1975;28:958.

95. Leaf A, Weber PC. Cardiovascular effects of n-3 fatty acids. *N Engl J Med* 1988;318:549.

96. Lee TH, Hoover RL, Williams D, et al. Effect of dietary enrichment with eicosapentaenoic acid and docosahexaenoic acids on in vitro polymorphonuclear and monocyte leucotriene generation and polymorphonuclear leucocyte function. *N Engl J Med* 1985;312:1217.

97. Levy RI. Causes of the decrease in cardiovascular mortatility. *J Cardiol* 1984;54:7c.

98. American Heart Association. Dietary guidelines for healthy adult Americans. *Circulation* 1986;74:1465A.

99. Ernst E. Effects of n-3 fatty acids on blood rheology. *J Int Med* 1989;225(Suppl 1):129.

100. Barcelli U, Glas-Greenwalt P, Pollack VE. Enhancing effect of dietary supplement with n-3 fatty acids on plasma fibrinolysis in normal subjects. *Thromb Res* 1985;39:307.

101. Lorenz R, Spengler U, Fischer S, Duhm J, Weber PC. Platelet function, thromboxane formation and blood pressure cotrol during supplementation of the Western diet with cod liver oil. *Circulation* 1983;67:504.

102. Singer P, Berger I, Lueck K, Taube C, Naumann E, Goedicke W. Long-term effect of mackerel diet on blood pressure, serum lipids and thromboxane formation in patients with mild essential hypertension. *Atherosclerosis* 1986;62:259.

103. Ross R. The pathogenesis of atherosclerosis—an update. *N Engl J Med* 1986;314:488.

104. Fuster V, Badimon J, Adams PC, Turitto V, Chesebro JH. Drugs interfering with platelet function: mechanisms and clinical relevance. In: Verstraete M, Vermylen J, Lijnen R, Arnout J, eds. *Thrombosis and haemostasis.* Leuven University Press; 1987;349.

105. Hamberg M, Svensson J, Samuelsson B. Thromboxanes: a new group of biologically active compounds derived from prostaglandin endoperoxide. *Proc Natl Acad Sci USA* 1975;72:2994.

106. Moncada S, Gryglewski RJ, Buting S, Vane JR. An enzyme from arteries transforms prostaglandin endoperoxides to an unstable substance that inhibits platelet aggregation. *Nature* 1976;263:663.

107. Dyerberg J. Linolenate derived polyunsaturated fatty acids and prevention of atherosclerosis. *Nutr Rev* 1986;44:125.

108. Saynor R, Verel D, Gilliott T. The long term effect of dietary supplementation with fish lipid concentration serum lipids, bleeding time, platelets and angina. *Atherosclerosis* 1984;50:3.

109. Kinsella JE. Effects of polyunsaturated fatty acids on factors related to cardiovascular disease. *Am J Cardiol* 1987;60:23G.

110. Simopoulos AP. Omega-3 fatty acids in health and disease and in growth and development. *Am J Clin Nutr* 1991;54:438.

111. Lewis RA, Austen KF. The biologically active leucotrienes: biosynthesis, metabolism receptor functions and pharmacology. *J Clin Invest* 1986;3:889.

112. Willis AL, Smith D, Austen F. Suppression of principal atherosclerotic mechanisms by prostacyclins and other eicosanoids. *Prog Lipid Res* 1986;25:645.

113. Hawthorne AB, Filipowicz BL, Edwards TJ, Hawkey CJ. High dose eicosapentaenoic acid ethyl ester: effects on lipids and neutrophil leucotriene production in normal volunteers. *Br J Clin Pharmac* 1990;30:187.

114. Fitzgerald GA, Braden G, Fizgerald DJ, Knapp R. Fish oils in cardiovascular disease. *J Int Med* 1989;225(Suppl 1):25.

115. Burr ML, Fehily AM, Gilbert JF. Effect of changes in fat, fish and fibre intakes on death and myocardial reinfarction: diet and reinfarction trial (DART). *Lancet* 1989;2:757.

116. Viehman GE, Ma XL, Lefer DJ, Lefer AM. Time course of endothelial dysfunction and myocardial injury during coronary arterial occlusion. *Am J Physiol* 1991;261:H874.

117. Shimokawa H, Vanhoutte PM. Dietary cod-liveroil improves endothelium dependent responses in hypercholesterolemic and atherosclerotic porcine coronary arteries. *Circulation* 1988;78:1421.

118. Fox PL, Dicorleto PE. Fish oils inhibit endothelial cell production of a plateled-derived growth factor-like protein. *Science* 1988;241:453.

119. Riemersma RA, Sargent CA. Dietary fish oil and ischemic arrhythmias. *J Int Med* 1989;225(Suppl 1):111.

120. McLennan PL, Abeywardena MY, Charnock JS. Dietary fish oil prevents ventricular fibrillation following coronary artery occlusion and reperfusion. *Am Heart J* 1988;116:709.

121. Gudbjarnason S. Dynamics of n-3 and n-6 fatty acids in phospholipids of heart muscle. *J Int Med* 1989;225(Suppl 1):117.

122. Swanson JE, Lokesh BR, Kinsella JE. $Ca^{2+}$-$Mg^{2+}$ATPase of mouse cardiac sarcoplasmic reticulum is affected by membrane n-6 and n-3 polyunsaturated fatty acid content. *J Nutr* 1989;119:364.

123. Charnock JS. Antiarrhythmic effects of fish oils. In: Simopoulos AP, Kifer RR, Martin RE, Barlow SM, eds. Health effects of n-3 polyunsaturated fatty acids in seafoods. *World Rev Nutr Diet* 1991;66:278.

124. Hock CE, Holahan MA, Reibel DK. Effect of dietary fish oil on myocardial phopsholipids and myocardial ischemic damage. *Am J Physiol* 1987;252:H554.

125. Mertens J, Noll T, Spahr R, Kruetzenfeldt A, Piper HM. Energetic response of coronary endothelial cells to hypoxia. *Am J Physiol* 1990;258:H689.

126. Tschudi M, Richard V, Buehler FR, Luescher TF. Importance of endothelium-derived nitric oxide in porcine coronary resistance arteries. *Am J Physiol* 1991;260:H13.

127. Palmer RMJ, Ferrige AG, Moncada S. Nitric oxide release accounts for the biological activity of endothelium-derived relaxing factor. *Nature Lond* 1987;327:524.

128. Palmer RMJ, Ashton DS, Moncada S. Vascular endothelial cells synthesize nitric oxide from L-arginine. *Nature Lond* 1988;333:664.

129. Richard V, Tanner FC, Tschudi M, Luescher TF. Different activation of L-arginine pathway by bradikinin, serotonin, and clonidine in coronary arteries. *Am J Physiol* 1990;259:H1433.

130. Rees DD, Palmer RMJ, Moncada S. The role of endothelium-derived nitric oxide in the regulation of blood pressure. *Proc Natl Acad Sci USA* 1989;86:3375.

131. Motz W, Vogt M, Rabenau U, Scheler S, Luckhoff A, Strauer BE. Evidence of endothelial dysfunction in coronary vessels in patients with angina pectoris and normal coronary angiograms. *Am J Cardiol* 1991;68:996.

132. Morris JJ Jr. Mechanisms of ischemia in coronary artery disease: spontaneous decrease in coronary blood supply. *Am Heart J* 1990; 120:746.

133. Huetter JF, Piper HM, Spieckermann PG. Effect of fatty acid oxidation on efficiency of energy production in rat heart. *Am J Physiol* 1985;249:H723.

134. Shryock JC, Rubio R, Berne RM. Release of adenosine from pig aortic endothelial cells during hypoxia and metabolic inhibition. *Am J Physiol* 1988;254:H223.

135. Buderus S, Siegmund B, Spahr R, Kruetzenfeldt A, Piper HM. Resistance of endothelial cells to anoxia-reoxygenation in isolated guinea pig hearts. *Am J Physiol* 1989;257:H488.

136. Schrader J. Mechanisms of ischemic injury in the heart. *Basic Res Cardiol* 1985;80(Suppl 2):135.

137. Triana JF, Bolli R. Decreased flow reserve in "stunned" myocardium after a 10-min coronary occlusion. *Am J Physiol* 1991;261:H793.

138. Kloner RA, Rude RE, Carlson N, Maroko PR, DeBoer LWV, Braunwald E. Ultrastructural evidence of microvascular damage and myocardial cell injury after coronary artery occlusion: which comes first? *Circulation* 1980;62:945.

139. Forman MB, Puett DW, Virmani R. Endothelial and myocardial injury during ischemia and reperfusion: pathogenesis and therapeutic implications. *J Am Coll Cardiol* 1989;13:450.

140. Nayler WG, Elz JS. Reperfusion injury: laboratory artifact or clinical dilemma? *Circulation* 1986;74:215.

141. Watanabe H, Kuhne W, Spahr R, Schwartz P, Piper HM. Macromolecule permeability of coronary and aortic endothelial monolayers under energy depletion. *Am J Physiol* 1991;260:H1344.

142. McCord JM. Oxygen-derived free radicals in postischemic tissue injury. *N Engl J Med* 1985;312:159.

143. Tsao PS, Aoki N, Lefer DJ, Johnson III G, Lefer AM. Time course of endothelial dysfunction and myocardial injury during myocardial ischemia and reperfusion in the cat. *Circulation* 1990;82:1402.

144. Eberli FR, Weinberg EO, Grice WN, Horowitz GL, Apstein CS. Protective effect of increased glycolytic substrate against systolic and diastolic dysfunction and increased coronary resistance from prolonged global underperfusion and reperfusion in isolated rabbit hearts perfused with erythrocyte suspensions. *Circ Res* 1991;68:466.

145. Opie LH. Metabolism of free fatty acids, glucose and catecholamines in acute myocardial infarction. *Am J Cardiol* 1975;36:938.

146. Hess ML, Okabe E, Poland J, Warner M, Stewart JR, Reenfield LJ. Glucose, insulin, potassium protection during the course of hypothermic global ischemia and reperfusion: a new proposed mechanism by the scavenging of free radicals. *J Cardiovasc Pharmacol* 1983;5:35.

147. Zucchi R, Limbruno U, DiVincenzo A, Mariani M, Ronca G. Adenine nucleotide depletion and contractile dysfunction in the "stunned" myocardium. *Cardiovasc Res* 1990;24:440.

148. Kusuoka M, Inoue M, Marban E. Decreased efficiency of energy utilization in stunned myocardium. *Circulation* 1988;78(Suppl II):II-261.

149. Aoki N, Matsukura T, Miyagawa M, Yanagisawa A, Ishikawa K. Protection of the coronary endothelium and the myocardium from ischemia-reperfusion injury by arginine. *Circulation* 1991;84(Suppl II):1093.

150. Zimmer HG, Ibel H, Suchner U. Beta-adrenergic agonists stimulate the oxidative pentose phosphate pathway in the rat heart. *Circ Res* 1990;67:1525.

151. Spolarics Z, Lang CH, Bagby GJ, Spitzer JJ. Glutamine and fatty acid oxidation are the maim sources of energy for Kupffer and endothelial cells. *Am J Physiol* 1991;261:G185.

152. Gudbjarnason S, Cowan C, Bing RJ. Increase in hexosemonophosphate shunt activity during tissue repair. *Life Sci* 1967;6:1093.

153. Newsholme P, Newsholme EA. Rates of utilization of glucose, glutamine and oleate and formation of end-products by mouse peritoneal macrophages in culture. *Biochem J* 1989;261:211.

*The Critically Ill Cardiac Patient,*
edited by V. Kvetan and D. R. Dantzker,
Lippincott-Raven Publishers, Philadelphia © 1996.

CHAPTER 7

# Renal Disorders in the Cardiac Care Patient

Richard Barnett, RoseMarie Pasmantier, and Michael Geheb

Disorders of renal function are among the most common conditions affecting patients with heart disease (1–7). The kidney is particularly sensitive to diminution in myocardial performance as manifested by a range of potentially adverse fluid and electrolyte abnormalities. The development of acute renal failure (ARF) in this setting carries a strikingly high mortality which has not been greatly reduced by the wide availability of dialysis. The goal of this section is to convey a basic understanding of the pathophysiology of cardiorenal syndromes and to provide a simplified framework for pursuing treatment options. We will also consider the special concerns of patients requiring coronary care who have preexisting kidney failure.

## The Kidney as a Sensitive Monitor of Cardiac Function

The kidneys are comprised of several million nephrons containing an extensive capillary network receiving one-quarter of the cardiac output. These leaky glomerular capillaries generate 100 to 200 L/day of ultrafiltrate. This large quantity of fluid is extensively modified by tubular reabsorption and secretion resulting characteristically in a urine output of 1% or less of glomerular filtration (1 to 2 L/day). A practical approach to this subject will be initiated by analyzing how heart failure alters glomerular filtration, sodium reabsorption, and water excretion.

## Glomerular Filtration

As with many other organs, kidney function remains relatively constant by employing many autoregulatory

R. Barnett and R. M. Pasmantier: Division of Nephrology and Hypertension, Stony Brook Health Sciences Center, Stony Brook, New York 11794.
M. Geheb: Department of Medicine, The University of Alabama at Birmingham, Birmingham, Alabama

responses. Decreases in renal perfusion which result from diminished cardiac output are matched by alterations in the vascular resistances of the renal microcirculation. It is important to understand however that heart failure represents only one example of the diverse conditions in which renal perfusion, conceptualized as effective arterial volume, is reduced (2, 3, 6, 7). Decreased effective arterial blood volume is seen in true volume depletion with normal cardiac function and in heart failure (both associated with low cardiac output), in sepsis (associated with increased cardiac output), and in other states such as liver failure and nephrotic syndrome. In each of these conditions, decreased effective arterial blood volume is manifested by the clinical signs of impaired renal perfusion. Successful treatment of the specific underlying condition is accompanied by normalization of renal parameters.

Glomerlular filtration is maintained when perfusion is compromised by altering the resistances of the renal microcirculation (2). Afferent dilation and efferent constriction serve to increase the pressure in the glomerular capillary ($P_{GC}$), thus augmenting the volume of ultrafiltrate when renal blood flow is compromised. A variety of factors influence renal vasoreactivity in heart failure, but prostaglandin-mediated afferent dilatation and angiotensin-II-mediated efferent constriction are perhaps most important. Use of nonsteroidal anti-inflammatory agents (which inhibit prostaglandin synthesis) in this setting can promote a marked increase in afferent tone with concurrent decrements in $P_{GC}$ and glomerular filtration rate (GFR) (8). Alternatively, if an angiotensin-converting enzyme inhibitor causes a large decline in efferent tone without a parallel increase in renal blood flow, then $P_{GC}$ will also be reduced.

## Sodium Reabsorption

Under normal circumstances 60% to 70% of filtered sodium is reabsorbed in the proximal tubule, 25% to 30% is reabsorbed in the loop of Henle, and 15% to 25% is reabsorbed in the distal nephron under the influence of aldosterone. In heart failure, the increase in $P_{GC}$ raises the filtration fraction in Bowman's space with a resultant increase in the oncotic pressure of the efferent arterioles, peritubular capillaries of the proximal tubule, and interstitium. This leads to enhanced reabsorption of the filtrate (sodium, water, and urea) in the proximal tubule (2, 5). These events present as a "prerenal state" giving rise to a blood urea nitrogen (BUN)-creatinine ratio > 20:1 (7, 9). Elevated levels of angiotensin II and norepinephrine further augment proximal tubular sodium reabsorption. These events (called "proximalization" of the nephron) limit sodium presentation to the distal nephron. Decreased effective arterial blood volume also increases circulating renin-angiotensin-promoting enhanced aldosterone secretion and increased distal tubular renal sodium reabsorption. This combination of proximal and distal forces can reduce urinary sodium excretion to very low levels (<10 mEq/L).

### Water Reabsorption

Few areas in clinical nephrology are as misunderstood as disorders of water balance. The experienced clinician need only recall the instances where a hyponatremic patient with heart failure is mistakenly treated for the syndrome of inappropriate secretion of antidiuretic hormone (ADH) with a saline infusion. Water handling by the kidney is complex and elegant pathophysiology. It is dependent upon sodium delivery from the proximal nephron to the loop of Henle where pumps along the thick ascending limb of the loop create the "countercurrent" which generates the hypertonicity of the medullary interstitium (2). The continued reabsorption of sodium in the distal convoluted tubule drives the tubular fluid from isosmolar to hypo-osmolar (urinary osmolality < 100 mosm/L). Variable concentrations of antidiuretic hormone [arginine vasopressin (AVP)] modulate osmotically driven water flow from the distal nephron into the medullary interstitium, with final urinary osmolality ranging from maximally concentrated ($U_{osm}$ = 1,200 mosm/L) or minimally dilute ($U_{osm}$ < 100 mosm/L) urine dependent on the presence or absence of ADH, respectively. In heart failure ADH is present in high levels stimulated by reduced effective arterial blood volume (nonosmolar release of ADH). Because of the "proximalization" of sodium handling in heart failure, which disrupts the countercurrent multiplier in the loop of Henle, the ability to maximally concentrate and minimally dilute the urine is compromised.

### Summary and Treatment Implications

The renal response to heart failure is mediated through a decrease in effective arterial blood volume. Through the mechanisms described above, urine output declines, urinary sodium falls (<20 mEq/L), urine osmolality increases (>400) but remains less than maximally concentrated, and BUN-creatinine ratio increases (>20:1). Edema and hyponatremia are common. The therapeutic goal is to improve cardiac output and increase effective arterial blood volume. This can be attempted by afterload reduction or inotropic therapy. Improved effective arterial blood volume decreases the stimuli for AVP and aldosterone secretion and improves renal perfusion. The result is diminished "proximalization" of the nephron, increased urinary excretion of salt and water, with a decline in the BUN-creatinine ratio, reduction in urinary osmolality, and increase in urinary sodium (7, 9).

### DIURETIC THERAPY

The goal of diuretic therapy is sodium removal (treatment of pulmonary and generalized edema) and improvement of cardiac output (Table 1). If volume (sodium) removal maximizes filling pressures, cardiac output, and effective arterial blood volume, then renal perfusion improves with normalization of renal parameters. If volume removal decreases cardiac output, worsened prerenal azotemia occurs. Thus normalization of renal parameters which include an increase in urinary output and a decline in the BUN-creatinine ratio indicates improved cardiac performance.

### Proximal Tubular Diuretics

Although the proximal nephron is responsible normally for 60% to 70% of sodium reabsorption, because the loop of Henle and distal nephron have substantial downstream reabsorptive capacity, drugs active in the proximal nephron alone are weak diuretics (2, 6). Agents active in the proximal nephron include osmotic agents (mannitol), carbonic anhydrase inhibitors (acetazolamide), and other drugs that have effects in both the proximal and distal nephron (metolazone). Mannitol is uncommonly used as therapy with other diuretics for the treatment of heart failure and is used principally in the prevention of or early therapy for ARF. Acetazolamide, which is a bicarbonaturic agent, is ordinarily a weak diuretic but can induce a profound diuresis in the alkalemic patient, especially those

**TABLE 1.** *Diuretics: site of action*

Proximal tubule: mannitol, carbonic anhydrase inhibitors, metolazone
Loop diuretics: furosemide, butenamide, ethacrynic acid
Distal nephron
   Chloriuretic: thiazides, metolazone
   Potassium sparing: amiloride, triamterene, aldactone

with high levels of serum bicarbonate. Chronic carbon dioxide retainers with elevated bicarbonate levels may also benefit by this approach. Used in combination with loop diuretics, acetazolamide can ameliorate the metabolic alkalosis induced by loop diuretics, but at the expense of further volume depletion. The bicarbonaturia induced by acetazolamide may obligate significant potassium and phosphate wasting. Acetazolamide can be given in doses of 250 to 500 mg, intravenously or orally, every 4 to 6 hours.

## Loop Diuretics

The most effective diuretic agents are those that inhibit a sodium-potassium-chloride cotransporter in the thick ascending limb of Henle's loop, where 30% to 40% of filtered sodium is reabsorbed under normal circumstances (3). These agents include furosemide and bumetanide (both sulfa derivatives) and ethacrynic acid. In individuals allergic to sulfa moieties, ethacrynic acid, which is structurally unrelated to furosemide, may be used. These agents are the first line of defense when treating heart failure. They are effective even in advanced chronic renal failure, but high doses may be required (>1 g/day). In contrast to proximal agents, the loop drugs promote sodium delivery to distal sites in excess of their reabsorptive capacities. Their effectiveness can lead to volume depletion, with secondary activation of the renin-aldosterone system, which exacerbates potassium and magnesium excretion in the distal nephron as sodium overwhelms distal tubular reabsorptive capacity. Because they are chloriuretic agents, metabolic alkalosis is common. This coupled with potassium and magnesium depletion fosters increased arrhythmogenic potential. Dosages of furosemide range from as little as 20 mg orally or intravenously to as much as 300 mg intravenously every 3 to 4 hours. Continuous infusion therapy in which an initial bolus of 40 mg is followed by 10 to 40 mg/hr may be more effective and less ototoxic. The onset of action is rapid, and any patient who has not responded within 1 to 2 hours should be considered for increased dosing.

## Distal Nephron Diuretics

Because the distal nephron only has the capacity to reabsorb 10% to 15% of the filtered sodium load, diuretics active at that site have only limited diuretic capabilities. However, they remain very useful clinical agents. There are two mechanisms of action: direct inhibition of chloride (and sodium) reabsorption and inhibition of sodium-potassium and/or $H^+$ exchange (so-called potassium-sparing agents). The thiazide diuretics and metolazone fall into the first category, while amiloride, triamterene, and aldactone fall into the latter. Thiazides and metolazone, because they impair the sodium handling at the distal diluting segment, are the diuretics most frequently associated with hyponatremia. Potassium and magnesium wasting and metabolic alkalosis are commonly observed as complications. Thiazides are ineffective when the GFR is less than 30 mL/min. Metolazone, however, in combination with loop diuretics, may be used even in advanced renal failure. The potassium-sparing drugs can be used to prevent inordinate potassium loss and metabolic alkalosis. As individual agents, however, they tend to have even less effect than the thiazide agents. None of the distal agents should be considered as primary drugs for severe edema or life-threatening heart failure. They are administered principally as oral agents and should be considered as adjunctive to loop diuretics and other interventions.

## Therapeutic Implications and Combination Therapy

Loop agents are the diuretics of choice in heart failure. However, in one extreme the use of these agents can be associated with minimal changes in cardiac output and renal perfusion when diastolic filling pressures are high (the flat portion of the cardiac Starling curve), while in the other extreme, continued administration can reduce central filling pressures to suboptimal levels which will be reflected in worsening renal function, mirroring end-organ hypoperfusion. The inability of a loop diuretic to typically reduce urine osmolality, elevate urine sodium, and induce a diuresis within a few hours may be observed in several other settings. Severe heart failure associated with bowel edema may reduce drug absorption. Indeed, low therapeutic levels of commonly used agents (digoxin, dilantin) may parallel ineffective diuretic gut absorption. In these cases, intravenous diuretic therapy is indicated. Additionally the ability of the diuretic to be delivered to the site of action in the tubular lumen is compromised when GFR is significantly impaired. Continuous infusion therapy may be particularly effective in this circumstance. Continuous infusion also appears to obviate the intense distal nephron salt and water conservation resulting from bolus diuretic therapy, which is mediated by activation of the renin-angiotensin-aldosterone and vasopressin systems.

When the patient is resistant to loop diuretics, the addition of proximal or distally active agents is often effective. The goal is to block sodium reabsorption at each site of reabsorption and thus reverse "proximalization." In the presence of metabolic alkalosis and alkalemia intravenous acetazolamide (250 to 500 mg every 4 to 6 hours) can be very effective in combination with a loop diuretic. However, the therapeutic effect of acetazolamide is dependent on elevated bicarbonate levels. Metolazone, 5 to 10 mg orally (intravenous form is not available), can be very effective, even in advanced renal failure when used with loop diuretics.

Major complications of loop and thiazide diuretics include the electrophysiologic consequences of hypokalemia and hypomagnesemia (7, 10, 11), particularly in the peri-infarct period. Magnesium deficiency attenuates renal reabsorption of potassium and thus may impair correction of hypokalemia. Hypomagnesemia (< 1.0 mg/dL) can be associated with hypocalcemia, which can have adverse effects on inotropy in susceptible individuals. In patients with normal renal function, magnesium clearance is considerable, and other than easily reversed hypotension, serious side effects associated with aggressive intravenous replacement (4 to 8 g/day of magnesium sulfate) are rare. Life-threatening hypokalemic arrhythmias should be aggressively treated with supplementation. The oral route is best, but hypokalemia-induced bowel dysmotility may require intravenous administration. Particularly when plasma levels are less than 2.0 to 2.5 mEq/L, 20 to 40 mEq/hr can be reasonably administered intravenously during continuous electrocardiographic monitoring. However, vigorous potassium chloride infusion after serum levels are sustained in the 3.5 to 4.0 mEq/L range can result in the rapid development of life-threatening hyperkalemia. In the setting of renal failure potassium excretion may be only mildly reduced unless associated with the tubulointerstitial processes which complicate diabetes mellitus and obstructive uropathy. Modifications in both potassium and magnesium replacement with close monitoring of serum levels are especially indicated in these settings.

The potassium-sparing agents, especially amiloride and triamterene, are invaluable adjunctive therapies in the diuretic treatment of heart failure. Their weak natriuretic effects are counterbalanced by promoting marked reductions in potassium and magnesium excretion in patients receiving loop thiazide diuretics. Furthermore, by increasing potassium levels and reducing hydrogen ion secretion, complications of diuretic-associated metabolic alkalosis are substantially reduced. They are thus useful in the prevention and treatment of these electrolyte abnormalities but need to be used cautiously in circumstances in which renal potassium and magnesium elimination is impaired.

## Other Agents

In hypotensive patients, vasodilators should obviously be used with caution to avoid worsening renal perfusion. Nonetheless, in selected individuals the resulting increment in cardiac output may actually improve renal perfusion and function (3). In patients with severe heart failure, angiotensin-converting enzyme inhibitors may worsen renal function dramatically in the face of improved cardiac output because of preferential efferent vasodilatation (5). Hyperkalemia is commonly observed in this setting. The natriuresis associated with inotropic

agents is largely consequent to improved cardiac output and "low-dose" dopamine (3 to 5 μg/kg/min) may also directly inhibit proximal tubular reabsorption of sodium and may selectively alter glomerular vasoreactivity. The use of low-dose dopamine in conjunction with diuretics is often effective in establishing a therapeutic diuresis. Atrial natriuretic factor, secreted by the cardiac atria in heart failure, promotes salt and water diuresis in selected patients, but its routine pharmacologic use in heart failure in place of less costly medications cannot be recommended at this time.

## DISORDERS OF TONICITY IN HEART FAILURE

### Definitions

Tonicity refers only to the effective osmolality (that which affects water distribution across the cellular membrane). Effective endogenous osmols include sodium and glucose. Hypotonicity occurs when the calculated tonicity falls below 280 mosm/L. It is generally indicated when the $pNa^+$ is below 135 mEq/L:

$$\text{Calculated tonicity} = 2 \times pNa^+ \text{ (meq/L)} + \text{glucose (mg/dL)}/18$$

Osmolality refers to the concentration of all osmotically active particles including effective and ineffective osmols. Ineffective osmols (urea) are those that do not affect water distribution. It can be directly measured or estimated from plasma chemistries:

$$\text{Calculated osmolality} = 2 \times (pNa^+ \text{ meq/L}) + (\text{glucose mg/dL}/18) + \text{BUN (mg/dL)}/2.8$$

There are also effective (mannitol) and ineffective (ethanol, isopropyl alcohol, methanol) exogenous osmols. Their impact on tonicity and osmolality will be noted as needed.

### Hypotonicity and Hyponatremia

Hyponatremia associated with hypotonicity is the most frequent electrolyte disorder observed in patients with cardiac disease. Calculated osmolality and tonicity and measured osmolality are all decreased in this clinical setting. It is essential to separate the evaluation of hyponatremia (water balance) from the evaluation of volume status (sodium balance). Sodium overload (as evidenced by generalized and pulmonary edema) associated with a disproportionately greater degree of water overload (as evidenced by hyponatremia) is common in heart failure. The pathophysiology of impaired renal water excretion described earlier, the nonosmotic release of ADH, combined with the water loading that commonly occurs in these patients make water retention in excess of sodium retention and the resulting true hyponatremia and hypotonicity a common occurrence (6). Ordinarily, secretion of ADH is completely inhibited at a tonicity below normal, with a resulting minimum urine osmolality (<100 mosm/L), so that the normal person excretes an excess water load (up to 10 to 20 L/day as free water). In heart failure, renal sodium retention occurs (U Na$^+$ < 10 mEq/L) and urine osmolality is relatively concentrated (>100 mosm/L). When renal failure complicates the picture, renal sodium- and water-excreting capability are further compromised.

Other nonosmotic stimuli for ADH release include stress and pain. The most potent nonosmotic stimulus is nausea with or without vomiting. Lists of pharmacotherapeutic agents associated with hyponatremia are lengthy, but in the coronary care unit (CCU) the major offenders include thiazide diuretics, narcotics, chlorpropamide, and to a lesser extent, nonsteroidal anti-inflammatory agents. The thiazides (by impairing function of the cortical diluting segment) may aggravate any tendency toward water retention. Narcotics, when used to treat myocardial-derived pain and postoperative discomfort, can induce hypotension and nausea, thereby inducing ADH release. The oral hypoglycemic, chlorpropramide, and nonsteroidal anti-inflammatory drugs enhance ADH effect at the renal collecting duct.

## Pseudohyponatremia

The widespread use of ion-specific electrodes (which measure the true water concentrations of ions) is relegating the entity of pseudohyponatremia to historical interest. However, when flame photometry is used to determine plasma sodium (pNa$^+$) concentration, less than 10 mosm difference between the measured and calculated plasma osmolality will exclude pseudohyponatremia. With pseudohyponatremia, calculated osmolality will be much less than measured osmolality, which may be normal. It is seen in patients with severe hyperlipidemia and hyperproteinemia.

## Hyponatremia without Hypotonicity

True hyponatremia without hypotonicity can be seen with both hyperglycemia and mannitol infusion. Both sugars led to the osmotic shift of water from the intra- to extracellular compartment with dilution of the plasma sodium. A good rule of thumb to use is for each 100 mg/dL of glucose above normal, pNa$^+$ will be reduced 1.6 mEq/L. Mannitol-induced hyponatremia is less common but can occur with the accumulation of mannitol, especially in renal failure. With glucose-induced hyponatremia, the normal osmolar gap (<10) between measured osmolality and calculated osmolality is preserved. Calculated tonicity and osmolality tend to be elevated, and plasma sodium can be normal or usually decreased. Because mannitol is not measured routinely, significant accumulation of mannitol is associated with increased measured osmolality and an increased osmolar gap. The magnitude of the osmolar gap is proportional to the accumulation of mannitol. Significant mannitol accumulation is uncommon except in the presence of significant renal failure and severe heart failure.

### Diagnostic Approach

Table 2 represents a rapid diagnostic and treatment schema for most hyponatremic patients without advanced renal failure. Most classifications have used standard clinical criteria for establishing the volume status of the patient (6, 7, 12). Note that the renal response in a true volume (sodium) depletion such as diarrhea is identical to that in heart failure with sodium overload (indicated by edema), because both are associated with a decrease in effective arterial blood volume. Both present with "prerenal" clinical pictures marked by urinary sodium and water retention. This is indicated by low urinary sodium concentration (U Na$^+$ < 20 mEq/L), concentrated urine (U$_{osm}$ > 100 and usually > 400), and elevated plasma creatinine and BUN concentrations with BUN-creatinine ratios generally greater than 20. Uric acid excretion is also volume sensitive and is elevated in states with low effective arterial blood volume. Although the syndrome of inappropriate

**TABLE 2.** *Evaluation of hyponatremia*

| Disease | SIADH[a] | Diarrhea | Heart failure |
|---|---|---|---|
| Sodium balance | Normal | Decreased | Increased |
| Edema | None | None | Present |
| Effective blood volume | Increased | Decreased | Decreased |
| Plasma creatinine | Decreased | Increased | Increased |
| Blood urea nitrogen | Decreased | Increased | Increased |
| Plasma uric acid | Decreased | Increased | Increased |
| Urine osmolality | Increased (>100 mosm/L) | Increased (>100 mosm/L) | Increased (>100 mosm/L) |
| Urine sodium | Normal (>20 meq/L) | Decreased (<20 meq/L) | Decreased (<20 meq/L) |

[a]Syndrome of inappropriate secretion of antidiuretic hormone.

secretion of antidiuretic hormone (SIADH) is part of the differential in hyponatremic patients, it cannot be reliably diagnosed in the presence of heart failure (since the absence of any nonosmotic stimulus to ADH release is a requirement for the diagnosis).

### Therapeutic Approach

The most difficult situation encountered in cardiac patients is the association of edematous cardiac failure in combination with severe hypotonicity ($pNa^+$ < 120 mEq/L and tonicity < 245 mosm/L), in whom the hypotonicity is thought to substantially contribute to altered mental status. In these cases the approach must be to remove hypotonic fluid from the patient, starting with therapies that improve cardiac performance including diuretic therapy. As fluid is removed, hypertonic saline can be administered carefully to correct hypotonicity. Ultrafiltration should be begun early if more conservative measures do not yield an early response in fluid removal, especially in patients with severe hypotonicity and who have or are in danger of seizures. In cases with clear volume depletion at the outset, normal or hypertonic saline can be recommended directly, if carefully monitored for impact on cardiac performance.

At a $pNa^+$ < 120 meq/L, especially in patients with neurologic manifestations, therapy should be aggressive with a goal to correct $pNa^+$ at the rate of 0.5 to 1.0 meq/hr until a $pNa^+$ of 125 to 130 meq/L is achieved.

To calculate the "sodium deficit" to raise a $pNa^+$ from 120 to 130 meq/L in a 70-kg patient would be

$$70 \text{ kg} \times 0.6 = 42 \text{ kg (liters total body water)}$$

$$130 \text{ meq/L} - 120 \text{ meq/L} = 10 \text{ meq/L sodium deficit}$$

$$10 \text{ meq/L} \times 42 \text{ liters} = 420 \text{ meq sodium deficit}$$

Since each liter of 3% saline contains 513 meq of sodium, infusion of 800 cc of 3% saline at a controlled rate would be desirable.

### Hypernatremia and Hypertonicity

Hypernatremia is always associated with hypertonicity and is present with a $pNa^+$ > 145 meq/L (2, 6, 7, 10, 12). It is uncommonly encountered in patients with heart failure, except in a few circumstances. Since sodium bicarbonate solution is the most hypertonic solution in the clinical armamentarium (50 meq/50 cc ampule; 1,000 mosm/L), its recurrent use commonly induces hypernatremia. Hyperglycemic induced osmotic diuresis as well as overzealous loop diuretic administration can result in losses of water greater than $Na^+$ and promote hypernatremia. Hypertonicity (>320 mosm/L) and hypernatremia ($pNa^+$ > 150 meq/L) is associated with major neurologic derangement and focal neurologic findings and confers

significant mortality. As a guide to treatment free water deficits are calculated by assuming that the elevated $pNa^+$ results from pure water loss. Free water deficits can be estimated by

$$\text{Water deficit} = [0.6 \times \text{body weight (kg)}] \times \text{current } pNa^+/140 - 1$$

Thus, to correct a $pNa^+$ from 160 meq/L in a 70 kg-patient, the free water deficit would be estimated to be

$$(0.6 \times 70 \text{ kg})(160/140 - 1) = 5.9 \text{ kg (liters) water}$$

Thus the water deficit should be approximately 6 L. While strict guidelines have not been established regarding the rate of correction, it is reasonable to provide half of the water deficit during the first 24 hr in addition to fluids provided for maintenance of ongoing sodium and water losses.

### Hyperglycemia and Hypertonicity

Hypertonicity with varying plasma concentrations of sodium occur with hyperglycemia. Poorly controlled diabetes with hyperglycemia promotes an osmotic diuresis, with water loss greater than electrolyte. The syndrome of hyperosmolar nonketotic hyperglycemia occurs in elderly patients (13), who frequently have underlying cardiac compromise. Volume depletion can be profound in these individuals and is better tolerated hemodynamically than in comparable hypotonic depletion because glucose-induced water shifts from the intracellular space to the extracellular compartment maintain intravascular volume. For this reason, in the hypotensive patient, volume depletion must be addressed prior to treating hyperglycemia. It is reasonable in the hemodynamically stable individual to treat with hypotonic fluid replacement, with slow correction of hypernatremia. Rapid insulin-induced shifts of glucose from extracellular to intracellular spaces may promote hemodynamic instability. The treatment of diabetic ketoacidosis (DKA) is detailed elsewhere, but the role of volume repletion prior to significant glucose correction also applies. In this entity potassium deficits may be large despite transient hypoinsulin-associated hyperkalemia. Administration of this cation as potassium phosphate may mitigate the decline in plasma phosphate levels as glucose is taken up by cells. Since significant conversion of ketone bodies by the liver regenerates bicarbonate, it is rarely necessary to infuse sodium bicarbonate unless pH levels approach 7.1 or less. Indeed, base administration for treatment of DKA may eventually lead to less well tolerated metabolic alkalosis.

### DIABETIC NEPHROPATHY

Diabetes is the most common cause of end-stage renal disease in the United States (2) and is commonly associated with patients with cardiac disease. Clinical findings of diabetic nephropathy (DN) include nephrotic range proteinuria, hypertension, and progressive renal failure. Current therapy includes glucose control, modest protein restriction, and judicious use of angiotensin-converting enzyme inhibitors. Patients with DN are more susceptible for developing ARF from radiocontrast and other factors. Additionally, this group of patients is unusually prone to the development of hyperkalemia in response to various therapies initiated.

Diabetics are particularly prone to hyperkalemia because of the high incidence of hyporeninemic hypoaldosteronism in this population (2, 7, 10). It is also the most common cause of true hyperkalemia in all hospitalized patients. This entity is usually associated with DN complicated by varying degrees of renal insufficiency. Most of these individuals have subclinical expansion of their blood volume, which suppresses renin and secondarily aldosterone release, while the remainder have damage to the site of renal synthesis of renin. These patients frequently have borderline hyperkalemia. In the CCU severe stress raises counterregulatory hormones, resulting in relative hypoinsulinemia. The patient is commonly hypertensive, may be placed on a low-sodium diet, and may have exacerbation of heart failure, all factors that limit distal tubular sodium delivery leading to worsening hyperkalemia. Additionally, angiotensin-converting enzyme inhibitors are frequently used for afterload reduction in heart failure and to limit the progression of DN. Usually these individuals are not treated with beta-blockers, but if they are used to treat ischemia, they can further exacerbate hyperkalemia. The revival of digoxin as a popular treatment for heart failure can also exacerbate any hyperkalemic tendency. Finally certain calcium channel blockers, particularly those with marked effects on the conduction system (verapamil, diltiazem), can aggravate the hyperkalemic alteration of the electrocardiogram.

The treatment of moderate hyperkalemia associated with hyporeninemic hypoaldosteronism consists of resin binders such as kayexalate used judiciously. While resin binders certainly have their role, diarrhea limits patient and nursing enthusiasm for this messy therapy. Theoretically, mineralocorticoid replacement is effective but may aggravate underlying hypertension. In a stepwise fashion we recommend dietary sodium liberalization followed by loop diuretic administration after other predisposing factors such as complicating drugs have been addressed. If hyperkalemia persists, sodium supplementation in the form of a bicarbonate precursor (Schohl's solution containing sodium citrate + citric acid) not only enhances distal sodium presentation but also increases luminal electronegativity and thus enhances potassium secretion. Additionally, the resulting acute alkalemia may modestly facilitate cellular potassium uptake as well as mitigate the mild metabolic acidosis associated with hyporeninemic hypoaldosteronism.

Acute therapy for life-threatening hyperkalemia is summarized in Table 3. Calcium is the most rapid agent but needs to be administered intravenously (3). Sodium bicarbonate also acts within minutes to reduce plasma potassium, especially in acidemic patients. Aerosolized beta-agonists used in the treatment of chronic obstructive pulmonary disease (COPD) are systemically absorbed and fairly rapidly promote potassium influx but can be arrythmogenic. Oral and/or rectal resin binding therapy is one of the most effective means for potassium disposal but requires several hours to work. Hemodialysis (but not other dialytic modalities) can be life saving, but the rapidity of the decline in potassium levels may precipitate hypokalemic arrhythmias, particularly if the patient is receiving digoxin. Digoxin is not dialyzable, and severe intoxications should be treated with the antibody preparation supplemented with dialysis to ameliorate hyperkalemia. In most hyperkalemic patients treated with hemodialysis we limit the rate of potassium decline by gradually reducing dialysate potassium levels. Hyperkalemia is a commonly overlooked cause of cardiac arrest and should be considered in any bizarre wide complex ventricular arrhythmia.

## ACUTE ARF

While no universally accepted definition of ARF exists, a rapid decrease in glomerular filtration by at least 50% from baseline constitutes a significant decrement in kidney function (2, 6, 7). Renal failure represents an inability to excrete both endogenously produced and exogenously administered solute, and the clinical sequelae are secondary to the effects of accumulation of these solutes. Isolated ARF is usually a reversible condition which has disparate causes that have been loosely classified into prerenal, postrenal, and intrinsic renal etiologies. The recognition of the high mortality of ARF associated with multiorgan system failure (1) should heighten the interest of the cardiac intensivist in early detection and treatment. This section will outline certain practical considerations in the evaluation and management of this entity.

### Clinical Signs

The clinical signs and symptoms of ARF can be conveniently categorized into electrolyte complications, those

**TABLE 3.** *Treatment of hyperkalemia*

| |
|---|
| Calcium |
| Bicarbonate |
| Insulin ± glucose |
| Aerosolized beta-agonist |
| Diuretics |
| Exchange resins |
| Dialysis |

related to volume (sodium) overload, intractable acid-base disturbances especially metabolic acidosis, and uremic signs and symptoms. Electrolyte complications include hyponatremia and occasionally hypernatremia, hyperkalemia, hypocalcemia, and hyperphosphatemia. Volume overload, especially in patients with preexisting heart disease, can be an early indication for dialytic or ultrafiltration therapy. General uremic signs and symptoms include pericardial and pleural friction rubs, mental status changes, and asterixis in later stages (2, 14). Nausea and vomiting are common in the early stages. Other complications include bleeding diatheses and sepsis. In fact, common causes of death in severe uremia are infection and bleeding.

In general, mortality is improved when BUN and creatinine levels are maintained below 100 and 10 mg/dL, respectively. A reasonable therapeutic goal is to maintain values less than these.

Acute renal failure can be oliguric (<400 cc/day) or nonoliguric. The mortality of nonoliguric renal failure is less than that of oliguric renal failure and is associated with less severe degrees of renal insufficiency. It is generally associated with toxin administration, especially aminoglycoside antibiotics.

### Initial Evaluation

Acute changes in renal function are often subtly manifested by an elevated plasma creatinine and/or BUN obtained from routine blood chemistries or an observed decline in urine output. Concurrent increases in creatinine and BUN above the normal range support the diagnosis of ARF. A rapid evaluation should be initiated since decrements in kidney function can mirror concurrent systemic and potentially lethal processes. Table 4 lists the common causes of ARF presenting in cardiac patients. Table 5 lists clinical settings in which BUN and creatinine measurements may be altered by nonrenal conditions.

### Prerenal and Postrenal Causes of ARF

Prerenal processes are observed most frequently (3). Diminished cardiac output from left-sided disease predominates, but right-sided heart failure from pulmonary emboli and respiratory failure can decrease renal perfusion. Hemorrhage from gastrointestinal sources is usually an obvious consideration while sizable internal bleeding into a thigh from a prior vascular procedure in the groin is frequently overlooked. Early sepsis associated with systemic vasodilatation can impair renal perfusion. Drugs may promote functional declines without pathologic injury. Renal hypoperfusion from overzealous diuretic use and antihypertensive therapy should be considered. Indeed, a rapid decrease in blood pressure to normotensive levels in a previously poorly controlled hypertensive

**TABLE 4.** *Common causes of acute renal failure*

Prerenal
  Heart failure (left sided or right sided)
  Hemorrhage
  Sepsis
  Volume (sodium) depletion
  Poor oral intake, gastrointestinal losses
  Diuretics
  Hypoperfusion (drug associated)
  vasodilators
  Antihypertensives, particularly ACE inhibitors
  Nonsteroidal agents
Postrenal
  Bladder outlet obstruction
  Unilateral obstruction in solitary kidney
Intrinsic renal
  Acute tubular necrosis (oliguric)
  Aminoglycosides (non-oliguric)
  Radiocontrast (oliguric)
  Shock (oliguric)
  Allergic interstitial nephritis: nonsteroidal agents, antibiotics, diuretics
  Atheroemboli
  Malignant hypertension

patient can contribute to renal compromise. Nonsteroidal anti-inflammatory agents (which inhibit vasodilatory prostaglandins) preferentially promote afferent vasoconstriction which can result in profound declines in glomerular filtration when renal perfusion is already compromised by heart failure or any other cause of diminished effective arterial blood volume (8). Urinary parameters (9) include oliguria (< 400 cc/day), low urinary sodium (< 20 mEq/L), and a low fractional excretion of sodium (< 1%). A BUN-creatinine ratio above 20 may be present but not invariably. Typically the urine is relatively concentrated (> 450 mosm/L).

Obstructive uropathy is a common entity with multiple causes. However, with the exception of bladder outlet

**TABLE 5.** *Limitations of plasma creatinine and blood urea nitrogen as markers of renal function*

Increases plasma creatinine (underestimates GFR[a])
Impaired tubular secretion
  Cimetidine, trimethoprim
  Assay interference
  Acetoacetate, flucytosine
Decreases plasma creatinine (overestimates GFR)
  Reduced muscle mass: malnutrition (particularly alcoholism), old age
  Enhanced secretion: advanced renal failure
Increases blood urea nitrogen
  Elevated production: gastrointestinal bleeding, corticosteroids
Decreases blood urea nitrogen: tetracyclines
  Reduced production: liver failure, protein malnutrition

[a]Gel filtration permeation.

obstruction, particularly in the setting of an enlarged prostate, acute postrenal disease rarely produces the bilateral impairment required for the development of significant ARF observed in the heart failure patient. Obstruction of a functional unilateral kidney can precipitate ARF. Urinary parameters are exceedingly variable in obstructive uropathy.

## Intrinsic Causes of ARF

Intrinsic renal causes of ARF generally reflect diseases which are not remediable by correction of prerenal or postrenal factors. A large literature now suggests that any cause of poor renal perfusion combined with additional factors such as sepsis, aminoglycoside use, and radiocontrast exposure sets the stage for the development of intrinsic ARF (acute tubular necrosis). Acute renal failure associated with multiple organ system failure carries a particularly poor prognosis (3). Acute renal failure commonly occurs after a prolonged period of hypotension and renal ischemia. Nearly half of the cases are postsurgical and are associated with repair of aortic aneurysms and open-heart surgery. Intrinsic renal failure of most etiologies presents with a high urinary sodium (>20 mEq/L), an elevated fractional excretion of sodium (>2%), an inability to concentrate or dilute the urine (osmolality that is generally in a range of 300 to 450 mosm/L), and a urine sediment that contains cellular and renal tubular casts. Notably, red cell casts are absent.

## Drug-related Nephrotoxicity

Aminoglycoside-related nephrotoxicity occurs in 10% to 26% of cases, even when monitoring of blood levels is appropriate. Pure aminoglycoside nephrotoxicity is nonoliguric and declines in GFR occur 7 to 10 days after the initiation of therapy (2, 15). Prophylaxis against renal failure is appropriate volume repletion and maintenance of normal magnesium and potassium levels. Amphotericin-B-related nephrotoxicity presents with elevated creatinine and may be associated with hyperchloremic acidosis and renal potassium wasting. It is typically nonoliguric. When the BUN rises over 50 mg/dL, most sources recommend reducing the dosage. Toxicity is unusual at low doses (>600 mg) but usual at higher doses (cumulative doses >2 g). Allergic interstitial nephritis is underdiagnosed, may represent more than 10% of ARF, and ensues from therapy with virtually any pharmacologic agent, particularly antibiotics of the penicillin/cephalosporin families.

## Atheroembolic Disease

An increasingly well recognized cause of renal insufficiency associated with cardiac care patients is atheroembolic disease (2, 4, 16). Most of these individuals are older than 60 years of age and have extensive atherosclerotic lesions in renal or suprarenal vessels when subjected to vascular catheterization or surgery. The distal shower of cholesterol emboli elicits a foreign body reaction with intimal thickening from cell proliferation in small and medium-size arterioles. The lesions may be patchy or a manifestation of a systemic illness characterized by lower extremity digital infarction, renal dysfunction, renin-mediated hypertension, peripheral eosinophilia, and complement activation. The depression in kidney function may be dramatic and acute, frequently accompanied by evidence of compromise to other organs, including brain, pancreas, bowel, and skeletal muscle. Other individuals may not exhibit renal impairment until weeks or months after the inciting episode. It is no longer believed that this entity inexorably leads to advanced renal failure and death. Diagnosis requires a high index of suspicion and a careful, directed physical exam including fundoscopy. Laboratory studies are usually not helpful, but increases in BUN, creatinine, amylase, creatinine phosphokinase, and eosinophils and elevated sedimentation rate and depressed complement may support the diagnosis. Since the disease primarily spares the glomeruli and tubules, there may be no alteration in the urine sediment or dipstick for protein.

There is no current therapy demonstrated to be effective in atheroembolic disease. Efforts at limiting subsequent arterial catheterization and control of hypertension are reasonable. Hypotension may have particularly adverse consequences in vascular beds with atheroembolic involvement.

## Radiocontrast and Renal Failure

Few areas in the coronary care and renal literature have been as extensively addressed as the issue of nephrotoxicity induced by radiocontrast material ((1, 2, 17–19). This entity, which occurs within 24 hours of dye administration, is manifested by low urinary sodium, progressive increases in creatinine, decline in urine output, and in most patients reversibility within several days after dye administration. Almost all individuals exhibit modest declines in GFR, paralleling small increases in serum creatinine after dye administration. Interestingly, a preliminary report suggested that greater than a 50% increase over baseline in peak plasma creatinine may identify individuals with severalfold higher cardiovascular mortality up to a year or more removed from their cardiac angiography (20). In the short term, however, the major concern is oliguric renal failure severe enough to require dialytic intervention (Table 6 details a list of potential risk factors). Preexisting renal disease from any etiology is the most consistent risk factor. At a baseline plasma creatinine between 2 and 4 mg/dL, the risk may be minimally higher than patients with "normal" kidney function

**TABLE 6.** *Radiocontrast risk factors*

Pre-existing renal disease
Diabetes mellitus
Multiple myeloma
Volume deletion
Decreased cardiac output
Multiple or large loads of contrast
Volume of contrast

(2% to 5%). However, in patients with plasma creatinine values above 4 mg/dL up to 50% may need to undergo dialysis. However, in almost all cases the potential benefits of angiographically directed bypass surgery or angioplasty outweigh the risks of reversible kidney failure.

To date there have been no significant renal advantages identified for the various contrast agents. The lower osmolar nonionic dyes promote less fluid shifts from the intracellular to extracellular (and vascular) compartments and may result in a lower incidence of ARF, especially in patients at high risk, although this remains unproven (17–19). The use of specific therapies, including calcium channel blockade, loop diuretics, and mannitol, has not been demonstrated consistently effective. Sentiment that improved effective arteriolar volume and the establishment of an ongoing diuresis (50 to 100 cc/hr) may limit the incidence of renal failure has been supported by a recent study utilizing infusion of half-normal saline (19). Addition of a loop diuretic and mannitol administered prior to the dye load may be indicated in individuals manifesting varying degrees of heart failure.

### Other Causes of ARF

Other causes of ARF include generalized rhabdomyolysis [associated with creatinine phosphokinase (CPK) values generally greater than 1,000 units/mL]. Renal failure rarely occurs as a result of the relatively mild increases in CPK associated with even severe myocardial infarction. Acute vasculitis, acute glomerulonephritis, and uric acid nephropathy are other uncommon causes of renal failure and are not generally seen in patients with uncomplicated cardiac disease.

### Diagnostic Approaches

Several diagnostic procedures are useful in the evaluation of ARF (Table 7). Placement of a urinary catheter will rule out obstruction and can be employed to monitor subsequent changes in urine output. Urinalysis is invaluable and, coupled with urine and serum chemistries, may delineate the causes listed in Table 6. Renal ultrasound may indicate the presence of obstruction (hydronephrosis), chronic renal failure (small kidneys), or renovascular abnormalities (disparate kidney size). Doppler techniques can indicate renal venous or arterial thrombosis, which is generally bilateral in severe ARF. In equivocal cases or under circumstances in which body habitus limits the value of such studies, magnetic resonance imaging visualization of the renal vasculature may obviate the use of potentially nephrotoxic contrast dye. Renal scan may define discrepancies in renal blood flow and aid in the identification of obstruction using a "lasix washout" technique in which the diuretic which is ineffective in obstruction will enhance excretion from the ectatic collecting system. The demonstration of preserved renal blood flow with poor excretion helps confirm the diagnosis of ARF. Response to a fluid challenge in the setting of ARF when low urinary sodium is present can help separate incipient ARF from prerenal causes. Swan-Ganz catheterization may be necessary to monitor fluid and cardiac performance during such a challenge.

### Management of ARF

Once prerenal or postrenal causes have been excluded, the underlying cause of kidney dysfunction needs to be addressed (2, 21). Initial steps include the discontinuation and avoidance of agents that can cause ARF or allergic interstitial nephritis. Acute renal failure associated with sepsis, multiorgan system failure, and other factors (Table 8) has a worse outcome, is often prolonged, and frequently requires dialytic therapy (21). To date there is no pharmacologic strategy which unequivocally hastens the return of function in established ARF.

Nonoliguric ARF is more easily managed than oliguric renal failure. Ideally fluid intake should not exceed

**TABLE 7.** *Urinary findings in acute renal failure*

| Condition | UNa | FENa | U$_{osm}$ | BUN/Cr | Urinalysis |
|---|---|---|---|---|---|
| Pre-renal azotemia | <20 | <1 | >400 | >20:1 | Normal, few hyaline casts |
| Acute obstruction | var | var | var | <20:1 | Normal |
| ATN: typical | >20 | >1 | <400 | <20:1 | Muddy brown casts |
| ATN: radiocontrast | <20 | <1 | >400 | var | Normal, some RT |
| Allergic interstitial nephritis | >20 | >1 | <400 | <20:1 | eos, WBC ± casts |
| Acute glomerulonephritis | <20 | <1 | >400 | var | RBC casts/ |
| Atheroembolic disease | var | var | var | var | var, often normal occ eos |

UNa; FENa; BUN, blood urea nitrogen; Cr, creatinine; var; ATN; eos; WBC, white blood cells; RBC, red blood cells.

**TABLE 8.** *High mortality in acute renal failure*

Mechanical ventilation
Malignancy
Malnutrition
Thrombocytopenia
Liver failure
Multiorgan system failure

output (urine, stool, drainage tubes) by more than 500 to 1,000 cc/day in the euvolemic individual. Urine output can often be augmented by continuous furosemide infusion in which an initial bolus injection of 40 mg is followed by gradually increasing doses of this agent (10 to 40 mg/hr). Increased urine output aids in management of electrolyte and acid-base problems and provides sufficient leeway to commence adequate enteral or parenteral nutrition. Hyponatremia may be treated with fluid restriction and occasional cautious sodium supplementation. Hypernatremia is less frequently observed and generally responds to water replacement. Significant hyperkalemia is seldom observed since most patients are usually managed by restricted diets and judicious resin binder therapy (kayexalate). Metabolic acidosis is ameliorated by careful oral or intravenous alkali therapy. Nasogastric suction can be used to generate substantial bicarbonate only if gastric pH is below 2, a circumstance that is seldom encountered if high-stress patients are treated with $H_2$ blockers.

It is our practice to initiate directed nutritional support early in the course of ARF. The overall strategy is to provide 25 to 35 kcal/kg/day, which may be adjusted dependent on stress level (1, 3). The Harris-Benedict equations are frequently used to estimate basal caloric requirements. Modest protein restriction of 0.6 to 1.0 g of protein/kg/day is provided in the form of essential and nonessential amino acids. Measurement of nitrogen balance is the best way to estimate protein requirements but may be difficult if there are large daily fluctuations in losses of protein from hemorrhage, wound sites, the gastrointestinal tract, or dialysis.

The administration of numerous intravenous medications and the volume requirements of patients with ARF who are nutritionally optimized may predispose to overload and even frank worsening of cardiac function. When these therapeutic requirements exceed the ability to manage ARF medically, dialytic therapy needs to be initiated.

## Renal Replacement Therapies

The development of different dialytic therapies over the past four decades has dramatically altered the therapeutic approach to ARF (2, 14). Today, dialysis is initiated early in the course of ARF, before heart failure, hyperkalemia, pericarditis, or seizures warrant emergent therapy. A general goal is to institute dialysis prior to severe azotemia (BUN > 100 mg/dL; plasma creatinine < 10 mg/dL). The advantages and disadvantages of three major types of renal replacement therapy are summarized in Table 9. Optimally a center should have significant experience with each modality, but institutional preferences and staffing frequently dictate the approach selected.

Hemodialysis is the oldest and most familiar technique and is particularly valuable for managing hypercatabolic or hyperkalemic patients and those with acute volume overload. As usually employed, hemodialysis is actually a combination of dialysis (removal of nitrogen and other waste products) and ultrafiltration (removal of sodium and water or volume). Indeed, the two processes can be separated using conventional equipment. Acute volume removal, combined with electrolyte and osmolar shifts, can promote rapid changes in systemic and central pressures, resulting in increased myocardial oxygen demand in unstable cardiac patients. Thus sequential techniques in which ultrafiltration for 1 to 2 hours precedes dialysis for 2 to 4 hours is recommended for hemodynamically unstable patients.

In patients who may require dialysis for more than a few days, preserving access sites becomes a major consideration, especially the selection site for placement of the standard double lumen catheter. The femoral vein is the safest approach, although its somewhat lower blood flow may limit clearances. It frequently becomes infected if left in place for greater than 1 week. The subclavian vein is the easiest site to maintain, provides high blood flows, but is associated with a high incidence of subsequent venous stenosis which may limit future forearm access placement. As a result, we recommend the internal jugular route, which has successfully been maintained in patients for several months.

The choice of dialyzer membrane has been the subject of recent attention (22). In general the standard cuprophane dialyzer promotes activation of complement and other factors which adversely influence pulmonary and systemic vascular resistances. While these phenomena may be well tolerated in stable, chronically dialyzed patients, more biocompatible membranes such as polyacrylonitrile and polysulfone should be employed in the

**TABLE 9.** *Indications for hemodialysis (HD), peritoneal dialysis (PD), and continuous arteriovenous hemofiltration (CAVH)*

|  | HD | PD | CAVH |
|---|---|---|---|
| Pulmonary edema | +++ | + | +++ |
| Hyperkalemia | +++ | + | + |
| Hypermetabolic | +++ | + | + |
| Overdose | +++ | + | + |
| Hemorrhage | – – | ++ | – – |
| Hypotension | – – | + | ++ |
| Large volume requirements | – – | ++ | ++ |

management of critically ill individuals. Such patients should also be treated with bicarbonate dialysate in order to minimize the hemodynamic instability and myocardial depression associated with acetate solutions.

Cardiac and critically ill patients with ARF frequently manifest gastrointestinal or other bleeding complications, making standard anticoagulation techniques problematic (14). Regional heparinization using protamine was an early attempt at limiting systemic effects. More recently, use of citrate, which provides regional anticoagulation, has become widespread. Its minor electrolyte and acid-base side effects are usually well tolerated. Alternatively, frequent flushing of the dialysis circuit with saline during a 4-hour session may totally obviate anticoagulation in selected patients. However, this approach cannot be utilized in patients requiring large amounts of volume removal.

The increasingly widespread use of continuous dialytic therapies (23, 24), including continuous arteriovenous hemofiltration (CAVH), continuous arteriovenous hemodialysis (CAVHD), continuous venous-venous hemofiltration (CVVH), and continuous venous-venous hemodialysis (CVVHD), represents an exciting advance in the ability to manage renal failure in hemodynamically compromised patients. Recent evidence indicates that a continuous approach is at least equivalent and may be preferable in selected critically ill patients.

In its simplest form CAVH employs two catheters placed typically in a femoral artery and vein, where the arteriovenous pressure difference drives blood across a "leaky" hemofilter. This device, which looks like a small kidney dialyzer, has an ultrafiltration port which can be attached to a Foley bag for drainage and can remove substantial amounts of extracellular fluid each hour. The quantity of volume removed can be augmented by connecting the ultrafiltration port to wall suction. In this fashion 20 to 30 L/day of fluid can be removed with "clearances" obtained by replacing the desired proportions of ultrafiltrate with a physiologic solution such as Ringer's lactate. Interestingly by adding the replacement fluid on the venous side, higher clearances and less clotting of the hemofilter are observed. Thus, in a patient who requires a great deal of volume for the delivery of nutrition and medications, a comparable amount of volume can be removed. If the ultrafiltration port is not connected to suction, volume depletion and hypotension progressively limit further ultrafiltration. Although conceptually simple, the technique requires trained nursing and physician personnel familiar with catheter placement and installation of lines and the hemofilter. In centers which do not have access to standard dialysis techniques it can be life saving and used for weeks at a time. Anticoagulation poses some risk, which may be mitigated by regional techniques but frequent filter clotting can become labor intensive. Individuals with platelet counts less than 50,000 mm$^3$ may be much less prone to clotting of the hemofilter.

Several advances in continuous dialytic techniques have increased its versatility but are somewhat more complex. Continuous arteriovenous hemodyalisis is one modification in which the hemofilter has two ports, permitting the infusion of "dialysate" or physiologic fluid to enhance clearances in addition to volume removal. Continuous venous-venous hemofiltration employs a blood pump to provide the pressure differential across a standard double lumen central venous catheter. An indwelling arterial catheter is thus avoided. However, unlike CAVH, CVVH requires specific monitoring equipment for air embolus. Large losses of extracellular fluid as ongoing ultrafiltration occurs are common with CVVH and require monitoring. Continuous Continuous venous-venous hemodyalisis is also being used in a few centers. In this technique, peritoneal dialysate solution infused at 500 cc/hr in the hemofilter dialysate ports increases clearances.

Acute peritoneal dialysis is frequently employed in cardiac patients with end-stage renal disease. Its obvious advantages include hemodynamic stability and the lack of an anticoagulation requirement. Clearances of nitrogenous wastes and potassium are inferior to standard hemodialysis (14), although the use of automated cycling equipment enhances clearance by permitting frequent exchanges of peritoneal dialysate with a reduced dwell time.

## REFERENCES

1. Barnett R. Renal function evaluation. In: Vlay SC, ed. *Medical care of the cardiac surgical patient.* New York: Blackwell Scientific; 1991.
2. Brenner BM, Rector FC. *The kidney.* Philadelphia, PA: WB Saunders; 1991.
3. Carlson RW, Geheb MA. *Principles and practice of medical intensive care.* Philadelphia, PA: WB Saunders; 1993.
4. Colt HG, Begg RJ, Saporito JJ. Cholesterol emboli after cardiac catheterization. Eight cases and a review of the literature. *Medicine* 1988;67:389.
5. Dzau VJ. Renal and circulatory mechanisms in congestive heart failure [Clinical Conference]. *Kidney Int* 1987;31:1402.
6. Rose BD. *Clinical physiology of acid-base and electrolyte disorders.* New York: McGraw-Hill; 1994..
7. Schrier RW. *Renal and electrolyte disorders.* Boston: Little, Brown; 1986.
8. Patrano C, Dunn MJ. The clinical significance of inhibitory renal prostaglandin synthesis. *Kidney Int* 1987;32:1.
9. Kamel KS, Ethier JH, Richardson RMA, Bear RA, Halperin ML. Urine electrolytes and osmolality: when and how to use them. *Am J Nephrol* 1990;10:89.
10. Arieff AI, DeFronzo RA. *Fluid, electrolyte, and acid-base disorders.* New York: Churchill Livingstone; 1985.
11. Krishna GG. Hypokalemic states: current clinical issues. *Sem Nephrol* 1990;10:515.
12. Narins RG, Jones ER, Stom MC, Rudnick MR, Basti CP. Diagnostic strategies in disorders of fluid electrolyte and acid-base homeostasis. *Am J Med* 1982;72:496.
13. Khardori R, Soler NG. Hyperosmolar, hyperglycemic nonketotic syndrome: report of 22 cases and brief review. *Am J Med* 1984;77:899.
14. Drukker W, Parsons FM, Maher JF. *Replacement of renal function by dialysqis.* Boston: Martinus Nijhoff; 1983.
15. Humes HD. Aminoglycoside nephrotoxicity. *Kidney Int* 1988;33:900.
16. Mannesse CK, Klankestijin PJ, Man in't Veld AJ, Schalekamp NADH. Renal failure and cholesterol crystal embolization: a report of 4 surviving cases and a review of the literature. *Clin Nephrol* 1991;36:240.

17. Lautin EM, Freeman NJ, Schoenfeld AH. Radiocontrast-associated renal dysfunction: incidence and risk factors. *Am J Roentgenol* 1991; 157:49.
18. Rudnick MR, Goldfarb S, Wexler L. Nephrotoxicity of ionic and non-ionic contrast media in 1196 patients: a randomized trial. *Kidney Int* 1995;47:254.
19. Solomon R, Werner C, Mann D. Effects of saline, mannitol and furosemide on acute decreases in renal function induced by radiocontrast agents. *N Engl J Med* 1994;331:1416.
20. Lange M, Muenz L, Clark C, Merritt A, Bucher T, Popma J. Unexpectedly high post-hospital discharge mortality following acute renal failure. *J Am Soc Nephrol* 1994;5:399(abst).
21. Lieberthal W, Levinsky NG. Treatment of acute tubular necrosis. *Sem Nephrol* 1990;10:571.
22. Hakim RM, Wingard RL, Parker RA. Effect of the dialysis membrane in the treatment of patients with acute renal failure. *N Engl J Med* 1994;331:1338.
23. Bellomo R, Boyce N. Acute continuous hemodiafiltration: a prospective study of 110 patients and a review of the literature. *Am J Kidney Dis* 1993;21:508.
24. Weiss L, Danielson BG, Wikstrom B. Continuous arteriovenous hemofiltration in the treatment of 100 critically ill patients with acute renal failure: report on clinical outcome and nutritional aspects. *Clin Nephrol* 1989;31:184.

The Critically Ill Cardiac Patient,
edited by V. Kvetan and D. R. Dantzker,
Lippincott-Raven Publishers, Philadelphia © 1996.

CHAPTER 8

# Abdominal Crises in the Cardiac Patient

Jonathan F. Critchlow and Mitchell P. Fink

Problems with the gastrointestinal (GI) tract plague the clinician involved in treating the cardiac patient for a number of reasons. First, disorders of the GI tract may mimic acute cardiac events, as symptoms may be similar and the physical examination and laboratory investigations are often not very helpful in distinguishing between these entities. Second, cardiac patients are likely to have arteriosclerotic lesions involving splanchnic vessels, other comorbid diseases, and a substantial risk of developing low-flow states. Accordingly, these patients are at risk for a number of intra-abdominal catastrophes, which result from poor organ perfusion. Such conditions include acalculous cholecystitis, nonocclusive mesenteric infarction, and bleeding from stress-related mucosal disease. Third, the diagnosis of coincident GI problems in patients with acute cardiac disease is often delayed, leading to increased morbidity and mortality. Fourth, therapeutic interventions in cardiac patients can increase the risk for GI complications. For example, vasopressors, though effective in raising blood pressure, may decrease global or local circulation and precipitate mesenteric and/or hepatic ischemia; heparin and thrombolytic agents, though helpful in lysing clots in the coronary circulation, may lead to bleeding complications in the GI tract; aspirin and other nonsteroidal anti-inflammatory agents, though helpful in keeping angioplasties and coronary stents open, may lead to gastric ulceration; intra-aortic balloon pumping and valve replacement may be life saving in certain patients but increase the risk of visceral embolization; and, though coronary artery bypass surgery may be essential for saving life or restoring quality of life, it may be associated with postoperative GI complications, such as pancreatitis, acalculous cholecystitis, or exacerbation of preexisting peptic ulcer disease.

It is difficult to estimate the true incidence of GI complications in patients treated for cardiac disease. The age of patients treated has increased, the spectrum of their comorbid diseases (particularly peripheral vascular disease, diabetes, and pulmonary dysfunction) has expanded, and therapies have become more invasive and complex. As a consequence, the incidence of intra-abdominal problems in this group of patients probably has increased. The best studied category of cardiac patients contains those who have undergone cardiac surgery. A number of series report complications involving the GI tract in 1% to 2% of patients undergoing cardiopulmonary bypass (1–5). Approximately half of these problems were due to bleeding, usually from the upper tract, with pancreatitis, mesenteric ischemia, intestinal perforation, and cholecystitis being less common but still potentially deadly complications (Table 1). The likelihood of these complications increases with age, valve surgery, use of vasopressors or intra-aortic balloon pump (IABP), and longer bypass times (1). Mortality occurs 20% to 60% of cases (1–5).

In this chapter, we will discuss the acute abdominal catastrophes which may complicate the course of the cardiac patient. We will focus on disorders which arise from preexisting medical conditions and disorders which are attributable to general or regional hypoperfusion.

## GASTROINTESTINAL BLEEDING

Acute GI bleeding is the most frequent abdominal complication of patients undergoing coronary artery bypass surgery (1–6). This complication occurs in 0.35% to 0.7% of cases, accounting for approximately 50% of all GI complications. Bleeding is most often from the stomach or duodenum, although occasionally lower tract bleeding from diverticula or arteriovenous malformations occurs.

Patients with acute cardiac disease are at risk for the development of hemorrhage from the upper GI tract due to several distinct problems. The most common of these is exacerbation of a preexisting ulcer diathesis or de novo

J. F. Critchlow and M. Fink: Department of Surgery and Multidisciplinary Critical Care Service, Beth Israel Hospital, Boston, Massachusetts; and Harvard Medical School, Boston, Massachusetts 02215.

**TABLE 1.** *Gastrointestinal complications following cardiopulmonary bypass from a series of 5,438 patients*

| Category | Incidence (no. of complications) | Mortality (no. of of deaths) |
|---|---|---|
| Acid/peptic disease | | |
|   Gastric erosion or ulceration with upper GI bleeding | 29 | 4 |
|   Penetration/perforation without bleeding | 3 | |
|   Duodenal erosion or ulceration with upper GI bleeding | 7 | 2 |
|   Penetration/perforation without bleeding | 4 | 2 |
| Total complications due to gastric/duodenal erosion or ulceration | 43 (in 41 patients) | 8 |
| Cholecystitis | 4 | |
| Pancreatitis | 2 | |
| Intestinal obstruction | | |
|   Small-bowel obstruction | 1 | |
|   Cecal volvulus | 2 | |
|   Ogilvie's syndrome | 3 | |
| Total intestinal obstruction | 6 | |
| Diverticular disease | | |
|   With inflammation only | 1 | |
|   With perforation | 3 | |
|   With hemorrhage | 5 | 1 |
| Total | 9 | |
| Intestinal infarction | 3 | 3 |
| Hepatic necrosis | 4 | 2 |
| Pseudomembranous colitis | 2 | |
| Total complications/mortality | 73 | 14 |

There were 73 complications in 69 patients. GI, gastrointestinal.

formation of peptic disease (7). The use of anticoagulants increases the risk of clinically significant hemorrhage from peptic disease. Administration of nonsteroidal anti-inflammatory drugs in the treatment of cardiac disorders increases the incidence of mucosal ulcerations of the stomach and duodenum (8). Patients developing acute respiratory failure and/or multiple-organ failure are at increased risk for stress-related mucosal erosions and so-called stress ulcers (9). As discussed below, it appears that the exacerbation of peptic disease and the contribution of nonsteroidal agents are clearly the most common causes of bleeding in these patients. Data suggesting that a high percentage of patients bleed from "stress ulceration" probably reflect misunderstanding of terminology rather than the true incidence of patients with this disorder (6).

Acute upper GI hemorrhage is a relatively common problem with an average mortality rate of up to 10% in large series involving all patients. Although 80% to 90% of patients stop bleeding spontaneously, a few die without appropriate therapy, usually as a complication of end-organ dysfunction following hemorrhagic shock. Mortality rates increase with age and concurrent illness (10).

Emergency operations to control bleeding from the GI tract carry significant mortality. The risk of death is reduced markedly if the procedure can be done electively. The high operative mortality associated with emergency operations may reflect that these patients are often older and have more severe bleeding than their medically treated counterparts and that mortality is high in those in whom therapy is unduly delayed (11). On the other hand, if medical therapy supplants surgery in less severe bleeding situations, mortality rates will fall (12). Thus, the logical approach is one of medical therapy with operation in selected cases.

The cornerstones of medical therapy are resuscitation, continuing correction of hypovolemia, blood transfusion, correction of coagulopathy, and close monitoring. In essence this is supporting the patient while giving nature its best chance to stem the hemorrhage. To date, there are no convincing data suggesting that any specific medical therapy decreases mortality, stops acute bleeding, or avoids surgery. The only possible exception to this statement is that the control of bleeding may be improved when endoscopic procedures are used to control hemorrhage (13).

Although it is recommended that patients with upper GI hemorrhage undergo early endoscopy, early controlled trials did not show that this lowered mortality (14). Any advantages conferred by the improvements and diagnostic accuracy were probably limited because most patients stop bleeding spontaneously, and during the era when these studies were completed, endoscopic therapeutic options were limited. However, endoscopy does identify certain groups of patients who are best treated with early surgery [e.g., patients with a "visible vessel at the base of the ulcer" (15)], medical therapy (e.g., patients with gastric erosions), or a specific approach (e.g., patients bleeding from varices).

More recent trials of endoscopic therapy also have not demonstrated a tremendous decrease in mortality (10). However, as these studies enrolled relatively small numbers of patients, it has been suggested that the failure to document benefit may be due to a type II statistical error. Meta-analyses *have* shown a significant decrease in mortality with endoscopic therapy (13). The endoscopic stigmata of hemorrhage such as red spot, adherent clot, visible vessel, or acute bleeding are clues to increased incidence of recurrent bleeding, as are findings of an ulcer size greater than 1 to 2 cm (10, 13). As techniques become more refined, patients with these stigmata are being treated endoscopically, probably with improved survival.

Gastric lavage is of value for the diagnosis of upper GI bleeding and in clearing the stomach of clots prior to endoscopy. However, it is unproven that gastric lavage has efficacy in causing cessation of hemorrhage. Although iced saline lavage decreases gastric blood flow in dogs as much as 50% (16), such reductions may be the result of diminished cardiac output rather than a local effect on gastric resistance vessels. Cooling also inhibits coagulation and causes generalized hypothermia. The addition of norepinephrine to iced lavage fluids has no added effect on gastric blood flow. The theoretical benefits of washing away extra clot and activated anticoagulants must be balanced against the possibility of disturbing a newly formed hemostatic plug. Therefore, it is recommended that only room temperature or warm lavage fluids be utilized as a diagnostic maneuver and as an aid to increasing visualization with the endoscopy.

Although the use of $H_2$ antagonists in acute hemorrhage is commonplace, there are no studies which offer clear-cut evidence of significant benefit. Randomized trials to assess the efficacy of these agents generally have been too small to evaluate the impact on the important, but relatively rare, end points of death, rebleeding, and necessity for surgical intervention. A meta-analysis of the compiled data from 27 randomized trials suggests that these agents may lower rates of rebleeding, surgery, and death by 10%, 20%, and 30%, respectively (17). However, even in this relatively large meta-analysis, the statistical significance for these effects is marginal. There are several possible reasons for the failure to document significant benefit from the use of these antisecretory agents:

a. There are relatively few patients at risk for these complications, as most patients stop bleeding spontaneously and identification of those at risk is not straightforward. Thus, many patients are needed to demonstrate significant efficacy.

b. On the one hand, it is unlikely that any medical therapy can "improve" on the usual favorable outcome in cases of acute upper GI hemorrhage. On the other hand, it is doubtful that treatment with $H_2$ antagonists can stop exsanguinating hemorrhage from a rent in the gastroduodenal artery. Thus, only select groups of patients may benefit. To date, these groups have not been clearly identified, although it has been suggested that gastric lesions may be more amenable to antisecretory therapy.

c. Early protocols employed regimens which do not consistently control gastric pH. Sustained achlorhydria was not achieved, especially in patients given intermittent boluses of $H_2$ antagonists. Continuous infusion regimens seem to be more effective in sustaining achlorhydria (18); however, improved success in preventing rebleeding or avoiding operation has not been demonstrated with continuous infusions of $H_2$ blockers or the use of more potent antisecretory agents such as the proton pump inhibitor Omeprazole (19). Whether a type II error is responsible for this is unclear. Studies utilizing intravenous vasopressin, prostaglandins, or somatostatin have shown little, if any, benefit (10, 20).

Despite medical and endoscopic therapy, some patients continue to bleed and require surgery. In a recent meta-analysis of patients receiving endoscopic therapy for acute upper GI hemorrhage, there was a rebleeding rate of 20% (13). Fifty percent of patients had a second episode of rebleeding despite another attempt at endoscopic control; surgery was therefore required in 10% of the cases in the series. A recent prospective randomized trial of early surgery based on minimal criteria (stigmata of hemorrhage or bleeding) versus delayed surgery for patients with severe continuing or recurrent bleeding suggested that early surgery benefits patients who are over 60 years old (21). This underscores the importance of age (60 years being the usual cut-off value) as an important predictor of survival in both operated and nonoperated patients (22). Patients under the age of 60 probably tolerate continued hemorrhage with fewer problems better than those over 60 do. Thus, older patients may actually benefit from earlier surgery because they are less able to compensate during sustained bleeding.

The choice of operation for bleeding *duodenal* ulcer depends primarily on the surgeon's preference, although this may be influenced by the patient's age, prior ulcer history, and hemodynamic stability. The choice of procedure also can be affected by the anatomic aspects of the ulcer itself. Vagotomy and pyloroplasty with oversewing of the ulcer is preferred by many surgeons because operative time is short and mortality tends to be low (23, 24). Rebleeding rates after vagotomy and pyloroplasty are relatively low but may approach 10% to 15% (23–25). Resectional therapy, including vagotomy and antrectomy, is thought to carry a higher mortality rate, but, in experienced hands, mortality after antrectomy may approach that seen with vagotomy and pyloroplasty. Rebleeding rates are lower with resectional therapy, especially when the ulcer is removed or excluded from the GI tract (25). Recurrent ulceration rates are also lower, and although antrectomy may be a more formidable operation in the emergency setting, it may be advantageous in patients with long-standing disease and those in whom no discrete vessel can be identified for ligation.

Emergency highly selective vagotomy and oversewing have been used with success in some series (26). Although this alternative procedure has a low incidence of long-term complications, concerns remain regarding efficacy both in the long and short term.

Treatment of bleeding from a discrete bleeding *gastric* ulcer is most often a formal gastric resection (27). Several factors guide this approach. Gastric ulcers frequently occur secondary to poor mucosal protection and may not heal rapidly if only oversewn. Bleeding from gastric ulcers is usually not quite as torrential as that from a duodenal ulcer with an open gastroduodenal artery at its base. Thus patients with bleeding gastric ulcers may be more stable during operation. Gastric ulcers also raise the concern for malignancy, which does not pertain in the duodenum. Vagotomy is not required, except in cases of pyloric channel ulcer, which is actually a variant of duodenal ulcer disease. The occasional gastric ulcer near the gastroesophageal junction, which is not amenable to a distal gastrectomy, is occasionally managed with biopsy or wedge resection, vagotomy, and gastric drainage.

Angiographic embolization of bleeding ulcers has been performed successfully in selected patients. This therapy may have a role for patients who continue to bleed despite medical and endoscopic therapy but are thought to be unable to tolerate laparotomy (usually because of pulmonary insufficiency). Although success with this approach has been reported, concerns remain over the adequacy of resuscitation in the angiography suite and dyeload required, which may have detrimental consequences for patients with marginal renal function.

Mucosal erosions in critically ill patients have been termed *stress ulcers* or *stress-related gastroerosive disease*. These erosions are extremely common after illness or trauma and are seen endoscopically in 75% to 90% of critically ill patients (9). These lesions cause bleeding in 5% to 15% of patients in the intensive care unit not receiving prophylaxis (28). These are superficial mucosal lesions which are most often found in the fundus of the stomach (28, 29). These erosions are thought to reflect a failure of gastric defense mechanisms rather than increased acid production except in rare cases of severe sepsis (29, 30). Gastric mucosal ischemia is probably a key instigator of this process, which can be perpetuated by gastric acidity and other noxious agents. Mucosal ulceration due to stress is a separate entity from discrete ulcers caused by increased acid production from peptic disease or secondary to head trauma (i.e., Cushing's ulcer). Bleeding is the only significant sequelae of the stress ulcer syndrome, as these superficial erosions do not perforate. Therefore, if perforation is seen, it is due to another entity.

Early studies in critically ill patients not receiving prophylactic therapy showed a 5% to 15% bleeding rate (9, 31). Mortality rates exceeded 50% in cases with significant overt bleeding. Therapy for this syndrome has focused on prophylaxis rather than treatment of established bleeding. Prophylaxis consists of neutralizing gastric acid and/or increasing gastric defense mechanisms. Several early studies found definite benefits of prophylaxis on overt bleeding and survival (28, 31). More recent studies comparing efficacy of different prophylactic strategies have shown a lower incidence of serious bleeding and mortality. Whether the lower incidence of serious bleeding is due to some form of prophylaxis or due to a lower incidence of this syndrome because of better resuscitation and fluid therapy is unclear.

Antacid prophylaxis, which aims to keep the gastric pH above 3, has been shown to significantly decrease the incidence of bleeding and possibly to stop that which has begun (31). This form of therapy, though effective, can be time consuming, be messy, and possibly produce aspiration or diarrhea.

Intravenous $H_2$ blockers, although providing less precise pH control, have efficacy very similar to antacids with respect to the prevention of severe hemorrhage (9,

28). Improved pH control may be obtained with primed infusions rather than bolus regimens (32). As cimetidine inhibits the cytochrome P-450 system, care must be taken in adjusting dosing regimens of drugs metabolized by this pathway, such as theophylline, warfarin, and lidocaine (33).

Sucralfate seems to have comparable efficacy to acid-reducing regimens for the prophylaxis of stress bleeding. Its mechanism of action is unclear but may be due to a local protective effect and augmentation of the effect of basic fibroblast growth factor (34). There have been recent concerns over the permissive effects of achlorhydria from acid reduction regimens on the overgrowth of enteric gram-negative organisms and the increased potential for nosocomial pneumonia (35). Although several studies have suggested higher nosocomial pneumonia rates in patients receiving acid-reducing prophylaxis with antacids or cimetidine compared to sucralfate, these differences have not reached statistical significance and several studies have failed to show a similar pattern (36). However, the concerns about the potential for nosocomial pneumonia still warrant further study.

Although prostaglandin analogues protect gastric mucosa against a variety of experimental injuries in animals, early human trials showed no benefit of a $PGE_2$ analogue for prevention of stress bleeding (37). However, more recent trials with misoprostil have shown this agent to be as effective as an antacid regimen (38).

Treatment of established bleeding from stress ulceration is similar to that for bleeding from other nonvariceal upper GI entities and includes hemodynamic support and correction of coagulopathy and hypothermia. Antacid therapy may be helpful in this entity (31). Surgical therapy has been reported as necessary in 10% to 40% of patients with severe ongoing bleeding from stress ulceration, but mortality is over 50% (39). The most common operation for massive bleeding is vagotomy and drainage and oversewing of bleeding sites. Near total or total gastrectomy has been utilized by some surgeons, because the incidence of rebleeding after this procedure is lessened. Stress-related bleeding also has been controlled with gastric devascularization, which is interesting considering that gastric hypoperfusion is thought to be central to the pathogenesis of this entity. Fortunately, the incidence of massive bleeding has decreased to the point where some view this as an entity of historical interest only. In our experience over the last 10 years, we have seen only one nonterminal patient bleed massively from stress ulceration. Some recent reports suggesting a high incidence of this entity probably have improperly classified cases of upper GI hemorrhage as due to erosive gastritis when the source of bleeding was a more common entity such as a gastric or duodenal ulcer (6). Bleeding from discrete ulcers in the duodenum is virtually always caused by peptic disease rather than stress-related mucosal erosion (7). As discussed before, bleeding from peptic disease or nonsteroidal agents certainly remains a serious and relatively common problem.

## PANCREATIC COMPLICATIONS

The incidence of acute pancreatitis and its sequelae are often difficult to determine in acutely ill cardiac patients. The best studied groups seem to be those patients who develop this complication following cardiopulmonary bypass. Even here, the relative incidence varies greatly between series and seems to be much higher in autopsy series than when identified prospectively (40). Pancreatic complications account for approximately 5% to 25% of the GI complications seen after open-heart surgery (1, 2, 41). However, in autopsy series following cardiac surgery, pancreatitis is reported in as many as 16% of patients examined (40). This suggests that pancreatic complications may be present commonly in severely ill patients but not suspected clinically. There are several possibilities for these discrepancies:

1. Patients who have multiple complications after open-heart surgery are both more likely to die and also to develop pancreatitis.
2. Pancreatitis in itself may contribute to death.
3. Pancreatitis is often difficult to diagnose, especially in critically ill patients, leading to underestimation of its incidence.

A number of factors have been implicated in the development of pancreatitis in patients with cardiac disease and after cardiac surgery. This complication is seen more frequently in patients with hypotension, patients treated with inotropes, and patients developing renal failure (41, 42). It is thought that hypotension and hypoperfusion, as a result of either general instability or cardiopulmonary bypass, are key elements in the development of ischemic injury to the pancreas. Compliment activation and platelet or white blood cell aggregation may also play a role (41). Some have suggested that postoperative formation of stones in lithogenic bile also may contribute (43). Some investigators (44) have found a correlation with the administration of calcium (>800 mg/m₂ body surface area), although others have not found this to be a factor (41).

The diagnosis in the awake patient often can be made on clinical grounds. Sudden development of abdominal pain and nausea, especially with back pain, is most common. The patient may develop fever. Physical examination often shows a quiet abdomen, which may be exquisitely tender in the epigastrium. Occasionally a mass may be palpated.

Laboratory investigations frequently disclose an elevated serum amylase concentration (45). Serum amylase levels are elevated in most, but not all, patients with acute pancreatitis. It should be kept in mind that an elevation of amylase concentration can be found in a number of other conditions other than pancreatitis, such as renal failure, bowel obstruction or perforation, salivary duct obstruction, pneumonia, macroamylasemia, or malignancy (46). In one study of patients developing pancreatitis postbypass, pancreatitis was sometimes found only at laparotomy for a complicated postoperative course, and only 50% of these patients manifested an elevated amylase (41). Other blood tests may be helpful in corroborating the diagnosis of pancreatitis and assessing its severity. Elevations of white blood cell count, serum glucose, and lactic dehydrogenase (LDH) levels may portend a poorer prognosis. These, in conjunction with advanced age and high fluid requirements, are predictors of severity of pancreatitis (47, 48).

Routine radiographs are used primarily to include or exclude other entities such as pneumonia and bowel perforation or obstruction in the development of a list of differential diagnoses. An ultrasound examination may be helpful, particularly if little bowel gas is present and it demonstrates pancreatic enlargement, gallstones, or a pseudocyst. A normal examination does not exclude pancreatitis, and often examinations may be suboptimal due to superimposed ileus and large amounts of bowel gas (49).

Computed tomography (CT) is much more useful than either plain films or ultrasound in evaluating patients with presumed pancreatitis (50). A normal CT scan in the face of deteriorating clinical findings suggests that the patient does not have pancreatitis and other diagnoses should be entertained. The CT scan also may suggest other processes. In particular, CT is an exquisitively sensitive way to detect small amounts of free air, and this finding, and/or contrast extravasation, supports the diagnosis of a bowel perforation. The extent of disease, especially nonperfused areas of pancreas on dynamic contrast-enhanced scan (51), and associated abnormalities, such as fluid collections, may be predictive of the severity of the clinical course of pancreatitis (50). Evidence of pancreatic necrosis or peripancreatic infection on scan may lead to earlier operative intervention and debridement.

The early therapy of pancreatitis involves adequate resuscitation of intravascular volume. Loss of circulating volume can be enormous due to the sequestration of fluid into "third spaces" (e.g., retroperitoneum, mesentery, bowel wall). The hemodynamic pattern during early pancreatitis may appear similar to that of blood loss, especially in cases of hemorrhagic pancreatitis, although the clinical picture more often resembles that of septic shock with elevated heart rate, high cardiac output, and low peripheral vascular resistance. Invasive monitoring, including Swan-Ganz catheterization, may be required to adequately gauge the adequacy of resuscitation.

A large number of pharmacologic agents have been studied in attempts to control the ravages of pancreatitis. Attempts to control pancreatic secretion (with agents such as somatostatin), inhibit proteolysis (with aprotinin), or reduce inflammation (with indomethacin or prostaglandin) all have been futile. Prophylactic antibiotics have not been shown to be of benefit, except possibly in cases of biliary pancreatitis, in which the possibility of cholangitis or infected bile exists (52).

As gallstones are thought to be a much less common factor in the development of pancreatitis in the cardiac patient than the general population, indications for specific investigations and therapy such as endoscopic retrograde cholangiopancreatography (ERCP) and surgery are not common. The timing of definitive therapy of gallstone-related pancreatitis with ERCP or surgery is extremely controversial (53, 54). As most patients respond with supportive measures alone, early intervention may have a role only in the most acute cases (55). Even in selected groups, the risks of intervention are always present and the benefits seem small when compared to delayed therapy.

Patients with severe pancreatitis can develop infected pancreatic necrosis, which is often inappropriately called "pancreatic abscess." This complication arises from super-infection of necrotic peripancreatic tissue and is not a localized, drainable abscess, but instead a mass of nonviable infected tissue which must be surgically debrided. A patient with increasing severity of symptoms, fever, and illness 1 to 2 weeks after the onset of acute pancreatitis should be suspected as having this serious complication. A CT scan may be helpful in demonstrating the presence of small amounts of air in the retroperitoneum or as a guide for a needle aspiration and gram stain of the peripancreatic phlegmon. If this aspirate is positive for white blood cells and organisms, then surgery is required involving one or many debridements. Despite all improvements in therapy, mortality rates for this complication still range from 20% to 50% with surgery and approximates 100% without operation (56).

## GASTROINTESTINAL PERFORATION

Although perforations of the GI tract occur in the cardiac patient less commonly than bleeding complications, they are still relatively frequent, representing approximately 15% of GI complications (1–3). These perforations are most frequently found in the stomach and duodenum as a consequence of gastric or duodenal ulceration. Perforated sigmoid diverticula are also reported but are relatively rare. Occasionally, segments of infarcted intestine may perforate as well, but this will be discussed under the section on intestinal ischemia.

Patients with gastroduodenal perforation seem to have an especially virulent form of peptic disease. This may be an exacerbation of preexisting peptic ulcer diathesis, which has been present for many years but has been quiescent and is only unmasked after a severe illness or surgery (7). By definition, true stress-related mucosal erosions or stress ulcerations do *not* perforate and, therefore, cannot be held responsible for gastric or duodenal perforations. Nonsteroidal anti-inflammatory drugs also seem to increase the incidence of perforation (8).

The diagnosis of perforation is most often signaled by the development of abdominal pain and tenderness several days to a week after an acute cardiac event or surgery. The patient may have a low-grade fever and vital signs may be stable, or hypotension may develop if peritoneal soilage is marked. Patients most often have upper abdominal tenderness and may have rigidity, guarding, rebound tenderness, and ileus. These typical findings of peritoneal irritation may be markedly blunted in patients who are receiving corticosteroids or who have been heavily dosed with analgesics and/or sedatives following cardiac surgery. The white blood cell count is usually somewhat elevated, although this abnormally may reflect a general stress response, and thus this finding may not be particularly useful. Hyperamylasemia is seen in approximately 15% of cases of upper intestinal perforation (57) and may lead to the misdiagnosis of the problem as acute pancreatitis.

Plain radiographs may be extremely helpful in the diagnosis of intestinal perforation. Free air is seen in approximately 70% of the cases on an upright chest film (58), but care must be taken to assure that the patient has had adequate time (5 to 10 min) in the upright position to allow air to accumulate under the diaphragm. Not infrequently, free air in the peritoneum may be the only clinical finding in the intubated and sedated patient. Computed tomography is much more sensitive than are plain films for detecting the presence of free air in the abdomen (58) and may be especially helpful in determining whether or not there is true free air present or whether the findings on the chest film are due to tracking of mediastinal or plural air into the subdiaphragmatic space following cardiac surgery, pneumothorax, or mechanical ventilation. An upper GI series (using gastrograffin as the contrast agent) is helpful in cases without free air, when the diagnosis is in question, or, if nonoperative therapy is being considered, to demonstrate that a perforation is sealed.

Most patients with a perforated ulcer will require surgical therapy (59). Nonoperative therapy may be considered when it is clear that there is no ongoing soiling of the peritoneum, the patient has adequate immune function, the patient is expected to have the ability to manifest clinical signs of deterioration, and cancer is not expected. Therefore, nonoperative management can be considered in patients with symptoms lasting more than 24 hours, no signs of diffuse peritonitis, and a sealed ulcer demonstrated by upper GI series or CT (60) (Table 2). Approximately 30% of patients with perforation are shown to be sealed on radiographic studies (61). If nonoperative therapy is to be pursued, surgical consultation is essential. The patient should have nasogastric suction and continuous infusion of an $H_2$ antagonist to suppress acid secretion and promote ulcer healing. Antibiotics active against

**TABLE 2.** *Selection of nonoperative therapy for perforated ulcer*

| Relative indications | Contraindications |
|---|---|
| Duodenal ulcer | Gastric ulcer |
| History > 25 hr | History < 24 hr |
| Localized findings | Generalized peritonitis |
| Sealed by contrast study | Free perforation on upper gastrointestinal tract |
| Improvement with time | Increasing symptoms |
| | Steroids |

gram-negative bacteria should be administered. Patients who have received antibiotics in the recent past should be considered for antifungal therapy with fluconazole. The patient should be monitored closely for deterioration of physical examination, vital signs, or symptoms in which case surgical therapy should be instituted immediately. The delayed complications of localized abscess may be searched for at approximately 1 week after perforation by CT scan and, if present, drained percutaneously. Patients with multiple medical problems are often considered for nonoperative therapy. However, it should be remembered that the somewhat complicated but compensated patient with multiple medical problems is much better able to withstand controlled surgery than uncontrolled sepsis.

The primary goal of surgical therapy is closure of the perforation. Additional benefits of operative therapy are the drainage of infected contents, lavage, and possibly surgical control of the underlying peptic disease. All patients with a perforated duodenal ulcer should have the ulcer sealed by suture closure or omental patch and the peritoneal cavity irrigated. Gastric ulcers, because of concerns about long-term healing and carcinoma, generally should be resected (5). Patients with a long history of duodenal ulcer disease (especially on therapy), obstruction, relative hemodynamic stability, and absence of flagrant peritonitis are good candidates for definitive therapy (parietal cell vagotomy, vagotomy and pyloroplasty, or vagotomy and antrectomy) (5, 62–64). Recently, laparoscopic repair of perforated duodenal ulcers with or without concomitant acid-lowering procedures has been reported (65, 66), but more experience with these techniques will need to be accrued before this approach gains wide acceptance.

As our understanding of the pathogenesis of peptic ulceration improves, the indications for definitive ulcer therapy in *duodenal* perforations are dwindling. Patients with perforations associated with nonsteroidal anti-inflammatory drug therapy probably do not require acid-lowering procedures. Those without preexisting symptoms may be well controlled postoperatively with medical therapy with $H_2$ antagonists or proton pump inhibitors and these agents may be helpful in the promotion of postoperative healing (67). With the identification of infection with *Helicobacter pylori* as the underlying cause for most cases of peptic ulceration not caused by nonsteroidal anti-inflammatory drugs and the ability to successfully eradicate this organism with antibiotics, very few patients are now candidates for more complicated surgical procedures.

## CHOLECYSTITIS

Acute cholecystitis is one of the surgical emergencies which may appear in the cardiac patient during recovery from complicated myocardial infarction or after cardiac surgery. Although relatively rare, acute cholecystitis certainly occurs in acutely ill patients and may cause a great deal of difficulty in diagnosis and therapy. Glenn et al. presented a series of cases of postoperative acute cholecystitis in 1947 (68), after which is became clear that many patients develop the syndrome in the absence of gallstones. Most series of acute cholecystitis occurring in critically ill patients report a high percentage of cases (35% to 85%) of acalculous cholecystitis (69, 70). This condition has been described after abdominal, orthopedic, and gynecologic surgery as well as after trauma burns and other causes of critical illness (71).

In the general population, acute cholecystitis is associated with the presence of gallstones in about 90% of cases (69). Diagnosis is often relatively easy on the basis of history and physical examination plus the finding of gallstones by ultrasound. The cardiac patient, however, often presents a similar constellation of symptoms. Moreover, it is sometimes difficult to obtain an adequate history from these patients, and they frequently have risk factors present for the development of biliary disease without stone formation. Over 50% of postoperative patients with acute cholecystitis have acalculous disease (69–71). The percentage is even higher among patients with critical illness (71). Acalculous cholecystitis is more frequent in males and patients with renal failure (69, 71). In one series of patients with acalculous cholecystitis, 50% of patients had cardiovascular disease and 25% had diabetes mellitus. Acalculous cholecystitis typically is a more serious problem than acute calculous cholecystitis. Ischemic necrosis and gangrene complicate acalculous disease appearing in 45% to 80% of patients, and perforation is reported in 40% of patients 48 hours after onset of symptoms (72).

Cholecystitis on the basis of stone disease is caused by cystic duct obstruction. The etiology of acalculous cholecystitis, however, is probably multifactorial (Table 3). Bile stasis often occurs due to fasting, parenteral nutrition, and anesthesia. Bile viscosity may be increased by dehydration and an increased pigment load from hemoglobin degradation products following transfusion or hemolysis. Several case reports have demonstrated cholesterol emboli to the gallbladder in patients who have had IABP in place (73). Ampullary constriction caused by narcotics may be worsened by generalized edema (74). Coloniza-

**TABLE 3.** *Factors influencing pathogenesis of acalculous cholecystitis*

| |
|---|
| Bile stasis: fasting, parenteral nutrition, ileus, anesthesia |
| Increased bile viscosity/concentration: dehydration, hemolysis/pigment load |
| Cystic duct/ampullary obstruction: anatomic variants, narcotics, edema |
| Ischemia of gallbladder wall: hypotension/shock, vasopressors, increased wall tension |
| Bacterial colonization: age, acquired immunodeficiency syndrome |

tion of bile by bacteria, which is more common in the elderly, may also contribute to infection. Cases of primary acalculous cholecystitis due to cytomegalovirus and cryptosporidium has been reported in patients with acquired immunodeficiency syndrome (AIDS) (75).

In many instances, a key factor in the development of alcalculous cholecystitis is an episode of hypotension or shock, leading to gallbladder ischemia (71). Hypoperfusion of the gallbladder may be exacerbated by the use of vasopressors. A concomitant increase in wall tension caused by inability of the gallbladder to empty may exacerbate poor perfusion. Orlando et al. (76) have developed the concept of gallbladder perfusion pressure, defined as cystic arterial pressure minus intraluminal gallbladder pressure. Low gallbladder perfusion pressure appears to play a central role in the development of acalculous cholecystitis.

The diagnosis of acalculous cholecystitis can be difficult. Patients can present with abdominal pain and right upper quadrant tenderness, which should alert the clinician to this diagnosis. A palpable gallbladder is sometimes, but not always, found. It is not always possible, however, to obtain reliable information by physical examination in critically ill patients who are sedated and narcotized.

Laboratory investigations are often difficult to interpret in this group of patients. Elevation of the white blood cell count is a frequent but nonspecific finding, as are abnormal liver enzymes. These laboratory abnormalities are usually due to other factors such as intrahepatic cholestasis rather than obstruction of either the cystic or common bile ducts.

Ultrasound examinations may be helpful but may be unreliable in the critically ill. Such examinations are frequently compromised by abdominal wounds and excessive bowel gas. In the absence of gallstones, one must rely on secondary sonographic signs to make the diagnosis of cholecystitis. Gallbladder distention, biliary sludge, subserosal edema, and wall thickening all support the diagnosis of cholecystitis, but the sensitivity of ultrasound is only 60% in the best of cases (77). False-positives are common due to distention from fasting or generalized edema. Intramural gas or sloughed mucosal membranes are much more specific findings but are less common. Computed tomography is no better than ultrasonography (78).

Attempts at performing functional studies of the gallbladder with radionuclide cholescintigraphy were originally of limited utility in the critically ill. The vast majority of these patients have dysfunction of the gallbladder as measured by standard scanning, and the incidence of false-positives is extremely high (60% to 90%) (79, 80). False-negatives were also seen in early series (81). Difficulties were also encountered in patients with severe hepatocellular dysfunction. More recent studies suggest that the addition of morphine to the scan, so-called morphine-cholescintigraphy, renders the test more sensitive and specific. Sensitivities and specificities as high 90% have been reported (82). More corroborating studies need to be done, but this approach seems quite promising.

Percutaneous aspiration of the gallbladder has been used as a diagnostic maneuver. However, inspection of the aspirate on gram stain and culture has a low sensitivity (40% to 50%), and this technique is best reserved as a therapeutic rather than a diagnostic modality (83).

The treatment of acalculous cholecystitis remains controversial. This entity is commonly associated with full-thickness gangrene and necrosis, leading ultimately to mortality. Because of a high rate of gangrene and the potential perforation, urgent cholecystectomy has been advocated as the procedure of choice. Parenteral antibiotics directed against gram-negative facultative and anaerobic organisms should be administered. Although information is not yet available, laparoscopic cholecystectomy is potentially useful in selected patients with nonperforated disease. However, concerns must be raised over the effect of carbon dioxide pneumoperitoneum in patients with respiratory failure. In those who are absolutely unable to withstand cholecystectomy, cholecystostomy has been utilized in several series (76, 80). In most early series, this procedure carried a fairly high mortality. It is unclear whether this was secondary to patient selection or to failure of cholecystostomy to adequately rid the patient of infection and disease. Other series noted that the majority of survivors were treated with open cholecystostomy rather than cholecystectomy.

Percutaneous cholecystostomy under local anesthesia is an emerging alternative that may be life saving in selected cases (84). Although there is some risk of failure in patients with a gangrenous gallbladder, the ultrasound-guided percutaneous transhepatic approach is probably useful in the majority of patients if they are treated early. Patients need to be watched extremely closely, and if signs of very rapid improvement are absent, then operative therapy should be instituted rapidly.

## INTESTINAL ISCHEMIA AND INFARCTION

The cardiac patient is at risk for the development of intestinal ischemia or infarction due to several factors (Table 4). First, these patients may be at risk for the

**TABLE 4.** *Risk factors for development of mesenteric ischemia*

| Arterial embolism | Mesenteric thrombosis | Nonocclusive mesenteric ischemia |
|---|---|---|
| Atrial fibrillation | Arteriosclerosis | Shock |
| Myocardial infarction | Dissection | Hypothermia |
| Mechanical valve | Angiography | Dialysis |
| Rheumatic valve | Hypercoagulable state | Digoxin |
| IABP[a] | | Diuretics |
| Angiography | | Beta blockers |

[a]Intra-aortic balloon pump.

development of mesenteric arterial embolism on the basis of cardiac arrhythmias, recent myocardial infarction, placement of prosthetic valves, or angiographic procedures. Second, underlying arteriosclerosis of visceral vessels, placement of an IABP, or an aortic dissection may predispose to mesenteric arterial thrombosis. Third, intestinal infarction frequently occurs in patients with low output syndromes and multiple-organ failure. Intestinal infarction is sometimes frequently associated with hepatic necrosis at operation or autopsy. Patients with nonocclusive mesenteric ischemia often are hypotensive, undergoing emergency procedures prior to development of these complications, which carry a mortality rate of over 70% and are frequently associated with long bypass times, necessity for intra-aortic balloon pumping, prolonged mechanical ventilation, hypotension, and use of vasopressors (1). It is tempting to say that an aggressive diagnostic and therapeutic approach offers a chance at lessening the high mortality of these syndromes, but early mesenteric ischemia is characterized by vague and non-specific symptoms and signs, and routine laboratory investigations and radiographs are often not diagnostic. However, a high index of suspicion and early diagnosis are the only chances for improving the high mortalities seen with intestinal ischemia.

Arterial emboli to the GI tract are much less common than are emboli to the brain or extremities. Embolization most commonly occurs at a bifurcation of the superior mesenteric artery, usually after the takeoff of the middle colic artery. Many patients with visceral emboli will have experienced prior or concomitant embolization to the brain or extremities. Clasically, visceral arterial embolization occurs in patients with atrial fibrillation or recent myocardial infarction. The patients present with acute onset of severe abdominal pain. Other risk factors include recent valve surgery, angiographic procedures, or placement of an IABP. Sir Zachary Cope warned that "any patient with an arrhythmia such as auricular fibrillation who complains of abdominal pain is highly suspect of embolization to the superior mesenteric artery until proved otherwise"(85). Patients with visceral emolization are often younger then

those suffering from arterial thrombosis or nonocclusive infarction and seem to derive more benefit from early aggressive angiography and surgery (86).

Mesenteric arterial thrombosis most often occurs very proximally on the superior mesenteric artery. The most common etiology is advanced arteriosclerosis of this artery with disease involving at least one of the other major visceral vessels of the abdominal aorta leading to decreased collateral flow. Trauma, aortic dissection (either spontaneous or induced by IABP placement), and hypercoagulable states may contribute to the development of this syndrome. A history of abdominal angina is present in approximately 50% of patients who develop ischemia secondary to arterial thrombosis. In these patients, the onset of abdominal pain typically is more insidious than is the case in patients with acute arterial thrombosis (87).

A nonocclusive mechanism accounts for 25% to 50% of patients with visceral ischemia and infarction. These patients usually exhibit evidence of low cardiac output and organ perfusion. Frequently they are receiving digitalis, diuretics, or vasopressors.

The critical event for development of nonocclusive mesenteric ischemia appears to be low cardiac output, which activates the renin-angiotensin axis leading to a marked increase in mesenteric resistance and a disproportionate decrease in blood flow to the gut (88).

Acute intestinal ischemia most often presents with abdominal pain which is frequently *out of proportion to physical findings*. The lack of persuasive physical findings or laboratory abnormalities unfortunately frequently continue to the point of frank infarction even under observation. This problem is as difficult today as it was earlier in this century when Zachary Cope observed that "the abdomen gradually becomes distended, but permanent tenderness and rigidity are absent until late in the course of the disease. Fever, leukocytosis, hypotension and tachycardia tend to be very late manifestations (too late!) and attempts to establish the correct diagnosis must antedate the time when the true state of affairs is evident even to the most inexperienced observer. Overt peritonitis occurs so late in the course of the disease, that it might well be regarded as a pre-morbid event"(85).

Physical findings and aberrations in laboratory and radiographic investigations are few in the early stages. With prolonged ischemia, pain increases and bowel sounds may decrease and abdominal distention may be present. At this stage, the signs of intravascular volume depletion may become manifest as fluid is sequestered in the bowel wall, bowel lumen, and peritoneal cavity. When ischemia continues to the point of transmural infarction, localized or generalized tenderness or peritoneal signs appear. Laboratory values lag behind symptoms. Elevation of the hematocrit can be a nonspecific finding indicative of intravascular volume depletion. Elevation of the white blood cell count is usually a later sign.

Elevation of the serum amylase activity also may be present, but this finding is nonspecific and unreliable and may add to the confusion of the situation by prompting misdiagnosis of the problem as pancreatitis. Impressive elevations of liver transaminases suggest hepatic hyperprofusion and necrosis. Lactic acidosis may be present but is a late finding. The absence of acidosis may occur when blood flow to the gut is so low that washout of protons and other metabolic end products virtually ceases.

In the earliest stages of nonocclusive ischemia, plain films of the abdomen are normal. Later, a nonspecific picture of distended small-bowel loops may develop. This pattern can be difficult to distinguish from early mechanical obstruction. "Thumb printing" or bowel wall thickening may be present. Gas in the bowel wall is a late finding. Gas bubbles in the mesenteric or portal veins are another late and very ominous sign.

Once intestinal ischemia is suspected, the patient must be resuscitated. A decision must be made whether to perform immediate surgery or arteriography. Patients demonstrating unequivocal evidence of peritonitis must undergo laparotomy. However, arteriography may be a useful diagnostic and even therapeutic maneuver in patients who have no signs of peritonitis and who are reasonably stable. The diagnosis of an embolus or thrombosis can be clearly made, and in those patients the surgeon is given a clear "road map" from which to plan embolectomy or revascularization of the gut. Arteriography also may identify vasoconstriction and evidence of nonocclusive disease. Arterial spasm and "pruning" and decreased filling of intramural vessels may be seen in patients with nonocclusive mesenteric ischemia.

Some authors have advocated aggressive management using preoperative arteriography and selective infusions of vasodialators such as papaverine and phenoxybenzamine. It is unclear whether their improved survival rates reflect their therapy or simply an increased awareness and earlier supportive treatment of patients with intestinal ischemia (89).

If clots can be demonstrated within the mesenteric system, lytic therapy may also be undertaken. There have been a few early encouraging reports (90); however, lytic therapy carries substantiated risks, including problems due to anaphylaxis, bleeding, and a delay in definitive therapy.

The primary initial therapy of intestinal ischemia is fluid resuscitation and restoration of blood flow to the intestine. Adequate fluid resuscitation may be all that is necessary in the mildest cases. Restitution of flow to the entire body and to the local circulation is of the utmost importance. Some laboratory evidence suggests that the use of angiotension-converting enzyme (ACE) inhibitors may be useful in increasing mesenteric blood flow by interrupting excessive activation of the renin-angiotensin axis (91). The efficacy of therapy with ACE inhibitors in clinical situations remains unproven, and one must worry about hypotension as a side effect of this strategy. The

judicious use of inotropes with beta activity used as a part of the total resuscitation of the patient is reasonable.

Systemic heparinization is instituted in cases of embolism or thrombosis to prevent clot propagation and further emboli. Occasional cases of emboli have been demonstrated to have lysed and migrated distally on angiography.

Broad-spectrum antibiotic therapy is useful not only for the treatment of possible systemic infection and bacterial translocation from the gut, but also because it may be helpful in salvaging locally ischemic areas from transmural infarction. Animal studies suggest that recovery of a damaged gut wall from an ischemic event is enhanced by antibiotic therapy.

The restoration of blood flow to ischemic areas may promote the production of oxygen free radicals. It has been suggested from animal data that this "reperfusion" injury may actually be more detrimental to the intestine than the ischemia itself (92). Mitigation of the ischemia/reperfusion damage with scavaging agents such as dimethyl sulfoxide (DMSO) or allopurinol may hold promise, but the timing of administration and delivery of these agents have frustrated clinical investigators.

Once resuscitation and early therapy have been completed, a decision regarding surgery must be made. Operation is performed to restore blood flow to the intestine and to resect obviously infarcted bowel. The diagnosis of arterial occlusion versus nonocclusive disease is often made at the time of surgery. In cases of vascular occlusion, attempts are made either by embolectomy or bypass to restore the viability of the intestine. After maximal attempts have been completed to restore visceral blood flow, the determination of intestinal viability is undertaken. The surgeon should attempt to minimize the amount of bowel resected, although extensive segments of the intestine may be ischemic. Viability and the limits of resection typically are determined by using a combination of clinical criteria such as presence of pulsation in the mesentery and the presence, peristalsis, and coloration of the intestinal wall. Additional data can be obtained via the use of a Doppler ultrasound to detect arterial flow in the wall and fluorescein injections to document perfusion (93, 94). In cases where large amounts of small intestine are of marginal viability, the surgeon may elect to return these areas to the peritoneal cavity, close the abdomen, and then return 24 hours later for a planned "second-look" operation in an effort to avoid massive enteric resections. For infarctions involving more limited sections of intestine, resection is performed with primary anastomosis in the most favorable cases and with the establishment of stomas in cases where intestinal viability is questioned or where there is involvement of the colon.

Despite the advances in intraoperative technique and postoperative care, mesenteric ischemia and infarction still carry a mortality rate of approximately 70%. Most deaths are due to delay in diagnosis, severe underlying disease, and the development of multiple organ failure.

# REFERENCES

1. Johnston G, Vitikainen K, Knight R, Annest L, Garcia C. Changing perspective on gastrointestinal complications in patients undergoing cardiac surgery. *Am J Surg* 1992;May(5):525.
2. Huddy SPJ, Joyce WP, Pepper JR. Gastrointestinal complications in 4473 patients who underwent cardiopulmonary bypass-surgery. *Br J Surg* 1991;78:293.
3. Aranha GV, Pickleman J, Pifarre R. The reasons for gastrointestinal consultation after cardiac surgery. *Am Surg* 1984;50(6):301.
4. Hanks JB, Curtis S, Hauks BB. Gastrointestinal complications following bypass. *Surgery* 1982;92:294.
5. Lawhorne TW, Davis JL, Smith GW. General surgical complications after cardiac surgery. *Am J Surg* 1978136:254.
6. Rosen HR, Vlahakes GJ, Rattner DW. Fulminant peptic ulcer disease in cardiac surgical patients: pathogenesis, prevention and management. *Crit Care Med* 1992;20(3):354.
7. Matthews JB, Tortella BJ, Silen W. Gastrointestinal hemorrhage and perforation in the postoperative period. *Surg Gynecol Obstet* 1988;167(5):389.
8. Gabriel SW, Jaakimainen L, Bombardier C. Risk for serious gastrointestinal complications related to use of non-steroidal anti-inflammatory drugs: a meta-analysis. *Ann Int Med* 1991;115:787.
9. Zuckerman GR, Cort D, Shuman RB. Stress ulcer syndrome. *J Int Care Med* 1988;3:21.
10. Laine L, Peterson WL. Bleeding peptic ulcer. *New Engl J Med* 1994;331:717.
11. Kim U, Ruick J, Aufses AH. Surgical management of acute upper gastrointestinal bleeding. Value of early diagnosis and prompt surgical intervention. *Arch Surg* 1978;114:1444.
12. Vellacott KD, Dronfield MW, Atkinson M, Langman MHS. Comparison of surgical and medical management of bleeding peptic ulcers. *Br Med J* 1982;284:548.
13. Cook DJ, Guyatt GH, Salena BT, Laine LA. Endoscopic therapy for acute non-variceal upper gastrointestinal hemorrhage: a meta-analysis. *Gastroenterology* 1992;102:139.
14. Peterson WL, Barnett CC, Smith HJ, Allen MH, Corbett DB. Routine early endoscopy in upper gastrointestinal tract bleeding: a randomized controlled trial. *N Engl J Med* 1981;304:925.
15. Griffiths WJ, Newman DA, Welsh JD. The visible vessel as an indicator of uncontrolled or recurrent gastrointestinal hemorrhage. *N Engl J Med* 1979;300:1441.
16. Waterman WG, Walker BA. The effect of gastric cooling on hemostasis. *Surg Gynecol Obstet* 1974;137:80.
17. Collins R, Langman M. Therapy with histamine H2-antagonists in acute gastrointestinal hemorrhage. *N Engl J Med* 1985;313:660.
18. Peterson WW, Richardson CT. Sustained fasting achlorhydria: a comparison of medical regimens. *Gastroenterology* 1985;88:666.
19. Daneshmend TK, Hawkey O, Langman MJS, et al. Omeprazole vs. placebo for acute upper gastrointestinal bleeding: randomized double blind control trial *BMJ* 1992;304:143.
20. Fogel MR, Knaver CM, Ljudevit LA, et al. Continuous intravenous vasopressin in active upper gastrointestinal bleeding: a placebo-controlled trial. *Ann Intern Med* 1982;96:565.
21. Morris DL, Kawker PC, Brearly S, et al. Optimal timing of operation for bleeding peptic ulcer: prospective randomized trial. *Br Med J* 1984;228:1277.
22. Branicki FJ, Coleman S, Fok J, et al. Bleeding peptic ulcer: a prospective evaluation of risk factors for re-bleeding and mortality. *World J Surg* 1990;14:262.
23. Stone AM, Stein R, McCarthy K, et al. Surgery for bleeding duodenal ulcer. *Am J Surg* 1978;136:306.
24. Bekada H, Charikhi M, Harcher R, et al. Bleeding peptic ulcer. *Am J Surg* 1989;147:375.
25. Welch CE, Rodkey GV, Gryska PV. A thousand operations for ulcer disease. *Ann Surg* 1986204:454.
26. Johnson D, Lyndon J, Smith RB, et al. Highly selective vagotomy without a drainage procedure in the treatment of hemorrhage, perforation and stenosis due to peptic ulcer. *Br J Surg* 1993;60:790.
27. Herrington JL, Davidson J. Bleeding gastrointestinal ulcers: choice of operations. *World J Surg* 1987;ll:204.
28. Puera D, Johnson LF. Cimetadine for prevention and treatment of gastroduodenal mucosal lesions in patients in an intensive care unit. *Ann Intern Med* 1988;103:173.
29. Silen W, Merhave A, Simpson JNL. The pathophysiology of stress ulcer disease. *World J Surg* 1981;5:165.
30. Stothert JC, Simonowitz DA, Dellinger EP, et al. Randomized prospective evaluation of cimetidine and antacid control of gastric pH in the critically ill. *Ann Surg* 1980;192:169.
31. Hastings PR, Skillman JJ, Bushell S, Silen W. Antacid titration in the prevention of acute gastrointestinal bleeding: a controlled randomized trial in 100 critically ill patients. *N Engl J Med* 1978;308:1041.
32. Ostro MJ, Russell JA, Solden SJ, et al. Control of gastric pH with cimetidine: boluses vs. primed infusions. *Gastroenterology* 1985;89:532.
33. Freston JW. Safety perspectives on parenteral H2 receptor antagonists. *Am J Med* 1987;83(Suppl 6A):58.
34. Folkman J, Weisz PB, Joullie MM, et al. Control of angiogenesis with synthetic heparin substitues. *Science* 1989;243:1490.
35. Driks MR, Craven DE, Cell BR, et al. Nosocomial pneumonia in intubated patients given sucralfate as compared with antacids or histamine type-2 blockers. *N Engl J Med* 1987;317:1376.
36. Karlstadt RG, Iberti TJ, Silverstein J, et al. Comparison of cimetidine and placebo for the prophylaxis of upper gastrointestinal bleeding due to stress-related gastric mucosal bleeding in the intensive care unit. *J Int Care Med* 1990;5:26.
37. Skillman JJ, Lisbon A, Long P, Silen W. 15(4)-15 methyl prostaglandin E2 does not prevent gastrointestinal bleeding in seriously ill patients. *Am J Surg* 1984;14:461.
38. Zinner MJ, Rypins LF, Martin O, et al. Misoprostil vs. antacid in the prevention of stress bleeding and lesions in ICU patients: a randomized prospective double-blind trial. *Gastroenterology* 1987;92:1711 (abst).
39. Hubert JP, Kiernan PD, Wech JJ, et al. The surgical management of bleeding stress ulcers. *Ann Surg* 1980;191:672.
40. Warshaw AL, O'Hara PJ. Susceptibility of the pancreas to ischemic injury in shock. *Ann Surg* 1978;188:197.
41. Lefor AT, Vuocolo P, Parker FB, Sillen LF. Pancreatic complications following cardiopulmonary bypass. *Arch Surg* 1992;127:1225.
42. Jacobs ML, Daggett WM, Civetta JM, et al. Acute pancreatitis: analysis of factors influencing survival. *Ann Surg* 1977;185:43.
43. Little JM, Avramovic J. Gallstone formation after major abdominal surgery. *Lancet* 1991;337:1135.
44. Fernandez-del-Castillo C, Harringer W, Warshaw A, et al. Risk factors for pancreatic cellular injury after cardiopulmonary bypass. *N Engl J Med* 1991;325:382.
45. Hass GS, Warshaw AL, Daggett WM, Aretz JHT. Acute pancreatitis after cardiopulmonary bypass. *Am J Surg* 1985;149:508.
46. Adams JT, Libertino JA, Schwartz SI. Significance of an elevated serum amylase. *Surgery* 1968;63:877.
47. Ranson JHC, Rifkind KM, Roses DF. Prognostic signs and the role of operative management in acute pancreatitis. *Surg Gynecol Obstet* 1974;138:69.
48. Sauven P, Playforth MJ, Evans M, Pollock AV. Fluid sequestration: an early indicator of mortality in acute pancreatitis. *Br J Surg* 1986;73:799.
49. McKay AJ, Imrie CW, O'Neill J, Duncan JG. Is an early ultrasound scan of value in acute pancreatitis? *Br J Surg* 1982;69:369.
50. Ranson JCC, Balthazar E, Caccuale R, et al. Computed tomography and the prediction of pancreatic abscess in acute pancreatitis. *Ann Surg* 1985;201:656.
51. Kivisarri L, Somer K, Standertskhold-Nordenstam CG, Schroder T, Kivilaakso E, Lempinen M. A new method for the diagnosis of acute hemorrhagic-necrotizing pancreatitis using contrast-enhanced CT. *Gastrointest Radiol* 1984;9:27.
52. Finch WT, Sawyers JL, Schenker S. A prospective study to determine the efficacy of antibiotics in acute pancreatitis. *Ann Surg* 1976;183:667.
53. Steer ML. Timing of surgery for gallstone pancreatitis. *Gastroenterology* 1986;91:780.
54. Rosseland AK, Solhuag JH. Early or delayed endoscopic papilotomy (EPT) in gallstone pancreatitis. *Ann Surg* 1984;199:165.
55. Neoptolemos JP, Carr-Locke DL, London NJ, et al. Controlled trial of urgent endoscopic retrograde cholangiopancreatography and endoscopic sphincterotomy versus conservative treatment for acute pancreatitis due to gallstones. *Lancet* 1988;II:979.

56. Beger HG, Krautzberger W, Bittner R, Block S, Buchler M. Results of surgical treatment of necrotizing pancreatitis. *World J Surg* 1985; 9:972.

57. Amerson JR, Howard JM, Vaules KDJ. The amylase concentration in serum and peritoneal fluid following acute perforation of gastroduodenal ulcers. Ann Surg 1958;147:245.

58. Madrazo BL, Halpert RD, Sander MA, Pearlberg JL. Computerized tomographic findings in penetrating peptic ulcer. *Radiology* 1984; 153:751.

59. Roso HL, Berne CJ. Acute perforation of peptic ulcer. In: Nyhus LM, Wastell C, eds. *Surgery of the stomach and duodenum.* 4th ed. Boston: Little Brown; 1986:457.

60. Kristersen ES. Conservative therapy of 155 cases of perforated peptic ulcer. *Acta Chir Scand* 1980;146:189.

61. Crofts TJ, Park KG, Stelle RJ, Chung SS, Li AK. A randomized trial of nonoperative treatment for perforated peptic ulcer. *N Engl J Med* 1989;320:970.

62. Tanphiphat C, Tanprayoon T, NaThalang A. Surgical treatment of perforated duodenal ulcer: a prospective trial between simple closure and definitive surgery. *Br J Surg* 1985;72:370.

63. Christiansen J, Anderson OB, Bonnesen T, Backgaard N. Perforated duodenal ulcer managed by simple closure versus closure and proximal gastric vagotomy. *Br J Surg* 1987;74:286.

64. Ceneviva R, de Castro e Silva A, Castelfranchi PL, Modena JLP, Santos RF. Simple suture with or without proximal gastric vagotomy for perforated duodenal ulcer. *Br J Surg* 1986;73:427.

65. Mouret P, Francois Y, Vignal J, Barth X, Lombard-Blatet R. Laparoscopic treatment of perforated peptic ulcer. *Br J Surg* 1990;77:1006.

66. Sunderland GT, Chisholm EM, Lau WY, Chung SC, Li AK. Laparoscopic repair of perforated peptic ulcer. *Br J Surg* 1992;79:785.

67. Simpson CJ, Lamont G, Macdonald I, Smith IS. Effect of cimetidine on prognosis after simple closure of perforated duodenal ulcer. *Br J Surg* 1987;74:104.

68. Glenn F. Acute cholecystitis following surgical treatment of unrelated disease. *Ann Surg* 1947;126:411.

69. Ottinger LW. Acute cholecystitis as a postoperative complication. *Ann Surg* 1976;184:162.

70. Devine RM, Farnell MB, Much P. Acute cholecystitis as a complication in surgical patients. *Arch Surg* 1984;119:1389.

71. Walden DT, Urrutia F, Soloway RD. Acute acalculous cholecystitis. *J Int Care Med* 1994;9:235.

72. Johnson LB. The importance of early diagnosis of acute acalculous cholecystitis. *Surg Gynecol Obstet* 1987;164:197.

73. Thomas W, Zaret P. Cholesterol emboli causing acute gangrenous cholecystitis. *Mt Sinai J Med* 1984;51:716.

74. Glenn F, Becker CG. Acute acalculous cholecystitis: an increasing entity. *Ann Surg* 1982;195:131.

75. Kauin H, Jonas RB, Chowdhury L, Kabins S. Acalculous cholecystitis and cytomegalovirus infection in the acquired immunodeficiency syndrome. *Ann Intern Med* 1986;104:53.

76. Orlando R, Gleason E, Drezner AD. Acute acalculous cholecystitis in the critically ill patient. *Am J Surg* 1983;145:472.

77. Carroll BA. Preferred imaging techniques for the diagnosis of cholecystitis and cholelithiasis. *Am J Surg* 1989;210:1.

78. Cornuell EE, Rodriguez A, Mirvis SW, Shorr RM. Acute acalculous cholecystitis in critically ill patients. Preoperative diagnostic imaging. *Ann Surg* 1989;210:52.

79. Garner WL, Marks MV, Fabri DJ. Cholescentigraphy does not work in the critically ill. *Crit Care Med* 1986;428:417(abst).

80. Flancbaum L, Majerns TC, Cor EF. Acute post-traumatic acalculous cholecystitis. *Ann Surg* 1985;150:252.

81. Lee AW, Proudfoot WH, Griffen WO. Acalculous cholecystitis. *Surg Gynecol Obst* 1984;159:33.

82. Flancbaum L, Choban PS, Sinha R, Jonasson O. Morphine cholescentigraphy in the evaluation of hospitalized patients with suspected acute cholecystitis. *Ann Surg* 1994;22:25.

83. McGahan JP, Lindfors KK. Acute cholecystitis: diagnostic accuracy of percutaneous aspiration of the gallbladder. *Radiology* 1988;167:664.

84. Werbel GB, Nahrwold DL, Joekl RJ, et al. Percutaneous cholecystostomy in the diagnosis and treatment of acute cholecystitis in the high-risk patient. *Arch Surg* 1989;124:782.

85. Silen W. *Cope's early diagnosis of the acute abdomen.* New York: Oxford University Press; 1983:192.

86. Ottinger LW. Mesenteric ischemia. *N Engl J Med* 1982;307:535.

87. Brandt LT, Boley SJ. Ischemic intestinal syndromes. *Adv Surg* 1981; 15:1.

88. Reemus JF, Brandt IJ, Boley SJ. Ischemic diseases of the bowel. *Gastroenterol Clin North Am* 1990;19:319.

89. Boley SJ, Feinstein FR, Sammartino R, et al. *Surg Gyneocol Obstet* 1981;153:561.

90. Flickenger EG, Johnsrode IS, Ogburn NJ. Local streptokinase infusion for superior mesenteric thromboembolism. *Am J Roentgenol* 1983;140:771.

91. Bailey RW, Bulker GB, Hamilton SR, et al. Protection of the small intestine from non-occlusive mesenteric ischemia due to cardiogenic shock. *Am J Surg* 1987;153:108.

92. Parks DA, Granger DN. Ischemia induced microvascular changes: role of xanthine oxidase and hydroxyl radicals. *Am J Physiol* 1983; 245:6285.

93. Katz S, Wahal A, Williams L. New parameters of viability in ischemic bowel disease. *Am J Surg* 1974;127:136.

94. Shah S, Anderson C. Prediction of small bowel viability using Doppler ultrasound. *Am Surg* 1985;194:97.

*The Critically Ill Cardiac Patient,*
edited by V. Kvetan and D. R. Dantzker,
Lippincott-Raven Publishers, Philadelphia © 1996.

CHAPTER **9**

# Neurologic Disorders and Heart Disease

Daniel Nyhan and Richard J. Traystman

Cardiovascular disease remains the leading cause of death in the Western world. Neurologic disease is also an important cause of death. Indeed, when one considers that the risk factors for the most prevalent disorders of both the cardiovascular and nervous systems are similar, it is not surprising that apparently independent disorders of these two systems may coexist. In fact, the presence of disease in either system should alert one to the possibility of concurrent disease in the other (e.g., the presence of coronary and cerebrovascular disease in the same patient and the association of bicuspid aortic valves and intracranial aneurysms). Moreover, primary diseases of the nervous system may actually result in disorders of a previously normal cardiovascular system (e.g., subarachnoid hemorrhage may result in cardiac conduction abnormalities, dysrhythmias, and neurogenic pulmonary edema). Conversely, primary cardiac disease frequently results in serious neurologic sequelae. This latter constitutes the basis of this chapter. The manifestation of any neurologic disorder occurring in the context of cardiac disease may span the spectrum of severity, ranging from mild and/or transient on the one hand to severe and life threatening on the other.

## CEREBRAL EMBOLISM

Emboli are an important cause of cerebral infarction, and a cardiac source for such emboli accounts for approximately 15% of all cerebral infarcts (1). Neurologic manifestations resulting from embolic compromise of cerebral blood flow tend to be of sudden onset, may resolve (a function of lysis of the embolic particle), often recur repeatedly over time, and frequently have protean clinical features (a function of embolization to differing cere-

brovascular distributions). However, the vast majority of cerebral emboli lodge within the distribution of the middle cerebral artery with less than 10% occurring within the vertebrobasilar system. The suspicion that emboli, rather than an atherothrombotic event, caused a neurologic insult is accentuated by the finding of a source (frequently cardiac) or risk factor for such emboli.

### Etiology of Cerebral Embolism

Cerebral emboli may arise from the great vessels (aorta, carotids), from the heart itself, or from the venous circulation (paradoxical emboli in the setting of right to left intracardiac or pulmonary shunts). Several cardiac conditions predispose to cerebral emboli; however, atrial fibrillation and myocardial infarction are the most common.

Atrial fibrillation predisposes to left atrial thrombus formation. Atrial fibrillation may be present permanently (chronic atrial fibrillation) or patients may have sinus rhythm interrupted by periods of fibrillation (paroxysmal atrial fibrillation). The two overlap and paroxysmal atrial fibrillation often progresses to chronic atrial fibrillation. Conversely, but much less frequently, chronic atrial fibrillation may revert to sinus rhythm. In addition, atrial fibrillation frequently occurs in the setting of valvular heart disease but sometimes may not be related to the latter (nonvalvular atrial fibrillation). In the Framingham Heart Study, the incidences of new atrial fibrillation were 21.5 and 17.1 per 1,000 males and females, respectively (2). In this same study, stroke rates for individuals 55 to 64 years of age were 37.9 and 29.9 per 1,000 for males and females, respectively. Cardiovascular mortality and morbidity were doubled in patients who had atrial fibrillation (3), and even among patients with nonvalvular atrial fibrillation the stroke rate was increased fourfold (3). This risk of ischemic stroke is thought by some to be even higher when one takes "silent" cerebral infarcts into account (3). In contrast to the above studies documenting the frequent occurrence of strokes in patients with atrial

D. Nyhan and R. J. Traystman: Department of Anesthesiology/Critical Care Medicine, The Johns Hopkins University School of Medicine, Baltimore, Maryland 21287-4965.

fibrillation, one study (4) described a low incidence of this complication. However, their definition of "lone" atrial fibrillation was extremely restrictive and even precluded patients over 60 years of age.

Left ventricular thrombus may form in patients following myocardial infarction. Thrombus formation is uncommon following an inferior myocardial infarction but is common following anterior infarction, especially if there is associated anterior or apical hypokinesis or akinesis. Recent advances in imaging technology have led to the recognition that mural thrombi may occur in up to 40% of patients with an anterior myocardial infarction (5). However, systemic emboli (including cerebral emboli) are relatively uncommon (<5%). Patients with infarction who develop atrial arrhythmias or cardiac failure and those who have had a prior stroke are at increased risk of a peri-infarction cerebral embolus, which usually occurs within 2 weeks of the infarction. Large, mobile mural thrombi that protrude into the left ventricular cavity are more likely to result in systemic embolization.

Several less frequently occurring cardiac diseases also predispose to cerebral embolism. Dysrhythmias other than atrial fibrillation may predispose to thromboembolic disease. The bradytachyarrhythmias related to the sick sinus syndrome may lead to embolic stroke and represent an indication for prophylactic anticoagulation. Systemic emboli occur in approximately 30% of patients with rheumatic valvular heart disease, and 40% of these are cerebral. The incidence of embolic complications increases severalfold if atrial fibrillation is present (1). Cardiac valve replacement can result in cerebral emboli and infarction. Prosthetic valves, especially those in the mitral position, are more frequently associated with systemic emboli. Septic emboli in patients with infective endocarditis and emboli from left atrial myxomata are relatively common manifestations of these less than common cardiac diseases. Mitral Valve Prolapse of varying severity is a relatively common finding (approximately 5% of adults) (6). However, cerebral infarction is rare in these patients.

## Management of Cerebral Embolism

In patients with suspected cardioembolic phenomenon, specialized investigations are directed toward (a) confirming the site and extent of the neurologic injury and (b) establishing a cardiac source. The former could include use of computerized axial tomography and cerebral angiography while the latter could involve use of echocardiography, continuous electrocardiographic monitoring, and cardiac angiography.

Treatment of patients with embolic cerebral infarcts is aimed at (a) treating the obstructed vessel with a view to alleviating the obstruction and reinstituting blood flow, (b) treating the cardiac cause or risk factor responsible for the neurologic complication, and (c) determining the

requirement for long-term treatment. In general, anticoagulation is indicated when a cardiac source of emboli has been demonstrated or is felt likely to be present. However, anticoagulation is contraindicated in patients who have had large cerebral infarcts, in those patients who have uncontrolled hypertension, and in those who suffered hemorrhagic infarcts, at least on a short-term basis. The decision to continue anticoagulants on a long-term basis is determined by the underlying cardiac disease. For example, life-long anticoagulation is indicated in patients with chronic atrial fibrillation. In contrast, the risk of emboli is low once 3 to 6 months have passed following a myocardial infarction.

## CEREBRAL HYPOPERFUSION

Cerebral hypoperfusion resulting from cardiac disease is a relatively common clinical problem. It may be transient or more prolonged, and its duration and thus the resultant neurologic injury are significantly influenced by the underlying cardiac disease and the relative success of any treatment intervention. In addition, the severity of any neurologic injury will also be influenced by the presence of coexistent cerebrovascular disease. The neurologic manifestations of hypoperfusion may be focal or diffuse and range in severity from dizziness to severe diffuse encephalopathy and death. Cerebral hypoperfusion due to a profound decrease in cardiac output may result from a profound depression in myocardial pump functions, from mechanical obstruction to blood flow, or from the development of dysrhythmias.

### Etiology of Cerebral Hypoperfusion

Cerebral hypoperfusion occurs only with profound compromise in myocardial pump function. This, obviously, is most frequently observed as a preterminal phenomenon. The neurologic manifestations observed result from cerebral hypoxia and acidosis.

Syncope is one of the three classic symptoms of severe aortic stenosis. It may be precipitated in aortic stenosis by peripheral vasodilation and resultant preferential shunting of blood away from the cerebral vasculature. Similar neurologic manifestations may occur in obstructive cardiomyopathies (where the pathophysiology is accentuated and symptoms may be precipitated by conditions that augment inotrophy) and in patients with primary pulmonary hypertension. An inappropriately positioned left atrial myxcoma may cause a precipitous decrease in cardiac output by obstructing blood flow between the left atrium and left ventricle. Any condition that results in profound bradycardia may cause dizziness and syncope (e.g., beta-blockers, calcium antagonists, the combination, hypersensitive carotid sinus).

Ventricular dysrhythmias are an important and relatively frequent cause of total cerebral hypoperfusion and sudden death. It is estimated that sudden death from cardiac causes accounts for more than 300,000 victims per year in the United States (7, 8). Rapid improvements in the out-of-hospital management of these patients has permitted the resuscitation of many of these patients and has provided the opportunity to provide long-term treatment for these patients. This latter includes the treatment of the malignant arrhythmias themselves [antiarrhythmic drugs, automatic internal cardiac defibrillators (AICDs)] and, where feasible, the treatment of the underlying cardiac pathology. The clinical picture of sudden death has been assumed to be due to the sudden onset of potentially lethal ventricular arrhythmias. Ambulatory electrocardiographic monitoring in 157 patients who suffered sudden death revealed ventricular tachycardia progressing to ventricular fibrillation in 62%, primary ventricular fibrillation in 8%, torsades de pointes in 13%, and bradyarrhythmias in 17% of patients (9). Patients with idiopathic dilated cardiomyopathy, hypertrophic cardiomyopathy, long QT syndrome, and right ventricular dysplasia may develop malignant ventricular arrhythmias and sudden death. Over 90% of patients who have had episodes of sudden death have coronary artery disease as the underlying cause. In patients who are resuscitated, there is high long-term mortality (26% at 1 year, 38% at 2 years).

### Management of Cerebral Hypoperfusion

The management of these cases consists of active and symptomatic treatment of the neurologic injury and the identification and treatment (where possible) of the underlying cardiac disease. For example, in patients who have had "sudden death" the management consists not only of a detailed electrophysiologic assessment but also the determination of the underlying etiology. Malignant arrhythmias and sudden death occur most frequently in patients who have advanced cardiac disease. In fact, patients with advanced left ventricular dysfunction and patients with myocardial damage and scar tissue formation are at increased risk of sudden death. However, it is also now recognized that sudden death may occur in patients with coronary artery disease who do not have extensive secondary myocardial damage. Recent studies (8) have highlighted the fact that sudden death may occur in patients who even after extensive noninvasive and invasive evaluation have no evidence of structural or anatomic abnormalities. It has been suggested and sometimes persuasively argued (7, 8) that such cases may be due to silent myocardial ischemia. The latter may occur not only in the presence of anatomic coronary artery disease but also as a result of coronary artery spasm.

### HYPERTENSION

Systemic hypertension is an established risk factor for both coronary artery and cerebrovascular disease. Accelerated hypertension is now a much less frequent occurrence because of routine screening for hypertension and the availability of effective antihypertensive medications. When accelerated hypertension does occur, it usually presents either with neurologic (hypertensive encephalopathy) or cardiac manifestations (hypertensive cardiac failure and pulmonary edema). Hypertensive encephalopathy is a clinical syndrome characterized by altered mental status without focal neurologic signs but usually with retinopathy, papilledema, and varying degrees of renal insufficiency. Nonaccelerated hypertension is associated with cerebral lacunar infarcts (secondary to diffuse microangiopathy) and intracerebral hemorrhage. The neurologic manifestations dominate the clinical picture, and although cardiac disease usually does coexist, the latter may not necessarily be an overriding, immediate clinical problem.

### CONCURRENT CEREBROVASCULAR AND CORONARY ARTERY DISEASE

As inferred at the outset, the risk factors for the development of vascular disease are similar and independent of the organ within which the vascular bed lies. Thus, it is not surprising that if degenerative vascular disease exists in one organ it may also exist elsewhere. The presence of both cerebrovascular (specifically extracranial carotid) disease and coronary artery disease is an extremely important example of such. Cardiac disease in patients requiring noncardiac surgery (including carotid endarterectomy) is discussed in Chapter 2. The possible contribution of cerebrovascular disease to the neurologic complications during and following cardiopulmonary bypass are discussed later in this chapter. Cerebrovascular disease may manifest itself as asymptomatic carotid bruits, transient ischemic attacks (TIAs), or cerebral infarcts, and any of these may occur in cardiac patients with coronary artery disease ranging from silent ischemia to cardiogenic shock requiring inotropic support and intra-aortic balloon pump assistance.

Asymptomatic carotid bruits are present in approximately 4% of the population over 45 years of age (10). They are more frequent among females and increase with age in both sexes. Individuals with carotid bruits do have an increased risk of both cerebral and myocardial infarction. Transient ischemic attacks are, as one might predict, associated with increased risks of both cerebral and myocardial infarction and overall mortality (11). Cerebral infarction due to atherostenosis and thrombus formation may sometimes be difficult to distinguish from that due to emboli (either cardiac or arterial to venous) since the clinical picture may often differ only in subtle ways. However, the differentiation may be important because of differential acute (with or without anticoagulation) and long-term treatments (long-term anticoagulation and digitalization in patients with atrial fibrillation, risk factor modification in patients with degenerative cerebral arterial disease).

## DIAGNOSTIC AND THERAPEUTIC CARDIAC PROCEDURES AND NEUROLOGIC DISORDERS

### Cardiac Catherization

This procedure is associated with a low, though well-recognized, incidence of neurologic complications. One prospective study revealed an incidence of less than 1% (12). The clinical features are protean, but seizures and hemiparesis are observed most frequently. It is likely that emboli arising either from the instruments used to perform the catherization or from catheter-induced injury to the diseased vessels are responsible for these neurologic complications.

### Cardiac Surgery

Neurologic complications of cardiac surgery are an extremely important cause of postoperative mortality and morbidity following this procedure. These complications are much more frequent following cardiac surgical procedures which utilize cardiopulmonary bypass than they are in true "closed" cardiac surgical procedures.

Cardiac surgery procedures requiring cardiopulmonary bypass are performed on more than 350,000 patients in the United States each year. The incidence of neurologic complications depends on the specific neurologic complication one is discussing. Indeed, the incidence of these protean complications (Table 1) is highly variable.

#### Incidence and Epidemiology

Focal neurologic deficits occur in 2% to 6% of patients placed on cardiopulmonary bypass for cardiac surgery (13, 14). Approximately three-quarters of these occur intraoperatively, the remainder occurring postoperatively (15). The majority of these patients make a good functional (though not necessarily complete neurologic) recovery. However, 1% to 3% of patients have a permanent neurologic deficit. Furthermore, when one examines this group as a whole, the length of time spent in the intensive care unit and in the hospital is considerably longer than for those who do not develop focal neurologic deficits. Subtle signs of neurologic injury occur more frequently (16). Such abnormalities include disturbances of gait, vibration sense, reflexes, sensory perception, and visual field defects. One investigator (17) has noted retinal abnormalities in up to 25% of patients undergoing cardiopulmonary bypass.

Neuropsychologic testing provides a means of detecting subtle abnormalities of central nervous system function. Such testing reveals abnormalities in 30% to 60% of adult patients undergoing cardiac surgery involving cardiopulmonary bypass (14). Many of these abnormalities in learning, memory, etc., persist, with 20% to 30% present 6 months postoperatively, one-third of these thought to be permanent.

Delirium and encephalopathy occur following cardiac surgery with a frequency which is directly related to how strictly one defines the syndrome. One study (18) suggests an incidence approaching 30%. Other psychiatric problems also occur following cardiopulmonary bypass. These may present for the first time postoperatively or represent an exacerbation of preexisting conditions (e.g., anxiety, depression, personality disorders).

Injuries to the peripheral nervous system are also well-recognized complications in cardiac surgery patients. Sternal retraction may cause stretching of the inferior cord of the brachial plexus, causing either motor or sensory signs in the distribution of the ulnar nerve. Phrenic nerve injury may be caused by "cold injury" due to iced solutions in the mediastinum, by direct surgical trauma, or by ischemia (in association with dissection of the internal mammary artery). Unilateral phrenic nerve paralysis does not usually cause clinical problems, in contrast to bilateral paresis, which may result in respiratory failure. Recurrent laryngeal nerve injury is rare and, when it occurs, is usually left sided. Injury to nerves in the lower limb are usually a function of improper positioning in a paralyzed patient.

Certain neurologic complications appear to occur more frequently in children following cardiac surgery. Seizures (of varying types) are not an uncommon manifestation of neurologic injury following cardiopulmonary bypass in children. Extrapyramidal syndromes (choreoathetosis) also occur with disturbing frequency in these patients. The issue of whether or not cardiac surgery with cardiopulmonary bypass causes developmental delay in these patients is controversial. It is unclear whether the disease for which the surgical procedure is being performed or the surgical procedure per se causes the developmental delay. The appropriate comparison to assess the effects of cardiac surgery with bypass on developmental function cannot be performed because the appropriate comparison group consists of patients with the disease to whom no surgical therapy would be offered.

**TABLE 1.** *Classification of neurologic complications following cardiac surgery*

Focal deficits
Neuropsychiatric
Neuropsychologic performance decrements
Peripheral nerve injury
Pediatric patients (seizures, extrapyramidal syndromes, ? developmental delay)

### Etiology

Each of the central nervous system complications associated with cardiac surgery and cardiopulmonary bypass probably has multiple causes which are not always well defined in an individual patient and interact in ways which are currently poorly understood. Moreover, factors that contribute to one neurologic complication (e.g., stroke) may or may not be important in the genesis of a different complication (e.g., a depressive psychosis). However, several studies over the last two decades indicate that certain characteristics or risk factors of both the patient population (Table 2) and the methodologic conduct of the surgical procedure (Table 3) influence the incidence of neurologic complications.

It is now generally accepted that atherodegenerative disease of the ascending aorta is the most important risk factor for the development of focal neurologic deficits following cardiopulmonary bypass (13, 19–21). This is due to embolization of atheroma which may occur at any time but occurs most frequently during aortic cannulation, at the initiation of cardiopulmonary bypass, during aortic cross-clamping or declamping, and during aortic side-biting clamp placement (to perform proximal saphenous vein anastomosis). This phenomenon (embolization) has been documented intraoperatively using transcranial Doppler studies (22–24). It has recently been suggested that ultrasound studies of the ascending aorta (conducted intraoperatively) allows one to identify patients with significant disease. The resultant modification in the surgical approach and technique decreased the incidence of neurologic complications in this subpopulation to that of the overall cardiac surgery patient population (25).

Concurrent cerebrovascular disease is associated with neurologic complications following cardiopulmonary bypass. However, the clinical manifestations of preexisting cerebrovascular disease are highly variable, ranging from asymptomatic carotid bruits to overt strokes, and even within any of these patients, it is unclear whether cerebrovascular disease is an independent risk factor for neurologic complications following cardiopulmonary bypass. Asymptomatic carotid bruits are not associated with acute neurologic complications after heart surgery, and studies which demonstrate an increased incidence of stroke showed no correlation with the side of the carotid bruits (15). Prophylactic carotid endarterectomy (CEA) in patients with transient ischemic attacks does decrease

**TABLE 2.** *Possible patient "risk factors" for neurologic complications following cardiac surgery*

Disease of ascending aorta
Carotid disease
  Asymptomatic bruits, transient ischemic attacks, prior cerebrovascular accident
Age
Poor left ventricular function
Female gender
Atrial fibrillation, left ventricular thrombus

**TABLE 3.** *Possible operative risk factors for neurologic complications following cardiac surgery*

Duration of cardiopulmonary bypass
Deep hypothermic circulatory arrest
Glucose levels
Hematocrit
Acid-base balance
Use/lack of use of neuroprotective agents
Filters
Open vs. closed procedure

the *long-term* incidence of stroke. However, there is no evidence that CEA in patients with TIAs decreases the incidence of strokes associated with cardiac surgery. Both those observations (in patients with asymptomatic carotid bruits and in those with TIAs) probably reflect the fact that cerebrovascular and ascending aortic disease frequently coexist and that emboli from the ascending aorta are the probable cause of strokes in these cardiac surgery patients. A history of prior stroke may similarly be an indication of generalized severe altherodegenerative disease.

Advanced age is associated with an increased incidence of stroke following cardiac surgery (26). However, it is unclear whether age per se or the relentless progression of degenerative disease associated with the aging process is responsible for this observation (27). Poor ventricular function is associated with neurologic complications probably due to perioperative (post- as well as intraoperative) hypotension and inadequate cerebral perfusion (15, 28).

True "open"-heart procedures (e.g., valve replacement) are associated with more frequent cerebral emboli than are "closed" procedures (e.g., coronary artery bypass grafting). However, this does *not* result in a greater incidence of neurologic complications. Indeed, patients presenting for bypass surgery now have a higher incidence of neurologic complications which probably reflects their age and more advanced atherodegenerative disease (29). Similarly, the use of "filters" in the cardiopulmonary bypass circuit does decrease evidence of embolization but does not reduce neurologic complications. The same comments apply to the use of bubble (versus membrane) oxygenators. [However, there may be other nonneurologic (e.g., respiratory, hematologic) clinical benefits to using a membrane oxygenator.]

It has recently been reported (30, 31) that females have a higher incidence of neurologic complications following heart surgery. Again this may reflect the age of the population since females are older when they require surgical intervention to attenuate coronary insufficiency. This reflects the "protective" effects of estrogens in premenopausal females.

Several intraoperative factors have the potential to influence the incidence of neurologic complications. Such factors include the duration of cardiopulmonary bypass, glucose levels, acid-base management, hematocrit levels, use of circulatory arrest, and use of pharmacologic agents that may confer cerebral protection (e.g., sodium thiopental). It is generally agreed that there is a direct relation between the duration of cardiopulmonary bypass and the incidence of neurologic complications. There is ample good theoretical evidence to indicate that hyperglycemia (by facilitating anaerobic glycolysis and intracellular acidosis) may accentuate neuronal injury. Studies of neurologic outcome and neuropsychologic function following cardiac surgery have thus far failed to demonstrate a benefit of euglycemia (32). Even so, some authors still recommend avoiding hyperglycemia during cardiac surgery (33). Blood gases can be manipulated in one of two ways during hypothermia. With a *pH-stat* method, the pH and $Pa_{CO_2}$ are kept at values that we conventionally view as normal for 37°C (i.e., they are kept at pH 7.4 and 40 torr, respectively). With an *alpha-stat* method, the pH increases and the $Pa_{CO_2}$ decreases during hypothermia. There is good theoretical and experimental evidence which indicates that oxygen utilization, intracellular acid-base status, and enzyme functions are favorably influenced by using an alpha-stat approach. Cerebral autoregulation is preserved during moderate hypothermia when alpha-stat is used but not when pH-stat is used (34). However, no neurologic outcome studies have compared these two approaches. Hemodilution is employed during cardiopulmonary bypass to attenuate the increase in viscosity that would otherwise occur with hypothermia. Increases in blood flow and increased oxygen extraction compensate for the decreased oxygen-carrying capacity of blood during hypothermia. However, ischemic areas, including such areas in the brain, may already be maximally dilated and thus unable to invoke these compensatory mechanisms. In fact, there is evidence that neurologic complications in cardiac surgery are worse in patients with the largest decrement in hematocrit (35). Deep hypothermic circulatory arrest (DHCA) is used in pediatric cardiac surgery and in adults undergoing repair of aortic arch aneurysms. Cerebral blood flow and cerebral oxygen consumption are abnormal following a period of DHCA. Low flow during cardiopulmonary bypass has been suggested as a possible means of favorably altering the abnormal physiology and adverse outcome associated with DHCA (36). Recent data seem to support this hypothesis (37). Barbiturates have been shown to attenuate brain injury following focal insults. Two separate studies have been conducted examining the efficacy of barbiturates in ameliorating the neurologic complications of cardiac surgery and cardiopulmonary bypass. The first study (38) demonstrated a favorable influence of barbiturates in patients undergoing true open-heart operations, but these patients were not subjected to hypothermia. The second study (39) failed to show a positive influence of barbiturates in patients who did not have a true open-heart procedure but who were subjected to hypothermia. It is likely that the differing results reflect the different populations and that hypothermia itself may have a neuroprotective effect. In view of the questionable benefits of barbiturates in the usual clinical setting and their recognized side effects (prolonged intubation, the requirement for inotropic support), these agents are not viewed as viable clinical tools in most clinical situations.

## OTHERS

Neurologic manifestations may be part of syndromes which also have cardiac features (e.g., glycogen storage diseases, the mucopolysaccharidoses, the muscular dystrophies). In these conditions, both systems are part of the disease or syndrome. In contrast, in the aforementioned situations cardiovascular pathophysiology actually results in or causes neurologic disease. Finally, while intracranial aneurysms are associated with bicuspid aortic valves, subarachnoid hemorrhage arising from these aneurysms cause cardiopulmonary dysfunction (dysrhythmias, neurogenic pulmonary edema) rather than vice-versa.

## REFERENCES

1. Cerebral Embolism Task Force. Cardiogenic brain embolism. *Arch Neurol* 1986;43:71.
2. Kannel WB, Abbott RD, Savage DD, McNamara PM. Epidemiologic features of chronic atrial fibrillation. *N Engl J Med* 1982;306:1018.
3. Pritchett ELC. Management of atrial fibrillation. *N Engl J Med* 1992; 326:1264.
4. Kopecky SL, Gersh BJ, McGoon MD, et al. The natural history of lone atrial fibrillation: a population-based study over three decades. *N Engl J Med* 1987;317:669.
5. Visser CA, Kan G, Meltzer RS, et al. Embolic potential of left ventricular thrombus after myocardial infarction: a two-dimensional echocardiographic study of 119 patients. *J Am Coll Cardiol* 1985;5: 1276.
6. Boughner DR, Barnett HJM. The enigma of the risk of stroke in mitral valve prolapse. *Stroke* 1985;16:175.
7. DiMarco JP. Coronary artery spasm, silent ischemia, and cardiac arrest. *N Engl J Med* 1992;326:1490.
8. Myerburg RJ, Kessler KM, Mallon SM, et al. Life-threatening ventricular arrhythmias in patients with silent myocardial ischemia due to coronary artery spasm. *N Engl J Med* 1992;326:1451.
9. Chang-Sing P, Peter CT. Sudden death: evaluation and prevention. *Cardiol Clin* 1991;9:653.
10. Sandok BA, Whisnant JP, Furlan AJ, Mickell JL. Carotid artery bruits: prevalence survey and differential diagnosis. *Mayo Clin Proc* 1982;57:227.
11. Candelise L, Vigotti M, Fieschi C, et al. Italian multicenter study on reversible cerebral ischemic attacks: VI—prognostic factors and follow-up results. *Stroke* 1986;17:842.
12. Weissman BM, Aram DM, Levinsohn MW, Ben-Shachar G. Neurologic sequelae of cardiac catheterization. *Cathet Cardiovasc Diagn* 1985;11:577.
13. Tuman KJ, McCarthy RJ, Najafi H, Ivankovich AD. Differential effects of advanced age on neurologic and cardiac risk of coronary artery operations. *J Thorac Cardiovasc Surg* 1992;104:1510.
14. Aris A, Solanes H, Camara ML, et al. Arterial line filtration during cardiopulmonary bypass: neurologic, neuropsychologic, and hematologic studies. *J Thorac Cardiovasc Surg* 1986;91:526.
15. Reed GL III, Singer DE, Picard EH, DeSanctis RW. Stroke following coronary-artery bypass surgery: a case-control estimate of the risk from carotid bruits. *N Engl J Med* 1988;319:1246.

16. Shaw PJ, Bates D, Cartlidge NEF, et al. Neurologic and neuropsychological morbidity following major surgery: comparison of coronary artery bypass and peripheral vascular surgery. *Stroke* 1987;18:700.
17. Shaw PJ, Bates D, Cartlidge NEF, Heavside, Julian DG, Shaw DA. Early neurological complications of coronary artery bypass surgery. *Br Med J* 1985;291:1384.
18. Smith LW, Dimsdale JE. Postcardiotomy delirium: conclusions after 25 years? *Am J Psychiatry* 1989;146:452.
19. Gardner TJ, Horneffer PJ, Manolio TA, Hoff SJ, Pearson TA. Major stroke after coronary artery bypass surgery: changing magnitude of the problem. *J Vasc Surg* 1986;3:684.
20. Mills NL, Everson CT. Atherosclerosis of the ascending aorta and coronary artery bypass. *J Thorac Cardiovasc Surg* 1991;102:546.
21. Lynn GM, Stefanko K, Reed JF III, Gee W, Nicholas G. Risk factors for stroke after coronary artery bypass. *J Thorac Cardiovasc Surg* 1992;104:1518.
22. Padayachee TS, Parson S, Theobold R, Linley TJ, Gosling RG, Deverall PB. The detection of microemboli in the middle cerebral artery during cardiopulmonary bypass: a transcranial doppler ultrasound investigation using membrane and bubble oxygenators. *Ann Thorac Surg* 1987;44:298.
23. van der Linder J, Casimir-ahn H. When do cerebral emboli appear during open heart operations? A transcranial doppler study. *An Thorac Surg* 1991;51:237.
24. Pugsley W, Klinger L, Paschalis C, et al. Microemboli and cerebral impairment during cardiac surgery. *Vasc Surg* 1990;24:34.
25. Wareing TH, Davila-Roman VG, Barzilai B, Murphy SF, Kouchoukos NT. Management of the severely atherosclerotic ascending aorta during cardiac operations. *J Thorac Cardiovasc Surg* 1992;103:453.
26. Gardner TJ, Horneffer PJ, Manolio TA, et al. Stroke following coronary artery bypass grafting: a ten-year study. *Ann Thorac Surg* 1985;40:574.
27. Stump DA, Tegeler CH, Newman SP, Wallenhaupt S, Roy RC. Older patients have more emboli during coronary artery bypass graft surgery. *Anesthesiology* 1992;77:A52(abst).
28. Slogoff S, Reul GJ, Keats AS, et al. Role of perfusion pressure and flow in major organ dysfunction after cardiopulmonary bypass. *Ann Thorac Surg* 1990;50:911.
29. Kuroda Y, Uchimoto R, Kaieda R, et al. Central nervous system complications after cardiac surgery: a comparison between coronary artery bypass grafting and valve surgery. *Anesth Analg* 1993;76:222.
30. slogoff S, Girgis KZ, Keats AS. Etiologic factors in neuropsychiatric complications associated with cardiopulmonary bypass. *Anesth Analg* 1982;61:903.
31. Staniemi KA, Juolasmaa A, Hokkanen ET. Neuropsychologic outcome after open-heart surgery. *Arch Neurol* 1981;38:2.
32. Frasco P, Croughwell N, Bluementhal J, et al. Association between blood glucose level during cardiopulmonary bypass and neuropsychiatric outcome. *Anesthesiology* 1991;75:A56(abst).
33. Hindman BJ. Neurologic complications of cardiac anesthesia and surgery. In: Hindman BJ, ed. *Neurological and psychological complication of surgery and anesthesia.* Boston: Little Brown; 1994:1
34. Murkin JM, Farrar JK, Tweed WA, McKenzie FN, Guiraudon G. Cerebral autoregulations and flow/metabolism coupling during cardiopulmonary bypass: the influence of $P_aCO_2$. *Anesth Analg* 1987;66:825.
35. Shaw PM, Bates D, Cartlidge NEF, et al. An analysis of factors predisposing to neurological injury in patients undergoing coronary bypass operations. *Q J Med* 1989;72:633.
36. Reves JG, Greeley WJ. Cerebral blood flow during cardiopulmonary bypass: some new answers to old questions. *Ann Thorac Surg* 1989;48:752.
37. Newburger JW, Jonas RA, Wernovsky G, et al. A comparison of the perioperative neurologic effects of hypothermic circulatory arrest versus low-flow cardiopulmonary bypass in infant heart surgery. *N Engl J Med* 1993;329:1057.
38. Nussmeier NA, Arlund C, Slogoff S. Neuropsychiatric complications after cardiopulmonary bypass: cerebral protection by a barbiturate. *Anesthesiology* 1986;64:165.
39. Zaidan JR, Klochany A, Martin WM, Ziegler JS, Harless DM, Andrews RB. Effect of thiopental on neurologic outcome following coronary artery bypass grafting. *Anesthesiology* 1991;74:406.

*The Critically Ill Cardiac Patient,*
edited by V. Kvetan and D. R. Dantzker,
Lippincott-Raven Publishers, Philadelphia © 1996.

# CHAPTER 10

# Septic Shock:

## Mechanisms, Cardiovascular Abnormalities, and New Therapeutic Approaches*

Waheedullah Karzai, Charles Natanson, and Bradley D. Freeman

In the last decade, two areas of investigation, in particular, have furthered our understanding of the pathophysiology of the sepsis syndrome. These include the identification and characterization of inflammatory mediators and the definition of the cardiovascular changes associated with septic shock. This chapter will review recent developments in these areas. First, we will provide an overview of septic shock with a particular emphasis on clinical trials examining anti-inflammatory agents. We will then summarize investigations from our own laboratories pertaining to the characterization of sepsis-associated cardiac abnormalities.

The sepsis syndrome and its associated cardiovascular abnormalities is believed to result from a profound host inflammatory reaction to a variety of pathogenic organisms (1). In an attempt to develop a unifying definition of this syndrome, participants of a recent consensus conference characterized sepsis as a systemic response to infection, manifested by tachycardia, tachypnea, leukopenia or leukocytosis, and marked alterations in temperature. Further, septic shock was defined as these findings accompanied by hemodynamic instability (2). Since patients with sepsis may have any number of these signs and symptoms, no single physiologic or laboratory parameter serves to universally identify this syndrome. The incidence of sepsis in U.S. hospitals during the last decade has increased by more than 100%, reflecting several trends in medical practice (3). These include the increased use of invasive medical procedures, the devel-

opment of more aggressive cancer chemotherapeutic regimens, the proliferation of medical centers providing bone marrow and solid organ transplantation, and the application of extraordinary life-support technologies in patients at the extremes of age.

Recent advances in molecular biology and immunology have increased our understanding of the pathogenesis of sepsis (1) (Fig. 1). Initially, a nidus of infection is established when invading pathogens circumvent host defensive barriers such as skin and mucosal membranes. Depending on both a given pathogen's virulence and the host's immune response, local defenses may be overwhelmed, leading to either bloodstream invasion by the pathogen or systemic release of pathogenic products. This results in heightened activation of systemic host defenses, including plasma factors (complement, clotting cascades) and cellular components (neutrophils, monocytes, lymphocytes, macrophages, endothelial cells), which in turn release potentially toxic host mediators (cytokines, kinins, eicosinoids, platelet-activating factor, nitric oxide, etc.) that augment the inflammatory response. Unchecked, this escalating immune response, in concert with microbial toxins, may lead to hemodynamic instability, organ dysfunction, and death.

Standard treatment of sepsis includes the use of broad-spectrum antibiotics, surgical eradication of the infectious nidus, and intensive life-support measures (e.g., dialysis, mechanical ventilation, vasoactive agents, etc.). Despite these approaches, sepsis-associated mortality remains high (25% to 75%) (4, 5). In a finite number of patients, myocardial depression appears to significantly contribute to lethality. To date, the mechanisms responsible for this myocardial depression and, for that matter, all forms of sepsis-induced organ injury have resisted clear definition.

W. Karzai, C. Natanson, and B. D. Freeman: Critical Care Medicine Department, National Institutes of Health, Bethesda, Maryland 20892.

*Modified in part from Nathanson L. et al. *Ann Intern Med* 1994;120(9):771, with permission.

*Treatment of Septic Shock*

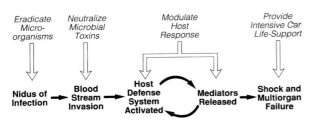

**Pathogenesis of Septic Shock**

**FIG. 1.** The pathogenesis and treatment of septic shock. Solid black arrows follow the pathogenesis of septic shock beginning with a nidus of infection and ending in shock and multisystem failure. Open arrows indicate potential treatment strategies. From Natanson C, et al. *Ann Intern Med* 1994; 120(9):771, with permission.

## MEDIATORS OF SEPSIS

Recent sepsis-related investigations have focused on characterizing the mediators involved in producing this syndrome. These substances are of interest not only because of their pathogenic importance but also because of

their potential as therapeutic targets (Fig. 2). Research pertaining to four principal mediators—endotoxin, cytokines, neutrophils, and nitric oxide—will be presented in this manuscript. These specific mediators are the subjects of both laboratory and human clinical investigations.

### Endotoxin

Gram-negative bacteria are frequent etiologic agents of septic shock. Endotoxin, a lipopolysaccharide present in the outer membrane of gram-negative bacteria, is believed to play a significant role in the pathogenesis of gram-negative infections (6). Endotoxin is composed of three structurally and functionally distinct components: a hypervariable outer surface carbohydrate, the O-side chain; a core sugar; and an outer membrane lipid-A moiety (Fig. 3). The lipid-A moiety, which is structurally conserved among diverse gram-negative species, appears to impart the toxicity to this molecule (6). There has been great interest in developing antibodies directed against the lipid-A moiety to treat sepsis. However, because it is deeply imbedded in the bacterial outer membrane, it is unclear if lipid A is structurally capable of binding antibody. Several initial clinical trials examining polyclonal antiserum directed against lipid-A and core sugars failed to show a consistent

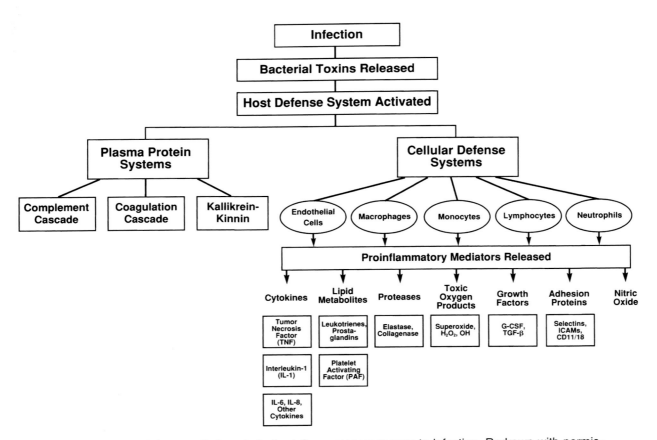

**FIG. 2.** Potential therapeutic targets in the inflammatory response to infection. Redrawn with permission from Bioworld Financial Watch, American Health Consultants Inc., Atlanta, GA.

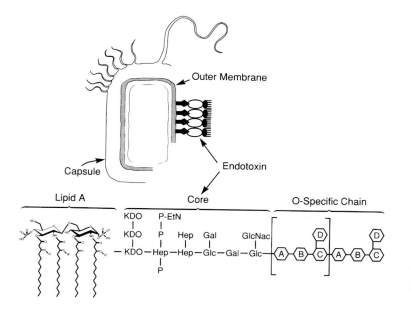

**FIG. 3.** The endotoxin molecule divided into its functional units. Refer to text for details. Modified, with permission, from Young LS, et al. *Ann Intern Med* 1977;86:456.

treatment benefit in patients with septic shock (1, 7–9). Subsequently, monoclonal antibodies were developed to produce a more specific anti–lipid A therapy with less risk of infection transmittal. HA-1A (Centocor Inc., Malvern, PA), a human IgM monoclonal antibody directed against lipid A, showed initially promising results in mice challenged with bacteria (10). When studied in a randomized clinical trial of 543 patients, HA-1A appeared to significantly decrease 28-day mortality in patients with gram-negative septic shock (11). However, subsequent analysis raised questions about the validity of these results (1) (Table 1). Our laboratory, using a canine *Escherichia coli* peritonitis model which simulates the cardiovascular abnormalities of human septic shock, evaluated the role of HA-1A in sepsis. Interestingly, HA-1A significantly decreased 28-day survival (12). Animals receiving HA-1A developed greater systemic illness and comparable degrees of endotoxemia relative to control-treated animals. In addi-

tion, diastolic cardiac function appeared adversely effected with HA-1A therapy, possibly the result of nonspecific binding of HA-1A to cardiolipin (9). A subsequent prospective human trial of HA-1A was performed because of questions raised about the validity of the initial clinical trial and the lethal effects of HA-1A in canines. This trial was terminated prematurely due to increased mortality in some patients treated with HA-1A (1, 13). The reason for this increased mortality has not been explained (1, 14). E5 (Xoma Inc., Berkely, CA), an IgM monoclonal antibody directed against lipid A, also failed to show a therapeutic benefit in patients with gram-negative infections in two large multicenter clinical trials (1, 15, 16).

To date, human trials of anti–lipid A antibodies in sepsis have been disappointing. Conceivably, these lipid-A-directed antibodies lack appropriate bioactivity. Alternatively, circulating endotoxin may not be a viable therapeutic target in septic shock. Newer agents are

**TABLE 1.** *Summary of four clinical trials with monoclonal endotoxin-core directed antibodies*

| Therapy | Diagnostic group | Treatment group | Mortality rate (%) | p-value[a] | Reference |
|---|---|---|---|---|---|
| E5[b] | Gram-negative bacteremia | Placebo | 41 | | |
| | | E5 | 38 | 0.72 | 15 |
| E5[b] | Gram-negative sepsis/ nonrefractory shock | Placebo | 26 | | |
| | | E5 | 30 | 0.21 | 1 |
| HA-1A[c] | Gram-negative bacteremia (14-day mortality) | Placebo | 34 | | |
| | | HA-1A | 24 | 0.12 | 11 |
| HA-1A | Gram-negative bacteremia (14-day mortality) | Placebo | 32 | | |
| | | HA-1A | 33 | 0.86 | 14 |

[a]p-value for mortality.
[b]Xoma Co.
[c]Centocor, Inc.

under study which may possess more potent antiendotoxin activity. These include high-density lipoprotein and bactericidal/permeability-increasing protein, both of which would theoretically function better than anti–lipid A antibodies to bind and neutralize endotoxin. Testing of these newer agents in both animal models and humans may clarify whether endotoxin is a useful therapeutic target in sepsis.

## Cytokines

Cytokines are peptides which function as cellular signals to regulate both the amplitude and duration of the host's inflammatory response (17). Two cytokines, tumor necrosis factor (TNF) and interleukin-1 (IL-1), have been most extensively studied because of their apparent central role in mediating the inflammatory response during infection. Tumor necrosis factor and IL-1 are released from cells of the monocyte-macrophage lineage in response to a variety of infectious stimuli (18–20). Upon release, these cytokines may act locally, in a paracrine fashion, or circulate systemically, where they bind to carrier proteins or extracellular receptors. Extracellular receptors that bind to TNF and IL-1 (i.e., soluble TNF and IL-1 receptors) are shed from neutrophils and vascular endothelium in response to acute inflammation (21, 22) (Fig. 4). It is hypothesized that these extracellular soluble receptors function to increase cytokine half-life and to modulate cytokine/cell-associated receptor interaction (23, 24). In addition, the function of IL-1 is also regulated by IL-1 receptor antagonist (IL-1ra), an acute phase cytokine which functions as a competitive antagonist of IL-1 at the target cell (21). During sepsis, the interplay between cytokine release, extracellular soluble receptor binding, and target cell interaction is complex and not fully understood.

Tumor necrosis factor and IL-1 appear to mediate both a proinflammatory and anti-inflammatory response during infections. Both recruit and activate neutrophils, macrophages, and lymphocytes and both increase gene

expression of acute-phase proteins and granulocyte colony-stimulating factors (25). The anti-inflammatory responses of TNF and IL-1 include increased gene expression for manganese superoxide dismutase and cyclo-oxygenase, release of acute-phase proteins and antiproteases, induction of anti-inflammatory cytokines (i.e., IL-4, IL-6, IL-10, TGF-β, IL-1ra), and downregulation of TNF and IL-1 receptors (25). These favorable, anti-inflammatory responses may partly explain the beneficial effect of low-dose IL-1 or TNF administration during endotoxin and intraperitoneal bacterial challenge in mice and rats and the adverse effect of TNF inhibition in animal models of *Legionella* or *Candida* infection and bacterial peritonitis (26–30).

Cytokine inhibition as a therapy in sepsis is predicated on the assumption that exaggerated inflammatory responses develop in some patients, perhaps because of failed normal inflammatory control mechanisms. Several clinical studies have examined the role of cytokine inhibition during sepsis (31–38) (Table 2). A multicenter phase II trial of a murine monoclonal anti-TNF antibody (CellTech Slough, United Kingdom) (31) as well as two larger multicenter clinical trials studying similar type agents, in both North America and in Europe (Bayer/Miles, Berkeley CA), failed to show benefit in patients with septic shock (32, 33). Perhaps more disturbing are the results of a randomized, blinded, phase II trial of human dimeric TNF receptor in sepsis syndrome. Patients receiving intermediate (0.45 mg/kg) and high (1.5 mg/kg) doses of this compound experienced significantly worse 28-day mortality, compared to placebo or low-dose (0.15 mg/kg) therapy (35) (Table 2).

Clinical studies of IL-1 inhibition during sepsis have also been disappointing. These trials have been limited primarily to the use of recombinant IL-1ra (Synergen Inc., Boulder, CO). This drug, in a randomized, open-label, phase II trial in 99 patients with sepsis or septic shock resulted in improved 28-day survival (36). However, two subsequent randomized, double-blind, phase III multicenter trials of IL-1ra in patients with sepsis or sep-

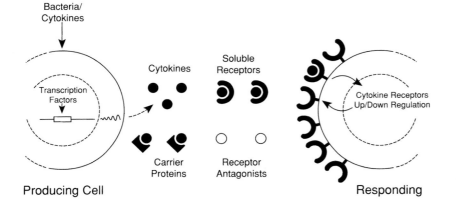

**FIG. 4.** Regulation of cytokine activity in vivo. From Natanson C, et al. *Ann Intern Med* 1994;120(9):771, with permission.

**TABLE 2.** *Summary of six clinical trials with cytokine inhibition in sepsis*

| Therapy | Diagnostic group | Dose (mg/kg) | Mortality rate (%) | p-value[a] | Reference |
|---|---|---|---|---|---|
| CBOO6[b] (anti-TNF Mab) | Sepsis or septic shock | 0.1 | no benefit with increasing dose | ns | 31 |
| Bay-x-1351[c] (anti-TNF Mab) | Sepsis or septic shock | 0 | 33 | ns | 32 |
|  |  | 7.5 | 30 |  |  |
|  |  | 15 | 31 |  |  |
| Bay-x-1351[c] (anti-TNF Mab) | Septic shock | 0 | 43 | ns | 33 |
|  |  | 3 | 37 |  |  |
|  |  | 14 | 45 |  |  |
| Dimeric TNF receptor[e] | Sepsis or septic shock | 0 | 30 | 0.016[d] | 35 |
|  |  | 0.15 | 30 |  |  |
|  |  | 0.45 | 48 |  |  |
|  |  | 1.5 | 53 |  |  |
| Antril (rhIL-1ra)[f] | Sepsis syndrome | 0 | 34 | ns | 37 |
|  |  | 1 | 31 |  |  |
|  |  | 2 | 29 |  |  |
| Antril (rhIL-1ra)[f] | Sepsis syndrome | g | g | ns | 38 |

[a]p-value for 28-day mortality.
[b]Celltech, Ltd.
[c]Bayer-Miles.
[d]p-value for dose-dependent harmful effect.
[e]Immunex.
[f]Synergen, Inc.
[g]Study terminated after 700 patients due to lack of efficacy.
ns, nonsignificant; anti-TNF Mab, anti–tumor necrosis factor monoclonal antibody; rhIL-1ra, recombinant human interleukin-1 receptor antagonist.

tic shock demonstrated no significant difference in 28-day mortality, comparing multiple doses of IL-1ra administration with placebo treatment (37, 38) (Table 2).

To date, inhibition of neither TNF nor IL-1 has been shown to improve outcome in the treatment of human sepsis or septic shock. In this setting, it appears that suppression of cytokine function has the potential not only to be not beneficial, but harmful, possibly due to impairment of cytokine-dependent bacterial clearance or disruption of cytokine-mediated tissue protection. It is apparent that the optimal timing and duration of this therapy are not yet defined. It is possible that this therapy may only be beneficial if limited to specific tissue compartments (e.g., lung, peritoneum) or to subgroups of patients manifesting an exaggerated cytokine response. Until these issues are more clearly delineated, the feasibility of inhibiting the harmful cytokine effect during sepsis, while preserving beneficial cytokine function, remains unknown.

## Inflammatory Cells

The neutrophil and its toxic byproducts are thought to participate in the tissue injury and organ dysfunction occurring during sepsis and septic shock (39–41). Consequently, inhibiting specific neutrophil function has appeal as a therapy for sepsis. Neutrophil inhibition has been demonstrated to improve outcome in animal models of hemorrhagic shock, infection, and hypothermic injury (42–44). A potential limitation of this approach is the development of significant immunocompromise. Consequently, successful therapies which inhibit neutrophil activity during sepsis must produce a beneficial anti-inflammatory effect without significant impairment of host defense.

To investigate the potential of neutrophil inhibition as a treatment strategy for sepsis, several investigators have examined the effects of monoclonal antibodies directed against neutrophil integrins, such as the CD11/18 adhesion complex. The CD11/18 complex is a cell surface glycoprotein that mediates neutrophil-endothelial cell adhesion, an initial step in neutrophil vascular transmigration (45–47). Several inflammatory mediators, such as endotoxin, IL-1, and TNF, stimulate neutrophil adherence to endothelium through this complex (48). Monoclonal antibodies against the CD11/18 complex in vitro and in vivo prevent endotoxin, TNF, and complement-induced neutrophil adhesion and injury to endothelial cells and neutrophil extravascular migration (49, 50). Use of such antibodies in various animal models of shock and infectious challenge have produced conflicting results (51, 52). We have examined anti-CD11/18 monoclonal antibody treatment in our canine model of septic shock (53). Animals pretreated with anti-CD11/18-directed monoclonal antibodies underwent placement of an infected peritoneal clot and subsequent antibiotic treatment. Relative to control animals, animals treated with anti-CD11/18 antibodies developed significantly lower mean arterial pressure, cardiac index, central venous pressure, and arterial pH and demonstrated greater serum endotoxemia. Further, anti-CD11/18-treated animals showed a trend toward poorer survival. These findings suggest that CD11/18 inhibition during sepsis results in impairment of cardiovascular function, tissue perfusion, and endotoxin clearance. If extrapolated to clinical practice, these results indicate that inhibition of CD11/18 function could worsen host defense and outcome during bacterial sepsis.

As an alternative strategy, our laboratory has also been interested in studying the effects of augmenting neutrophil function during sepsis. The prophylactic administration of recombinant granulocyte colony-stimulating factor (rG-CSF) (Amgen, Thousand Oaks, CA), a potent stimulator in vitro and in vivo of immature and mature neutrophil function (54), has previously been shown to have beneficial effects in immunocompromised models of infection (55). However, the effects of this therapy in the normal, nonneutropenic host during sepsis are not fully defined. We pretreated canines with rG-CSF, beginning 9 days before and continuing for 3 days after infected peritoneal clot implantation (56). The rG-CSF pretreatment produced a severalfold increase in peripheral neutrophil counts (e.g., 50,000 to 60,000 cells/mm$^3$) prior to infection. After infected clot placement, rG-CSF pretreatment was associated with prolonged survival times, higher mean arterial blood pressure, improved left ventricular ejection fraction (LVEF), and more rapid endotoxin clearance. These findings suggest that treatment with rG-CSF at doses sufficient to increase the number of circulating neutrophils may favorably effect host defense and survival in certain types of sepsis.

On the basis of in vivo models, the effect of neutrophil inhibition with monoclonal antibodies directed against CD11/18, its ligands, or other integrin complexes on organ injury and outcome in sepsis is unclear. In specific circumstances, such as animal models of bacterial meningitis or hemorrhagic shock, inhibition of integrin function appears to have a beneficial effect on organ injury and survival (42, 43, 57). In contrast, our findings, as well as those of other investigators, failed to show benefit with this type of therapy (53, 58–60). Inhibition of neutrophil function as a therapy for sepsis may only be beneficial in certain types or routes of infections where compromise of host defense does not negate the favorable effects of neutrophil inhibition. In contrast, augmentation of neutrophil function had a favorable effect on outcome in our peritonitis model (56). Together, these findings indicate the inherent difficulty in inhibiting inflammation, a necessary response to clear infection, and suggest that, in certain circumstances, increasing the inflammatory response may be beneficial.

### Nitric Oxide

Nitric oxide (NO·) is a ubiquitous intracellular messenger in mammalian systems. It is involved in neurotransmission, immune cell function, hormone secretion, cardiovascular regulation, and endothelial-cell leukocyte interaction (61–63). Nitric oxide is synthesized from the amino acid L-arginine by the enzyme nitric oxide synthase (NOS). Nitric oxide mediates its vascular effects through the activation of soluble guanylate cyclase, which in turn increases the intracellular concentration of cyclic guanidine monophosphate (cGMP), resulting in smooth muscle relaxation (61) (Fig. 5). There exist at least two isoforms of NOS which are distinct in their structure, tissue distribution, and activity state. Constitutive nitric oxide synthase (cNOS) is calcium dependent and cell surface receptor regulated. The cNOS isoform in vascular endothelium is activated by a variety of substances (acetylcholine, bradykinin, histamine, and adenosine) and is essential to the maintenance of vasomotor homeostasis. Inducible nitric oxide synthase (iNOS) is calcium independent and not regulated by cell surface receptors. It is expressed in vascular smooth muscle and phagocytic cells after stimulation by a variety of substances, including endotoxin and proinflammatory cytokines (61, 62). It is postulated that the NO· generated from iNOS is markedly increased during sepsis. However, the full role of NO· during sepsis is still unknown. Increased production of NO· may be largely responsible for sepsis-induced hypotension (64) and myocardial

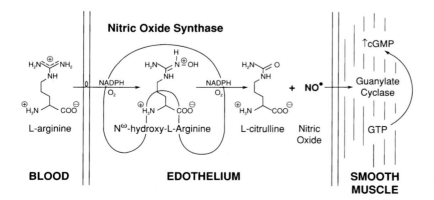

**FIG. 5.** Nitric oxide synthetic pathway. Refer to text for details. From Natanson C, et al. *Ann Intern Med* 1994;120(9):771, with permission.

depression (65). Nitric oxide also has well-documented cytotoxic effects (66), and its overproduction in this setting may lead to direct tissue injury and organ dysfunction. Finally, recent evidence has shown that nitric oxide may exert a proinflammatory effect during septic shock by enhancing cytokine release from phagocytic cells (67). Despite potentially harmful effects, NO· may also play a beneficial role in sepsis. Nitric oxide appears important in maintaining visceral and microvascular blood flow and in inhibiting platelet aggregation and leukocyte adhesion (68, 69). In addition, NO· has been described as having antimicrobial activity and immunomodulating effects (70).

Inhibition of NOS represents an appealing therapeutic strategy, since as many as 50% of patients who succumb to septic shock develop hypotension refractory to conventional vasopressor therapy (71). However, the use of NOS inhibitors in animal models of sepsis has produced conflicting results. Nitric oxide synthase inhibition has been demonstrated to restore vascular responsiveness to catecholamines and to correct hypotension in animal models of TNF and endotoxin challenge (72). In other animal models, inhibition of nitric oxide production is clearly harmful. Administration of $N$-methyl-L-arginine (L-NMA), a nonselective nitric oxide synthase inhibitor, to anesthetized rats and dogs increased renal vascular resistance and decreased renal blood flow (73, 74). Further, in models of sepsis using endotoxin challenge, L-NMA increased capillary leak and intestinal damage in rats and depressed cardiac output in anesthetized dogs (75, 76). High doses of L-NMA in anesthetized, endotoxin-challenged rats caused cardiovascular collapse and death (77). These data suggest that complete inhibition of nitric oxide synthase may be undesirable. Despite these conflicting results, NOS inhibitors have been used to treat hypotension in patients with sepsis and in those receiving cytokine therapy for cancer (78, 79).

To examine the role of nitric oxide in sepsis, we challenged canines with endotoxin and treated them with several doses (1, 2, 4, and 10 mg/kg/hr) of L-$N$-methyl-arginine (L-NMA), a nitric oxide synthase inhibitor (80). In endotoxemic animals, L-NMA increased the systemic vascular resistance index but decreased cardiac index and oxygen delivery index, worsened lactic acidosis, produced hepatic toxicity, and, at the highest dose examined (10 mg/kg/hr), increased the mortality rate. Another NOS inhibitor, $N$-amino-L-arginine had similar effects in this model (81). The effects of NOS inhibition on the cardiac index observed in these studies were similar to those found in other animal models and in patients with sepsis (78, 79, 82). These findings raise concern that NOS inhibition may decrease tissue perfusion in septic shock.

Nitric oxide appears to mediate both harmful and beneficial effects during sepsis. Nonselective NOS inhibitors, which block both cNOS and iNOS, have not yet proven beneficial in the treatment of sepsis or septic shock. The nonselective inhibition of NOS as a treatment strategy for septic shock may be harmful, particularly at high doses, because of blockade of necessary nitric oxide functions. The use of nonselective NOS inhibitors in low doses or selective NOS inhibitors in high and low doses deserves further study in sepsis.

## CARDIOVASCULAR ABNORMALITIES OF SEPSIS

As stated previously, myocardial depression contributes to the morbidity and mortality in some patients with sepsis and septic shock. Over the past several years, our laboratory has investigated the cardiovascular abnormalities of sepsis. Specifically, we have described the profile of the cardiovascular response in sepsis and have evaluated the role of bacterial factors, host response, and potential mechanisms of injury in an attempt to better understand this abnormality.

### Physiologic Response of the Heart in Sepsis

Our early investigations of the cardiovascular abnormalities of sepsis focused on describing both the nature of these abnormalities and the time course of their occurrence. In a canine model of peritonitis and in humans fulfilling the criteria for septic shock, we sequentially measured LVEF using radionuclide cineangiography. Simultaneously, cardiac output (CO) was determined using pulmonary arterial thermodilution catheters. From these measurements, LV end-diastolic volume index (LVEDVI) could be derived [LVEDVI = CO/(HR × LVEF × weight)]. We found that by 24 hours after the onset of septic shock, a decrease in LVEF and, with adequate volume replacement, an increase in LVEDVI occurred (Figs. 6 and 7) (4, 83). Cardiac output was either unchanged or increased. Similar changes were demonstrated in right ventricular function. In survivors, these derangements returned to normal in 7 to 10 days (4, 84, 85). Thus, radionuclide studies demonstrated evidence of myocardial depression not revealed by measurements of cardiac output alone. It appears that preservation of CO in septic shock occurs by sepsis-induced tachycardia and preservation of stroke volume through left ventricular (LV) dilatation (i.e., Frank-Starling mechanism) (86) (Fig. 7).

### Determinants of Cardiovascular Dysfunction

#### Role of the Infecting Agent

Our studies of the cardiovascular dysfunction of sepsis next centered on identifying pathogenic features of

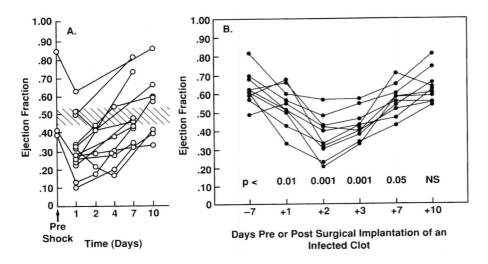

**FIG. 6.** Serial left ventricular ejection fraction (LVEF) vs. Time in **(A)** humans and **(B)** canines with septic shock. The hatched region in Fig. 1A is the normal range. Individual ejection fractions are indicated by circles. Lines connect days. In both humans with septic shock and animals challenged with bacteria the LVEF markedly decreases over 1 to 2 days and recovers in 7 to 10 days. Modified, with permission, from Parker MM, et al. *Ann Intern Med* 1984;100:483; and Natanson C, et al. *J Clin Invest* 1986;78:259.

bacterial organisms, specifically examining the influence of bacterial dose, type, and viability. In addition, we investigated the importance of specific bacterial products such as endotoxin in producing these cardiovascular abnormalities.

### Dose of Bacteria

To study the role of bacterial dose in producing cardiovascular dysfunction, we examined the relationship between the size of the inoculum and degree of cardiovas-

cular abnormality. Increasing colony counts of *E. coli* incorporated into an intraperitoneal fibrin-thrombin clot in our canine model produced progressive decreases in cardiac function and lethality in a dose-dependent fashion. These cardiac abnormalities included decreases in LVEF, progressive LV enlargement, and shifts on LV function curves (EDVI vs. LV stroke work index and peak systolic pressure vs. end-systolic volume index) (Figs. 6 and 8). Of interest, the time course of cardiovascular abnormality was independent of dose. Cardiovascular abnormalities were most pronounced at 2 to 3 days after clot implantation, and full recovery occurred by 10 days. It appears that

## SERIAL CHANGES IN LEFT VENTRICULAR FUNCTION DURING SEPTIC SHOCK

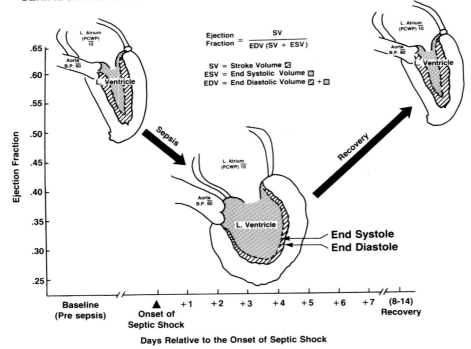

**FIG. 7.** Illustration of how cardiac output is maintained during septic shock despite a depressed LVEF. The hearts are shown at end diastole, or maximum filling, at three separate time points, presepsis (baseline), days 1 to 4 of sepsis, and postsepsis (recovery). The shaded area corresponds to end-systolic volume; the hatched area corresponds to stroke volume. These two areas combined are the end-diastolic volume. On days 1 to 4 of sepsis the LVEF decreases, but because the heart increases in size (large end-diastolic volume), stroke volume is maintained or increased. From Natanson C, et al. *Anesth Clin North Am* 1988;6:73, with permission.

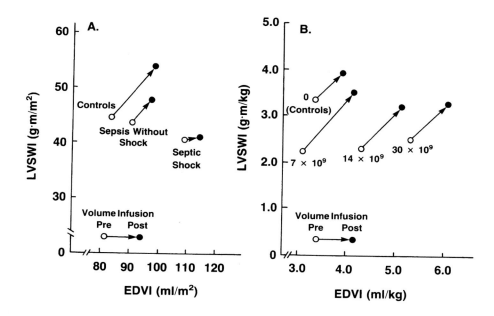

**FIG. 8.** Frank-Starling left ventricular (LV) function curves in **(A)** humans with septic shock (as compared to critically ill controls and patients with sepsis without shock) and **(B)** canines with septic shock (comparing increasing doses of intraperitoneal bacteria). Mean end-diastolic volume index (EDVI) and LV stroke work index (LVSWI) are plotted pre- and postvolume challenge. In both humans and animals with septic shock, Frank-Starling curves are shifted progressively downward and to the right with increasing severity of disease. From Natanson C, et al. *Am J Physiol* 1988;254:H558; and Ognibene FP, et al. *Chest* 1988;93:903, with permission.

the size of the bacterial inoculum is a significant factor in influencing the severity, but not the time course, of sepsis-related cardiovascular abnormalities (86).

### Type of Bacteria and Role of Endotoxin

Our attention turned next to examining the role of bacterial type in producing cardiovascular abnormality during sepsis. We initially compared the relative abilities of gram-positive and gram-negative organisms to produce both endotoxemia and cardiovascular changes. Using our peritonitis model, we challenged animals with *S. aureus,* a gram-positive organism lacking endotoxin, and *E. coli,* a gram-negative organism which contains endotoxin in its outer membrane. *S. aureus* and *E. coli* produced an identical profile of cardiovascular change (Fig. 9). Additionally, when comparing identical colony counts, *S. aureus* was more potent at producing these changes than *E. coli.* Thus, we demonstrated that gram-positive organisms lacking endotoxin could fully produce the cardiovascular changes of septic shock (87). This finding is of particular interest because endotoxemia has been proposed as a central mechanism in all forms of shock (88). According to this model, serious illness compromises gastrointestinal mucosal integrity, allowing endogenous enteric flora to produce systemic endotoxemia. However, no serum endotoxin could be detected in animals infected with *S. aureus,* even when measured shortly prior to death (Table 3). Together, these data suggest that neither the presence of endotoxin nor of endotoxemia is necessary to produce these cardiovascular abnormalities. Further, it appears that endotoxin is not the common pathway of injury or the central mechanism of all septic shock.

We next studied the relationship between endotoxin, virulence, and cardiovascular abnormalities during gram-negative infection. We challenged animals with three distinct gram-negative bacteria: a strain of *E. coli* containing virulence factors associated with human disease (encapsulation, serum resistance, and ability to produce hemolysis), a strain of *E. coli* without these factors, and *Pseudomonas aeruginosa,* an unrelated gram-negative organism (89, 90). Virulence factors are present in pathogenic bacteria and function to circumvent host defense. All three of these bacteria produced the distinct profile of cardiovascular abnormalities seen over a 7- to 10-day period in septic shock in humans. However, comparing similar colony counts, the virulent *E. coli* and *P. aeruginosa* were more potent in producing cardiovascular abnormalities and lethality than the nonvirulent *E. coli.*

Unexpectedly, the nonvirulent *E. coli* produced greater endotoxemia than virulent organisms (89, 90). To determine if this disparity between level of endotoxemia and lethality resulted from the production of a more potent endotoxin by virulent organisms, we challenged animals intraperitoneally with purified endotoxin obtained from both the virulent and nonvirulent *E. coli* strains (91). Intraperitoneal challenge with purified endotoxin resulted in the same pattern of cardiovascular changes seen with viable bacteria. In addition, equal amounts of endotoxin from virulent and nonvirulent organisms produced similar degrees of hemodynamic abnormalities and lethality. Thus, a more potent endotoxin did not explain the lack of concordance between the degree of endotoxemia and lethality. It appears that while endotoxin alone can produce all of the cardiovascular abnormalities which occur with gram-negative infection, it is not the sole mediator. Further, among gram-negative bacteria, the level of endotoxemia produced by a specific

## Type of Clot

## Ejection Fraction

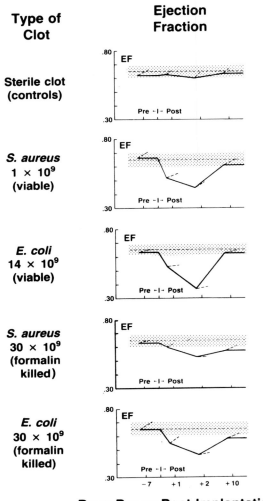

Sterile clot (controls)

S. aureus 1 × 10⁹ (viable)

E. coli 14 × 10⁹ (viable)

S. aureus 30 × 10⁹ (formalin killed)

E. coli 30 × 10⁹ (formalin killed)

**Days Pre or Post Implantation of Infected or Sterile Clot**

**FIG. 9.** Plot of time course of LVEF for sterile or infected clot. The dashed horizontal line within the shaded area is a mean based on 100 other dogs; the shaded area is a normal range adjusted to the number in the comparison group; the solid line is a serial mean change between days; and the dashed line originating from the solid line is a response to volume infusion each day. In data from dogs receiving both viable and formalin-killed *S. aureus* and *E. coli*, similar patterns of hemodynamic change as measured by LVEF from baseline to day 10 occurs. The graphs from control dogs *(top row)* demonstrate no serial changes in hemodynamic parameters from baseline to day 10 postsurgery. Modified, with permission, from Natanson C, et al. *J Clin Invest* 1989;83:243.

bacterial strain does not appear as important as the virulence factors associated with that bacterial strain in producing these abnormalities.

### Viability

We next examined the role of organism viability in producing cardiovascular abnormalities. We challenged canines with formalin-killed and heat-killed bacteria (87, 91). Compared to viable organisms, killing of gram-positive and gram-negative bacteria resulted in lower mortality and less cardiovascular dysfunction. However, viable, formalin-killed, and heat-killed organisms produced an identical time course of cardiovascular dysfunction (i.e., greatest myocardial depression at 2 to 3 days with recovery by day 10) (Fig. 9). These experiments suggest that while viable bacteria are more potent at producing cardiovascular injury, viability is not essential to the production of cardiovascular dysfunction during sepsis.

### Summary of Bacterial Factors

These series of experiments suggest that dose, type, and viability of bacteria affect the severity, but not the time course, of sepsis-induced cardiovascular abnormalities. Further, while endotoxin may play a role at mediating sepsis during some gram-negative infections, it is neither essential to producing these manifestations, nor is it the common mediator in all types of shock. It appears that structurally and functionally distinct bacteria and bacterial products interact with the host to produce similar patterns of cardiovascular dysfunction, suggesting a common pathway of injury.

### Host Factors

Since a diversity of bacteria and bacterial products produce a qualitatively similar pattern of cardiovascular changes, we next examined the host response to infection as a potential common pathway of injury. As previously stated, a central defect in the sepsis syndrome appears to be derangement in normal control mechanisms and an "excessive" host inflammatory response. Tumor necrosis factor, IL-1, and the complement system are proinflam-

**TABLE 3.** *Level of endotoxemia during* S. aureus *and* E. coli *septic shock in canines*

| Endotoxin concentration (EU/mL)[a] | Sterile clots (controls) | S. aureus (1 × 10⁹ CFU/kg BW) | E. coli (14 × 10⁹ CFU/kg BW) |
|---|---|---|---|
| Median | 0.8 | 0 | 45.5 |
| Range | 0.0–1.7 | 0.0–06.4 | 3.72–74.8 |

From Natanson C, Danner RL, Elin RJ, et al. Role of endotoxemia in cardiovascular dysfunction and mortality. *Escherichia coli* and *Staphylococcus aureus* challenges in a canine model of human septic shock. *J Clin Invest* 1989;83:243; with permission.
[a]One endotoxin unit (EU) = activity of 100 pg of U.S. standard endotoxin.
CFU, colony-forming unit; BW, body weight.

matory mediators directly implicated in the pathogenesis of sepsis (17, 92–99). In two separate sets of experiments, we examined the cardiovascular effects of TNF and IL-1 administration (100–102). In addition, we examined whether animals congenitally deficient in the third component of complement (C3) would have attenuated cardiovascular response to endotoxin challenge (103). We chose C3-deficient animals to study this question because C3 is essential to the function of both the classical and alternative pathways of complement activation.

We challenged canines with the intravenous administration of TNF over a 30-minute period. This resulted in the distinct pattern of cardiovascular changes of sepsis occurring over 7 to 10 days in humans and animals challenged with viable bacteria. In contrast, intravenous challenge with IL-1, even in high doses, did not produce these changes in cardiac function. Further, C3 deficiency did not alter the cardiovascular effects of endotoxin challenge. Our findings suggest that TNF, but not IL-1 or complement, is a necessary factor in producing these cardiac abnormalities. Tumor necrosis factor may be an essential component of the host response in producing this common profile of cardiovascular abnormality.

## Mechanisms of Myocardial Depression in Septic Shock

The mechanisms by which bacterial toxins and host mediators interact to produce the cardiovascular abnormalities of sepsis are, to date, unknown. In sequential experiments, we have examined coronary perfusion, myocardial metabolic derangements, microscopic structural abnormalities, alterations in systemic catecholamine homeostasis, and nitric oxide as possible causes of cardiovascular dysfunction.

### Coronary Perfusion

It has been suggested that the myocardial dysfunction of sepsis is a result of inadequate coronary perfusion. One of our initial investigations examined coronary blood flow during sepsis. Coronary sinus thermodilution catheters were placed in patients with septic shock to measure coronary sinus flow and sample coronary sinus venous blood. Despite a reduction in LVEF, coronary sinus blood flow was normal or increased in all septic patients. Further, no significant increase in net myocardial lactate production was observed (104). Our findings were consistent with those reported by Dhainaut et al., who also demonstrated increased coronary sinus flow in patients with sepsis (105). These findings suggest that myocardial depression occurring during septic shock is not the result of gross alteration in myocardial perfusion.

### Energy Metabolism

A potential limitation of studies examining perfusion abnormalities during sepsis is the inability to exclude shunting in the coronary circulation. Thus, blood sampled from the coronary sinus might not be representative of events occurring at the cellular level. Consequently, we next examined whether impairment of oxygen utilization contributes to impaired myocardial performance at the tissue level.

In vivo $^{31}$P magnetic resonance spectroscopy (P-MRS) techniques have been developed to determine cellular high-energy phosphate levels (106–109). Using the phosphocreatine-to-adenosine triphosphate ratio (PCr:ATP) as an estimate of intracellular free energy, P-MRS analysis has proven to be a sensitive indicator of abnormalities of myocardial energy metabolism (106). We performed a study in which canines underwent median sternotomy 2 days following septic clot implantation, the time of maximal myocardial depression in our model. At the time of surgery, an extracorporeal coronary sinus to superior vena cava shunt was created to measure myocardial oxygen consumption. In addition, an epicardial 3-cm P-MRS surface coil was placed to assay high-energy phosphate levels in LV myocardium. Animals were then challenged with increasing doses of catecholamines to enhance myocardial metabolic demand.

We hypothesized that impaired cellular oxygen utilization with concomitant decrease in intracellular free-energy stores was the basis of myocardial dysfunction in sepsis. As a consequence, catecholamine-induced increase in myocardial metabolic demand should have resulted in a decrease in intracellular high-energy phosphate levels, as measured by P-MRS. We found that catecholamine challenge did significantly increase myocardial oxygen consumption. However, no abnormalities in oxygen extraction, lactate production, or intracellular concentration of high-energy phosphate compounds in the myocardium of septic canines was found (Table 4;

**TABLE 4.** *Change in myocardial high-energy phosphate store with maximal increase in myocardial oxygen consumption (MVO$_2$)$^a$*

| Study group | Maximum percent increase in MVO$_2$ (mean ± SE)$^b$ | Percent mean change in PCr/β-ATP ratio |
|---|---|---|
| Septic | 135 (±31) | 3.7 (±2.2)* |
| Control | 524 (±83) | 2.7 (±2.7)* |

From Solomon MA, Correa R, Alexander HR, et al. Myocardial energy metabolism and morphology in a canine model of sepsis. *Am J Physiol* 1994;266:H757; with permission.

$^a$For each maximum MVO$_2$ the corresponding percent change from baseline in phosphocreatine/adenosine triphosphate ratio (PCr/β-ATP).

$^b$Maximum percent increase from baseline (before catecholamine infusion) in MVOC$_2$ was determined for each animal.

*$p$ = ns.

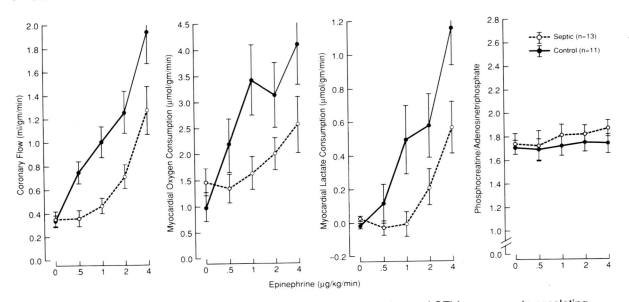

**FIG. 10.** Assessing myocardial work. Each graph displays mean change (-SE) in response to escalating doses of epinephrine for coronary flow, myocardial oxygen consumption, myocardial lactate consumption, and phosphocreatine/adenosine triphosphate, in septic *(open circles)* and control *(closed circles)* animals 2 days after infected and sterile clot implantation. Note, despite increasing metabolic demands, septic hearts maintain high energy phosphate levels (phosphocreatine-adenosine triphosphate ratios) and always consume lactate. From Solomon MA, et al. *Am J Physiol* 1994;266:H757, with permission.

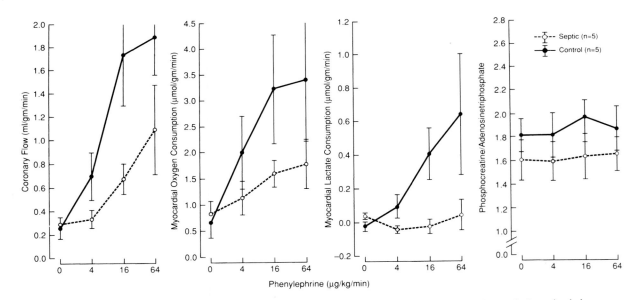

**FIG. 11.** Assessing myocardial work. Format similar to Fig. 6 except escalating dose of phenylephrine are now plotted on the *X*-axis. From Solomon MA, et al. *Am J Physiol* 1994;266:H757, with permission.

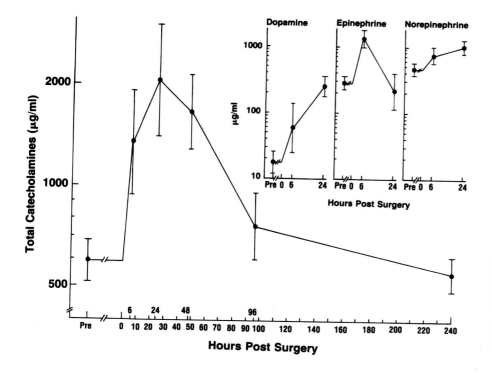

**FIG. 12.** Serial mean total catecholamine levels in canines infected with an *E. coli*-infected clot. *Inset:* Data from individual catecholamines plotted from only 0 to 24 hr postsurgery. Note the similarity in time course of increases in catecholamine levels with decreases in LVEF shown in Fig. 2B. From Natanson C, et al. *Am J Physiol* 1990;259:H1440, with permission.

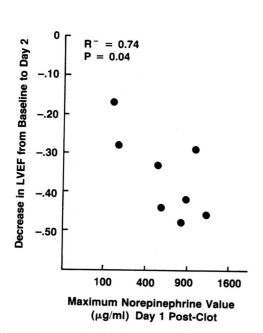

**FIG. 13.** Comparison of decrease in LVEF from baseline to day 2 postsurgery and maximum norepinephrine value (pg/mL) on day 1 postsurgery in septic-canines. From Natanson C, et al. *Am J Physiol* 1990;259:H1440, with permission.

Figs. 10 and 11) It appears that sepsis-induced cardiac dysfunction is not caused by inadequate myocardial oxygen delivery or deficiency of high-energy phosphate stores (110).

### Role of Catecholamines

It has been proposed that the cardiac dysfunction of sepsis may be due to abnormalities in catecholamine homeostasis. In in vivo models, supraphysiologic doses of norepinephrine are capable of producing myocardial depression in a dose-dependent fashion (111). We have examined the relationship between circulating catecholamines and cardiac dysfunction in our canine peritonitis model. We serially measured serum catecholamine levels following infected clot placement. We found that increases in total and individual catecholamines paralleled the time course of abnormalities in myocardial function, with catecholamine levels being maximally elevated when myocardial depression was most pronounced (112) (Fig. 12). In addition, increased levels of catecholamines were associated with more severe decreases in LVEF (Fig. 13). Catecholamine levels and cardiovascular abnormalities normalized over a period of 7 to 10 days.

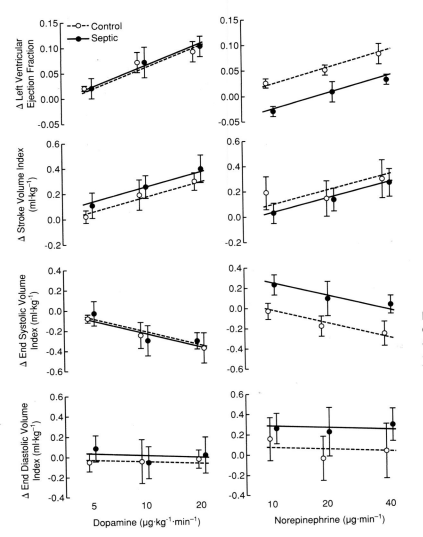

**FIG. 14.** Days 2 and 3 after clot implantation; changes in left ventricular performance and size after increasing doses of dopamine *(left panels)* and norepinephrine *(right panels)*, comparing control animals *(open circles)* and septic animals *(closed circles)*. Despite the septic animals having a significantly decreased LVEF (data not shown) the LVEF and SVI response to catecholamines shown above is relatively preserved. Note, data are plotted from a common origin to compare changes in response to catecholamines in septic and control animals. The LVEF in septic animals was significantly depressed; if these data were plotted from absolute values, a significant downward shift in the LVEF response of septic animals would be evident. From Karzai W, et al. *Am J Physiol [in press]*, with permission.

To determine whether these increases in levels of circulating catecholamines associated with myocardial disease were related to altered myocardial catecholamine sensitivity, we measured the cardiovascular response to escalating doses of both dopamine and norepinephrine in our canine peritonitis model. In noninfected control animals, both dopamine and norepinephrine increased cardiac performance, as determined by LVEF and stroke volume index (SVI). This was associated with a decrease in end-systolic volume index (ESVI) and no alteration in end-diastolic volume index (EDVI) (113). Dopamine and norepinephrine also increased LVEF and SVI in septic and control animals (Fig. 14). However, in the presence of sepsis, the blood pressure and LVEF dose-response curves for dopamine and norepinephrine respectively were shifted downward. These findings suggest that while the qualitative actions of both agents during sepsis

are unchanged, catecholamine sensitivity is decreased. Elevated catecholamine levels and altered catecholamine sensitivity may partly explain the cardiovascular abnormalities of septic shock.

### Structural Abnormalities

In an effort to identify a structural basis to explain the cardiovascular abnormalities of sepsis, we next microscopically examined myocardium taken from canines during sepsis-induced cardiac depression (110). Light microscopy of LV tissue obtained from canines 2 days after infected peritoneal clot implantation, the time of maximal myocardial depression, revealed only minimal neutrophil infiltration. However, electron microscopic analysis showed evidence of both microvascular and

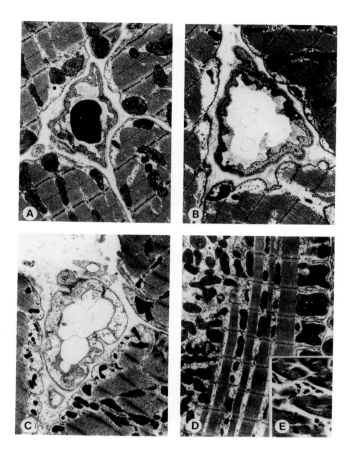

**FIG. 15.** Cardiac tissue from control **(A)** and septic **(B–E)** animals. A–C: Electron micrographs, original magnification ×13,000. D: Electron micrograph, original magnification ×10,500. A: Normal, compact myofibrils and mitochondria. In the center is a capillary containing a red blood cell. In B, note dark black deposits over the upper two-thirds of capillary endothelial surface. These represent nonocclusive fibrin deposition. In C, note the marked intracellular edema of endothelial cell comprising the capillary. D: Myofibrillar bands running vertically. Note, particularly, on left, disruption and loss of the myofibrillar bands. E: Minimal neutrophil infiltration. From Solomon MA, et al. *Am J Physiol* 1994;266: H757, with permission.

myocyte injury. This included myocyte edema and necrosis, sarcolemmal scalloping, endothelial cell swelling, perivascular edema, and nonocclusive fibrous bands within endothelial cell lumens (110) (Fig. 15). These findings suggest that bacterial toxins, in conjunction with endogenous mediators, produce endothelial and myocyte damage which may ultimately contribute to myocardial depression.

### Role of Nitric Oxide

The role of NO· in sepsis was previously described. Several lines of evidence suggest that NO· contributes to sepsis-induced cardiac dysfunction (64, 114). Specifically, in vitro NOS inhibition has been demonstrated to block the negative inotropic effects of TNF-α, IL-1, and IL-6 in a beating papillary muscle preparation (65). We have studied the role of two NOS inhibitors on cardiac function in vivo using our canine model. During endotoxin challenge, two separate inhibitors of nitric oxide production, *N*-amino-L-arginine and *N*-methyl-L-arginine, did not alter the decrease in LVEF characteristic of septic shock. This lack of benefit could not be

explained by alteration in afterload or preload (Fig. 16) (80, 81). These findings argue against a direct role for NO· in mediating myocardial depression during septic shock.

### CONCLUSION

Sepsis and septic shock refer to a syndrome in which a diversity of pathogenic organisms elicit an excessive release of proinflammatory mediators, ultimately resulting in cardiovascular dysfunction, hemodynamic instability, and multiorgan failure. Conventional therapy of this syndrome has included eradication of the infectious nidus, appropriate antimicrobial therapy, and hemodynamic support with fluid resuscitation and vasopressor agents. However, despite these measures, the morbidity and mortality of the sepsis syndrome remains excessive (1,2,3,115,116). Newer antisepsis therapies have focused on neutralizing specific bacterial toxins or blocking the effects of endogenous proinflammatory mediators. To date, the use of antiendotoxin monoclonal antibodies in multiple clinical trials has proven ineffective at improving outcome in sepsis and septic shock. Likewise, inhibi-

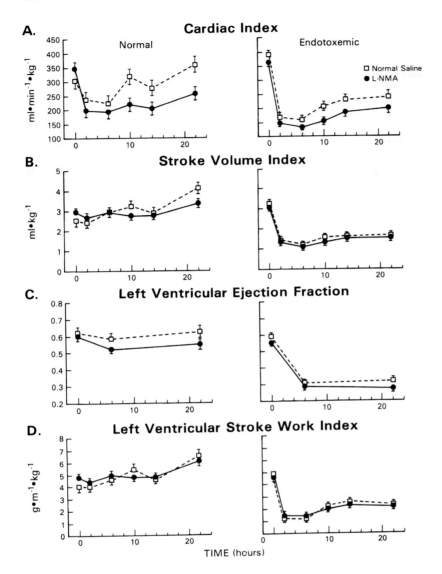

**FIG. 16.** Serial changes (mean - SE) in **(A)** CI, **(B)** SVI, **(C)** LVEF, and **(D)** LVSWI in normal and endotoxemic dogs. Animals were treated with a 22-hr infusion of either normal saline *(squares)* or L-NMA *(circles)*. From Cobb JP, et al. *J Exp Med* 1992;176:1175; with permission.

tion of proinflammatory cytokines has similarly been inefficacious, or harmful, in multiple human trials. Other potential strategies, including modulation of neutrophil function and inhibition of NO· production, have yielded conflicting results in animal models and are largely untested in humans. These disappointing results may be explained by the fact that there is a potential limitation inherent in any therapy designed to suppress host response in sepsis. While inhibition of inflammatory mediators (e.g., with cytokine antagonists, antineutrophil antibodies, or NOS inhibitors) may limit systemic inflammation, many essential functions (e.g., host defense) may be impaired, resulting in an overall detrimental effect (Fig. 17).

Our investigations into the cardiac abnormalities of sepsis have included the role of bacterial factors, spe-cific components of the host inflammatory response, and several potential mechanisms of myocardial dysfunction (4,83,84,86,87,110,117). It appears that functionally and structurally distinct bacterial factors interact with the host to produce a singular profile of cardiovascular injury. Abnormalities in oxygen utilization, inadequate coronary perfusion, and dysregulation of NO· production do not appear to be factors in mediating this cardiac dysfunction. Mechanisms which may contribute to this common pathway include abnormalities in catecholamine homeostasis and disruption of the coronary microcirculation leading to edema and myocyte damage. While these findings enhance our knowledge and partly explain the myocardial derangements occurring during sepsis, a full understanding of this complex process remains to be elucidated.

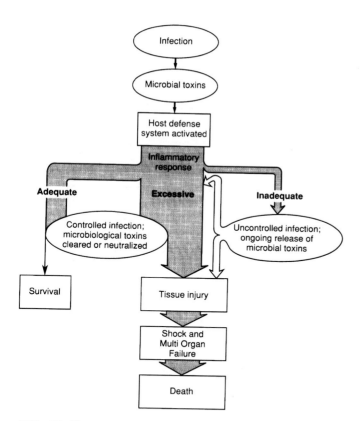

**FIG. 17.** The pathogenesis of septic shock divided by the level of the inflammatory response. Some patients likely produce an adequate inflammatory response which effectively controls infection, resulting in survival. Other patients, possibly immunocompromised, respond with an inadequate inflammatory response which is unable to control infection. Consequently, sepsis results in shock, multiorgan failure, and death. There also may be a subgroup of patients who develop an exaggerated inflammatory response. This response may be effective at controlling infection but results in generalized tissue injury and multiorgan dysfunction. To be effective, therapeutic strategies may need to be tailored to these three individual responses. From Natanson C, et al. *Ann Intern Med* 1994;120(9):771; with permission.

## REFERENCES

1. Natanson C, Hoffman WD, Suffredini AF, Eichacker PQ, Danner RL. Selected treatment strategies for septic shock based on proposed mechanisms of pathogenesis. *Ann Intern Med* 1994;120(9):771.
2. Bone RC, Balk RA, Cerra FB, Dellinger RP, Fein AM, Knaus WA. Definitions for sepsis and organ failure and guidelines for the use of innovative therapies in sepsis. The ACCP/SCCM Concensus Conference Committee. *Chest* 1992;101:1644.
3. Increase in National Hospital Discharge Survey Rates for Septicemia-United States, 1979–1987. *MMWR* 1990;39:31.
4. Parker MM, Shelhamer JH, Bacharach SL, et al. Profound but reversible myocardial depression in patients with septic shock. *Ann Intern Med* 1984;100:483.
5. Danner RL, Eln RJ, Hosseini JM, Wesley RA, Reilly JM, Parrillo JE. Endotoxemia in human septic shock. *Chest* 1991;99:169.
6. Westphal O, Jann K, Himmelspach K. Chemistry and immunochemistry of bacterial lipopolysaccharide as cell wall antigens and endotoxins. *Prog Allergy* 1983;33:9.
7. Baumgartner JD. Immunotherapy with antibodies to core lipopolysaccharide: a critical appraisal. *Infect Dis Clin North Am* 1991;5:915.
8. Calandra T, Glauser MP, Schellekens J, Verhoef J. Treatment of gram-negative septic shock with human IgG antibody to *Escherichia coli* j5: a prospective, double-blind, randomized trial. *J Infect Dis* 1988;158:312.
9. Baumgratner JD, Glauser MP, McCutchan JA, Ziegler EJ, van Melle G, Klauber MR. Prevention of gram-negative shcok and death in surgical patients by antibody to endotoxin core glycolipid. *Lancet* 1985;2:59.
10. Teng NN, Kaplan HS, Hebert JM, Moore C, Douglas H, Wunderlich A. Protection against gram-negative bacteremia and endotoxemia with human monoclonal IgM antibodies. *Proc Natl Acad Sci* 1985;82:1790.
11. Ziegler EJ, Fisher CJ, Sprung CL, Straube RC, Sadoff JC, Foulke GE. Treatment of gram-negative bacteremia and septic shock with HA-1A human monoclonal antibody against endotoxin. A randomized, double-blind, placebo-controlled trial. The HA-1A Sepsis Study Group. *N Engl J Med* 1991;324:429.
12. Quezado ZMN, Natanson C, Alling DW, et al. A controlled trial of HA-1A in a canine model of gram-negative septic shock. *JAMA* 1993;269:17:2221.
13. Luce JM. Introduction of new technology into critical care practice: a history of HA-1A human monoclonal antibody against endotoxin. *Crit Care Med* 1993;21:1233.
14. McCloskey RV, Straube RC, Sanders C, Smith SM, Smith CR, and the CHESS Trial Study Group. Treatment of septic shock with human monoclonal antibody HA-1A. A randomized, double-blind, placebo-controlled trial. *Ann Intern Med* 1994;121:1.
15. Greenman RL, Schein RM, Martin MA, Wenzel RP, MacIntyre NR, Emmanuel G, and the XOMA Sepsis Study Group. A controlled clinical trial of E5 murine monoclonal IgM antibody to endotoxin in the treatment of gram-negative sepsis. *JAMA* 1991;266:1097.
16. Bone RC, Balk RA, Fein AM, et al. A second controlled clinical study of E5, a monoclonal antibody to endotoxin: results of a prospective, multicenter, randomized clinical trial. *Crit Care Med* 1995;23:994–1006.
17. Nathan C, Sporn M. Cytokines in context. *J Cell Biol* 1991;113:981.
18. Endres S, Cannon JG, Ghorbani R, Dempsey RA, Sisson SD, Lonnemann G. In vitro production of IL-1 beta, IL-1 alpha, TNF and IL-2 in healthy subjects: distribution, effect of cyclooxygenase ingibition and evidence of independent gene regulation. *Eur J Immunol* 1989;19:2327.
19. Hesse DG, Tracey KJ, Fong Y, Manogue KR, Palladino MA, Cerami A. Cytokine appearance in human endotoxemia and primate bacteremia. *Surg Gynecol Obstet* 1988;166:147.
20. Canon GC, Tompkins RG, Gelf JA, Michie HR, Stanford GG, van der Meer JW. Circulating interleukin-1 and tumor necrosis factor in septic shock and experimental endotoxin fever. *J Infect Dis* 1990;161:79.
21. Dinerrello CA, Wolff SM. The role of interleukin-1 in disease. *N Engl J Med* 1993;328:106.
22. Ding AH, Porteu F. Regulation of tumor necrosis factor receptors on phagocytes. *Proc Soc Exp Biol Med* 1992;200:458.
23. Aderka D, Engelmann H, Maor Y, Brakebusch C, Wallach D. Stabilization of the bioactivity of tumor necrosis factor by its soluble receptors. *J Exp Med* 1992;175:323.
24. Fernandez-Botran R. Solube cytokine receptors: their role in immunoregulation. *FASEB J* 1991;5:2567.
25. Dinarello CA. The proinflammatory cytokines interleukin-1 and tumor necrosis factor and treatment of septic shock syndrome. *J Infect Dis* 1991;163:1177.
26. Alexander HR, Sheppard BC, Jensen JC, Langstein HN, Buresh CM, Venzon D. Treatment with recombinant human tumor necorsis factor-alpha protects rats against the lethality, hypotension, and hypothermia of gram-negative sepsis. *J Clin Invest* 1991;88:34.
27. van der Meer JW, Barza M, Wolff SM, Dinarello CA. A low dose of recombinant interleukin-1 protects granulocytopenic mice from lethal gram-negative infection. *Proc Natl Acad Sci* 1988;85:1620.
28. Nakane A, Minagawa T, Kato K. Endogenous tumor necrosis factor (cachectin) is essential to host resistance against *Listeria monocytogenes* infection. *Infect Immunol* 1988;56:2563.
29. Allendoerfer R, Magee DM, Smith JG, Bonewald L, Graybill JR.

Induction of tumor necrosis factor-alpha in murine *Candida albicans* infection. *J Infect Dis* 1993;167:1168.

30. Echtanger B, Falk W, Mannel DN, Krammer PH.. Requirement of endogenous tumor necrosis factor/cachectin for recovery from experimental peritonitis. *J Immunol* 1990;145:3762.

31. Fisher CJ, Opal SM, Dhainaut JF. Influence of an anti-tumor necrosis factor monoclonal antibody on cytokines in patients with sepsis. *Crit Care Med* 1993;21:318.

32. Abraham E, Wunderink R, Silverman H, et al. Efficacy and safety of monocolonal antibody to human tumor necrosis factored in patients with sepsis syndrome. *JAMA* 1995;273:934–941.

33. Carlet J, Cohen J, Anderson J. Intersept: an international efficacy and safety study of monoclonal antibody (MAb) to human tumor necrosis factor (hTNF) in patients with the sepsis syndrome. Interscience Conference on Antimicrobial Agents and Chemotherapy. New Orleans, USA 1994;34:7(abst).

34. Van Zee KJ, Kohno T, Fischer E, Rock CS, Moldawer LL, Lowry SF. Tumor necrosis factor soluble receptors circulate during experimental and clinical inflammation and can protect against excessive tumor necrosis factor in vivo and in vitro. *Proc Natl Acad Sci* 1992;89:4845.

35. Sadoff J. Soluble TNF receptors. Presented at the Third International Congress of the Immune Consequences of Trauma, Shock and Sepsis: Mechanisms and therapeutic approaches, Munich, Germany, March 5, 1995.

36. Fisher CJ, Slotner GJ, Opal SM, Pribble JP, Bone RC, Emmanuel G. Initial evaluation of human recombinant interleukin-1 receptor antagonist in the treatment of sepsis syndrome: a randomized, open-label, placebo-controlled multicenter trial. *Crit Care Med* 1994;22:12.

37. Fisher CJ, Dhainaut J-F, Pribble JP, Knaus WA, IL-1 Receptor Antagonist Study Group. A study evaluating the safety and efficacy of human recombinant interleukin-1 receptor antagonist in the treatment of patients with sepsis syndrome: preliminary results from a phase III multicenter trial. *Clin Intens Care* 1993;4:8S(abst).

38. Press Release. Synergen stops clinical trial of Antril for severe sepsis. Interim results do not demonstrate efficacy. PR Newswire, New York, 1994;

39. Zimmerman JJ, Ringer TV. Inflammatory host responses in sepsis. *Crit Care Clin* 1992;8:163.

40. Rinaldo JE, Christman JW. Mechanisms and mediators of the adult respiratory distress syndrome. *Clin Chest Med* 1990;11:621.

41. Bersten A, Sibbald WJ. Acute lung injury in septic shock. *Crit Care Clin* 1989;5:49.

42. Vedder NB, Winn RK, Rice CL, Chi EY, Arfors KE, Harlan JM. A monoclonal antibody to the adherence-promoting leukocyte glycoprotein, CD18, reduces organ injury and improves survival from hemorrhagic shock and resuscitation in rabbits. *J Clin Invest* 1988;81:939.

43. Saez-Llorens X, Jafari HS, Severien C, et al. Enhanced attenuation of meningeal inflammation and brain edema by concomitant administration of anti-CD18 monoclonal antibodies and dexamethasone in experimental *Haemophilus* meningitis. *J Clin Invest* 1991;88:2003.

44. Mileski WJ, Raymond JF, Winn RK, Harlan JH, Rice CL. Inhibition of leukocyte adherence and aggregation for treatment of severe cold injury in rabbits. *J Appl Physiol* 1993;74(3):1432.

45. Malik AB. Endothelial cell interactions and integrins. *New Horizons* 1993;1:37.

46. Smith CW, Marlin SD, Rothlein R, Toman C, Anderson DC. Cooperative interactions of LFA-1 and Mac-1 with intercellular adhesion molecule-1 in facilitating adherence and transendothelial migration of human neutrophils in vitro. *J Clin Invest* 1989;83:2008.

47. Arfos KE, Lundberg C, Lindbom L, Lundberg K, Beatty PG, Harlan JM. A monoclonal antibody to the membrane glycoprotein complex CD18 inhibits polymorphonuclear leukocyte accumulation and plasma leakage in vitro. *Blood* 1987;69(1):338.

48. Pohlman TH, Stanness KA, Beatty PG, Ochs HD, Harlan JM. An endothelial cell surface factor(s) induced in vitro by lipopolysaccharide, interleukin-1, and tumor necrosis factor-alpha increases neutrophil adherence by a CDw18-dependent mechanism. *J Immunol* 1986;136:4548.

49. Doerschuk CM, Winn RK, Coxson HO, Harlan JM. CD18-dependent and -independent mechanisms of neutrophil emigration in the pulmonary and systemic microcirculation of rabbits. *J Immunol* 1990;14(6):2327.

50. Mulligan MS, Smith CW, Anderson DC, et al. Role of leukocyte adhesion molecules in complement-induced lung injury. *J Immunol* 1993;150:6:2401.

51. Sharrar SR, Winn RK, Nurry CE, Harlan JM, Rice CL. A CD18 monoclonal antibody increases the incidence and severity of subcutaneous abscess formation after high-dose *Staphylococcus aureus* injection in rabbits. *Surgery* 1991;110:213.

52. Walsh CJ, Carey PD, Cook DJ, Bechard DE, Fowler AA, Sugerman HJ. Anti-CD18 antibody attenuates neutropenia and alveolar-capillary membrane injury during gram-negative sepsis. *Surgery* 1991; 110:205.

53. Eichacker PQ, Hoffman WD, Farese A, et al. Leukocyte CD18 monoclonal antibody worsens endotoxemia and cardiovascular injury in canines with septic shock. *J Appl Physiol* 1993;74(4):1885.

54. Golde DW, Baldwin GC. Myeloid growth factors. In: Gallin JI, Goldstein IM, Snyderman R, eds. *Inflammation: basic principles and clinical correlates.* New York: Raven Press; 1992:291.

55. Mooney DP, Gamelli RL, O'Reilley M, Hebert JC. Recombinant human granulocyte colony-stimulating factor and *Pseudomonas* burn wound sepsis. *Arch Surg* 1988;123:1353.

56. Eichacker PQ, Waisman Y, Natanson C, et al. Cardiopulmonary effects of granulocyte colony-stimulating factor in a canine model of bacterial sepsis. *J Appl Physiol* 1994;77(5):2366.

57. Tuomanen EI, Saukkonen K, Sande S, Cioffe C, Wright SD. Reduction of inflammation, tissue damage, and mortality in bacterial meningitis in rabbits treated with monoclonal antibodies against adhesion-promoting receptors of leukocytes. *J Exp Med* 1989;170:959.

58. Eichacker PQ, Farese A, Hoffman WD, et al. Leukocyte CD11b/18 antigen-directed monoclonal antibody improves early survival and decreases hypoxemia in dogs challenged with tumor necrosis factor. *Am Rev Respir Dis* 1992;145:1023.

59. Sharar SR, Winn RK, Murray CE, Harlan JM, Rice CL. A CD18 monoclonal antibody increases the incidence and severity of subcutaneous abscess formation after high-dose *Staphylococcus aureus* injection in rabbits. *Surgery* 1991;110:213.

60. Rosen H, Gordon S, North RJ. Exacerbation of murine listeriosis by a monoclonal antibody specific for the Type 3 complement receptor of myelomonocytic cells. Absence of monocytes at infective foci allows *Listeria* to multiply in nonphagocytic cells. *J Exp Med* 1989;170:27.

61. Lorente JA, Landin L, De Pablo R, Renes E, Liste D. L-Arginine pathway in the sepsis syndrome. *Crit Care Med* 1993;21(9):1287.

62. Cobb JP, Cunnion RE, Danner RL. Nitric oxide as a target for therapy in septic shock. *Crit Care Med* 1993;21(9):1261.

63. Nathan C. Nitric oxide as a secretory product of mammalian cells. *FASEB J* 1992;6:3051.

64. Kilbourn RG, Jubran A, Gross SS, et al. Reversal of endotoxin-mediated shock by *N*-methyl-L-arginine, an inhibitor of nitric oxide synthesis. *Biochem Biophys Res Commun* 1990;172:1132.

65. Finkel MS, Oddis CV, Jacob TD, Watkins SC, Hattler BG, Simmons RL. Negative inotropic effects of cytokines on the heart mediated by nitric oxide. *Science* 1992;257:387.

66. Estrada C, Gomez C, Martin C, Moncada S, Gonzalez C. Nitric oxide mediates tumor necrosis factor-alpha cytotoxicity in endothelial cells. *Biochem Biophys Res Commun* 1992;186:475.

67. Van Dervort AL, Yan L, Madara PJ, Cobb JP, Wesley RA, Tropea MM. Nitric oxide increases endotoxin (LPS)-induced cytokine production by human neutrophils (PMNs). *Clin Res* 1993;41:281(abst).

68. Radomski MW, Palmer RM, Moncada S. An L-arginine/nitric oxide pathway present in human platelets regulates aggregation. *Proc Natl Acad Sci* 1990;87:5193.

69. Kubes P, Suzuki M, Granger DN. Nitric oxide: an endogenous modulator of leukocyte adhesion. *Proc Natl Acad Sci* 1991;88:4651.

70. May GR, Crook P, Moore PK, Page CP. The role of nitric oxide as an endogenous regulator of platelet and eutrophil activation within the pulmonary circulation of the rabbit. *Br J Pharmacol* 1991;102:759.

71. Parker MM, Shelhamer JH, Natanson C. Serial cardiovascular variables in survivors and non-survivors of human septic shock. *Crit Care Med* 1987;15:923.

72. Hollenberg SM, Cunnion RE, Zimmerberg J. Nitric oxide synthase inhibition reverses arteriolar hyporesponsiveness to catecholamines in septic rats. *Am J Physiol* 1993;264:H660.

73. Tollins JP, Raij L. Modulation of systemic blood pressure and renal hemodynamic responses by endothelium-derived relaxing factor (nitric oxide). In: Moncada S, Higgs EA, eds. *Nitric oxide from L-arginine.* New York: Elsevier Science; 1990:463.

74. Walder CE, Thiemermann C, Vane JR. The involvement of endothelium-derived relaxing factor in the regulation of renal cortical blood flow in the rat. *Br J Pharmacol* 1991;102:967.

75. Hutcheson IR, Whittle BJR, Boughton-Smith NK. Role of nitric oxide in maintaining vascular integrity in endotoxin-induced acute intestinal damage in the rat. *Br J Pharmacol* 1990;101:815.

76. Klabunde RE, Ritger RC. *N*-amino-L-arginine restores arterial blood pressure but reduces cardiac output in a canine model of endotoxic shock. *Biochem Biophys Res Commun* 1991;178:1135.

77. Nava E, Palmer RM, Moncada S. The role of nitric oxide in endotoxin shock: effects of $N_3$-monomethyl-L-arginine. *J Cardiovas Pharmacol* 1992;20(Suppl 12):S132.

78. Petros A, Lamb G, Leone A, Moncada S, Bennett D, Vallance P. Effects of a nitric oxide synthase inhibitor in humans with septic shock. *Cardiovasc Res* 1994;28:34.

79. Kilbourn RG, Belloni P. Endothelial cell production of nitrogen oxides in response to interferon gamma in combination with tumor necrosis factor, interleukin-1, or endotoxin. *J Natl Cancer Inst* 1990; 82:772.

80. Cobb JP, Natanson CO, Quezado ZMN, et al. Differential hemodynamic effects of L-NMMA in endotoxemic and normal dogs. *Am J Physiol* 1995;268 (*Heart Circ Physiol* 37):H6134–H642.

81. Cobb JP, Natanson C, Hoffman WD, et al. *N*-amino-L-Arginine, an inhibitor of nitric oxide synthase, raises vascular resistance but increases mortality rates in awake canines challenged with endotoxin. *J Exp Med* 1992;176:1175.

82. Kilbourn RG, Gross SS, Jubran A. *N*-methyl-L-arginine inhibits tumor necrosis factor-induced hypotension: implications for the involvement of nitric oxide. *Proc Natl Acad Sci* 1990;8:3629.

83. Natanson C, Fink MP, Ballantyne HK, MacVittie TJ, Conklin JJ, Parillo JE. Gram-negative bacteremia produces both severe systolic and diastolic cardiac dysfunction in a canine model that simulates human septic shock. *J Clin Invest* 1986;78:259.

84. Parker MM, McCarthy KE, Ognibene FP, Parrillo JE. Right ventricular dysfunction and dilatation, similar to left ventricular changes, characterize the cardiac depression of septic shock in humans. *Chest* 1990;97:126.

85. Kimchi A, Ellrody AG, Berman DS. Right ventricular performance in septic shock: a combined radionuclide and hemodynamic study. *J Am Coll Cardiol* 1984;4:945.

86. Natanson C, Danner RL, Fink MP, et al. Cardiovascular performance with *E. coli* challenges in a canine model of human sepsis. *Am J Physiol* 1988;254:H558.

87. Natanson C, Danner RL, Elin RJ, et al. Role of endotoxemia in cardiovascular dysfunction and mortality. *Escherichia coli* and *Staphylococcus aureus* challenges in a canine model of human septic shock. *J Clin Invest* 1989;83:243.

88. Fine J. The bacterial factor in traumatic shock. In: Page IH, Corcoran AC, eds. Springfield, IL: Thomas; 1954.

89. Danner RL, Natanson C, Elin RJ, et al. *Pseudomonas aeruginosa* compared with *Escherichia coli* produces less endotoxemia but more cardiovascular dysfunction and mortality in a canine model of septic shock. *Chest* 1990;98:1480.

90. Hoffman WD, Natanson C, Danner RL, et al. Bacterial organism virulence factors may be more important than endotoxemia in determining cardiovascular dysfunction and mortality in canine septic shock. *Clin Res* 1989;37(2):344A(abst).

91. Hoffman WO, Danner RL, Quezado ZMN, et al. Role of endotoxemia in cardiovascular dysfunction and lethality: virulent and nonvirulent Escherichia coli challenges in a canine model of septic shock. *Infection and Immunity* 1996;64:406–412.

92. Endres S, Cannon JG, Ghobani R, Dempsey RA, Sisson SD, Lonnemann G. In vitro production of IL-1 beta, IL-1 alpha, TNF and IL-2 in healthy subjects: distribution, effect of cyclooxygenation inhibition and evidence of independent gene regulation. *Eur J Immunol* 1989;19: 2327.

93. Okusawa S, Gelfand JA, Ikejuima T, Connolly RJ, Dinarello CA. Interleukin-1 induces a shock-like state in rabbits. Synergism with tumor necrosis factor and the effect of cyclooxygenase inhibition. *J Clin Invest* 1988;81:1162.

94. Tracey KJ, Beutler B, Lowry SF, Merryweather J, Wolpe S, Milsark IW. Shock and tissue injury induced by recombinant human cachectin. *Science* 1986;234:470.

95. Micie HR, Spriggs DR, Manogue KR, Sherman ML, Revhaug A, O'Dwyer ST. Tumor necrosis factor and endotoxin induce similar metabolic responses in human beings. *Surgery* 1988;104:280.

96. Fischer E, Marano MA, Van Zee KJ, Rock CS, Hawes AS, Thompson WA. Interleukin-1 receptor blockade improves survival and hemodynamic performance in *Esherichia coli* septic shock, but fails to alter host responses to sublethal endotoxemia. *J Clin Invest* 1992; 89:1551.

97. Beutler B, Milsark IW, Cerami AC. Passive immunization against cachectin tumor necrosis factor protects mice from lethal effect of endotoxin. *Science* 1985;229:869.

98. Fearon DT, Ruddy S, Schur PH, McCabe WR. Activation of the properdin pathway of complement in patients with gram-negative bacteremia. *N Engl J Med* 1975;292:937.

99. Sprung CL, Schultz DR, Marcial E, et al. Complement activation in septic shock patients. *Crit Care Med* 1986;14:525.

100. Natanson C, Eichenholz PW, Danner RL, et al. Endotoxin and tumor necrosis factor challenges in dogs simulate the cardiovascular profile of human septic shock. *J Exp Med* 1989;169:823.

101. Eichenholz PW, Eichacker PQ, Hoffman WD, et al. Tumor necrosis challenges in canines: patterns of cardiovascular dysfunction. *Am J Physiol* 1992;263:H668.

102. Eichacker PQ, Hoffman WD, Farese A, et al. TNF but IL-1 in dogs causes lethal lung injury and multiple organ dysfunction similar to human sepsis. *J Appl Physiol* 1991;71(5):1979.

103. Quezado ZMN, Hoffman WD, Winkelstein JA, et al. The third component of complement protects against *Escherichia coli* endotoxin-induced shock and multiple organ failure. *J Exp Med* 1994;179:569.

104. Cunnion RE, Schaer G, Parker MM, Natanson C, Parillo JE. The coronary circulation in human septic shock. *Circulation* 1986;73: 637.

105. Dhainaut JF, Huyghebaert MF, Monsallier JF, et al. Coronary hemodynamics and myocardial metabolism of lactate, free fatty acids, glucose, and ketones in patients with septic shock. *Circulation* 1987;3:533.

106. Heinemen FW, Balaban RS. Phophorous-31 nuclear magnetic resonance analysis of transient changes of canine myocardial metabolism in vivo. *J Clin Invest* 1990;85:843.

107. Katz LA, Swain JA, Portman MA, Balaban RS. Relation between phosphate metabolites and oxygen consumption of the heart in vivo. *Am J Physiol* 1989;256:H265.

108. Portman MA, James S, Heineman FW, Balaban RS. Simultaneous monitoring of coronary blood flow and 31P-NMR detected myocardial metabolites. *Magn Reson Med* 1988;7:243.

109. Robitaille PM, Merkle H, Lew B, et al. Transmural high energy phosphate distribution and response to alterations in workload in the normal canine myocardium as studied with spatially localized 31P NMR spectroscopy. *Magn Reson Med* 1990;16:91.

110. Solomon MA, Correa R, Alexander HR, et al. Myocardial energy metabolism and morphology in a canine model of sepsis. *Am J Physiol* 1994;266:H757.

111. Reichenbach DD, Benditt EP. Catecholamines and cardiomyopathy: the pathogenesis and potential importance of myofibrillar degeneration. *Hum Pathol* 1970;1:125.

112. Natanson C, Danner RL, Reilly JM, et al. Antibiotics versus cardiovascular support in a canine model of human septic shock. *Am J Physiol* 1990;259:H1440.

113. Karzai W, Reilly JM, Hoffman WD, et al. Hemodynamic effects of dopamine, norepinephrine, and fluids in a dog model of sepsis. *Am J Physiol [in press]*.

114. Nava E, Palmer RMJ, Moncada S. Inhibition of nitric oxide synthesis in septic shock: How much is beneficial? *Lancet* 1991;338:1555.

115. Young LS, Martin WJ, Meyer RD, Weinstein RJ, Anderson ET. Gram-negative rod bacteremia: microbiologic, immunologic, and therapeutic considerations. *Ann Intern Med* 1977;86:456.

116. Natanson C, Parillo JE. Septic shock. *Anesth Clin North Am* 1988; 6:73.

117. Ognibene FP, Parker MM, Natanson C, Shelhamer JH, Parrillo JE. Depressed left ventricular performance. Response to volume infusion in patients with sepsis and septic shock. *Chest* 1988;93:903.

*The Critically Ill Cardiac Patient,*
edited by V. Kvetan and D. R. Dantzker,
Lippincott-Raven Publishers, Philadelphia © 1996.

# CHAPTER 11

# Transport of Critically Ill Cardiac Patients

Kenneth Greer, David Crippen, and John Hoyt

There are many aspects of "transport" which might be considered when reviewing the delivery of health care services to patients with cardiac disease. First would be "scene rescue," to put it in the language of the paramedic and emergency medical services (EMS) community. Next would be the interhospital transport of patients from a community hospital facility to high-technology tertiary referral centers. Finally would be intrahospital transport when a critically ill patient, dependent on life support such as the intra-aortic counterpulsation balloon (IACB) and mechanical ventilation, must leave the intensive care unit (ICU) to go to radiology or the operating room or the cardiac catheterization laboratory. All of these are important aspects of transport, but the focus of this chapter will largely be on the interhospital transport of cardiac patients as might be associated with regionalized cardiac care services.

First a few brief comments on scene rescue. Cardiac events such as chest pain, congestive heart failure, myocardial infarction, life-threatening arrhythmias occur in the community. They may occur at home or on the street or in a restaurant or any of a number of other places. Bystander support and skilled EMS community rescue squads are essential to survival. The EMS personnel must know life support and be able to diagnose and initiate treatment in communication with medical command. The better the EMS personnel and their equipment for prehospital support, the better the outcome from an acute cardiac event. This is not a particularly controversial statement in the 1990s, and an entire network of EMS personnel and emergency medicine departments provide a safety net system of life support for patients with cardiac disease in the United States.

The interhospital transport of patients with cardiac disease turns out to be somewhat more controversial. Should transport be done by an ambulance or helicopter? Should

the crew have a paramedic or a nurse or a physician? How does one handle mechanical ventilation or IACB or pacemaker or left ventricular assist device (LVAD)? Not all hospitals have cardiac catheterization laboratories or cardiac surgery operating suites. Not all hospitals do cardiac transplantation. And yet patients with cardiac disease get sick at home or on the street or in a restaurant or at a number of other places. These patients are commonly taken to community hospitals where initial stabilization occurs. Transfer to a cardiac center may take place at that time or after several days in the ICU. This transfer from the community hospital to the tertiary referral hospital will be the focus of this chapter.

In the subsequent sections of this chapter we will look at the history of interhospital transport of critically ill patients and many of the issues that surround that expensive activity. When the general public and much of the medical community sees a medical evacuation helicopter cruising the skies, they instantly think of trauma. In fact, the 1994 statistics for medical evacuation show that the majority of transports (57%) are medical, such as the patient with cardiac disease (1). In most cases these helicopters are staffed by an emergency medicine trained nurse and paramedic or two nurses. Physicians on flight teams, even resident physicians, are rare. And yet many of the cardiac patients, replete with endotracheal tubes, arterial catheters, pulmonary artery catheters, and an intra-aortic balloon in the case of cardiogenic shock, are much more ICU patients than emergency medicine patients. Appropriate standards for the transport of such patients are not well delineated, but a review of the history of transport and considerations for transport of cardiac patients may shed some light on this question.

## HISTORY

The transport of the critically ill has its origins in the evacuation of wounded soldiers. Man's conflict on the battlefield resulted in many severely wounded soldiers who

K. Greer, D. Crippen, and J. Hoyt: St. Francis Medical Center, University of Pittsburgh, Pittsburgh, Pennsylvania 15201.

would die if they did not receive proper advanced medical attention. During World War II it took 1 to 2 days to transport an injured soldier from the front lines to a medical station. In the subsequent Korean Conflict of the 1950s the time of transport was decreased to 2 to 3 hours. During the Vietnam War this time was shortened to 1 to 2 hours. In most cases patient transport was completed less than 1 hour after the time of injury. This rapid decrease in transport time was in large part due to the advent of the helicopter for medical evacuation from the scene of injury.

The helicopter was the conceptual brainchild of Leonardo da Vinci, but it was not until the late 1930s that a helicopter successfully completed multiple flights. This was the work of Igor Sikorsy. By the late 1940s Bell Helicopters had a single-rotor helicopter that was licensed in the United States for commercial use (2). The helicopter has the unique quality of vertical flight, which eliminates long runways for takeoff and landing. The helicopter can quickly travel to remote areas and land at the scene of an accident or adjacent to a hospital. Patients can be quickly evacuated from an accident scene or small hospital and sent to a tertiary care facility for regionalized medical services.

In 1966 the U.S. Congress (3) addressed the issue of accidents on the highway system. The result was the Highway Safety Act, which stated that many victims of highway accidents die needlessly or are permanently disabled due to their inability to receive appropriate medical attention. There was a national call to mobilize every available resource to save lives and limit injury to those who were in highway accidents. The helicopter was identified as an excellent means of transporting accident victims. It could avoid all ground congestion caused by the accident, land at almost any site no matter how remote or otherwise inaccessible, and quickly transport the victim to a hospital.

In 1967 the state of Maryland established the first plan for a statewide helicopter evacuation program. The plan was put into effect in 1969 (4) by a combined effort of the Maryland State Police and the University of Maryland. This system had a statewide communication network in which the police officer at the scene of an accident could be in communication with the trauma center. If needed, a helicopter could be dispatched to the accident scene and rapid and expert medical care could be delivered in a matter of minutes. As a result of this program, the Maryland Center for the Study of Trauma noted a significant decrease in mortality rate, from almost 50% in 1969 to approximately 20% in 1972. There was a fourfold increase in patient admissions.

With the success of the Maryland Trauma Program in the late 1960s and early 1970s and the development of other trauma transport systems, a large number of children were also being transported. It soon became clear that the needs of children were quite different from their adult counterparts. The Denver Pediatric Emergency Transport System emerged in 1975. It was composed of three hospitals in Denver. This was the first system in the country devoted solely to the transport of the pediatric and neonatal patient (5). This system had three goals: first to increase the utilization of ICU beds of the three hospitals that joined to make up the program, second to provide a transport system that would service critically ill and injured children, and third to coordinate the skills and facilities of the member hospitals to assure optimal and comprehensive care of the patient without significant duplication of services. The system covered over 500,000 square miles and transported over 250 patients in the first 6 months. Currently pediatric transport and pediatric specialty transport teams have flourished throughout the country.

In the last 10 years there has been a significant increase in other patients that are transported to a tertiary care facility. Trauma and pediatric patients currently do not represent the majority of patients that are evacuated via helicopter. According to the 1994 annual transport statistics for hospital-based helicopter programs (6), 46.1% of all patients transported are adult patients with a medical diagnosis. Approximately 38.9% are adult trauma patients and the remainder are pediatric medical and trauma patients. It appears that of the adult patients, the vast majority have a cardiac diagnosis.

Approximately 60% to 75% of adult, nontrauma transports are secondary to a cardiac disease (7). This is due, in part, to many new technologic advancements which have developed in the last decade that are not available at all hospitals. These include cardiac catheterization, angioplasty, level 1 critical care, hemodynamic support, cardiac transplantation, and the use of artificial hearts.

## PHILOSOPHY OF TRANSPORT

The philosophy of the medical evacuation system will significantly affect team function and composition. The historical philosophy of medical evacuation was developed from trauma care and was known as "scoop and run."

It was the goal of transport to move the patient as quickly as possible from the accident scene where treatment was inadequate to a facility where the necessary level of therapy was readily available.

Initially this philosophy centered on getting the patient to the tertiary care trauma center with substantial speed and minimal delay. The emphasis was on speed of transport. The scoop-and-run philosophy was supported by the trauma concept of the "Golden Hour." The time interval from injury to stabilization and arrival of the patient in the trauma center operating room had to be minimal. Mortality rate increases with delay. This initial philosophy was expanded and modified to promote rapid stabilization in the field and transport to a tertiary care trauma hospital. Still the time at the scene is kept at a minimum.

Since the evaluation of regionalized trauma services, another transport philosophy has developed centered on extending the bedside time and bringing intensive care services to the patient in the community hospital. These are transports that are physician guided and rely upon stabilization of the patient prior to medical evacuation. This is sometimes known as "stay and play," and this system has been developed by critical care departments and is employed mainly for patients with unstable cardiac disease (8, 9). The medical evacuation philosophy of a transport program will thus determine team composition, bedside time, equipment available on the helicopter, and the level of care given prior to the transport.

## CRITICAL CARE TRANSPORT TEAM

Medical evacuation team composition is an important issue for the safe interhospital transport of a patient with a life-threatening cardiac problem. The recommendation of the Association of Air Medical Services (AAMS) for helicopter transport teams is two crew members one of which is a flight nurse. Fifty-three percent of all programs provide a nurse/paramedic team, 11% a nurse/physician team, 11% a nurse/nurse team, 20% a nurse/other team, and 5% are some other combination (10). The composition of the team depends on the philosophy of the program, the patient population being transported, and the availability of personnel. One other factor has a great influence. This is the Consolidated Omnibus Budget Reconciliation Act (COBRA) of 1986. COBRA requires that the transferring hospital assume full liability for the adequacy of patient stabilization prior to transport. This law places the transferring hospital in a position of guaranteeing the adequacy of transport to the receiving institution. The transport must be provided by individuals trained and qualified to provide whatever treatment is necessary to maintain the patient's condition and prevent complications (11). Transport teams should provide a level of service that is equal to or greater than that which is provided at the transferring institution.

There has been great debate over the optimal composition of the transport team (12–14). In particular, the question is whether a transport physician can significantly impact the morbidity and mortality of patients when compared to a well-trained nonphysician team. It appears there is no clear answer to this question. Certain subgroups of patients may benefit from a physician on the transport team. One study (14) found that the clinical judgment and skill level of the physician was significantly contributory to the patient management in certain populations. The physician role was most contributory in transport for pediatric cardiac disease (82%) and adult cardiac disease (44%). It was also noted in the same study that as the severity of illness increased, as indicated by an increasing Therapeutic Intervention Scoring System (TISS) score, the physician contribution increased significantly. As TISS increased to over 20, physician contribution was seen in over 50% of the cases, however; this is a small patient population. In fact, there has never been a study comparing an attending critical care physician based team to the common nurse/paramedic team for the transport of cardiac patients.

The use of the physician for the transport of cardiac patients has significant support in the literature. Patients with acute myocardial infarction have more frequent complications during transport. It has been reported (15) that of cardiac patients who are described as unstable prior to transport, approximately one-third will experience some life-threatening complication during transport. Patients who exhibit cardiogenic shock have been found to have an even higher incidence of complications, many of which require physician intervention (16).

It is reasonable to conclude that adult cardiac patients and those patients with a high severity of illness score will benefit from physician transport. The physician accompanying the transport team should be an expert in medical emergencies with excellent life support skills. Sending an intern or an inexperienced resident will not be beneficial for the care of the patient.

The personnel who transport the unstable cardiac patient should be qualified to provide the expertise necessary for initial stabilization and management of sophisticated life support systems. This includes expertise in the intra-aortic balloon pump (IABP), pulmonary artery (PA) pressure monitoring, pacemakers, ventilatory modes, advanced airway skills, and a working familiarity with all inotropic, vasoactive, and antiarrhythmic drugs. For the critically ill cardiac transport the ideal team consists of a critical care nurse with extensive ICU experience, a critical care technologist who is familiar with all forms of monitoring and IABP support, and a physician who is trained in critical care medicine. This team should be able to manage all adverse patient situations (9).

## EQUIPMENT

The medical equipment required for a critical care transport varies significantly with the type of patient. The helicopter or ground ambulance should mimic a small portable ICU. Limitations of space and weight will dictate the type of equipment. The crew should be familiar with the use and location of all equipment which should be inspected daily for signs of malfunction.

The helicopter, airplane, or ground vehicle should be equipped with an inverter to convert the DC power produced by the engine to AC power employed by standard medical equipment. This is essential for the transport of power-consuming equipment such as an IABP. When several pieces of equipment are drawing power from the inverter, the power requirement may exceed the output of the inverter, leading to equipment malfunction. The medical evacuation team must be aware of the power needs of all equipment utilized during transport. Total power consumed must be below the maximum rated power output of the inverter. If the inverter becomes overloaded, the system will cease to function. If a transport requires high power output, some of the equipment may be run intermittently off the battery system and be switched back and forth during the transport to avoid overload.

The transport vehicle should be equipped with inboard oxygen. The oxygen should be stored outside the cabin in the helicopter with flow control managed internally. Oxygen may be stored internally or externally in ground vehicles. The volume of stored oxygen should supply the patient adequately for twice the time of a normal or average transport at the highest oxygen flow rates. It is important to keep in mind that while transporting in an unpressurized helicopter or fixed-winged aircraft, oxygen requirements will increase as one ascends to higher altitude. In particular, ventilator pressure settings will have to be adjusted to maintain the tidal volume during ascent.

Suctioning equipment, cardiac monitor, and a defibrillator should all be mounted in the aircraft within easy reach and be clearly visible during transport. By adding other equipment to the basic equipment on board, the team can tailor the aircraft or ground vehicle for its particular mission and the needs of the patient.

## SPECIALTY EQUIPMENT

Conceptually, the transport equipment should have several common features:

1. Equipment should be lightweight, portable, and self-contained. Any exposed critical elements should be well protected.
2. The equipment should be mounted or secured during flight. The equipment should be readily accessible in flight if the patient's condition deteriorates. Equipment should not block access to the patient during transport.
3. All equipment should be able to run on battery power and have AC capabilities. Larger equipment (such as an IABP) should be capable of recharging during transport.
4. All electrical equipment should run without electromagnetic interference with navigation or communication radios.
5. Secondary battery backup should be available for all electrical equipment.
6. The equipment performance should be monitored during transport, withstand changes in pressure and temperature, and be able to function under extreme vibration.
7. All alarms should have visual analogues and all monitor panels should be lighted for visualization at night.

## MEDICATIONS

Medications taken on transport must be well organized into a very compact carrying apparatus. Each class of drug utilized in the ICU should be represented. For example, there are currently three thrombolytic agents available in the United States. All three should not be taken but instead one member of this class of drugs should be available on the flight. All drugs that are required for resuscitation should be available.

In addition to medications, adequate intravascular volume expanders should be available with an infusion pump system. Almost yearly the infusion devices become more compact and more exact. All inotropic, vasoactive medications should be infused by a pump with a controlled flow rate. Initially transport pumps were single-medication, pumps but now multichannel infusion systems are available (Fig. 1). One that is commonly employed is the MiniMed, which allows for three separate intravenous (IV) drips to be infused by one pump. It is lightweight (3 pounds) and small. The delivery range varies from 0.1 to 999 mL/hr. Such systems can be powered by batteries for 6 to 8 hours. A compact, highly accurate infusion system is desirable for interhospital transport.

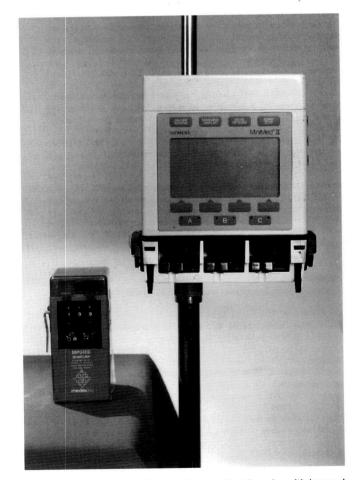

**FIG. 1.** Single-channel Roller Pump *(right)* and multichannel MiniMed Pump *(left)*.

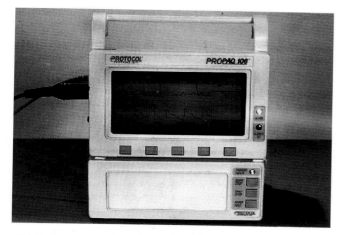

**FIG. 2.** ProPaq transport monitor. Electrocardiographic invasive and noninvasive blood pressure monitoring, pulmonary artery waveform, and Sao2 monitoring can be provided simultaneously.

## MONITORING

Monitoring is paramount during the transport. Electrocardiographic and oxygen saturation by pulse oximeter should be standard for every cardiac patient. Blood pressure monitoring should be available for both invasive and noninvasive techniques. Capability for all invasive monitored pressures should be available during the transport. Pulmonary artery pressures should be monitored when a Swan Ganz catheter is in use. A rapid change in PA pressures may be an indication of a patient decompensation. It is best if each one of these parameters is monitored on one piece of equipment. One monitoring system that is currently popular with transport teams is the Propaq System (Fig. 2). The monitor is lightweight, only 6 pounds. It is battery powered and can be operational for up to 30 hours once charged to full battery capacity. A printer is available to provide a record of the patient's condition during transport. The monitoring system must allow the clinician to follow all patient trends under any adverse environmental condition.

## VENTILATORS

The critical care team should be able to provide the full range of respiratory support. Intubation equipment must be available on all transports and separate from other equipment (Fig. 3). It should be accessible for use at any time. The laryngoscope should be a high-intensity fiberoptic system that allows for maximum visualization during poor lighting conditions. This may include the cabin of a helicopter at night or a hallway in the hospital.

The modes of ventilation on transport have changed significantly from hand ventilation bags to complex mechanical ventilators. The transport ventilator should, like all equipment, be both compact and reliable. Most transport ventilators are time cycled. Ventilator rate ranges from 0 to 30 breaths per minute.

A rate control of zero will allow for spontaneous breaths in some equipment. Tidal volume will vary from 50 to 1,500 mL. One problem with some transport ventilators is a limit of peak pressure to 45 to 50 cm $H_2O$. Oxygen concentration is usually 100%. Typically inverse ratio ventilation and pressure control are not available on most transport ventilators.

## MODE OF TRANSPORTATION

There are currently three modes of patient transport utilized in the United States: ground ambulance, rotor-wing aircraft (helicopter), and fixed-wing aircraft. Each method has distinct advantages and disadvantages (17).

In general, ground ambulances travel at rates of 55 miles per hour or greater and provide 220 to 270 cubic feet of patient care space. The ground vehicle can provide port-to-port service with minimal transfers of the patient between vehicles. Transport is hampered by only a few weather restrictions. Ground ambulance charges are less than helicopter transport charges. However, the ground vehicle has a high incidence of producing motion sickness, longer transport times, and a breakdown in communications when the vehicle is in a valley or surrounded by mountains.

The helicopter provides a faster speed (130 to 170 miles per hour). It's vertical takeoff and landing capabilities allow for easy access to most hospitals. In general, the helicopter has a better communication system and is free of ground interference. The helicopter has a small cabin space, usually 80 to 220 cubic feet, which makes patient care more difficult during a patient decompensa-

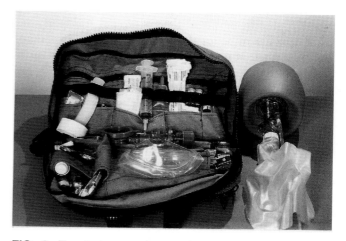

**FIG. 3.** Respiratory equipment bag. Airway management tools should be kept separate with easy accessibility.

tion. In addition to the space limitation there is a weight limit of approximately 2,000 pounds of payload. Effective lift is decreased by increasing temperature, altitude, and humidity (18). The crew requires special helicopter safety training and helicopter familiarization, which limits the individuals that may be employed acutely as crew members. The accident rate is lower for helicopters than ground vehicles, but helicopter accidents are usually more dangerous.

Fixed-wing aircraft can provide effective transport for distances of over 150 to 200 miles. This type of aircraft is capable of flying with a predesignated flight plan and above inclement weather conditions. The cabin space of the fixed-wing aircraft is larger than most helicopters, but there is usually greater difficulty in loading and unloading the patient. The major disadvantage of this type of aircraft is the requirement for an airport. The result is considerable time spent in multiple transfers of the patient that may involve both ground vehicles and helicopters. It is during these transfers that IV lines and other equipment can become disconnected.

Many factors must come into play in the consideration of the best method of transport for a particular patient. The decision on mode of transport will be based on the following:

1. *Distance and time to reach the receiving institution.* There is a general feeling that helicopter transport is faster than ground transport due to the high speed of the aircraft (130 to 170 miles per hour). However, most helicopters are based at a central location while ambulances are scattered throughout the community. In many situations the helicopter has to leave the hospital base and fly to the referring hospital, while most ambulances have a much shorter first leg of the journey. In addition to the actual flight time, there is the time spent on ground transfer and preparing for lift-off and shutdown at both the referring and receiving institution. This time significantly increases the total time from request for transport to the actual arrival at the tertiary care center. For most helicopter flights to be faster than a ground transport, the flight time has to be greater than 15 minutes (39 miles). This translates into a 40-minute ground transport time from the referring hospital (19).

At times, the patient is too far from the receiving institution. The helicopter becomes a relatively slow and ineffective means of transport. At a distance of greater than 150 to 200 miles from the receiving institution, helicopter transport becomes ineffective. In this case fixed-wing transport should be considered. Local factors such as the distance from the airport to the hospital and type of available helicopter will also determine the most effective means of medical evacuation.

2. *Level of care and patient stability.* The level of care that the patient is receiving will also determine the urgency and need for speed of transport. If the patient is in a tertiary care facility, stabilized on current modes of therapy, and is being referred for more definitive therapy, i.e., heart transplant evaluation, speed of transport may be a low priority. If the patient is hemodynamically unstable in a small community hospital and requires therapies that are not available at the referring hospital, then speed is a significant issue.

3. *Geography.* Certain terrain will also limit the mode of transport. Mountainous terrain is a good justification for helicopter transport. Remote areas with few roads will also shift the decision toward the helicopter. High-altitude regions may favor the use of specialty aircraft with high lift and fixed-wing aircraft that require shorter takeoff distances. These are fixed conditions, and the local transport service can be designed to meet these needs.

4. *Weather.* In general, ground transport units are far more weather resistant than rotor-wing aircraft. Most helicopters fly under Visual Flight Regulations (VFR) conditions. These are regulations set forth by the Federal Aviation Administration (FAA) (20). Under conditions of poor visibility and low cloud ceilings, flight is not permitted. If the pilot and aircraft are certified for Instrument Flight Rules (IFR), the pilot may fly with the use of advanced navigational aids by using a predesignated and assigned route under constant control of the air traffic controller. Many aeromedical flight services are not currently licensed to fly under the IFR rules; therefore ground backup is the only alternative. The IFR rules will increase the preparation time for the flight by 15 minutes or more. The flight must originate and end at an airport. This too will increase the length of time required to complete the medical evacuation.

There are some environmental conditions in which rotor flight is not permissible and ground transport is the only viable option. In conditions of severe icing, rotor-wing flight should not be attempted. The ice that would form on the rotor blades would make lift difficult and safe flight almost impossible. Severe wind and local weather conditions such as lake effect, snow fall as seen on the Great Lakes, in which heavy deposits of snow can occur within a short period, would also make safe rotor flight impossible. In these instances a ground support backup is desirable (21).

5. *Availability of mode of transport.* At times the ideal mode of transport for a patient may not be available. All helicopter or ground vehicles may be in use. In this case a decision is made on the urgency of the transport and the team goes with whatever mode of transport is available.

6. *Unusual events hampering transport.* There are certain conditions when ground travel becomes almost impossible. This is seen during high urban traffic (rush hour). In major cities, ground transport can be almost impossible. Air transport will be advantageous even though the actual distance may be only a few miles. Certain natural disasters may limit one mode over the other. Earthquakes will limit ground transport while hurricanes will limit air transport.

The transport service must be able to adapt to these conditions and relocate personnel to other transport vehicles during these times.

7. *Special equipment or personnel needs that are required to transport a patient.* On a rare occasion the equipment or personnel needed for patient care will not fit into the standard ambulance or medical transport aircraft. This is usually the case when the patient requires mechanical ventilation, and IABP, and a LVAD. In addition to the equipment requirement, the personnel required for patient life support include a physician, perfusionist, critical care nurse, and respiratory therapist depending upon the length of the transport. In these cases the requirement for size of vehicle is the determining factor. A ground ambulance with an extended module (which can be furnished by local fire companies or some ambulance services) can be employed for transport. When the distance is great, more than several hundred miles, a military or large cargo plane can be converted and utilized for the transport of patients requiring multiple modalities of advanced life support (22). This type of transport is extremely labor intense and requires extended periods of preparation in order to make certain that all equipment and personnel are present and all transfers are accomplished with minimal difficulty.

8. *Cost.* In this age of ever-increasing awareness of cost containment, air transport has come under scrutiny. Most helicopter transport charges are in the range of 2,200 to 3,500 dollars per hour (1994 dollars) (6, 23), and ground transport is approximately 350 dollars per hour (23). This factor should enter into the equation when arranging a transport. The higher cost of flight has to be justified by patient need, not just convenience.

It is usually not one particular factor that determines the mode of transport but rather weighing the relative merits of each. A well-designed transport service for cardiac patients must have both rotor- and fixed-wing aircraft plus a dedicated ground system. The ground system is essential for short transports and as a backup for severe weather conditions.

The ground unit should have the same level of staffing and equipment as the aircraft. This should complement the air service and represent the same level of medical expertise.

## TYPES OF PATIENTS TO BE TRANSPORTED

Patient selection is an important consideration for the cardiac transport team. Patients should be transported to a tertiary referral center when their medical needs are not adequately met at the primary institution. It is evident that this will vary from hospital to hospital depending on staff and resources. Cardiac patients are most commonly transported for a procedure or intervention that is not available in the community hospital. The procedures most commonly offered to cardiac patients include percutaneous transluminal coronary angioplasty (PTCA), cardiac catheterization, electrophysiologic studies (EPSs), coronary artery bypass graft, valvular surgery, pacemaker implantation, or support with an intra-aortic balloon counterpulsation. In one study by Fromm (7) 69.3 % of all transported cardiac patients received at least one of these procedures. The procedures were usually done soon after arrival at the tertiary care center with over 54% occurring within the first 72 hours. The patient may also be transferred from one tertiary care hospital to another for special treatment such as LVAD, extracorporeal membrane oxygenation (ECMO), or transplantation evaluation.

Patients inappropriate for interhospital transport are also a dilemma. Those patients with progressive multiple system organ failure who are not transplant candidates will not benefit from transport. Patients in cardiac arrest who cannot be stabilized by the transport team should not be considered for transport. The severity of illness should not necessarily be used to justify avoiding transport. Even patients with very high APACHE II scores (greater than 20) have been reported to survive using aggressive hemodynamic support (24).

## SEVERITY OF ILLNESS

Several techniques of severity of illness scoring have been tested to evaluate transport patients. Each system attempts to provide a rapid assessment of the patient's illness to facilitate medical evacuation planning. For years the APACHE II score has been utilized as a gold standard in critical care for severity of illness scoring (25). APACHE II has problems as a method of assessing severity of illness before and after transport. First it is difficult to obtain the score over the phone. There are a substantial number of variables that must be collected. Second, APACHE II predictive powers are based on the condition of the patient in the ICU in the first 24 hours of admission, not over several hours, as seen with transport medicine.

The Rapid Acute Physiology Score (RAPS) (26) is another scoring system utilized in transport patients. The RAPS uses elements of APACHE II that are readily available. It consists of only four variables. They are pulse, blood pressure, respiratory rate, and the Glasgow Coma Scale (GCS). The scoring system is identical to APACHE II for all parameters except for GCS. The point value for the GCS is scaled down so that its proportional contribution to RAPS is the same as that to the APACHE II system. The RAPS has been found to have a very high correlation to APACHE II and a similar predictive power for mortality rate.

The SAPS has also been utilized as a predictor of mortality for transport patients. The SAPS is more complex than RAPS in that it employs 14 variables. It requires both clinical evaluation and one venous blood sample.

This may not be ideal for all transport but may be utilized for extended air transport, such as those by fixed-wing (27). The SAPS, like RAPS, has been found to be comparable to the APACHE system. There is one severity of illness scoring system that is quite different than those previously described. This is a system developed for the cardiac patient by the Stanford Medical Center (8). Patients are placed in a classification 0 to IV based on the level of monitoring and life support. Those at level 0 require no monitoring and are hemodynamically stable. Class IV patients are hemodynamically unstable, requiring invasive monitoring and respiratory and inotropic support. Survival decreased as classification number increased. This system allows for a very rapid assessment of the relative degree of patient illness. Severity of illness systems can be utilized for rapidly predicting patient problems in transport, a generalized level of mortality, and determination of the team composition for the transport. It may also be used to evaluate the success of the care rendered during transport.

## IABP TRANSPORTS

One of the most challenging problems of transport medicine is the cardiac patient requiring IABP support. The IABP was introduced to clinical medicine over 20 years ago. It was first used as a means to wean patients off the cardiopulmonary bypass pump after cardiac surgery. In the late 1970s and early 1980s the role of the IABP expanded outside the operating room. The IABP was used to treat unstable angina, cardiogenic shock, and recurrent ventricular tachycardia secondary to ischemia and to stabilize patients with acute ventricular septal defect (VSD) and severe mitral regurgitation prior to surgery (28, 29). With the advent of percutaneous insertion techniques, the IABP has been more available to community hospitals (30, 31). The transport dilemma is the difficulty of moving the cardiac patient on the IACB from a community hospital to a tertiary care center for definitive cardiac therapy. Air transport facilitates this transport process, but space is limited. This has been successfully accomplished by a number of aeromedical services (24, 32, 33).

The authors' institution has extensive experience in the transport of patients on the IACB. We utilize a unique team consisting of a critical care physician, a critical care nurse, and a technologist all expert in the use of advanced life support. The team received 245 requests to transport IACB patients from 1986 until the end of 1994. Of these 245 requests, 5 patients expired prior to the arrival of the critical care transport team. Three additional patients expired while the team was at the bedside aiding in their care and subsequently were not transported. The remaining 237 patients were all transported safely to the receiving hospital.

Upon review of the patients transported with an intraaortic balloon pump, 229 cases were available for review. The diagnosis of cardiogenic shock was by far the most common. Seventy-nine patients were safely transported with cardiogenic shock as the primary diagnosis. Intractable angina or severe coronary artery disease was the diagnosis in 61 patients. Acute myocardial infarction was the primary diagnosis in 56 patients. Severe cardiomyopathy was the precipitating cause for the IACB in 24 patients. Acute VSD with hemodynamic instability was present in 3 patients, and 6 patients had severe congestive heart failure for which an IACB was inserted to prevent further decline.

In addition to the transport of the patient already on the IACB, the team, due to its unique composition, was able to insert the IACB at the referring hospital prior to transport in 50 patients. This unique concept of bedside stabilization at the referring hospital bedside has enabled medical evacuation of patients who previously could not be transported due to their hemodynamic instability.

## EQUIPMENT

In order to successfully transport a patient on an IABP, the equipment has to be compact and light. The monitor has to be easily visible during transport and the IABP must function in an uninterrupted fashion during the transport. In the late 1980s, new transport IABP equipment became much more compact and portable. There are several portable IABPs that are currently on the market, the Kontron Kaat II and the Datascope 90 T (Fig. 4). While relatively small, both have considerable weight—130 and 149 pounds, respectively. This weight includes the balloon pump and mounting equipment needed to secure the IABP in the aircraft or ambulance. Currently the FAA does not certify the IABP unless it is originally mounted on the aircraft. An IABP falls under the category of cargo which must be restrained in such a way as to prevent shifting in any direction. The balloon may be secured with tie-down devices or fit into a mount already in place in the aircraft. Mounting devices may be built onto preexisting transport IABPs (Fig. 5).

The IABP console should be visible throughout the flight. The IABP should be powered by the helicopter inverter (see equipment). Most models have 90 minutes to 3 hours of battery operational time. One of the key problems with air IABP transports is controlling the balloon volume with changes in altitude and atmospheric pressure. According to Boyle's law, at a constant temperature the volume of a gas varies inversely with pressure. As the pressure in the aircraft decreases during assent, the volume of gas in the balloon will increase. Barometric pressure changes about 40 mm Hg for every 2,000 feet. During an assent of 2,000 feet, the volume of the balloon will increase 2.5 cc if no change or purging is initiated.

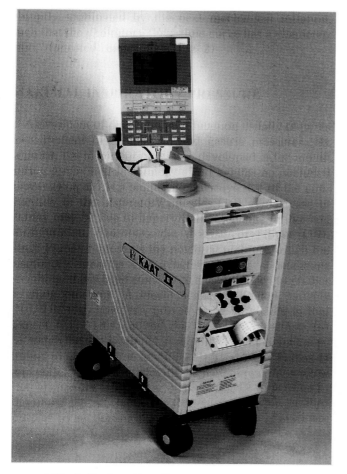

**FIG. 4.** Kontron Kaat II transport balloon pump.

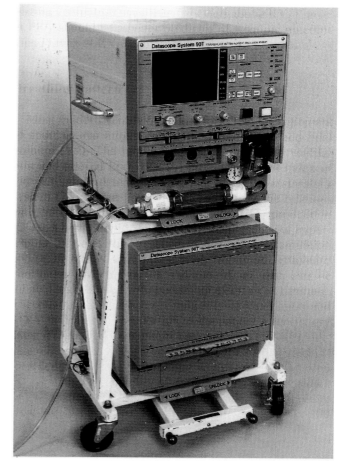

**FIG. 5.** An older model from DataScope; the 90T required the construction of a lower mounting device which provides stabilization security during transport.

During an assent the IABP can be purged, which will reference the transducer to the changing pressure and prevent possible balloon expansion and rupture. One must remember that the volume that is removed during an assent must be replaced on descent or the IABP will have a lower volume and ineffective counterpulsation (32).

## TREATMENT OF SHOCK

The onset of shock secondary to myocardial infarction or dysfunction carries a high mortality, 40 to 80 percent. The mortality rate depends on two factors, reversibility of the problem as by angioplasty or surgery and the speed of physiologic interventions such as IABP (30, 34). Once a patient has developed shock, measures must be implemented to reverse the physiologic disturbance or death is almost certain. The IABP has been demonstrated to decrease mortality. In some community hospitals this procedure is not available. Frequently these patients are candidates for transport to a tertiary care hospital. Those who cannot be readily stabilized by medical management in the community hospital should have the IABP placed prior to transport. This treatment will commonly reverse the ischemia and improve the safety of the trip. If these patients are not stabilized prior to transfer, deterioration of the patient's condition may arise en route when resuscitation is difficult.

In certain regions of the country cardiac teams have developed for the insertion of the IABP prior to transport (34). By utilizing a ground ambulance and specially trained individuals, the first group formulated for this function was able to complete 14 of 16 insertions of the IABP at the referring hospital and to successfully discharge 8 of the 14 patients (34). Such teams require extensive training and personnel resources. They require a physician skilled in IABP insertion and complex hemodynamic problem management. The teams require one to two critical care nurses who must be experienced in IABP function. Such teams permit centralization and regionalization of cardiac care services so that patients with advanced and unstable cardiac disease may be safely transported to tertiary care centers for definitive therapy.

Interhospital transport of critically ill cardiac patients is part of a philosophy of regionalized cardiac services. Regionalization of trauma, burns, neonatology, and pediatrics is relatively well accepted by the medical community. Regionalzation of cardiac services with clear guidelines for triage and transport of cardiac patients is not well accepted. As a matter of fact, many small community hospitals in this country have gotten into the business of cardiac catheterization in the absence of an on-site program for cardiac anesthesia and surgery. This leads, from time to time, to a critical situation where a cardiologist discovers unsuspected critical left main coronary artery disease during cardiac catheterization or has a life-threatening complication of the procedure in a primary care community hospital. Stabilization of the patient with an IACB is needed with rapid transport to a tertiary referral hospital with cardiac surgical services. The final section of this chapter with deal with the difficult issue of regionalization of medical services.

## REGIONALIZATION OF CRITICAL CARE SERVICES

A facility offering academic resources, monitoring technology, round-the-clock skilled personnel, invasive diagnostic capability, and comprehensive medical/surgical care defines a tertiary medical care center. Anecdotal but logically compelling evidence suggests that critical care services provided by tertiary centers improves outcome for selected patient populations by matching scarce and expensive resources with the patient population most likely to benefit from them. In August of 1994, a select panel of interested members of the Society for Critical Care Medicine reviewed the existing literature concerning regionalization of critical care services (35). A total of 146 English language manuscripts were reviewed by the panel to determine the feasibility and problems concerning regionalization for adult medical/surgical patients in today's sociopolitical climate. Existing data elucidated several major issues.

1. Would improved outcome result from regionalization of critical care services? The literature suggests that, on a generalized basis, outcomes should be expected to be improved with regionalized care (36, 37). Not all hospitals offer the dedicated facilities, staff, and technology for hemodynamic monitoring during thrombolytic therapy, intra-aortic balloon counterpulsation support, cardiac catheterization, and cardiac surgery. Likewise, advanced technology for neurosurgery, management of respiratory failure, and nutritional support cannot exist at all hospitals in the face of growing cost restraints. For a facility not possessing such necessary attributes to attempt the same level of care as a tertiary center may promote inefficiency, resulting in increased length of stay, cost of treatment, and possibly increased morbidity and mortality. However, most of this evidence refers to trauma or neonatal pediatrics, very defined areas of medicine, and to adult medical-surgical patients with unstable hemodynamics. There were no papers suggesting a worse outcome when patients were regionalized.

2. Would regionalization of critical care services reduce the cost of medical care? There was no firm scientific evidence that cost was reduced in areas where regionalization had been implicated. However, possible savings realized from avoidance of duplicated services and shortened length of stay due to enhanced efficacy are difficult to detail in scientific inquiries. This is especially true since regionalization of critical care services has not yet effectively occurred. Therefore, all facets of this question are speculative.

3. What kinds of patients may benefit from regionalized critical care services? The task force felt that certain clinical syndromes in adult patients might benefit more than others from regionalization:

a. There has been believably improved outcomes when patients with the adult respiratory distress syndrome are treated in centers specially equipped to deal with it (38).

b. For patients with cardiac decompensation requiring coronary artery bypass or angioplasty, the volume of patients and the volume of patients treated (39) and experience of the surgical staff appear to be important (40).

However, convincing evidence of the efficacy of regionalization was lacking for other kinds of disorders commonly treated in the critical care environment, such as decompensated, ventilator-dependent chronic obstructive pulmonary disease, severe systemic sepsis, neurologic disorders, liver failure, renal failure, acquired immunodeficiency syndrome, and multiple organ system failure.

There was also no significant evidence that patients requiring over 4 days of intensive care would benefit from regionalization. This suggests that prospective severity of illness scoring might help to identify patients most likely to benefit from regionalized care and to avoid those who would clearly not benefit. There is a wealth of anecdotal evidence that we can accurately select patient populations most likely to benefit from critical care technology based on severity of illness scoring systems. No severity of illness assessment is perfect, but the APACHE III system increases in credibility as its data base enlarges. Current APACHE III data suggest that within 24 hours of admission, a risk estimate for death is accurate within 3% of actual predicted rates for 95% of hospital ICU admissions (41). If early triage (within 24 hours) based on such scores could reliably identify those patient populations most likely to benefit, this would improve the overall efficacy of regionalization. However, much study remains to be done in this area before severity of illness scores are refined to the point where they are selective and sensitive enough for practical use.

4. What is the ideal model of regionalization for adult medical-surgical patients? Standards will probably have to be revamped from those of trauma and pediatric models, to include number and quality of specialized personnel, sophistication of hardware available to stabilize and treat critically ill patients, and the availability of 24-hour-per-day services. In addition, if improved outcome is to be expected from earlier intervention by critical care teams, improved modes of interhospital transfer must be examined carefully (42). The establishment of a highly efficient and safe interhospital transport system bringing the benefit of miniaturized monitoring and ventilation modalities from the tertiary center to the field must be integral to the entire concept of regionalization (43).

5. What are the possible downsides to regionalization of critically ill adult patients? Ironically, regionalization has the potential to create an overload on current tertiary medical centers, most of which are stressed maximally. This is the kind of stress that precipitates staff unrest and high personnel turnover. Conversely, if hospitals at the community level transport all their sick patients to tertiary referral centers, their level of expertise needed to identify and stabilize such patients may deteriorate to the point where their overall competence may be threatened.

6. Future issues needing to be addressed:

a. Triage skills must be standardized at the level of referring hospitals so that accurate identification of patients who would benefit from regionalization would occur in a timely fashion.

b. Reimbursement schedules must reflect an incentive to move sicker patients when appropriate. Regionalization will never come to pass as long as physicians have a financial incentive to treat critically ill patients at the primary facility level rather than transfer them to tertiary centers.

c. Interhospital patient transport systems would need to be available in each tertiary referral center, fully equipped and staffed with skilled personnel 24 hours a day to safely effect interhospital regionalization. This would require adequate reimbursement from insurers in order to maintain team readiness in all conditions.

Following this extensive review, the majority of task force members felt that regionalization of critical care services for adult medical-surgical patients was probably beneficial but stopped short of an open endorsement. The vast majority of evidence supporting regionalization was intuitive and logically compelling but lacking in hard scientific evidence. Unfortunately, no controlled data exist comparing delivery logistics of critical care services because regionalization has not effectively occurred in this country. Continuing study and data building are needed before a definitive answer is available.

## CONCLUSION

Regionalization of cardiac services appears to be an appropriate task for the medical community in the same way that regionalization of trauma services occurred under the guidance of the American College of Surgeons. For that regionalization to occur, as in the case of trauma, there must be excellent medical evacuation systems. The authors of this chapter believe that the trauma-based medical evacuation helicopter systems cannot be applied in their present form to the regionalzation of cardiac services. Interhospital transport of cardiac patients requires a much higher level of skill and technology and falls much more in the realm of critical care. Scoop-and-run speed is not as important to cardiac patients as stay-and-play stabilization by the transport team at the referring hospital bedside. Expert life support and invasive monitoring are more important to the cardiac patient during interhospital transport than the blinding speed sought by the trauma team at a motor vehicle scene rescue. One of the solutions to this dilemma is the use of specialty teams for cardiac patients. This has worked well for pediatric and neonatal patients and should be a cost-effective solution to interhospital transport of patients with life-threatening cardiac disease.

## REFERENCES

1. Mayfield T. 1994 annual transport statistics and transport fees survey. *Air Med J* 1994;April(13):132.
2. Schneider C, Gomez M, Lee R. Evaluation of ground ambulance, rotor-wing, and fixed-winged aircraft services. *Crit Care Clin* 1992;8 (3):533.
3. U.S. Congress. Highway Safety Act of 1966, Pub L 89-564 89 Congress, 2nd Session, S 3052.
4. Cowley RA, Hudson F, Scanlan E, et al . An economical and proven helicopter program for the transporting the emergency critically ill and injured patient in Maryland. *J Trauma* 1973;13(12):1029.
5. Dobrin RS, Block B, Gilman JI, Massoro TA. The development of a pediatric emergency transport system. *Pediat Clin North Am* 1980;27 (3):633.
6. Mayfield T. 1994 Annual transport statistics and transport fees survey. *Air Med J* 1994;April(13):132.
7. Fromm RE, Haider R, Schlieter P, Cronin L. Utilization of specialized services by air transported cardiac patients: an indicator of appropiate use. *Aviat Space Environ Med* 1992;Jan(63):52.
8. Ehrenwerth J, Sorbo S, Hackel A. Transport of critically ill adults. *Crit Care Med* 1986;14:543.
9. Crippen D, Bonetti MM, Hoyt JW. Cost survival results of critical care regionalization for Medicare patients. *Crit Care Med* 1989;17: 601.
10. Collett HM. Annual transport statistics. *J Air Med Transport* 1991;10: 11.
11. Frew I, Roush WR, Lagreca K. CORBA: implications for emergency medicine. *Ann Emerg Med* 1988;17:835.
12. Burney RE, Passini L, HubertD, Maio R. Comparison of aeromedical crew performance by patient severity and outcome. *Ann Emerg Med* 1992;21:4:375.
13. Macnab AJ. Optimal escort for interhospital transport of pediatric emergencies. *J Trauma* 1991;31:(2):205.
14. Rhee KJ, Strozeski M, Burney R, Mackenzie JR, LaGreca-Reibling K. Is the flight physician needed for helicopter emergency medical services? *Ann Emerg Med* 1986;15(26):174.
15. Gore JM, Haffajee CL, Goldberg RJ. Evaluation of an emergency cardiac transport system. *Ann Emerg Med* 1983;12:675.

16. Kaplan L, Wash D, Burney RE. Emergency aeromedical transport of patients with myocardial infarction. *Ann Emerg Med* 19876;16:55.
17. Scheider C, Gomez M, Lee R. Evaluation of ground ambulance, rotor-wing, and fixed-wing aircraft services. *Crit Care Clin* 1992;8(3):533.
18. Jeppesen Sanderson Inc. Englewood, CA. Private pilot manual. 1984: sects 1-32 to 1-35.
19. Smith JS, Bradley JS, Pletcher SE, et al. When is air medical service faster than ground transportation. *Air Med J* 1993;12:258.
20. Aviation Supplies. Renton, WA. Federal Aviation Regulations and Airman's Information Manual. Pt 91, Sect 151.
21. Gentry S. Enhancement of a critical care transport services. *J Air Med Trans* 1992;Feb(11):17.
22. Troiani T. When routine transport is not enough. *MedicAir* 1991;Oct: 26.
23. Franc D. Ground ambulance: a viable alternative. *MedicAir* 1992; Winter:34.
24. Greer K, Hoyt JW, Rafkin HS, Bonetti MM. Experience with inter-hospital transport of 107 patients receiving intra-aortic counterpulsa-tion therapy: a call for regionalization of cardiac care. *Crit Care Med* 1993;March(21):(abst).
25. Knaus WA, Draper EA, Wagner DP, et al. APACHE II: a severity of disease classification system. *Crit Care Med* 1985:13(10):818.
26. Rhee KJ, Mackenzie JR, Burney RE, et al. Rapid acute physiology scoring in transport system. *Crit Care Med* 1990;18(10):1119.
27. Spittal MJ, Hunter SJ, Spencer I, Blake D, McLaren CAB. Secondary patient transfer by air. An audit of 3 years experience of the Royal Air Force in the world-wide transport of the critically ill patients. *Intens Care World* 1993;Dec(10):S21.
28. Bergman D, Cohen SR, Kaskel PS: Intra-aortic balloon pumping: indications and benefits. *Primary Cardiol* 1982;Oct(8):1–11.
29. Sturm JT, McGee MG, Fuhrman TM, et al. Treatment of postopera-tive low output syndrome with intra-aortic balloon pumping: experi-ence with 419 patients. *Am J Cardiol* 1980;45:1033.
30. Alcan KE, Stertzer SH, Wallash E, et al. The expanding role of the intra-aortic balloon counterpulsation in critical care cardiology in A Community-based hospital. *Cardiovasc Revie Rep* 1982;3(3):61.
31. Vignola PA, Swaye PS, Gosselin AJ. Guidelines for effective and safe percutaneous insertion and removal intraaortic balloon pump. *Am J Cardiol* 1981;48:660.
32. Mertlich G, Quaal S. Air transport of the patient requiring intra-aortic balloon pumping *Crit Care Clin North Am* 1991;11(3):443.
33. Holdefer WF, Diethelm AG, Bradshaw M, WeimarS. Long-distance aeromedical transport of patients requiring intra-aortic balloon pump support *Hosp Aviat* 1989;July(11):22.
34. Califf RM, Bengtson JR. Cardiogenic shock. *New Engl J Med* 1994; 330(24):1724.
35. Thompson DR, Clemmer TP, Applefield JJ, et al. Regionalization of critical care medicine: task force report of the American College of Critical Care Medicine. *Crit Care Med* 1994;22:1306.
36. Clemmer TP, Orme JF, Thomas FO, et al. Outcome of critically injured patients treated at level 1 trauma centers versus full-service community hospitals. *Crit Care Med* 1985;13:861.
37. Hannan E, O'Donnell J, Kilburn H. Investigation of the relationship between volume and mortality for surgical procedures performed in New York State hospitals. *JAMA* 1989;262;503.
38. Suchyta MR, Clemmer TO, Orme JF Jr, et al. Increased survival of ARDS patients with severe hypoxemia (ECMO criteria). *Chest* 1991; 99:951.
39. Showstack J, Rosenfeld K, Garnick D, et al. Association of volume with outcome of coronary artery bypass graft surgery. *JAMA* 1987; 257;785.
40. Williams SV, Nash DB, Goldfarb N. Difference in mortality from coronary artery bypass graft surgery at five teaching hospitals. *JAMA* 1991;226;810.
41. Knaus WA, Wagner DP, Draper EA, et al. The APACHE III prognos-tic system: risk prediction of hospital mortality for critically ill hospi-talized patients. *Chest* 1991;100:1619.
42. Rappoport J, Teres D, Lemeshow S, et al. Timing of intensive care unit admissions in relation to ICU outcome. *Care Med* 1990;18:1231.
43. Crippen D. Critical are transportation medicine: New concepts in pre-hospital stabilization of the critically ill patient. Am J Emerg Med 1990;8:551.

*The Critically Ill Cardiac Patient,*
edited by V. Kvetan and D. R. Dantzker,
Lippincott-Raven Publishers, Philadelphia © 1996.

# CHAPTER 12

# Pharmacologic Cardiovascular Support

John F. Butterworth IV, Richard C. Prielipp, Drew A. MacGregor, and Gary P. Zaloga

Pharmacologic support of the critically ill cardiac patient involves optimization of cardiac output and of vascular tone in systemic and pulmonary vascular beds. The goal of vasoactive and inotropic therapy is to restore delivery of blood flow and nutrients to critical organs which are at risk during circulatory failure. With the advent of the pulmonary artery catheter in the 1970s, physicians gained the ability to titrate inotropic and vasoactive drugs to specific physiologic endpoints. This chapter will review the pharmacologic agents available for support of the cardiovascular system in the critically ill cardiac patient, including inotropes, vasopressors and vasodilators, and drugs which regulate heart rate.

By definition, positive inotropic agents improve the mechanical performance of the heart. Some also directly reduce pulmonary and peripheral vascular resistances and directly reduce right- and left-sided heart filling pressures. In critical illness, inotropic drugs increase cardiac function to increase cardiac output and oxygen delivery during disorders such as myocardial ischemia or infarction, cardiomyopathy, post-cardiopulmonary bypass low-output syndrome, and sepsis. The many adverse actions of positive inotropic drugs demand that prescribing physicians be goal oriented when they infuse these agents. Many clinicians attempt to produce specific cardiovascular endpoints (e.g., cardiac index, $O_2$ delivery) or other physiologic endpoints (e.g., urine output, resolution of metabolic acidosis, etc); such an approach is preferable to administering set doses of drugs without regard to specific patient-defined goals.

Many clinical applications of inotropic drugs are unrelated to congestive heart failure and fall outside current package inserts indications. Many other classes of drugs are commonly administered to patients with circulatory failure, including nutritional supplements, electrolyte solutions, sedatives, narcotics, and neuromuscular blocking drugs. These adjunctive agents may have profound actions on the cardiovascular system. Likewise, the various "cardiac" drugs may have actions on organ systems other than the heart and vasculature, complicating the management of these critically ill patients. To underscore the ways that the underlying cause of myocardial depression determines the appropriate therapeutic intervention, we will review the settings and conditions in which inotropic and vasoactive agents are often prescribed to patients with critical illness.

## CHARACTERISTICS OF PATIENTS REQUIRING DRUG SUPPORT

### Chronic Heart Failure

Congestive heart failure is characterized by beta-adrenergic receptor downregulation (1) and decreased intracellular cAMP concentrations (2). Patients with chronic heart failure respond well to inotropic agents that are not cyclic adenosine monophosphate (cAMP) dependent and to afterload reduction. Thus, digoxin, diuretics, and captopril may be particularly effective. In randomized studies, mortality increased when positive inotropes other than digoxin were given to ambulatory patients with chronic heart failure despite lessened symptoms and improved quality of life (3, 4). Digoxin has recently been shown to improve cardiac function and symptoms in recent randomized studies (5, 6). Curiously, beta-adrenergic receptor blockers may prolong the lives of patients with chronic cardiomyopathy (7). Some patients with severe chronic heart failure require continuous infusion of positive inotropes (commonly phosphodiesterase inhibitors) for days to weeks while awaiting cardiac transplantation. Finally, patients with chronic heart failure may present with signs and symptoms of fluid overload, including gallop rhythms, peripheral and pul-

J. Butterworth, R. C. Prielipp, D. A. MacGregor, and G. P. Zaloga: Department of Anesthesia, Bowman Gray School of Medicine of Wake Forest University, Winston-Salem, North Carolina 27157-1009.

monary edema, hypoxemia, and weight gain, which requires short-term inotropic support to speed diuresis and weight loss and relieve pulmonary congestion.

## Acute Myocardial Infarction

A minority of patients admitted to the hospital after acute myocardial infarction require hemodynamic support with inotropes. Although there is controversy as to whether these patients benefit from placement of a pulmonary artery catheter (8), many clinicians believe that patients presenting to hospital after acute myocardial infarction with hypotension, oliguria, and pulmonary edema will benefit from peripheral and pulmonary arterial catheterization, intravenous positive inotropic drugs to supplement interventions aimed at reperfusion, and supportive care. In this setting, the goal is to improve systemic (particularly renal and cerebral) perfusion and coronary perfusion and eliminate pulmonary edema by "recruiting" viable but hypocontractile myocardium and increasing the contribution of nonischemic regions of the ventricle (9–11), without unduly increasing metabolic demand, permitting ischemic myocardium to have a better opportunity for recovery.

## Trauma and Sepsis Syndrome

Patients with acute traumatic injury or sepsis may demonstrate signs of inadequate tissue perfusion (i.e., mixed venous oxygen desaturation, elevated blood lactate concentrations, and oliguria) despite having a cardiac index that would be considered adequate under "normal," unstressed conditions (12). Such patients may receive positive inotropic drug support specifically to improve oxygen delivery to tissues (13). Whether this approach truly improves outcome remains highly controversial (14–18).

## Cardiac Surgery

The low cardiac output syndrome occurring after cardiopulmonary bypass (CPB) differs from both chronic congestive cardiomyopathy and the acute heart failure associated with myocardial infarction. Unlike patients in other settings, patients emerging from CPB demonstrate hemodilution, moderate hypocalcemia and hypomagnesemia, kaliuresis, and tissue thermal gradients and, depending on temperature and depth of anesthesia, may demonstrate low, normal, or high systemic vascular resistance (19). These patients, unlike those with congestive heart failure, usually do not demonstrate signs of fluid overload or pulmonary congestion. Increasing age, female sex, decreased left ventricular ejection fraction, and increased duration of extracorporeal perfusion are associated with a greater likelihood that inotropic drug support will be needed after elective coronary surgery (20) (Table 1). The degree and significance of adrenergic

**TABLE 1.** *Factors associated with need for inotropic drug support*

| Factor | P-value |
| --- | --- |
| Decreasing left ventricular ejection fraction | 0.002 |
| Increasing duration of cardiopulmonary bypass | 0.004 |
| Increasing age | 0.005 |
| Increasing duration of aortic clamping | 0.009 |
| Radiographic cardiac enlargement | 0.021 |
| Female | 0.027 |

Adapted from Royster RL, et al. *Anesth Analg* 1991;72:729, with permission.

receptor downregulation and uncoupling in patients emerging from CPB remain unclear (21, 22).

Inotropic drug therapy is given to patients undergoing cardiac surgery to increase the contractile function of the heart, increase cardiac output, and increase oxygen delivery to peripheral tissues and to the myocardium. This perioperative low-cardiac-output syndrome frequently includes hypotension, so it will usually not respond to vasodilator therapy. Fortunately, in patients with comparable risk factors, inotropic drug support after CPB does not significantly impair outcome, as such treatment does in medical congestive heart failure (20).

## POSITIVE INOTROPIC AGENTS

### Digoxin

Cardiac glycosides, including digoxin, inhibit $Na^+,K^+$ adenosinetriphosphatase (ATPase), an integral membrane protein responsible for $Na^+$ movement out of and $K^+$ movement into the cell. Inhibition of this enzyme increases intracellular $[Na^+]$. In response, the $Na^+/Ca^{2+}$ exchange protein in the plasma membrane increases $Na^+$ extrusion and $Ca^{2+}$ influx (23). Increased availability of $Ca^{2+}$ ions promotes their binding to tropinin-C and actin-myosin cross-bridging, increasing cardiac inotropy (23, 24). Cardiac glycosides increase vascular smooth muscle tone and transiently increase peripheral vascular resistance, which may partially offset the increase in cardiac inotropy (25).

Digoxin also slows atrioventricular (AV) nodal conduction to control atrial tachyarrhythmias. Digoxin sensitizes arterial baroreceptors in the carotid sinus, activates the vagal nuclei, and increases parasympathetic tone to the heart. These autonomic changes decrease sinoatrial and AV nodal activity and prolong the effective refractory period. Inhibition of $Na^+/K^+$ ATPase enhances automaticity by depolarizing the membrane and increasing the slope of phase 4 depolarization. Thus, digoxin prolongs the R-R interval, shortens the QT interval, produces ST-T segment depression along with diminished or inverted T waves, and increases cardiac cell automaticity.

In patients with chronic heart failure, digoxin reduces clinical symptoms and improves exercise capacity, increases left ventricular shortening and ejection fraction, and reduces catecholamine concentrations in blood (24, 26). Digoxin results in significant hemodynamic improvement, even in patients with "well-compensated" heart failure already receiving diuretics and angiotensin-converting enzyme inhibitors (5, 6, 27). In patients with left ventricular systolic dysfunction after cardiac surgery, 1 mg of intravenous digoxin significantly increased cardiac index within 2 hours and decreased pulmonary artery occlusion pressure within 4 hours while maintaining myocardial oxygen supply (28, 29).

Beneficial inotropic effects from administration of digitalis in sepsis have been reported in both animal (30, 31) and human studies (32, 33). Nasraway et al. (33) showed that in patients with sepsis, digoxin (10 µg/kg) increased left ventricular stroke work index (LVSWI) by 74%, while dopamine (5 to 12 µg/kg/min) increased LVSWI by 13%. Increased catecholamine concentrations in the blood of septic patients (34) may result in beta-adrenergic receptor downregulation (35), limiting the effectiveness of beta-adrenergic agonists and related drugs (such as dopamine) in this setting.

Because of the narrow margin between therapeutic and toxic doses, acute loading with digoxin requires consideration of concomitant disease (e.g., renal insufficiency), concurrent drug therapy (e.g., quinidine, amiodarone), and the specific digitalis preparation being prescribed (36). Digoxin toxicity is common and may result from its primary mechanism of action (increased intracellular $[Ca^{2+}]$). The relationship between plasma digoxin concentrations and clinical toxicity is obscured by the inconsistent relationship between plasma and myocardial digoxin concentrations. For instance, despite marked hemodilution, digoxin concentrations decrease minimally during extracorporeal circulation (37, 38), then return to preoperative levels immediately following bypass (38–40), with virtually no change in myocardial digoxin concentrations (37). Digoxin "rebound" may actually temporarily increase plasma levels 12 hours after bypass, which has been linked to cardiac arrhythmias (41). Thus, no additional perioperative digoxin supplementation is routinely required in digitalized patients undergoing CPB.

## Calcium

In addition to determining the contractile state of the heart muscle, intracellular calcium regulates secretion, hormonal release, cell division, clotting, enzyme activation, cell movement, ciliary motion, and neurotransmitter release (42). Calcium for muscle contraction is mostly released from intracellular sarcoplasmic reticulum; only small amounts enter the cell during depolarization. Maintenance of a constant circulating ionized calcium concentration (1 to 1.3 mM) is accomplished through the combined actions of parathyroid hormone and vitamin D; calcitonin, thyroid hormone, and catecholamines also effect calcium metabolism to a minor extent.

Calcium circulates in the blood in three forms: free (ionized calcium), protein-bound, and chelated calcium. Only the ionized form is hemodynamically active and regulated by hormones. Increasing the extracellular ionized calcium concentration will increase the contractile function of isolated cardiac or skeletal muscle. However, in order to increase contractile function significantly, ionized calcium concentrations must increase dramatically above normal values (1, 43). Moreover, administration of calcium salts to intact patients will increase systemic vascular resistance, offsetting the calcium effect on contractile function.

Carlon and colleagues (44) gave a calcium chloride bolus (10 mg/kg) and infusion (20 µg/kg/min) to critically ill patients, increasing mean arterial pressure throughout the calcium infusion but increasing cardiac index only for the first minute after the calcium bolus. Maynard and colleagues (45) varied the calcium concentrations of the dialysate in patients undergoing hemodialysis. Blood pressure was higher in patients with an increased ionized calcium concentration. Similarly, Henrich et al. (46) and Lang et al. (47) used echocardiography to demonstrate that cardiac contractility increased significantly when increased ionized calcium was increased in the dialysate. None of these studies evaluated cardiac output or oxygen delivery to tissues; thus, cardiac contractility could have been increased by calcium without improving oxygen delivery. In a group of patients with sepsis we observed that calcium (1 mg/kg/min for 20 minutes) significantly improved mean arterial blood pressure but had no effect on cardiac output (48).

Bolus administration of calcium salts has long been popular during and after cardiac surgery because it causes small, transient increases in cardiac output (49–51). We have shown, however, that the calcium-parathyroid hormone-vitamin D axis in adults and children undergoing cardiac surgery (52, 53) remains intact and returned their ionized calcium concentrations to normal without treatment.

We have also compared calcium chloride with placebo in two randomized blinded trials in patients emerging from CPB (54, 55). In the first study, 40 patients received either calcium chloride (5 mg/kg) as a bolus or placebo. Calcium increased mean arterial pressure and ionized calcium concentration but had no effect on cardiac output. In the second study, 36 patients undergoing bypass received three doses of calcium chloride (200 mg/dose), ephedrine (500 mg/dose), or placebo. Only ephedrine significantly increased cardiac output relative to placebo. Calcium had no effect on cardiac index. Two other randomized, placebo-controlled studies failed to show any increase in cardiac output with 5 or 10 mg/kg boluses of calcium chloride (56–58).

Calcium may interact with other vasoactive agents. We observed no increase in the hypertensive response to phenylephine after administration of calcium to patients recovering from coronary artery surgery (56). In a study of patients recovering from aortocoronary bypass surgery, we observed that calcium attenuated the increased cardiac output and glucose levels caused by epinephrine (57). Calcium administration after CPB may predispose patients for pancreatitis (58). There is similar inhibition of the response to dobutamine after calcium (59). This inhibition is likely the result of direct calcium inhibition of adenylyl cyclase (60), since calcium inhibition could be prevented *in vitro* by block of calcium channels or substitution of barium ions for calcium (61). In summary, calcium increases mean arterial pressure but does not reliably increase cardiac output in patients.

## Thyroid Hormone

Thyroid hormone has profound direct and indirect actions on the cardiovascular system. Clinical hypothyroidism is manifested by a reduced heart rate, cardiac index, stroke volume index, and peripheral vascular resistance, which are rapidly reversed with administration of thyroid hormone.

The *sick euthyroid syndrome*, characterized by low circulating $T_3$ concentrations and inappropriately low thyroid-stimulating hormone (TSH) concentrations, commonly seen in critically ill patients after CPB and sepsis, is also common in brain-dead patients awaiting organ donation. We have shown that administration of thyroid hormone will increase contractile function of ischemic reperfused myocardium (as after cardiac surgery) as potently as isoproterenol, even in the presence of overwhelming beta-adrenergic receptor blockade (62). Moreover, thyroid hormone did not increase intracellular cAMP. Two recent trials suggest that prophylactic $T_3$ neither improves cardiac index nor reduces the likelihood that other positive inotropic drugs will be required after cardiac surgery (63, 64).

The appropriate role for thyroid hormone as an inotropic agent in critical care medicine remains unclear. Intravenous $T_3$ is expensive and may have no clear advantage over other positive inotropic drugs.

## Phosphodiesterase Inhibitors

Phosphodiesterase enzyme (PDE) inhibition prevents metabolism of cAMP, increasing myocardial contractility. The PDE inhibitors (PDEIs) may also increase the sensitivity of contractile proteins to calcium, increase calcium influx via the Na/Ca exchange mechanism, and antagonize adenosine. The PDEI drugs provide an alternative to catecholamines in patients with beta-adrenergic receptor downregulation (e.g., chronic heart failure). Currently two bipyridine derivatives, amrinone and milri-

**TABLE 2.** *Comparison of amrinone and milrinone*

|  | Amrinone | Milrinone |
|---|---|---|
| Relative potency | 1 | 15–20 |
| Usual loading dose (mg/kg) | 0.75–1.5[a] | 0.05 |
| Maximum loading dose (mg/kg) | 3.0 | 0.075 |
| Usual infusion rate (µg/kg/min) | 5–10 | 0.375–0.75 |
| Thrombocytopenia[b] (%) | 2.6 | 0.4 |
| Incidence of ventricular arrhythmias[b] (%) | 0.8 | 3.6 |

[a]Larger dose (1.5 mg/kg) is used after cardiac surgery and extracorporeal circulation.
[b]In patients with chronic heart failure.

none (Table 2), are the only PDEIs approved for clinical use in the United States.

Positive inotropic effects of amrinone and milrinone have been shown in patients with chronic congestive heart failure which exceed the effects of afterload reduction by sodium nitroprusside (65, 66). Intracoronary milrinone markedly increased cardiac contractility without altering mean arterial pressure or systemic vascular resistance (67).

Amrinone is at least as effective as dobutamine for short-term management of severe congestive heart failure due to dilated cardiomyopathy. Following amrinone, cardiac filling pressures were reduced to a greater extent, diuresis was more consistent, and the dose-response relationship more predictable than with dobutamine (68). Moreover, in patients with severe heart failure, amrinone combined with dobutamine produced greater increases in stroke volume than either drug alone (69).

The PDEI drugs improve contractile function during emergence from CPB. Administration of amrinone (1.5 mg/kg + 10 µg/kg/min) prior to removal from CPB was equally effective to epinephrine (30 to 100 ng/kg/min) in maintaining cardiac output and the drugs had additive effects when combined (70, 71) (see Fig. 1). Dupuis et al. found that amrinone was more effective and associated

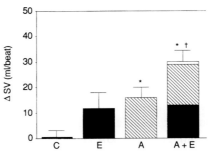

**FIG. 1.** Effects of control (C), epinephrine (30 ng/kg/min, E), amrinone (1.5 mg/kg, A), or amrinone + epinephrine (A+E) on stroke volume in patients just separated from cardiopulmonary bypass. The effects of A+E were significantly greater than those of either A, E, or C. Rrom Royster RL, et al. *Anesth Analg* 1993;77:662, with permission.

with fewer complications than dobutamine during separation from CPB (72). It is not yet clear whether combined PDEI and beta-adrenergic agonists yield true synergism in main.

Amrinone, a potent pulmonary artery vasodilator, improves right-sided heart function in patients with pulmonary hypertension (73, 74). Studies have shown that amrinone increases stroke volume and cardiac index, decreases systemic and pulmonary vascular resistances, and increases right ventricular ejection fraction (59, 74). We also found amrinone produced a dose-dependent increase in intrapulmonary shunt and decrease in $PaO_2$ in patients recovering from cardiac surgery (75) (Fig. 2A and B). Thus, like other pulmonary vasodilators, PDEI drugs may alter ventilation-perfusion matching in the lung.

Milrinone has inotropic and vasodilator effects similar to amrinone (76). Milrinone is 15 times more potent and one-sixth as likely to produce thrombocytopenia as amrinone. Milrinone produces dose-dependent increases in cardiac index and oxygen delivery in patients with congestive heart failure (77), patients undergoing cardiac surgery (78), a mixed population of critically ill patients (79), and patients awaiting cardiac transplantation (80). After coronary artery surgery, we determined that a 50 μg/kg loading dose was preferable to either 25 or 75 μg/kg (81). Both we (81) and others (82) have studied milrinone pharmacokinetics after CPB. A loading dose of 50 μg/kg plus 0.5 μg/kg/min infusion maintains plasma concentrations above 100 ng/mL in cardiac surgical patients and in other critically ill patients (83), producing 30% to 40% increases in cardiac index.

The PDEI drugs increase oxygen delivery with minimal thermogenic and metabolic effects in humans (84), a major difference from the catecholamines (85). In two animal models of sepsis, amrinone improved cardiac output and oxygen delivery without changing oxygen consumption (86, 87). Scalea administered either dobutamine or amrinone to septic patients (88), showing that both drugs increased oxygen delivery and consumption and were equally likely to produce hypotension. Vasodilation and afterload reduction caused by PDEIs are generally well tolerated with mean arterial blood pressure reductions of 10 to 15 mm Hg.

## Beta-Adrenergic Receptor Agonists

Catecholamines, defined by the 3,4-hydroxyl-ß-phenylethylamine structure (Fig. 3), bind specifically to beta-adrenergic receptors on the cell surface, activating a membrane-bound guanine nucleotide binding ($G_s$) protein. The $G_s$ protein activates adenylyl cyclase, generating cAMP (89). Cyclic AMP activates the cAMP-dependent protein kinases, which phosphorylate intracellular proteins including calcium channels, phospholambin, and troponin I. The net result is increased calcium influx through calcium channels and increased calcium sensitivity of certain regulatory proteins. Paradoxically, beta-adrenergic agonists *decrease* the sensitivity of the contractile myofilaments to intracellular calcium, an effect opposite to phosphodiesterase inhibitors or alpha-adrenergic receptor agonists (90). The net result of beta-adrenergic receptor activation is enhanced tension development (inotropy) and diastolic relaxation (lusitrophy).

Continuous exposure to catecholamines desensitizes beta-adrenergic receptors (91), an effect noted clinically in congestive heart failure (1, 92), after periods of reversible myocardial ischemia (93), after thoracic and abdominal surgical operations (94, 95), CPB (22, 96), and during sepsis (97–100). The number of beta-1-adrenergic receptors has been reported to decrease (99, 101, 102) or remain unchanged (103, 104) during sepsis. In

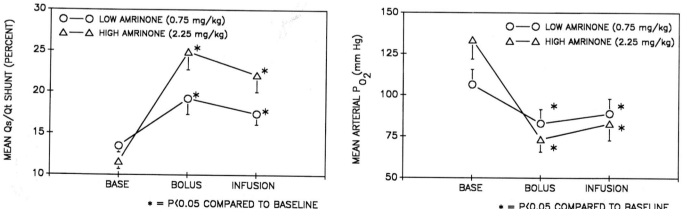

**FIG. 2. A:** Effects of amrinone loading doses and infusions on percent shunt in extubated patients recovering from aortocoronary bypass surgery. *$p < 0.05$ compared to baseline. **B:** Corresponding decrease in arterial $PaO_2$ after amrinone was given to the same group of patients. From Prielipp RC et al. *Chest* 1991;99:820, with permission.

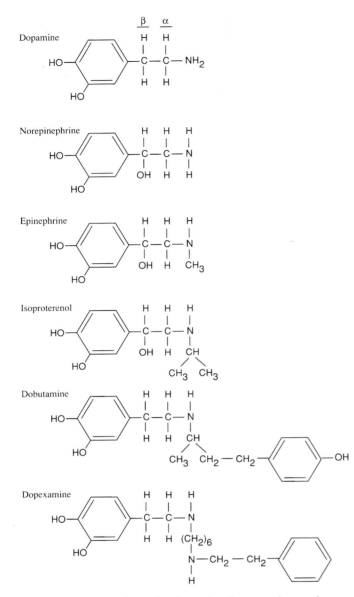

**FIG. 3.** Chemical formulas for naturally occurring and synthetic catecholamines.

heart failure, the neurohormonal-induced desensitization produces severe reduction in the density of beta-1-adrenergic receptors (105). While the number of beta-2-adrenergic receptors is maintained, decreased function may occur from "uncoupling" at the G-protein level (22, 106). Uncoupling of the receptor may be mediated by increased intracellular calcium concentrations (60, 107–108) or cellular mediators released during shock (e.g., lysophosphatidyl choline) (109). Thus, while the failing heart becomes more of a mixed beta-1/beta-2 responsive organ, both beta-1 and beta-2 pathways are compromised and may lead to "catecholamine resistance," hypotension, and, indirectly, multiple-organ failure (110).

## Dopamine

Dopamine, an important transmitter in the central and peripheral nervous systems, activates dopamine, beta-, and alpha-adrenergic receptors. Activation of $DA_1$ receptors, located postsynaptically, produces vasodilation in renal, mesenteric, coronary, and cerebral arteries. Activation of presynaptic $DA_2$ receptors inhibits release of norepinephrine and prolactin and may also produce nausea and vomiting in awake patients. At low rates of dopamine infusion, the combination of vasodilation ($DA_1$) and inhibition of norepinephrine release ($DA_2$) may produce systemic hypotension (111).

### Renal Dose Dopamine

Dopamine (0.2 to 3.0 µg/kg/min) is frequently employed to increase renal perfusion and urine output. The $DA_2$ receptors are activated in the lowest dose range (0.2 to 0.4 µg/kg/min); slightly higher doses recruit $DA_1$ receptors (0.5 to 3.0 µg/kg/min). Dopamine selectively increases renal blood flow more than cardiac output (112). In addition, $DA_1$ directly inhibits tubular solute reabsorption (113). Thus, dopamine is frequently infused during periods of renal "stress" such as during vascular surgery, sepsis, resuscitation, and CPB (114, 115). In animals, coinfusion of dopamine may attenuate the detrimental actions of vasopressors; however, this has not been confirmed in humans (106). In a recent study in critical illness, renal dose dopamine induced a diuresis without changing creatinine clearance, while dobutamine increased the creatinine clearance without any change in urine output (116). Selective $DA_1$ agonists such as fenoldopam may represent an improvement over nonselective dopamine agonists to control hypertension and preserve renal perfusion (117).

### Inotropic Dose Dopamine

As dopamine infusion rates increase to over 3 µg/kg/min, beta-1-, alpha-1-, and alpha-2-adrenergic receptors are recruited. Part of the inotropic response to dopamine depends on the release of endogenous norepinephrine; this may limit dopamine's effectiveness in catecholamine-depleted states such as chronic heart failure. The infusion rate of dopamine which will increase blood pressure ("alpha range") is variable but usually is considered to be at least 6 µg/kg/min. In cardiac surgery patients both dopamine and dobutamine increase heart rate, but dopamine increases left ventricular wall stress while dobutamine decreases left ventricular wall stress (118, 119). Combined, such changes (increased heart rate and ventricular wall stress) may contribute to increased myocardial lactate production, which has been documented in patients with cardiogenic shock treated with dopamine (107). Our experience has been that higher doses of dopamine frequently cause progressive tachycardia and increase diastolic ventricular filling pressure (secondary to venoconstriction and increased afterload), which is deleterious to ischemic or compromised myocardium. Therefore, our preference is to infuse dopamine at doses <5 μg/kg/min.

### Dopexamine

Dopexamine, a synthetic analog of dopamine, lacks any direct alpha-adrenergic agonist activity but expresses beta-2-adrenergic and dopaminergic (DA$_1$) agonist activity (120, 121), with the beta-2/beta-1 receptor affinity ratio estimated at 100:1. Dopexamine also exhibits significant indirect effects, including inhibition of presynaptic reuptake of norepinephrine (122). Moreover, the DA$_1$ and beta-2 arterial vasodilation produced by dopexamine reduce cardiac afterload while simultaneously increasing blood flow to the kidneys, intestines, liver, and spleen (120). Similar to low-dose dopamine, dopexamine increases urinary sodium and water excretion (123).

Dopexamine (1 to 4 μg/kg/min) significantly increased cardiac index and heart rate, while decreasing systemic and pulmonary vascular resistances after cardiac surgery (124, 125), with variable effect on stroke volume. Creatinine clearance was unchanged. Dopexamine with dobutamine in patients with low cardiac index (CI <2.5 L/min/m$^2$) after CPB (126) were equally effective at increasing cardiac index and inducing diuresis and urine sodium excretion, although tachycardia [heart rate (HR) > 120] was more common with dopexamine.

Other investigations of dopexamine frequently focus on its ability to increase oxygen delivery and improve splanchnic perfusion in critical illness. In endotoxic dogs, Cain showed dopexamine temporarily increased systemic oxygen delivery and consumption and improved mucosal gut blood flow (127). In 107 "high-risk" surgical patients, dopexamine titrated to increase oxygen delivery above 600 mL/min/m$^2$ was associated with a reduced 1-month surgical mortality from 22% in the control group to 6% (128) (Fig. 4).

### Epinephrine

Epinephrine stimulates beta-2-, beta-1-, and alpha-adrenergic receptors in a dose-dependent fashion. Epinephrine's potency raises concern over the effect of tachycardia, vasoconstriction, and possible myocardial ischemia. However, the sympathoadrenal (endogenous) secretion of epinephrine is critical to support cardiac contractility, exert tonic control of vascular beds, increase tissue plasminogen activator release (129), and modulate the "stress response."

Leenen found that epinephrine doses of 10, 20, and 40 ng/kg/min increased stroke volume by 2, 12, and 22%, respectively, and increased cardiac index by 0.1, 0.7, and

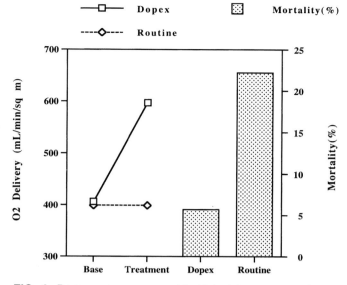

**FIG. 4.** Dopexamine was used in high-risk surgery patients (N = 53) to increase oxygen delivery (treatment goal: ≥600 mL/min/m$^2$), compared to routine perioperative care (N = 54). Mortality at 28 days was significantly reduced (p = 0.015) in the dopexamine treatment group. Derived from Boyd O, et al. *JAMA* 1993;270:2699.

1.2 L/min/m$^2$ (124). Heart rate also increased, but to <10 beats/min at all doses. Epinephrine is frequently used after cardiac surgery to support the function of "stunned," reperfused heart. During emergence from CPB, we showed epinephrine (30 ng/kg/min) increased both cardiac index and stroke volume by 14% without increasing heart rate (54). Similarly, epinephrine (20 and 40 ng/kg/min) increased stroke volume by 11% and 20%, respectively, without increasing heart rate after repair of cardiac septal defects (130). In septic patients with refractory hypotension, even higher doses of epinephrine have been used successfully. Bollaert infused epinephrine in 13 septic patients and increased cardiac index 34% and oxygen delivery 30%, without significantly increasing heart rate (131).

Epinephrine and virtually every other positive inotrope may induce myocardial ischemia in patients with coronary artery disease. Chronic exposure to catecholamines promotes platelet aggregation, perhaps leading to ischemia or infarction. Nonetheless, acute administration appears well tolerated. Sung infused epinephrine (60 to 240 ng/kg/min) to 22 patients with coronary artery disease. Adverse events (arrhythmias, ST-segment depression, or chest pain) were observed at infusion rates above 120 ng/kg/min (132). In a recent study of epinephrine in sheep, Bersten found that renal blood flow decreased only transiently, returning to baseline 30 to 60 minutes later (133). Thus, in normal volunteers, cardiac surgery patients, and septic patients, epinephrine infusion (20 to 100 ng/kg/min) effectively increases cardiac output, minimally increases heart rate, and has an acceptable incidence of side effects.

### Dobutamine

Dobutamine, a synthetic catecholamine released in 1978, is formulated as a racemic mixture of two stereo-isomers in which the alpha-adrenergic activity resides in the *levo* isomer and beta-adrenergic activity in the *dextro* isomer. Dobutamine generally produces dose-dependent increases in cardiac output and reductions in diastolic filling pressures. Venous return, augmented by adrenergic reduction of venous capacitance, likely contributes to the increase in cardiac output induced by dobutamine (126, 134).

"Conventional wisdom" often recommends dobutamine as an agent to increase cardiac output *without* increasing heart rate (135–137). This assumption is based on studies in patients with chronic heart failure (137), a population noted for beta-adrenergic receptor downregulation (91, 93), and severe metabolic disturbances (97). Other patient populations may have different hemodynamic profiles. We compared the effects of epinephrine (30 ng/kg/min) with dobutamine (5.0 µg/kg/min) in 52 patients recovering from coronary artery surgery. Both drugs significantly and similarly increased stroke volume index, but epinephrine increased heart rate by only 2 beats/min while dobutamine increased heart rate by 16 beats/min (138).

Dobutamine has been widely used to increase oxygen delivery to tissues in patients with critical illness (13, 17, 18). Recently, dobutamine was infused in doses from 5 to 200 µg/kg/min to increase oxygen delivery to greater than 600 mL/min/m² in 109 intensive care unit (ICU) patients (14). Despite having a significantly higher cardiac index and oxygen delivery, the treatment group in-hospital mortality was *higher* (54%) than the control group's (34%). This confirms that overly aggressive use of catecholamines may be detrimental to critically ill patients.

### Isoproterenol

Isoproterenol is a potent, nonselective beta-adrenergic agonist, devoid of alpha-adrenergic agonist activity. Isoproterenol dilates skeletal, renal, and mesenteric vascular beds and decreases diastolic blood pressure. Isoproterenol's potent chronotropic action, combined with its propensity to decrease coronary perfusion pressure, limits its usefulness in most patients with coronary artery disease. Current applications include treatment of bradycardia (especially after orthotopic transplantation), pulmonary hypertension and right ventricular failure, and heart failure after pediatric cardiac surgery (138).

Pulmonary hypertension associated with right ventricular dysfunction may be responsive to combined vasodilator/inotrope therapy. We found isoproterenol and

PGE₁ have greater specificity as pulmonary vasodilators than other vasoactive agents, as they significantly increased cardiac output and decreased pulmonary vascular resistance in experimental pulmonary hypertension in sheep (140). However, acute pulmonary hypertension and shock secondary to pulmonary embolus may not be responsive to isoproterenol. Molloy et al. reported that all acutely embolized animals treated with isoproterenol died, while all dogs treated with norepinephrine survived (141). Acute right ventricular ischemia and failure may require the higher coronary perfusion pressures provided by norepinephrine (vs. isoproterenol) in this situation.

### Vasopressors

Normal vascular tone is dependent upon the flux of calcium and potassium in and out of vascular smooth muscle, the local concentration of nitric oxide, the degree of alpha- and beta-adrenergic stimulation, and the influence of circulating vasoconstrictive chemicals such as angiotensin. Pharmacologic control of vascular tone therefore depends upon the manipulation of one or more of these variables.

Alpha-adrenergic agonists bind to alpha-receptors on the plasma membrane and, via a coupling G-protein, stimulate phospholipase C, then the intracellular messengers inositol triphosphate (IP₃) and diacylglycerol (DAG). Diacylglycerol activates protein kinase C, leading to an increased influx of calcium into the cell as well as an increased sensitivity of the contractile proteins to calcium. Inositol triphosphate enhances calcium release from the sarcoplasmic reticulum.

Alpha-receptor activity modulates peripheral vasomotor tone, coronary vasoconstriction (142), myocardial contractility, and medullary output. These receptors are known to exist in two basic subtypes (alpha-1 and alpha-2). Classically, activation of postsynaptic vascular alpha-1-adrenergic receptors produces vasoconstriction; activation of presynaptic alpha-2-adrenergic receptors reduces neurotransmitter concentration in the synaptic cleft through feedback inhibition. Alpha-1-adrenergic receptors exist on both presynaptic and postsynaptic membranes. Both alpha-1 and alpha-2-adrenergic agonists (indicating postsynaptic location of both receptor subtypes) may produce vasoconstriction. While alpha-1-adrenergic receptors are generally confined to the synaptic junction, alpha-2-adrenergic receptors may be located extrajunctionally.

Unlike several animal species, human ventricular contractility probably is not maintained by alpha-adrenergic receptors. Stimulation of these receptors does produce positive inotropic effects (143); however, myocardial alpha-adrenergic receptors may (143) or may not (144) be downregulated during chronic catecholamine exposure, as in chronic heart failure. Schwinn found alpha-1-adrenergic desensitization of peripheral vascular receptors in cardiac surgery patients with reduced (<40%) ejection fractions (145). Resistance to alpha-adrenergic agonists results from a decrease in alpha-adrenergic receptor number (104, 146, 147) or decreased coupling of receptors to phosphoinositide generation (104, 146).

Alpha-1-adrenergic receptors are distributed throughout the coronary microcirculation, whereas alpha-2-receptors are preferentially distributed in small arterioles (142). The potential for alpha-adrenergic agonist-induced coronary vasoconstriction raises concern about whether infusions of phenylephrine or norepinephrine might precipitate myocardial ischemia. In animals, phenylephrine-induced increases in blood pressure were accompanied by proportionate increases in myocardial blood flow (148), indicating that the myocardium is not at risk when phenylephrine is used to treat hypotension, because coronary autoregulation can override alpha-adrenergic agonist-induced constriction at the arteriolar level. The "paradoxical" cardiac benefit of alpha-adrenergic agonists can be explained by adrenergically mediated distribution of transmural blood flow and local metabolic autoregulation (149). Moreover, in cardiac surgery patients, when we infused phenylephrine to produce modest increases in mean arterial pressure, cardiac output was maintained (56). Phenylephrine titrated to reverse hypotension increases oxygen delivery, oxygen consumption, and urine output and decreases blood lactate concentrations in septic shock (150).

Norepinephrine, after a long period of unpopularity, is experiencing renewed interest during resuscitation. Meadows et al. (151) treated 10 patients with severe sepsis and hypotension unresponsive to volume expansion, dopamine, and dobutamine. Norepinephrine infusion (0.03 to 0.89 µg/kg/min) improved arterial blood pressure, left ventricular stroke work index, urine output, and, in most cases, cardiac index.

Desjars et al. (152) studied the renal effects of prolonged norepinephrine infusion in hypotensive patients with sepsis. Norepinephrine (0.5 to 1.5 µg/kg/min) plus low-dose dopamine improved urine flow and renal function compared to dopamine alone (mean dosage 14 µg/kg/min). Enhanced renal blood flow has been demonstrated in dogs with the combination of norepinephrine and low-dose dopamine compared to norepinephrine alone (106). Fukuoka et al. (153) found that norepinephrine (0.05 to 0.24 µg/kg/min) improved blood pressure and urine output in patients with serum lactate concentrations below 20 mg/dL but failed to improve urine output in sicker patients with lactate levels above 20 mg/dL.

Alpha-adrenergic agonists benefit certain patients with septic shock. Cardiovascular performance must initially be optimized by intravenous fluid. Inotropic drugs are then infused to optimize cardiac output, perfusion, and oxygen delivery. If hypotension is refractory, we often will add phenylephrine or norepinephrine to restore mean arterial pressure to over 60 mm Hg. In most patients, we administer dopamine (0.5 to 2 µg/kg/min) concomitantly to maintain renal perfusion (106, 152).

Calcium salts, which have been previously discussed, could also be considered primarily vasoconstrictors, given their limited effects on cardiac output.

## VASODILATORS

Vasodilators increase the diameter of blood vessels. From a physiologic modification of Ohm's law, we know that the pressure drop across a particular vascular bed equals the flow of blood multiplied by the vascular resistance:

$$\text{Pressure change} = \text{flow} \times \text{resistance}$$

or

$$\Delta P = Q \times R$$

where $\Delta P$ is the pressure change across the vascular bed, Q is the flow, and R is the resistance. From Poiseuille's law we know that

$$\text{Resistance} = (\text{viscosity} \times \text{vessel length} \times 8)/(\text{radius})^4$$

so small changes in radius cause much larger changes in resistance for any vascular bed, thus dramatically altering either blood flow or pressure.

Vasodilators are usually subdivided into primarily arterial, venous, or "mixed" agents (Table 3). Arterial dilators function to decrease arterial pressure, reduce left ventricular afterload, and, to a limited extent, decrease effective circulating blood volume, thus reducing left ventricular preload. Venodilators increase the volume of blood within venous capacitance vessels, reducing central blood volume (left ventricular preload) and blood pressure. Mixed vasodilators affect both arterial and venous capacitance vessels. Unfortunately, individual drugs rarely display absolute specificity toward either venous or arterial beds, and the effects on arterial or venous vessels depend upon numerous clinical parameters, including intravascular volume status.

There are at least four mechanisms by which vasodilating drugs may act: (a) direct relaxation of vascular smooth muscle, (b) inhibition of the renin-angiotensin vasoconstrictive pathway, (c) blockade of sympathetic stimulation, and (d) inhibition of normal cation flux in vascular smooth muscle. Direct relaxation of vascular

**TABLE 3.** *Primary classification of vasodilators*

Primarily arterial dilators: calcium channel blockers, hydralazine, phentolamine
Primarily venous dilators: nitroglycerin, other nitrate preparations
Mixed arterial and venous vasodilators: nitroprusside, prazosin, angiotensin-converting enzyme inhibitors

smooth muscle by local generation of nitric oxide (NO, formerly known as endothelium-derived relaxing factor) is the mechanism by which nitrates appear to exert their effect. Inhibition of angiotensin-converting enzyme (ACE) blocks the production of angiotensin II, a potent endogenous vasoconstrictor. Modulation of the peripheral vascular effects of adrenergic stimulation is the mechanism by which most alpha- and beta-adrenergic antagonists exert their vasodilating effects. Calcium and potassium channel antagonists interrupt the ion-flux-dependent vasoconstrictive tone present in all peripheral vessels.

Table 4 highlights common clinical conditions for which vasodilators are indicated in critically ill patients. Control of acute hypertension usually involves the use of an arterial or combined vasodilator such as nitroprusside, calcium channel blockers, or adrenergic antagonists. Controlled hypotension with vasodilators is used to reduce blood loss during surgery or to reduce the risk of rupturing aneurysms prior to surgery. Hemodynamic management of patients with myocardial dysfunction represents an expanding area for the use of vasodilators in critical illness. Reducing left ventricular afterload reduces wall tension and myocardial oxygen demand and, potentially, myocardial ischemia. It also improves "forward flow" in cardiac failure or mitral regurgitation.

Vasodilators have become the mainstay of therapy for chronic congestive heart failure. Arterial vasodilators improve cardiac output and may reduce symptoms of exercise intolerance; venodilators decrease symptoms of pulmonary congestion and hypoxemia (154, 155). Despite these beneficial effects, neither group of vasodilators has been shown to improve overall survival (156). Balanced vasodilators not only improve the symptoms associated with congestive heart failure but also prolong life (154, 157). In addition to ACE inhibitors, the combination of hydralazine and isosorbide dinitrate proves balanced vasodilation with improved survival in patients with congestive heart failure (154, 157, 158).

Separate from the venous and arterial dilating effects of vasodilators, there are a number of other changes that occur with these drugs. Lee et al. (159) found an acute reduction in the rate of diastolic filling of the left ventricle with administration of arterial vasodilators. There is also evidence showing that vasodilator therapy promotes cardiac muscle remodeling (155, 160). Alterations of

neurohumoral response of the heart, including reductions in atrial natriuretic factor concentrations and myocardial norepinephrine levels, have also been recognized as important components of the improved mortality from vasodilator therapy (161–163). These changes may preserve the myocardial response to stresses, limiting episodes of pulmonary congestion.

Rather than try to provide a comprehensive list of all vasodilator drugs currently available to the clinician, this discussion will concentrate on parenteral agents available for the more common clinical conditions listed previously.

## Magnesium

Magnesium, the second most abundant intracellular cation, is, similar to calcium, essential for many metabolic pathways (42). In addition to a variety of magnesium actions on cardiac contractility, magnesium also is required for normal regulation of ionized calcium, neuronal excitability, neuromuscular transmission, and skeletal muscle contraction. Magnesium relaxes vascular smooth muscle by functioning as a calcium channel antagonist and through its actions on the resting membrane potential (42). As with calcium, magnesium exists in three forms: ionized, protein bound, and chelated; similar to calcium, ionized magnesium is the physiologically active form. Since ionized magnesium electrodes are not readily available, clinicians use total serum magnesium concentrations as a marker for ionized magnesium concentrations. Moreover, since magnesium is primarily an intracellular cation, circulating magnesium concentrations may not reflect intracellular stores. Circulating magnesium concentrations are regulated primarily by the kidneys; there is no hormonal system for maintenance of magnesium. When large amounts of magnesium salts are infused, most of the magnesium dose is excreted in the urine; thus, repeated doses may be necessary to maintain normal magnesium concentration.

Magnesium has a variety of electrophysiologic actions on the heart and is widely used for its antiarrhythmic effects in critically ill patients, an action beyond the scope of this chapter (164). Magnesium also is a vasodilator and will interact with epinephrine infusion (Fig. 5A and B). In 22 patients recovering from coronary bypass surgery magnesium (10 mg/kg) reduced the increase in blood pressure after epinephrine without changing the response of cardiac output (165).

## Nitrates and Nitroprusside

Organic nitrates (e.g., nitroglycerin) have been the cornerstone therapy for angina pectoris and have been used to treat heart failure due to their ability to increase the volume of the venous capacitance vessels, reducing preload of a failing left ventricle. Nitroprusside has been the primary agent used to treat emergent hypertension since

**TABLE 4.** *Clinical indications for vasodilators*

Hypertensive urgency/emergency
Controlled hypotension
Reduction of left ventricular (LV) afterload: acute myocardial infarction, congestive heart failure, mitral regurgitation, cardiac surgery
Reduction of LV preload: congestive heart failure, acute myocardial infarction, sepsis, trauma

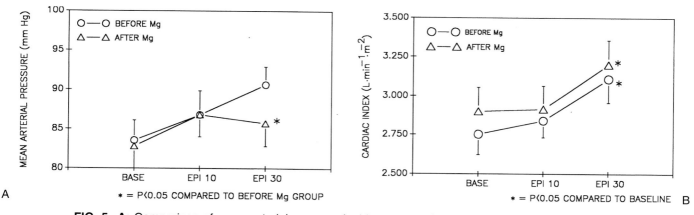

**FIG. 5. A:** Comparison of mean arterial pressure in 11 postoperative cardiac surgery patients before and after magnesium administration following concurrent epinephrine infusion at 10 and 30 ng/kg/min. Administration of magnesium significantly blunted the hypertensive response to epinephrine infusion. **B:** Comparison of cardiac index in 11 postoperative cardiac surgery patients before and after magnesium administration during concurrent epinephrine infusion at 10 and 30 ng/kg/min. Cardiac index significantly increased compared to baseline both before and after magnesium administration. From Prielipp RC, et al. *Anesthesiology* 1991;74:973, with permission.

its introduction over 20 years ago (166). Both nitroglycerin and nitroprusside are titratable parenteral solutions that have their effects through release of nitric oxide, resulting in direct vascular relaxation. Nitroprusside has effects on both arterial and venous beds, while the primary effects of nitroglycerin are on the venous system.

In contrast to the organic nitrates, sodium nitroprusside spontaneously generates nitric oxide; thus, it serves as a prodrug (167). Nitric oxide activates guanylate cyclase in vascular smooth muscle, producing increased intracellular concentrations of cyclic guanosine monophosphate (cGMP). Cyclic GMP reduces intracellular calcium concentration, producing vasodilation. Nitroprusside is also spontaneously broken down to cyanide (five cyanide ion radicals per sodium nitroprusside molecule). These will immediately react with methemoglobin to produce cyanomethemoglobin. Remaining cyanide radicals are converted to thiocyanate within the liver by the rhodanase enzyme.

When sodium nitroprusside infusions exceed 2 µg/kg/min, cyanide radicals may accumulate producing toxicity. The exact relationship between sodium nitroprusside infusion rates and toxicity are variable; therefore, any patient receiving sodium nitroprusside who exhibits central nervous system (CNS) dysfunction, cardiovascular instability, or metabolic acidosis should be suspected of having cyanide toxicity (168). When severe tissue hypoxemia develops, inhalation of 100% oxygen and administration of sodium bicarbonate (to correct metabolic acidosis), sodium nitrite (4 to 6 mg/kg IV), and sodium thiosulfate (150 to 200 mg/kg IV) are the usual treatments. Sodium nitrite promotes conversion of hemoglobin to methemoglobin to compete with cytochromes for cyanide radicals. Some practitioners administer hydroxocobalamin (vitamin $B_{12a}$) to prevent or treat

cyanide toxicity; however, the evidence that this is efficacious is unclear (167, 168).

Sodium nitroprusside is a potent vasodilator with immediate onset and a short half-life (measured in minutes). In congestive heart failure sodium nitroprusside reduces systemic vascular resistance, pulmonary vascular resistance, and central venous pressure. Cardiac output will usually increase (169–171). Nonhypovolemic patients without cardiovascular disease will experience variable changes in cardiac output. Sodium nitroprusside is frequently used during and after cardiac surgery, particularly after coronary artery bypass grafting or aortic valve replacement (171, 172). Sodium nitroprusside remains a common treatment for postoperative hypertension, often in combination with beta-adrenergic receptor blockers, calcium channel blockers, or nitroglycerin.

Nitroglycerin and other nitrates promote the release of nitric oxide within vascular endothelium. Nitric oxide activates guanylyl cyclase, increasing the intracellular concentration of cGMP. Cyclic GMP decreases cytosolic calcium, relaxing vascular smooth muscle (173).

Nitroglycerin's many vascular effects are particularly useful in myocardial ischemia. Intracoronary injection of nitroglycerin during cardiac catheterization will increase systolic diameter of coronary arteries. Although nitroglycerin and sodium nitroprusside have similar hemodynamic effects in myocardial ischemia, Chiariello and colleagues found that patients receiving nitroglycerin showed electrocardiographic improvement in marked contrast to those receiving sodium nitroprusside (174). Nitroglycerin may promote flow through collateral circulation (around a stenosis), whereas an equivalent dose of sodium nitroprusside will lower mean arterial pressure, possibly reducing collateral flow. Intravenous nitroglycerin appears to have a greater effect on the venous than the arterial circulation, resulting in pooling of blood in large-capacity venous beds (175). In acute myocardial infarction, studies have shown that nitroglycerin-treated patients have reduced infarct size and improved postinfarction left ventricular function compared to patients who received control therapy (176). Yusuf and colleagues (177) conducted a meta-analysis of randomized trials of intravenous nitroglycerin in acute myocardial infarction, finding that nitroglycerin treatment was associated with a clear reduction in the extent of infarction even in the absence of thrombolytic therapy.

Prophylactic nitroglycerin has been widely used perioperatively in patients with coronary artery disease, but the results have been variable. Kaplan and colleagues found a decreased incidence of ischemia and hypertension with prophylactic nitroglycerin (178). Other studies have shown no reduction in myocardial ischemia or infarction with this treatment (179). Nitroglycerin improves blood flow through internal mammary artery grafts (180). Nitroglycerin is also widely used perioperatively for control of hypertension. Many clinicians prefer it to nitroprusside due to the lack of risk of cyanide toxicity and its favorable effects in coronary artery disease.

There have been a number of studies evaluating the hemodynamic effects of nitroglycerin in patients with normal myocardial function as well as patients with congestive heart failure (181–184). Haber et al. showed how bolus doses of nitroglycerin reduced left ventricular end-diastolic volume (preload) in normotensive patients with normal left ventricular function, while patients with hypertension and preserved myocardial function exhibited a reduction in afterload (182). In this study, patients with congestive heart failure demonstrated reductions in both preload and afterload, with increases in stroke volume suggesting more of an afterload effect. Imai et al. have shown that the reduction in right atrial pressure is similar in patients with near normal ventricular function and patients with left ventricular dysfunction, and this reduction in right atrial pressure (RAP) is paralleled by a reduction in cardiac index (183). This study also noted that nitroglycerin infusions resulted in significant increases in the circulating concentrations of adrenaline and noradrenaline. Finally, Resakovic and colleagues demonstrated how the current hemodynamic status of patients in the acute phase of myocardial infarction determined the magnitude of the hemodynamic changes induced by intravenous nitroglycerin (184). In each of these studies, the primary reproducible effect of nitroglycerin was a reduction in filling pressures [RAP, pulmonary artery occlusion pressure (PAOP)], with less predictable decreases in arterial pressures and cardiac output.

### Angiotensin-converting Enzyme Inhibitors

In the absence of chronic heart failure, ACE inhibitors reduce blood pressure without altering cardiac output. Patients with chronic heart failure may experience an increase in cardiac output (185). Enalaprilat is the first parenteral ACE inhibitor. An initial dose of 1.25 mg over 15 minutes usually reduces arterial pressure promptly. Although rarely is more than 2.5 mg every 6 hours required, doses up to 20 mg per day have been administered safely. Combining ACE inhibitors with a diuretic usually augments the antihypertensive effect. As with all ACE inhibitors, caution must be used in patients with possible renal artery stenosis, due to drug-induced increases in angiotensin I.

### Hydralazine

Hydralazine is a direct-acting arterial vasodilator that relaxes vascular smooth muscle. Parenteral administration of hydralazine generally results in reduction of blood pressure within 15 minutes, and the effects last 3 to 4 hours in the presence of normal renal excretion. Because of potential reflex tachycardia and/or fluid retention, hydralazine is commonly administered with an adrenergic blocker or a diuretic for maximal antihypertensive efficacy.

### Calcium Channel Blockers

The calcium channel blockers all reduce calcium entry in cardiac and vascular smooth muscle, effecting vascular tone, cardiac contractility, and intracardiac electrical conduction. Sublingual nifedipine, 10 to 20 mg per dose, remains a common antihypertensive in critical illness. Intravenous nicardipine, a rapid-onset, high-potency, titratable agent dilates peripheral, coronary, and cerebral arteries and has shown promise in critical care settings where nitroglycerin and nitroprusside have been traditionally used (186, 187). Nicardipine and nimodipine may be useful in the management of cerebral vasospasm associated with subarachnoid hemorrhage, as well as hypertension following coronary bypass grafting. Other calcium channel blockers formulated for intravenous administration, including diltiazem and verapamil, are used primarily as antiarrhythmics. Chronic use of calcium channel blockers as antihypertensives has become highly controversial (187).

### Phentolamine and Phenoxybenzamine

Phentolamine and phenoxybenzamine, alpha-adrenergic receptor antagonists which reduce blood pressure by dilating both systemic arteries and veins, are used to treat hypertension due to an excess of circulating catecholamines. Prior to the introduction of labetalol, phentolamine was the primary agent used for the perioperative management of patients with pheochromocytoma. Phentolamine continues to be widely used during pediatric cardiac surgery to improve the uniformity of cooling prior to circulatory arrest (189). Orthostatic hypotension, reflex tachycardia, and increased myocardial oxygen demand limit the use of these agents in other circumstances.

## PHARMACOLOGIC REGULATION OF HEART RATE

In critical illness, the goal is not necessarily restoration of sinus rhythm but to achieve a rate and rhythm that will provide adequate blood flow to vital organs. Any arrhythmia accompanied by life-threatening hemodynamic compromise should be treated with the guidelines set forth by the American Heart Association in the Advanced Cardiac Life Support algorithms (190). Critically ill patients commonly develop tachyarrhythmias associated with less severe hemodynamic compromise, which may be corrected with drugs. This discussion will focus on two such rhythm disturbances: sinus tachycardia and sustained supraventricular tachycardia (SVT) with rapid ventricular response (including paroxysmal SVT, atrial fibrillation, and atrial flutter).

### Physiologic Control of Heart Rate

The resting heart rate results from the interaction of numerous factors acting on the electrical properties of myocardial cells, including age, disease, drugs, and emotional factors. In the absence of any sympathetic or vagotonic activity (i.e., in the denervated heart), the resting intrinsic adult heart rate averages approximately 100 beats per minute (191). Alterations in autonomic system activity (either direct or indirect) are the primary physiologic mechanisms involved in both the generation and treatment of sinus tachycardia and SVT.

Sinus tachycardia is the most common "arrhythmia" seen in the ICU. Most intensivists agree with a stepwise approach to diagnosis and treatment of this rhythm, based on the history and physical examination. Common physiologic causes of sinus tachycardia include pain, anxiety, agitation, hypoxemia, hypercarbia, fever, and hypovolemia. Less common etiologies include endocrine abnormalities, increased sympathetic nervous system activity, and decreased vagal tone. Malignant hyperthermia, poisoning, and neuroleptic malignant syndrome are rarer causes of sinus tachycardia. Pharmacologic intervention, if chosen, should correct the underlying physiologic abnormality and might include analgesia, anxiolysis, sedation, oxygen and pulmonary toilet, antipyretics, and restoration of intravascular volume, where appropriate. If sinus tachycardia is associated with adrenergic stimulation, thyrotoxicosis, myocardial infarction, or accelerated hypertension, intervention with a beta-adrenergic receptor antagonist may be beneficial.

Arrhythmias which originate above or within the AV node are commonly associated with ventricular rates above 120 beats per minute and hemodynamic instability. These rhythms include atrial fibrillation and flutter, paroxysmal SVT, and multifocal atrial tachycardia. The ultimate goal would be to restore normal sinus rhythm, but the immediate goal is to reduce ventricular rate to ensure adequate stroke volume. The ventricular response can be slowed through direct (intrinsic) activity, by antagonizing sympathetic function, or by increasing the vagal tone (Table 5). The primary drug classes used for this purpose include adenosine, calcium channel blockers, beta-adrenergic receptor blockers, digoxin, and alpha-adrenergic agonists, either alone or in combination.

### Adenosine

Adenosine is the first line of therapy for SVT with rapid ventricular response. Not only is adenosine effective at terminating most SVT, it does so with minimal significant side effects. The transient AV nodal block induced by adenosine may help identify the underlying rhythm in those cases not corrected by the drug (192).

### Calcium Channel Blockers

Verapamil was the first calcium channel blocker to be used to delay anterograde AV node conduction in SVT. Bolus injections of 2.5 to 5 mg achieve therapeutic concentrations within 5 to 10 minutes, with conversion to sinus rhythm in nearly all patients with AV nodal reentrant tachycardia (193). The most troublesome side effects of verapamil are vasodilation and hypotension. Verapamil has become a second-line agent to adenosine for the treatment of SVT.

Diltiazem, another calcium channel blocker available in parenteral form, is usually administered as a bolus of 15 to 25 mg followed by infusions of 10 to 20 mg per hour. Relative to verapamil, diltiazem accentuates activity at the AV node but causes less peripheral vasodilation. Intravenous diltiazem is an effective way to keep the ventricular rate under control for 24 to 48 hours, with perhaps a better response in patients with atrial fibrillation than with atrial flutter (194). There is also recent evidence that diltiazem given to coronary bypass patients will result in fewer ventricular and atrial tachyarrhythmias, less vasospastic ischemia, lower blood pressure, and lower resting heart rate (195, 196). In addition to its actions on the AV node, diltiazem also appears to modulate arrhythmias through CNS-mediated receptors (197).

**TABLE 5.** *Mechanisms and intravenous drugs used to treat supraventricular tachycardia*

Intrinsic atrioventricular nodal activity: adenosine, calcium channel blockers (diltiazem, verapamil)
Sympathetic antagonism: beta-adrenergic antagonists (esmolol, metoprolol, labetalol)
Increased vagal tone: digoxin, alpha-adrenergic agonists (phenylephrine)

Intravenous diltiazem is readily followed by its oral form, to provide protection from recurrence of SVT (198). While complete AV blockade rarely occurs with diltiazem alone, the risk is considerably higher if diltiazem is given concomitantly with a beta-adrenergic receptor antagonist (199).

## Beta-adrenergic Receptor Antagonists

Antagonism of the beta-1-receptor subtype results in reduction of heart rate and reduced myocardial contractility, especially in patients with elevated sympathetic tone (200). Clinically available beta-adrenergic receptor blockers all act through competitive inhibition; that is, their effects can be overcome by increased amounts of agonist. While beta-adrenergic receptor blockade has very little effect on resting normal hearts, beta-adrenergic receptor blockade can have profound effects on the cardiac and vascular systems in critically ill patients.

There are a number of beta-adrenergic antagonists available for parenteral use, including esmolol, metoprolol, and labetalol. Esmolol is a beta-1-selective antagonist with rapid onset (6 minutes to peak effect) and very short duration of action (half-life 9 minutes) that is used to treat tachycardia and hypertension in critically ill patients. Esmolol has no intrinsic sympathetic activity (ISA). Metoprolol is also a beta-1-selective antagonist without ISA that is commonly used to treat hypertension and lower myocardial oxygen demands in critically ill patients. Titrated intravenous doses of 5 to 15 mg will rapidly decrease arterial pressure. Esmolol and metoprolol have negative inotropic effects which may limit their usefulness in patients with compromised myocardial function.

Labetalol is a combined alpha- and nonselective beta-adrenergic receptor antagonist that inhibits neuronal uptake of norepinephrine and may also have direct vasodilating activity (201). Labetalol has some ISA at the beta-2-receptor, thus the alpha antagonism and beta-2 agonism allows for vasodilation while the beta-1 antagonism prevents the reflex tachycardia (202). Intravenous bolus doses of 5 to 20 mg, repeated at 10-minute intervals until the desired blood pressure is achieved, can be followed by a continuous infusion to allow tight control of the antihypertensive effects of the drug.

Beta-adrenergic receptor antagonism causes a reduction in conduction velocity throughout the heart, with decreased automaticity (including the sinus node), prolongation of the PR interval, AV nodal conduction, and QRS duration. For this reason, beta-blockers are excellent choices for the treatment of supraventricular tachyarrhythmias. Perhaps the best initial choice of parenteral beta-blocker is esmolol, as the onset of action is very rapid and the duration of action is only 9 minutes, thus providing a margin of safety above other parenteral beta-adrenergic receptor blockers. Bolus doses of up to 500 µg/kg followed by infusion of 50 to 250 µg/kg/min are indicated for treatment of paroxysmal SVT, atrial fibrillation, and atrial flutter either as initial therapy or when adenosine has failed to convert the rhythm. Esmolol is effective at controlling the signs and symptoms of thyrotoxicosis and the perioperative management of toxic goiter (203). Esmolol has also been used to control blood pressure and heart rate in patients with chronic pulmonary disease without causing bronchospasm (204). The primary side effect of esmolol is hypotension, exacerbated in patients with underlying volume depletion.

## Drugs to Increase Vagal Tone

If the speed at which sinus rhythm is restored is not critical, digoxin may be appropriate, especially if there are signs of left ventricular dysfunction or hypotension (193). The combination of digoxin with a rapid-acting beta-adrenergic receptor blocker, such as esmolol (see below), is very safe and can be very effective at converting patients in atrial fibrillation or flutter to sinus rhythm (205). Alpha-adrenergic agonists such as phenylephrine cause peripheral vasoconstriction and increase systemic blood pressure. The higher pressure sensed by the carotid body will result in a reflex increase in vagal activity. The net effect of this increased autonomic activity is a reduction in sinoatrial firing and AV conduction rate. While vagal reflex activation occurs when phenylephrine is given to patients with normal blood pressure, it is unclear if a similar response occurs in patients who are acutely hypotensive in whom the drug returns blood pressure to normal levels.

## SUMMARY

The availability of newer and better inotropic agents has led to their widespread application in critically ill medical and surgical patients. While the elective use of inotropic drugs has been associated with adverse outcomes in patients with cardiomyopathy and chronic heart failure, inotropic drugs used as part of treatment protocols designed to optimize oxygen delivery to tissues have been shown to improve outcome in critical illness. Future research must be aimed toward better definition of those clinical settings in which outcome can be improved with vasoactive drugs and toward identifying safer agents with fewer adverse side effects.

## ADDENDUM

Pharmacologic agents used to treat critically ill patients possess actions on many organ systems (206, 207). Some of these effects are therapeutic while many others are unwanted and detrimental. At times it may be difficult to sort out drug effects from alterations in organ function created by underlying disease. In addition, many patients receive multiple drugs and it may be difficult to determine which drug is producing which effects. Table 6

**TABLE 6.** *Noncardiac and cardiovascular actions of commonly used drugs*

| Drug | Noncardiac effects | Cardiovascular effects |
|---|---|---|
| **Alpha-adrenergic agonists:** phenylephrine (alpha-1), methoxamine (alpha-1), epinephrine[a] (alpha + beta), norepinephrine[a] (alpha + beta). *INDICATIONS:* hypotension; shock; nasal decongestant; local vasoconstriction; paroxysmal atrial tachycardia | Hypertension may result in cerebral hemorrhage, angina, myocardial infarction; headache; inhibits insulin secretion; contracts trigone and sphincter muscles of bladder (may cause urinary retention) | *Alpha-adrenergic effects:* increases systemic vascular resistance (vasoconstriction); hypertension; decreased mesenteric, cutaneous, renal blood flow; reflex bradycardia; increases myocardial oxygen consumption; may cause myocardial ischemia/infarction. |
| **Alpha-adrenergic receptor antagonists:** prazosin, phentolamine, phenoxybenzamine, terazosin. *INDICATIONS:* hypertension, pheochromocytoma, benign prostatic hypertrophy, congestive heart failure. | Decreased contraction of trigone and sphincter muscles of bladder resulting in increased urinary flow; nasal congestion; inhibits ejaculation; decreased platelet aggregation; increased insulin secretion; lipolysis; nausea; abdominal pain; increased gastric acid secretion (may exacerbate peptic ulcer disease); headache; dizziness; drowsiness. | *Alpha-1 receptor blockade:* inhibits catecholamine-induced vasoconstriction resulting in vasodilation; decreases blood pressure; hypotension; reduces arteriolar resistance; increases venous capacitance; reflex tachycardia and arrhythmias may occur; fluid retention may occur; increases cardiac output; postural hypotension; syncope. *Alpha-2 receptor blockade:* increases sympathetic output; decreases vagal tone; increases release of norepinephrine and acetylcholine from nerve endings; inhibits vascular contraction. |
| **Beta-adrenergic agonists:** isoproterenol (beta-1, beta-2), terbutaline (beta-2), albuterol (beta-2), metaproterenol (beta-2), pirbuterol (beta-2), ritodrine (beta-2), dobutamine[b] (beta > alpha), epinephrine[b] (alpha, beta-1, beta-2), norepinephrine[b] (alpha, beta-1). *INDICATIONS:* cardiac insufficiency, shock; bradycardia, bronchospasm; COPD; allergic reactions; premature labor. | Fear, anxiety, restlessness; headache; flushing; nausea; sweating; increases renin secretion; increases glucose output; stimulates glycogenolysis; hyperglycemia; enhances insulin and glucagon secretion; increases lipolysis; decreases circulating potassium; bronchodilation (beta-2); inhibits release of inflammatory mediators from mast cells (beta-2); enhances mucociliary clearance; inhibits uterine tone and contraction (beta-2); relaxes detrusor muscle of bladder (may cause urinary retention); increases WBC counts; muscle tremor (beta-2). | *Beta-adrenergic effects:* increases myocardial contractility (beta-1; positive inotropic effect); increases heart rate (beta-1; positive chronotropic effect); palpitations; increases cardiac output; increases myocardial oxygen consumption; may precipitate myocardial ischemia; decreases systemic vascular resistance (beta-2); hypotension may occur; arrhythmias may occur; increases automaticity; shortens refractory period of AV node; enhances AV and intraventricular conduction. |
| **Beta-adrenergic receptor antagonists:** nonselective (propranolol, timolol, nadolol, pindolol), selective beta-1 (esmolol, atenolol, metoprolol), partial agonists (pindolol, acebutolol), alpha and beta antagonist (labetalol). *INDICATIONS:* hypertension; myocardial ischemia and infarction; supraventricular and ventricular arrhythmias; tachycardia; aortic dissection; migraine; pheochromocytoma; hyperthyroidism; glaucoma. | Decrease renin release; bronchoconstriction; decrease glucose mobilization; blunt recognition of hypoglycemia; attenuate release of free fatty acids; decrease K uptake into cells; CNS effects—fatigue, sleep disturbances, depression. | Decreases myocardial oxygen consumption; negative chronotropic effect (reduces sinus rate, induces bradycardia); negative inotropic effect; reduction in systemic vascular resistance and blood pressure; decreases spontaneous depolarization rates of ectopic pacemakers; slows conduction in atria and AV node; increases functional refractory period of AV node. May cause hypotension and bradycardia; exacerbation of heart failure; exacerbation of symptoms of vascular insufficiency; rebound tachycardia, hypertension or myocardial ischemia following acute withdrawal. |
| **Amphotericin B:** *INDICATION:* Systemic fungal infection with susceptible organism. | Antifungal activity against *Candida* species, *Cryptococcus, Blastomyces, Histoplasma, Torulopsis, Coccidioides, Aspergillus, Mucormycosis.* Fever; chills; dyspnea; headache; nausea/vomiting; malaise; anorexia; phlebitis; bronchospasm; anemia (reduced erythropoietin); leukopenia; thrombocytopenia. Nephrotoxicity common; renal tubular acidosis; renal wasting of K and Mg; hypokalemia and hypomagnesemia may occur. | Hypotension; tachycardia; anaphylaxis. |
| **Angiotensin-converting enzyme inhibitors:** captopril, enalapril, lisinopril. *INDICATIONS:* hypertension, congestive heart failure. | Increases renal blood flow secondary to vasodilation; GFR unchanged or decreases; mild reduction in aldosterone secretion; potassium retention; renal insufficiency in patients with bilateral renal artery stenosis; angioedema; skin rash, loss of taste, cough; rare proteinuria or neutropenia. | Lowers systemic vascular resistance and blood pressure (hypotension may occur); blunts postural reflexes; greater effect in Na-depleted states (i.e., diuretic use); stroke volume and cardiac output may increase; little effect on heart rate; venodilation; decreases preload and afterload; decreases pulmonary artery pressures. |

**TABLE 6.** *Continued.*

| Drug | Noncardiac effects | Cardiovascular effects |
|---|---|---|
| **Antiarrhythmics—class IA:** quinidine, procainamide, disopyramide. *INDICATIONS:* supraventricular and ventricular arrhythmias | *Quinidine:* gastrointestinal effects (nausea, vomiting, diarrhea); hypersensitivity reactions, fever, bronchospasm, thrombocytopenia; cinchonism (tinnitus, loss of hearing, blurred vision, GI upset, headache, diplopia, photophobia, altered color vision, confusion, delirium, nausea, vomiting, diarrhea, abdominal pain). *Procainamide:* anorexia, nausea, vomiting, diarrhea, psychosis, hallucinations, depression, hypersensitivity reactions, fever, rash, myalgias, agranulocytosis, SLE-like syndrome (arthralgias, pericarditis, pleuritis, fever, antinuclear antibodies). *Disopyramide:* anticholinergic effects (dry mouth, constipation, blurred vision, urinary retention), nausea, vomiting, diarrhea, abdominal pain. | Block sodium channels; depress sinus node in patients with sick sinus; decrease firing rate of Purkinje fibers; increase fibrillation threshold in atria and ventricles; decrease phase 0 of action potential; increase duration of action potential; slow conduction; prolong repolarization; increase effective refractory period; abolish reentrant arrhythmias; therapeutic levels produce little change in heart rate or P-R, H-V, and QRS intervals; may prolong Q-T interval and widen QRS complex. *Quinidine toxicity:* QRS and Q-T interval widening, SA block, AV block, ventricular arrhythmias, asystole, torsades de pointes, abnormal automaticity may develop; may increase ventricular rate when treating atrial fibrillation; hypotension (vasodilation); blocks alpha-adrenergic receptor; syncope; cardiac arrest; blocks muscarinic cholinergic receptors (may increase sinus rate); increases digoxin levels. *Procainamide toxicity:* may cause hypotension after rapid intravenous administration; similar ECG changes as quinidine; paradoxical increase in ventricular response during treatment of atrial fibrillation; myocardial depression and hypotension may occur. *Disopyramide toxicity:* cardiac depression; increase in systemic vascular resistance; blocks muscarinic cholinergic receptors (tends to nullify direct cardiac depressant effects on SA and AV nodes); blocks calcium channels. |
| **Antiarrhythmics—class IB:** lidocaine, tocainide, mexiletine, phenytoin. *INDICATIONS:* ventricular arrhythmias, digitalis-induced arrhythmias. | *Lidocaine:* CNS effects include both excitatory and depressant effects; feelings of dissociation; paresthesias; drowsiness; stupor; coma; lightheadedness; agitation; anxiety; euphoria; confusion; disorientation; tinnitus; blurred or double vision; decreased hearing; nausea/vomiting; muscle twitching; convulsions; respiratory depression or arrest; rare allergic reactions. *Tocainide and mexiletine:* CNS effects include dizziness and tremor; gastrointestinal effects include nausea, vomiting, anorexia; agranulocytosis and bone marrow depression are reported with tocainide. *Phenytoin:* CNS effects include drowsiness, nystagmus, vertigo, ataxia, nausea. See phenytoin. | Block sodium channels; minimal effects on conduction in normal tissue; slows conduction in ischemic tissue; little effect on repolarization; decrease automaticity; increases fibrillation threshold; little effect on action potential or refractory period of atria; decrease duration of action potential in Purkinje fibers and ventricles; increases effective refractory period; abolish ventricular reentry; negligible ECG changes. *Lidocaine:* bradycardia; hypotension; myocardial depression; cardiac arrest. *Phenytoin:* See Phenytoin. |
| **Antiarrhythmics—class IC:** flecainide. *INDICATIONS:* ventricular arrhythmias, paroxysmal supraventricular tachycardias. | Visual disturbances (i.e., blurred or double vision); rare hepatic toxicity; malaise; fever; nausea; vomiting; diarrhea; anorexia; rash; paresthesias; dizziness; headache; paresis; ataxia; somnolence; anxiety; depression. | Sodium channel blockers; depress phase 0; markedly slow conduction; increase in P-A, A-H, and H-V intervals; little effect on repolarization; increase refractory period of AV node; little effect on refractory period of Purkinje fibers; therapeutic levels have little effect on heart rate; may increase ventricular rate in patients with atrial fibrillation; dose-related increases in P-R, QRS, Q-T intervals; heart block may occur; increase plasma digoxin levels. *Toxicity:* proarrhythmic effects may occur in 8–15%; may aggravate sinus node dysfunction (bradycardia, sinus arrest) and heart failure (negative inotropic effect). |

**TABLE 6.** *Continued.*

| Drug | Noncardiac effects | Cardiovascular effects |
|---|---|---|
| **Antiarrhythmics—class III:** bretylium, amiodarone. *INDICATIONS:* refractory ventricular arrhythmias. | *Bretylium:* nausea, vomiting, vertigo, dizziness. *Amiodarone:* pulmonary toxicity (hypersensitivity pneumonitis, interstitial/alveolar pneumonitis, fibrosis); hepatic injury; corneal microdeposits; blurred vision; cutaneous photosensitivity; blue discoloration; neurologic problems (malaise, fatigue, tremor, poor coordination and gait, peripheral neuropathy); GI complaints (nausea, vomiting, anorexia, constipation); inhibits peripheral conversion of thyroxine to triiodothyronine; may precipitate hypothyroidism; release of iodine may precipitate hyperthyroidism; increases LDL cholesterol; increases plasma levels of digoxin, warfarin, quinidine, procainamide, phenytoin, encainide, flecainide, diltiazem. | Delay membrane repolarization; prolong refractory period of Purkinje fibers and ventricular tissue; prolong duration of action potential; prolongs Q-T, J-T, P-A, and A-H intervals; increase threshold for ventricular fibrillation; myocardial contractility maintained. *Amiodarone:* decreases automaticity of sinus node and His-Purkinje system; decreases AV conduction and prolongs the P-R interval; heart block may occur; possess beta-adrenergic and alpha-adrenergic antagonistic properties; at therapeutic levels amiodarone decreases heart rate (symptomatic sinus bradycardia may develop); decreases vascular resistance; may aggravate arrhythmias in some patients. *Bretylium:* briefly increases automaticity, arrhythmias, and blood pressure after injection by releasing norepinephrine; hypotension common (up to 50%); blocks release of norepinephrine in response to neuron stimulation; peripheral adrenergic blockade; postural hypotension; syncope; may aggravate digitalis toxicity; enhances pressor effects of catecholamines. |
| **Antihypertensives:** clonidine (alpha-2-adrenergic agonist). *INDICATIONS:* hypertension; narcotic and alcohol withdrawal. | Salt and water retention; xerostomia (dry mouth); sedation; impotence; nausea; dizziness; postural hypotension; rare sleep disturbance, depression, and restlessness; potentiate analgesia and sedation from narcotics. *Withdrawal syndrome:* headache, apprehension, tremor, abdominal pain, sweating, tachycardia, hypertension (may lead to myocardial ischemia). | Reduces CNS sympathetic outflow; decreases systemic vascular resistance and blood pressure; transient hypertension with overdose (vascular alpha-2 effect); reduces heart rate and stroke volume; orthostatic hypotension (decreases venous return); rebound after acute withdrawal; increases parasympathetic outflow: bradycardia may occur. |
| **Antihypertensives:** hydralazine. *INDICATIONS:* hypertension; afterload reduction in patients with heart failure. | Salt and water retention; headache; nausea; flushing; dizziness. *Immune reactions:* lupuslike syndrome (i.e., arthralgia, arthritis, fever, pleuritis, pericarditis), serum sickness syndrome, hemolytic anemia, vasculitis, glomerulonephritis, polyneuropathy (pyridoxine responsive). | Vasodilator (arteries > veins); decreases systemic vascular resistance and blood pressure; hypotension may occur; reflex tachycardia and increased cardiac contractility; palpitations; may precipitate myocardial ischemia in patients with coronary artery disease. |
| **Antihypertensives:** methyldopa. *INDICATION:* hypertension. | Salt and water retention; sedation; decreased mental acuity (forgetfulness); depression; dry mouth; nasal stuffiness; headache; sleep disturbances; impotence; diarrhea; blurred vision; Parkinsonian signs. *Uncommon:* hemolytic anemia, leukopenia, positive Coombs test, thrombocytopenia, hepatitis, lupuslike syndrome, hyperthermia. | Decreases systemic vascular resistance (sympatholytic agent); decreases blood pressure; little change in heart rate or cardiac output; postural hypotension; rare bradycardia with first-degree heart block. |
| **Antihypertensives:** minoxidil. *INDICATIONS:* severe hypertension. | Renal vasodilator; stimulates renin release; fluid and salt retention may occur; hypertrichosis. | Relaxes vascular smooth muscle (primarily arteriolar dilator; little venous effect); reduces systemic vascular resistance and blood pressure; reflex increase in heart rate and cardiac contractility; may exacerbate myocardial ischemia; rare pericardial effusion. |
| **Antihypertensives:** sodium nitroprusside. *INDICATIONS:* hypertension, afterload reduction in patients with heart failure. | Inhibits platelet aggregation; thiocyanate toxicity (i.e., anorexia, nausea, fatigue, disorientation, psychosis); cyanide toxicity, ventilation/perfusion mismatch in lung (may cause hypoxemia). | Nonselective vasodilator; decreases systemic vascular resistance and blood pressure; hypotension common; cardiac output may increase due to afterload reduction; cardiac output may decrease due to diminished preload; modest reflex increase in heart rate; decreases myocardial oxygen consumption. |

**TABLE 6.** *Continued.*

| Drug | Noncardiac effects | Cardiovascular effects |
|---|---|---|
| **Antimuscarinic agents:** atropine (little CNS effect), scopolamine (penetrates CNS), belladonna alkaloids, pirenzepine, ipratropium (little CNS effect). *INDICATIONS:* bradycardia (atropine); preanesthesia medication (atropine, scopolamine); treatment of Parkinsonism; motion sickness (scopolamine); antispasmodic agents for GI tract (belladonna alkaloids); peptic ulcer disease (pirenzepine); bronchospasm (atropine-like drugs); mydriasis and cycloplegia; poisoning with choline ester or anticholinesterase. | Low doses depress salivary and bronchial secretion and sweating; dry mouth; pupillary dilation; inhibits accommodation; blurred vision; may increase intraocular pressure in patients with narrow angle glaucoma; large doses inhibit parasympathetic control of the bladder and GI tract (inhibits micturition and intestinal motility); inhibits gastric secretion and motility (pirenzepine inhibits gastric acid secretion at doses that have little effect on salivation or heart rate); bronchodilation. *CNS effects:* atropine: central excitation (restlessness, irritability, disorientation, hallucinations, delirium, seizures); with larger doses, stimulation is followed by depression, circulatory collapse, and respiratory failure. *Scopolamine:* CNS depression (drowsiness, amnesia, fatigue, dreamless sleep); may cause euphoria; large doses may cause central excitation (similar to atropine); prevents motion sickness. | *Atropine:* blocks vagal effects on heart (increases heart rate); atrial arrhythmias and AV dissociation may occur; AV conduction usually increased; shortens refractory period of AV node; may increase ventricular rate in patients with atrial fibrillation/flutter; dilates cutaneous blood vessels (atropine flush). *Scopolamine:* low doses cause cardiac slowing; large doses increase heart rate. |
| **Benzodiazepines:** midazolam, lorazepam, diazepam, chlordiazepoxide, flurazepam, oxazepam, triazolam. *INDICATIONS:* sedation, anxiety, seizures, muscle spasm, preanesthesia, anesthesia. | *CNS effects:* sedation, hypnosis, decreased anxiety, amnesia; may progress to stupor and coma; lightheadedness; lassitude; motor incoordination; ataxia; impaired mental and psychomotor functions; disorganized thought; confusion; dysarthria; dry mouth; bitter taste; weakness; headache; blurred vision; vertigo; nausea and vomiting; epigastric distress; diarrhea; may increase the occurrence of nightmares; disinhibitory effects; occasional CNS stimulation (i.e., euphoria, restlessness, hallucinations, irritability). Respiratory depression (small with normal hypnotic doses); decreases hypoxic drive; muscle relaxation; anticonvulsant. | Cardiovascular effects usually minor; may decrease blood pressure and cause tachycardia. |
| **Calcium channel blockers (L-type channels):** diltiazem, nicardipine, nifedipine, nimodipine, verapamil. *INDICATIONS:* myocardial ischemia (i.e., angina pectoris and myocardial infarction); hypertension; supraventricular tachyarrhythmias. | Excessive vasodilation may lead to dizziness, headache, flushing, and digital dysesthesia; nausea; peripheral edema; cough; wheezing; pulmonary edema; rash; somnolence; increase in serum digoxin levels; metabolism decreased in patients with hepatic dysfunction. | Vasodilation (primarily arterial): nicardipine = nifedipine = nimodipine > verapamil > diltiazem; hypotension may occur. Decreases cardiac contraction: verapamil > diltiazem > nifedipine = nimodipine > nicardipine; may exacerbate heart failure. Suppression of automaticity (SA node); diltiazem = verapamil >> nimodipine = nifedipine = nicardipine. Suppression of conduction (AV node); verapamil > diltiazem >> nicardipine = nifedipine = nimodipine. Decreases coronary vascular resistance; improves coronary flow; reflex increase in adrenergic tone (tachycardia may occur); bradycardia and asystole may occur. Additive effects with beta-blocker: verapamil and diltiazem. |
| **Carbonic anhydrase inhibitors:** acetazolamide. *INDICATIONS:* metabolic alkalosis, alkalinization of urine, mountain sickness, weak diuresis, glaucoma. | Metabolic acidosis; reduces intraocular pressure; renal calculi; drowsiness; paresthesias; weak diuresis. | Weak diuretic; may affect cardiovascular system via effects on acid-base status. |
| **Cyclosporine.** *INDICATIONS:* immunosuppression for transplants. | Immunosuppression; inhibits activation of T cells; inhibits IL-2 production by helper T cells; reduces production and release of lymphokines; does not cause myelosuppression; increases risk of infection. Nephrotoxicity common; neurotoxicity (i.e., tremor, seizures); hepatotoxicity; malignancies may develop; hirsutism; gingival hyperplasia; headache; paresthesias; flushing; sinusitis; gynecomastia; conjunctivitis; tinnitus; increases circulating prolactin levels. | Hypertension. |

**TABLE 6.** *Continued.*

| Drug | Noncardiac effects | Cardiovascular effects |
|---|---|---|
| **Digitalis:** digoxin. *INDICATIONS:* congestive heart failure; atrial fibrillation/flutter. | Hyperkalemia with toxicity; GI toxicity—anorexia, nausea/vomiting, diarrhea; neurologic toxicity—headache, fatigue, malaise, drowsiness, muscle weakness, neuralgic pain, paresthesias, disorientation, confusion, delirium, seizures; visual toxicity—blurred vision, halos, altered color vision, diplopia, neuritis; gynecomastia; levels increased by quinidine, verapamil, diltiazem, amiodarone; vagotonic. | Increases cardiac contractility; may increase blood pressure; slows ventricular rate in patients with atrial fibrillation/flutter; decreases resting membrane potential (slows phase 0 depolarization and conduction velocity); decreases action potential duration; enhances automaticity and arrhythmias; decreases refractory period of ventricular muscle; vagotonic; depresses conduction through AV node; increases refractory period of AV node; AV block may occur; reduces sympathetic activity; decreases sinus rate (vagal effect); sensitizes sinus node to Ach; ST and T wave ECG changes; Prolongs PR interval; may increase rate in patients with Wolff-Parkinson-White syndrome and is contraindicated. |
| **Dipyridamole.** *INDICATION:* Prophylaxis of angina pectoris. | Gastrointestinal intolerance (i.e., nausea, vomiting, diarrhea); headache; vertigo. | Vasodilator (decreases coronary vascular resistance, increases coronary blood flow, acts on small resistance vessels); rare hypotension. |
| **Diuretics-loop:** furosemide, bumetanide, ethacrynic acid. *INDICATIONS:* hypertension; fluid retention (i.e., edema, CHF); hypercalcemia. | Natriuresis; hypercalciuria; loss of potassium and magnesium in urine (may cause hypokalemia and hypomagnesemia); hyperuricemia; hyperglycemia; hyperlipoproteinemia; decreases lithium clearance; metabolic alkalosis; ototoxicity; rare hepatic and renal toxicity. | Decreases intravascular volume (may cause hypovolemia and hypotension); vasodilation. |
| **Diuretics—osmotic:** mannitol. *INDICATIONS:* fluid retention, increased intracranial pressure. | Increases serum osmolality; fluid and electrolyte depletion. | Acutely expands intravascular volume; may cause intravascular volume depletion. |
| **Diuretics—potassium sparing:** triamterene, amiloride, spironolactone. *INDICATIONS:* hypertension; fluid retention (i.e., edema, CHF). | May cause hyperkalemia; nausea, vomiting, leg cramps, dizziness may occur. *Spironolactone:* androgen-like effects, gynecomastia, increases calcium excretion, minor GI effects. *Triamterene/amiloride:* natriuresis, decreases calcium excretion, megaloblastic anemia may occur with triamterene (folate antagonism). | Decreases intravascular volume; hypovolemia and hypotension may occur. |
| **Diuretics—thiazides (distal tubule):** hydrochlorothiazide, metolazone. *INDICATIONS:* hypertension, fluid retention (edema, CHF). | Natriuresis; dilutional hyponatremia; loss of potassium in urine (may lead to hypokalemia); loss of magnesium in urine (may lead to hypomagnesemia); hyperuricemia; hyperlipoproteinemia; hyperglycemia; metabolic alkalosis; hypocalciuria (may exacerbate hypercalcemia); decreases lithium clearance. | Decreases intravascular volume; may lower blood pressure; hypovolemia may occur. |
| **Dopamine:** mediates effects via dopamine (0.5–3 mcg/kg/min), beta (3–7 mcg/kg/min), and alpha (> 7 mcg/kg/min) receptors. *INDICATIONS:* improve renal blood flow; diuresis; cardiac insufficiency; shock; hypotension. | *Dopamine receptors:* increases urinary sodium excretion; increases urine output; hypopituitarism with decreased secretion of thyroid stimulating hormone, growth hormone, prolactin, luteinizing hormone, and androgens. See beta- and alpha-adrenergic agonists for effects on beta- and alpha-receptors. | *Dopamine receptors:* low doses (0.5–3 mcg/kg/min) activate $D_1$ receptors in the vasculature; vasodilation of renal and mesenteric vessels; increases renal blood flow and GFR. Positive inotropic and chronotropic effect (beta-1); tachycardia; increases cardiac output; increases myocardial oxygen consumption; increases blood pressure (alpha). See beta- and alpha-adrenergic agonists for effects on beta- and alpha-receptors. |
| **Flucytosine.** *INDICATION:* fungal infection with susceptible organism. | Antifugal activity against *Candida* species, *Cryptococcus, Torulopsis.* Depresses bone marrow (leukopenia, thrombocytopenia, anemia); rash; nausea/vomiting; diarrhea; enterocolitis; hepatotoxicity. | |
| **H₂-receptor antagonists:** cimetidine, ranitidine, famotidine. *INDICATIONS:* peptic ulcer disease, esophageal reflux disease, stress ulcer prophylaxis. | Inhibit gastric acid secretion (competitive antagonist of $H_2$ receptors); secretion of intrinsic factor reduced ($B_{12}$ absorption little affected); predisposes to gastric colonization with microorganisms and pneumonia; no effect on LES or gastric emptying; small increases in serum creatinine (competition for tubular secretion). *CNS:* sedation, confusion, disorientation, dizziness. Occasional nausea, headache, skin rashes, itching, cytopenias, diarrhea, hepatotoxicity. Loss of libido, impotence, gynecomastia may occur with cimetidine (antiandrogenic effects). | Rapid intravenous infusion may cause bradycardia, hypotension, arrhythmias, and histamine release. |

**TABLE 6.** *Continued.*

| Drug | Noncardiac effects | Cardiovascular effects |
|---|---|---|
| **Heparin.** *INDICATIONS:* anticoagulation. | *Anticoagulation:* action mediated via antithrombin III (inhibits thrombin, kallikrein, and factors IX, X, XI, XII); high doses interfere with platelet aggregation. Bleeding may occur; thrombocytopenia; thrombotic complications may occur and lead to stroke, myocardial infarction, and other ischemic injuries; hepatic abnormalities (elevated enzymes); osteoporosis; inhibits aldosterone synthesis; hyperkalemia may occur; releases lipoprotein lipase (hydrolyzes triglycerides). | |
| **Neuromuscular blocking agents (nicotinic cholinergic receptor antagonists):** depolarizing agent (succinylcholine), competitive agents (tubocurarine, pancuronium, atracurium, metocurine, vecuronium. *INDICATION:* muscle paralysis. *Metabolism:* renal (tubocurarine, metocurine), hepatic (pancuronium), plasma esterase and nonenzymatic (atracurium), plasma and liver cholinesterase (succinylcholine). | Relaxation, weakness, and paralysis of skeletal muscle. Histamine release may occur with tubocurarine, metocurine, succinylcholine, atracurium (may cause hypotension and bronchospasm). Ganglionic blockade may decrease tone and motility of the gastrointestinal tract (usually mild). *Competitive agents:* can be antagonized with anti-ChE agents such as neostigmine, pyridostigmine, and edrophonium (usually given with a muscarinic antagonist to prevent stimulation of muscarinic receptors). Depolarizing agents: transient muscle fasciculations immediately following administration; muscle soreness or pain; elevation in circulating potassium (may be life threatening in patients with underlying muscle disease/injury, trauma, burns, or denervation); increased intraocular pressure; malignant hyperthermia. | *Competitive agents:* fall in blood pressure and tachycardia (autonomic ganglia blockade and histamine release) (varies with each agent); tubocurarine produces largest drop in blood pressure; pancuronium usually increases heart rate and may increase blood pressure; little change in heart rate or blood pressure with metocurine, atracurium, or vecuronium. Depolarizing agents: bradycardia (stimulation of vagal ganglia) or hypertension/tachycardia (stimulation of sympathetic ganglia). |
| **Nitrates:** nitroglycerin, isosorbide dinitrate. *INDICATIONS:* myocardial ischemia (anginal pectoris and infarction), congestive heart failure, hypertension. | Headache; facial and neck flushing; pallor; weakness; dizziness; inhibits platelet aggregation; relaxes bronchial smooth muscle, biliary tract smooth muscle, gastrointestinal tract smooth muscle, ureteral and uterine smooth muscle. | Relaxes smooth muscle; vasodilation (vein > artery); hypotension and syncope may occur; decreased right and left heart pressures (i.e., preload); decreases pulmonary vascular resistance; reflex tachycardia may occur; cardiac output may decrease unless preload is maintained; coronary vasodilation (especially large epicardial vessels); reduces myocardial work secondary to decreased preload and afterload; redistributes blood flow to subendocardial regions. |
| **Opioids:** morphine, fentanyl, sufentanil, alfentanil, meperidine, codeine, paregoric, loperamide. *INDICATIONS:* analgesia, anesthesia, sedation, cough, diarrhea; cardiogenic pulmonary edema. | *CNS effects:* analgesia, drowsiness, changes in mood, decreased mentation, euphoria, respiratory depression, blunts respiratory response to hypercarbia, depress cough reflex, obtundation, coma, hypothermia, nausea/vomiting, constriction of the pupil, lowers intraocular pressure, seizures may occur at very high doses. Decreases gastrointestinal motility; ileus; constipation; usually decreases gastric acid secretion; decreases biliary, pancreatic, and intestinal secretions; constriction of the sphincter of Oddi and elevation in bile duct pressures; biliary colic; may increase tone and contractions of the ureter; urinary retention; prolong labor; muscle rigidity may occur; noncardiogenic pulmonary edema may occur with overdose. | Peripheral vasodilation (arterial and venous); inhibit baroreceptor reflexes; hypotension may occur (especially orthostatic hypotension); may cause histamine release (especially morphine); does not significantly depress myocardial contractility; effects on cardiac output relate to changes in preload and afterload. Dilation of cutaneous blood vessels; flushing; histamine release (urticaria, flushing, puritis, bronchospasm). |
| **Oral anticoagulants:** warfarin, dicumarol. *INDICATIONS:* anticoagulation. | Antagonists of vitamin K; decreases production of factors II, VII, IX, X; decreases production of anticoagulant proteins C and S; bleeding may occur. *Infrequent reactions:* skin lesions and necrosis; thrombotic state may develop early following initiation of therapy in patients with protein C and S deficiency; purple toe syndrome; alopecia; urticaria; dermatitis; fever; nausea; diarrhea; abdominal cramps; anorexia. | |

**TABLE 6.** *Continued.*

| Drug | Noncardiac effects | Cardiovascular effects |
|---|---|---|
| **Phenobarbital.** *INDICATIONS:* seizure disorder, sedation, anesthesia. | Anticonvulsant; hypnosis; sedation; CNS depression; impaired mental and psychomotor functions; disorganized thought; confusion; depress respiratory drive and hypoxic drive; respiratory depression; hypothermia; nystagmus and ataxia at high doses; vertigo; nausea/vomiting; diarrhea; may produce irritability, agitation, and confusion; skin rash; hypersensitivity reactions; megaloblastic anemia; osteomalacia; may depress gastrointestinal tone; enhance porphyrin synthesis; laryngospasm; cough. | Hypotension (decreased systemic vascular resistance); myocardial depression at high doses; decreases cardiac output; decreases renal blood flow; decreases cerebral blood flow and intracranial pressure; tachycardia may occur. |
| **Phenytoin.** *INDICATIONS:* seizures, cardiac arrhythmias; neuralgias. | Antiepileptic activity (generalized and partial seizures); elevates seizure threshold; inhibits Na currents; rapid intravenous administration or high levels may cause CNS depression; cerebellar effects (nystagmus, ataxia, atrophy with high doses); vestibular effects (vertigo); diplopia; blurred vision; may cause hyperactivity, confusion, drowsiness, hallucinations; peripheral neuropathy; gingival hyperplasia; osteomalacia; hypocalcemia; inhibits insulin secretion; hyperglycemia; nausea/vomiting; anorexia; epigastric pain; megaloblastic anemia; hirsutism; rare bone marrow, hepatic, and skin toxicity. | Rapid intravenous administration may precipitate arrhythmias (i.e., fibrillation), depress conduction, and cause hypotension. Also see antiarrhythmics—class IB. |
| **Phosphodiesterase III inhibitors:** amrinone, milrinone. *INDICATIONS:* heart failure. | *GI toxicity:* nausea, vomiting, anorexia, abdominal pain, rare hepatotoxicity. Fever, thrombocytopenia (amrinone > milrinone). | Increases cardiac contractility (positive inotrope); moderate increase in heart rate; occasional arrhythmias; relaxes vascular smooth muscle; reduces systemic vascular resistance and blood pressure; reduces preload and afterload; may cause hypotension. |
| **Protamine.** *INDICATIONS:* reversal of heparin effect. | Hypersensitivity reactions; pulmonary edema; heparin rebound associated with anticoagulation and bleeding; bleeding may also result from protamine overdose; dyspnea, lassitude, nausea, vomiting, back pain. | Hypotension; bradycardia; flushing; pulmonary hypertension; anaphylaxis (associated with respiratory distress, circulatory collapse, capillary leak); hypertension less common. |
| **Thrombolytic agents** streptokinase (SK), urokinase (Uro), tissue plasminogen activator (t-PA). *INDICATIONS:* myocardial ischemia, pulmonary embolism, vascular occlusion. | Fibrinolysis and thrombolysis; increase formation of plasmin from plasminogen; hemorrhage may occur. Allergic reactions (i.e., rash, fever, anaphylaxis) common in patients with SK antibodies (i.e., from previous streptococcal infections). | |
| **Tricyclic antidepressants:** imipramine, amitriptyline, desipramine, nortriptyline, doxepin. *INDICATIONS:* depression, sleep disturbances. | Antidepressant; sleepiness; sedation; lightheadedness; weakness; fatigue; difficulty concentrating; confusion; may cause euphoria, manic excitment, and insomnia; tremor; increased risk of seizures. *Anticholinergic effects:* dry mouth, blurred vision, loss of accommodation, constipation, urinary retention, rare glaucoma. *Overdose:* brief phase of excitment (seizures, excitment) followed by depression (coma, respiratory depression, hypoxia, hypotension, hypothermia), tachycardia and other anticholinergic effects, arrhythmias. | Slight fall in blood pressure with normal doses; hypotension with overdose; postural hypotension (alpha-adrenergic receptor blockade); sinus tachycardia; myocardial depression; arrhythmias; prolongs cardiac conduction. *ECG changes:* inversion or flattening of T waves, prolonged conduction times (i.e., prolonged QRS). |

*a*Combines alpha- and beta-adrenergic effects (see beta-adrenergic agonists).
*b*Combines beta-adrenergic and alpha-adrenergic effects (see alpha-adrenergic agonists).
COPD, chronic obstructive pulmonary disease; WBC, white blood cell; AV, atrioventricular; CNS, central nervous system; GFR, glomenular filtration rate; GI, gastrointestinal; SLE, systemic lupus erythematosus; SA, sinoatrial; ECG, electroencephalographic; LDL, low-density lipoprotein; IL-2, interleukin-2; Ach, acetylcholine; CHF, congestive heart failure; LES, lower esophageal sphincter; ChE, cholinesterose.

is provided to assist the practitioner in assessing drug effects in critically ill patients. We have divided drug actions into noncardiac and cardiovascular effects.

## REFERENCES

1. Bristow MR, Ginsburg R, Minobe W, et al. Decreased catecholamine sensitivity and beta-adrenergic receptor density in failing human hearts. *N Engl J Med* 1982;307:205.
2. Feldman MD, Copelas L, Gwathmey JK, et al. Deficient production of cyclic AMP: pharmacologic evidence of an important cause of contractile dysfunction in patients with end-stage heart failure. *Circulation* 1987;75:331.
3. Curfman GD. Inotropic therapy for heart failure—an unfulfilled promise. *N Engl J Med* 1991;325:1509.
4. Packer M, Carver JR, Rodeheffer RJ, et al. Effect of oral milrinone on mortality in severe chronic heart failure. The PROMISE Study Research Group. *N Engl J Med* 1991;325:1468.
5. Uretsky BF, Young JB, Shahidi FE, Yellen LG, Harrison MC, Jolly MK. Randomized study assessing the effect of digoxin withdrawal in patients with mild to moderate chronic congestive heart failure: results of the PROVED trial. PROVED Investigative Group. *J Am Coll Cardiol* 1993;22:955–62.
6. Packer M, Gheorghiade M, Young JB, Costantini PJ, Adams KF, Cody RJ, Smith LK, Van Voorhees L, Gourley LA, Jolly MK. Withdrawal of digoxin from patients with chronic heart failure treated with angiotensin-converting-enzyme inhibitors. RADIANCE Study. *N Engl J Med* 1993;329:1–7.
7. Paolisso G, Gambardella A, Marrazzo G, et al. Metabolic and cardiovascular benefits deriving from beta-adrenergic blockade in chronic congestive heart failure. *Am Heart J* 1992;123:103.
8. Robin ED. Defenders of the pulmonary artery catheter. *Chest* 1988; 93:1059.
9. Bolli R, Hartley CJ, Rabinovitz RS. Clinical relevance of myocardial "stunning." *Cardiovasc Drugs Ther* 1991;5:877.
10. Conti CR. The stunned and hibernating myocardium: a brief review. *Clin Cardiol* 1991;14:708.
11. Tan LB. Evaluation of cardiac dysfunction, cardiac reserve and inotropic response. *Postgrad Med J* 1991;67(Suppl 1):S10.
12. Parrillo JE. Management of septic shock: present and future. *Ann Intern Med* 1991;115:491.
13. Shoemaker WC, Kram HB, Appel PL. Therapy of shock based on pathophysiology, monitoring, and outcome prediction. *Crit Care Med* 1990;18:S19.
14. Hayes MA, Timmins AC, Yau EHS, Palazzo M, Hinds CJ, Watson D. Elevation of systemic oxygen delivery in the treatment of critically ill patients. *N Engl J Med* 1994;330:1717.
15. Berlauk JF, Abrams JH, Gilmour IJ, O'Connor SR, Knighton DR, Cerra FB. Preoperative optimization of cardiovascular hemodynamics improves outcome in peripheral vascular surgery. A prospective, randomized clinical trial. *Ann Surg* 1991;214:289.
16. Schremmer B, Dhainaut JF. Heart failure in septic shock: effects of inotropic support. *Crit Care Med* 1990;18(1,Pt 2):S49.
17. Shoemaker WC, Appel PL, Kram HB. Oxygen transport measurements to evaluate tissue perfusion and titrate therapy: dobutamine and dopamine effects. *Crit Care Med* 1991;19:672.
18. Shoemaker WC, Appel PL, Kram HB, Duarte D, Harrier HD, Ocampo HA. Comparison of hemodynamic and oxygen transport effects of dopamine and dobutamine in critically ill surgical patients. *Chest* 1989;96:120.
19. Butterworth JF IV. Therapeutic choices in separation from cardiopulmonary bypass. *J Drug Devel* 1991;4(Suppl 2):16.
20. Royster RL, Butterworth JF IV, Prough DS, et al. Preoperative and intraoperative predictors of inotropic support and long-term outcome in patients having coronary artery bypass grafting. *Anesth Analg* 1991;72:729.
21. Brodde O-E, Zerkowski HR, Borst HG, Maier W, Michel MC. Drug- and disease-induced changes of human cardiac ß1- and ß2-adrenoceptors. *Eur Heart J* 1989;10(Suppl B):38.
22. Schwinn DA, Leone BJ, Spahn DR, et al. Desensitization of myocardial ß-adrenergic receptors during cardiopulmonary bypass. Evidence

for early uncoupling and late downregulation. *Circulation* 1991;84: 2559.
23. Heller M. Cardiac glycosides: new/old ideas about old drugs. *Biochem Pharmacol* 1990;40:919.
24. Fozzard HA, Sheets MF. Cellular mechanism of action of cardiac glycosides. *J Am Coll Cardiol* 1985;5:10A.
25. Ross J Jr, Waldhausen JA, Braunwald E, Lewis R. Studies on digitalis: I. Direct effects on peripheral vascular resistance. *J Clin Invest* 1960;39:930.
26. Kulick DL, Rahimtoola SH. Current role of digitalis therapy in patients with congestive heart failure. *JAMA* 1991;265:2995.
27. Gheorghiade M, Hall V, Lakier JB, Goldstein S. Comparative hemodynamic and neurohormonal effects of intravenous captopril and digoxin and their combinations in patients with severe heart failure. *J Am Coll Cardiol* 1989;13:134.
28. Cook LS, Johnson RG, Elkins RC. Cardiovascular time course after digoxin administration in left ventricular dysfunction after coronary artery bypass grafting. *Am J Cardiol* 1987;59:74.
29. Sethna D, Moffitt E, Gray R, et al. Effects of digoxin on myocardial oxygen supply and demand in patients following coronary artery bypass surgery. *Anesthesiology* 1982;56:356.
30. Cann MS, Stevenson T, Fiallos EE, Thal AP. Effect of digitalis on myocardial contractility in sepsis. *Surg Forum* 1971;22:1.
31. McDonough KH, Lang CH, Spitzer JJ. Effect of cardiotropic agents on the myocardial dysfunction of hyperdynamic sepsis. *Circ Shock* 1985;17:1.
32. Loeb HS, Cruz A, Teng CY, et al. Haemodynamic studies in shock associated with infection. *Br Heart J* 1967;29:883.
33. Nasraway SA, Rackow EC, Astiz ME, Karras G, Weil MH. Inotropic response to digoxin and dopamine in patients with severe sepsis, cardiac failure, and systemic hypoperfusion. *Chest* 1989;95:612.
34. Groves AC, Griffiths J, Leung F, Meek RN. Plasma catecholamines in patients with serious postoperative infection. *Ann Surg* 1973;178: 102.
35. Myers ML, Jacobson A, Finley R, Sibbald W. Beta receptor dysfunction in sepsis? *Crit Care Med* 1980;8:231(abst).
36. Lambert C, Rouleau JL. How to digitalize and to maintain optimal digoxin levels in congestive heart failure. *Cardiovasc Drugs Ther* 1989;2:717.
37. Carruthers SG, Cleland J, Kelly JG, Lyons SM, McDevitt DG. Plasma and tissue digoxin concentrations in patients undergoing cardiopulmonary bypass. *Br Heart J* 1975;37:313.
38. Arakaki F, Kumar MS, Deodhar SD, Welch CC. Digoxin level in digitalis intoxication and after surgery involving cardiopulmonary bypass. *Cleve Clin Q* 1973;40:133.
39. Molokhia FA, Beller GA, Smith TW, Asimacopoulos PJ, Hood WB Jr, Norman JC. Constancy of myocardial digoxin concentration during experimental cardiopulmonary bypass. *Ann Thorac Surg* 1971;11: 222.
40. Coltart DJ, Chamberlain DA, Howard MR, Kettlewell MG, Mercer JL, Smith TW. Effect of cardiopulmonary bypass on plasma digoxin concentrations. *Br Heart J* 1971;33:334.
41. Morrison J, Killip T. Serum digitalis and arrhythmia in patients undergoing cardiopulmonary bypass. *Circulation* 1973;47:341.
42. Butterworth JF, Zaloga GP. Calcium and magnesium as vasoactive drugs. *Baillieres Clin Anaesthesiol* 1994;8(1):109.
43. Erdmann E, Reuschel-Janetschek E. Calcium for resuscitation? *Br J Anaesth* 1991;67:178.
44. Carlon GC, Howland WS, Kahn RC, Schweizer O. Calcium chloride administration in normocalcemic critically ill patients. *Crit Care Med* 1980;8:209.
45. Maynard JC, Cruz C, Kleerekoper M, Levin NW. Blood pressure response to changes in serum ionized calcium during hemodialysis. *Ann Intern Med* 1986;104:358.
46. Henrich WL, Hunt JM, Nixon JV. Increased ionized calcium and left ventricular contractility during hemodialysis. *N Engl J Med* 1984; 310:19.
47. Lang RM, Fellner SK, Neumann A, Bushinsky DA, Borow KM. Left ventricular contractility varies directly with blood ionized calcium. *Ann Intern Med* 1988;108:524.
48. Zaloga GP, Roberts P, Black K, et al. The hemodynamic effects of calcium and dobutamine are additive in patients with sepsis. *Anesthesiology* 1992;77:A223(abst).
49. Shapira N, Schaff HV, White RD, Pluth JR. Hemodynamic effects of

calcium chloride injection following cardiopulmonary bypass: response to bolus injection and continuous infusion. *Ann Thorac Surg* 1984;37:133.

50. Lappas DG, Drop LJ, Buckley MJ, Mundth ED, Laver MB. Hemodynamic response to calcium chloride during coronary artery surgery. *Surg Forum* 1975;26:234.

51. Auffant RA, Downs JB, Amick R. Ionized calcium concentration and cardiovascular function after cardiopulmonary bypass. *Arch Surg* 1981;116:1072.

52. Robertie PG, Butterworth JF IV, Royster RL, et al. Normal parathyroid hormone responses to hypocalcemia during cardiopulmonary bypass. *Anesthesiology* 1991;75:43.

53. Robertie PG, Butterworth JF IV, Prielipp RC, Tucker WY, Zaloga GP. Parathyroid hormone responses to marked hypocalcemia in infants and young children undergoing repair of congenital heart disease. *J Am Coll Cardiol* 1992;20:672.

54. Royster RL, Butterworth JF IV, Prielipp RC, et al. A randomized, blinded, placebo-controlled evaluation of calcium chloride and epinephrine for inotropic support after emergence from cardiopulmonary bypass. *Anesth Analg* 1992;74:3.

55. Johnston WE, Robertie PG, Butterworth JF IV, Royster RL, Kon ND. Is calcium or ephedrine superior to placebo for emergence from cardiopulmonary bypass? *J Cardiothorac Vasc Anesth* 1992;6:528.

56. Butterworth JF IV, Strickland RA, Mark LJ, Kon ND, Zaloga GP. Calcium does not augment phenylephrine's hypertensive effects. *Crit Care Med* 1990;18:603.

57. Zaloga GP, Strickland RA, Butterworth JF IV, Mark LJ, Mills SA, Lake CR. Calcium attenuates epinephrine's ß-adrenergic effects in postoperative heart surgery patients. *Circulation* 1990;81:196.

58. Fernandez-del Castillo C, Harringer W, Warshaw AL, Vlahakes GJ, Koski G, Zaslavsky AM, Rattner DW. Risk factors for pancreatic cellular injury after cardiopulmonary bypass. *N Engl J Med* 1991;325:382–387.

59. Butterworth JF IV, Zaloga GP, Prielipp RC, Tucker WY Jr, Royster RL. Calcium inhibits the cardiac stimulating properties of dobutamine but not on amrinone. *Chest* 1992;101:174.

60. Prielipp RC, Hill T, Washburn D, Zaloga GP. Circulating calcium modulates adrenaline induced cyclic adenosine monophosphate production. *Cardiovasc Res* 1989;23:838.

61. Abernethy WB, Butterworth JF IV, Prielipp RC, Leith JP, Zaloga GP. Calcium entry attenuates adenylyl cyclase activity: a possible mechanism for calcium-induced catecholamine resistance. *Chest [in press]*.

62. Ririe DG, Butterworth JF IV, Royster RL, MacGregor DA, Zaloga GP. Triiodothyronine increases contractility independent of ß-adrenergic receptors or stimulation of cyclic-3´,5´-adenosine monophosphate. *Anesthesiology* 1995;82:1004–1012.

63. Bennett-Guerrero E, Jimenez JL, White WD, D'Amico EB, Baldwin BI, Schwinn DA. Cardiovascular effects of intravenous triiodothyronine in patients undergoing coronary artery bypass graft surgery. A randomized, double-blind, placebo-controlled trial. *JAMA* 1996;275:687–692.

64. Klemperer JD, Klein I, Gomez M, Helm RE, Ojamaa K, Thomas SJ, Isom OW, Krieger K. Thyroid hormone treatment after coronary-artery bypass surgery. *N Engl J Med* 1995;333:1522–1527.

65. Kass DA, Grayson R, Marino P. Pressure-volume analysis as a method for quantifying simultaneous drug (amrinone) effects on arterial load and contractile state in vivo. *J Am Coll Cardiol* 1990;16:726.

66. Jaski BE, Fifer MA, Wright RF, Braunwald E, Colucci WS. Positive inotropic and vasodilator actions of milrinone in patients with severe congestive heart failure. Dose-response relationships and comparison to nitroprusside. *J Clin Invest* 1985;75:643.

67. Colucci WS, Denniss AR, Leatherman GF, et al. Intracoronary infusion of dobutamine to patients with and without severe congestive heart failure. Dose-response relationships, correlation with circulating catecholamines, and effect of phosphodiesterase inhibition. *J Clin Invest* 1988;81:1103.

68. Marcus RH, Raw K, Patel J, Mitha A, Sareli P. Comparison of intravenous amrinone and dobutamine in congestive heart failure due to idiopathic dilated cardiomyopathy. *Am J Cardiol* 1990;66:1107.

69. Gage J, Rutman H, Lucido D, LeJemtel TH. Additive effects of dobutamine and amrinone on myocardial contractility and ventricular performance in patients with severe heart failure. *Circulation* 1986;74:367.

70. Butterworth JF IV, Royster RL, Prielipp RC, Lawless ST, Wallen-

haupt SL. Amrinone in cardiac surgical patients with left-ventricular dysfunction. A prospective, randomized placebo-controlled trial. *Chest* 1993;104:1660.

71. Royster RL, Butterworth JF IV, Prielipp RC, et al. Combined inotropic effects of amrinone and epinephrine after cardiopulmonary bypass in humans. *Anesth Analg* 1993;77:662.

72. Dupuis J-Y, Bondy R, Cattran C, Nathan HJ, Wynands JE. Amrinone and dobutamine as primary treatment of low cardiac output syndrome following coronary artery surgery: a comparison of their effects on hemodynamics and outcome. *J Cardiothorac Vasc Anesth* 1992;6:542.

73. Hess W, Arnold B, Veit S. The haemodynamic effects of amrinone in patients with mitral stenosis and pulmonary hypertension. *Eur Heart J* 1986;7:800.

74. Petry A, Dutschke P. Effects of amrinone on left and right ventricular function in patients with impaired myocardial performance during general anaesthesia. *Br J Anesth* 1994;72:567.

75. Harris MN, Daborin AK, O'Dwyer JP. Milrinone and the pulmonary vascular system. *Eur J Anaesth* 1992;5:27.

76. Prielipp RC, Butterworth JF IV, Zaloga GP, Robertie PG, Royster RL. Effects of amrinone on cardiac index, venous oxygen saturation and venous admixture in patients recovering from cardiac surgery. *Chest* 1991;99:820.

77. Benotti JR, Grossman W, Braunwald E, Carabello BA. Effects of amrinone on myocardial energy metabolism and hemodynamics in patients with severe congestive heart failure due to coronary artery disease. *Circulation* 1980;62:28.

78. Feneck RO. Effects of variable dose milrinone in patients with low cardiac output after cardiac surgery. *Am Heart J* 1991;121:1995.

79. Prielipp RC, Coursin DB, Wood WE, MacGregor DA, Meredith JW. Milrinone dose response study of $O_2$ transport, hemodynamics, and pharmacokinetics in ICU patients. *Anesthesiology* 1994;81:A344 (abst).

80. Sakanashi M, Tomomatsu E, Takeo S, et al. Effect of dobutamine on coronary circulation and cardiac metabolism of the dog. *Drug Res* 1978;28:798.

81. Butterworth JF IV, Hines RL, Royster RL, James RL. A pharmacokinetic and pharmacodynamic evaluation of milrinone in adults undergoing cardiac surgery. *Anesth Analg* 1995;81:783–792.

82. Bailey JM, Levy JH, Kikura M, Szlam F, Hug CC Jr. Pharmacokinetics of intravenous milrinone in patients undergoing cardiac surgery. *Anesthesiology* 1994;81:616.

83. Prielipp RC, MacGregor DA, Butterworth JF IV, Meredith JW, Levy JH, Wood KE, Coursin DB. Pharmacodynamics and pharmacokinetics of milrinone administration to increase oxygen delivery in critically ill patients. *Chest* 1996;109:1291–1301.

84. Ruttimann Y, Chioléro R, Revelly J-P, Jeanprêtre N, Schutz Y. Thermogenic effect of amrinone in healthy men. *Crit Care Med* 1994;22:1235.

85. Sjostrom L, Schultz Y, Gudinchet F, Hegnell L, Pittet PG, Jequier E. Epinephrine sensitivity with respect to metabolic rate and other variables in women. *Am J Physiol* 1983;245:E431.

86. Hermiller JB, Mehegan JP, Nadkarni VM, et al. Amrinone during porcine intraperitoneal sepsis. *Circ Shock* 1991;34:247.

87. Vincent JL, Domb M, Van der Linden P, et al. Amrinone administration in endotoxin shock. *Circ Shock* 1988;25:75.

88. Scalea TM, Donovan R. Amrinone as an inotrope in managing hypermetabolic surgical stress. *J Trauma* 1992;32:372.

89. Levitzki A. From epinephrine to cyclic AMP. *Science* 1988;241:800.

90. Morgan JP. Mechanism of action of inotropic drugs. *A textbook of cardiovascular medicine*, Supplement 6. Philadelphia: Saunders; 1989:136.

91. Liggett SB. Desensitization of the ß-adrenergic receptor: distinct molecular determinants of phosphorylation by specific kinases. *Pharmacol Res* 1991;24:29.

92. Fowler MB, Laser JA, Hopkins GL, Minobe W, Bristow MR. Assessment of the beta-adrenergic receptor pathway in the intact failing human heart: progressive receptor down-regulation and subsensitivity to agonist response. *Circulation* 74:1290.

93. Strasser RH, Marquetant R, Kubler W. Adrenergic receptors and sensitization of adenylyl cyclase in acute myocardial ischemia. *Circulation* 1990;82:II-23.

94. Marty J, Nimier M, Rocchiccioli C, et al. ß-Adrenergic receptor function is acutely altered in surgical patients. *Anesth Analg* 1990;71:1.

95. Smiley RM, Pantuck CB, Morelli JJ, Chadburn A, Knowles DM. Alterations of the ß-adrenergic receptor system after thoracic and abdominal surgery. *Anesth Analg* 1994;79:821.

96. Smiley RM, Pantuck CB, Chadburn A, Knowles DM. Downregulation and desensitization of the ß-adrenergic receptor system of human lymphocytes after cardiac surgery. *Anesth Analg* 1993;77:653.

97. Goldfarb RD. Cardiac mechanical performance in circulatory shock: a critical review of methods and results. *Circ Shock* 1982;9:633.

98. Sibbald WJ. Myocardial function in the critical ill: factors influencing left and right ventricular performance in patients with sepsis and trauma. *Surg Clin North Am* 1985;65:867.

99. Shepherd RE, McDonough KH, Burns AH. Mechanism of cardiac dysfunction in hearts from endotoxin-treated rats. *Circ Shock* 1986; 19:371.

100. Romanosky AJ, Giaimo ME, Shepherd RE, Burns AH. The effect of in vivo endotoxin on myocardial function in vitro. *Circ Shock* 1986; 19:1.

101. Eisinger MR, Jones SB, Westfall MV, Sayeed MM. Myocardial beta adrenergic receptors in *E. coli* induced septic shock. *Prog Clin Biol Res* 1988;264:319.

102. Silverman HJ, Lee NH, el-Fakahany EE. Effects of canine endotoxin shock on lymphocyte beta-adrenergic receptors. *Circ Shock* 1990;32: 293.

103. Beno DM, Jones SB. Cardiac beta-adrenergic receptors in septic peritonitis. *Circ Shock* 1986;18:370(abst).

104. Roth BL, Suba EA, Carcillo JA, Litten RZ. Alterations in hepatic and aortic phospholipase-C coupled receptors and signal transduction in rat intraperitoneal sepsis. In: Roth BL, Nielsen TB, McKee AE, eds. *Molecular and cellular mechanisms of septic shock.* New York: Alan R. Liss; 1989:41.

105. Bristow MR, Hershberger RE, Port JD, et al. ß-Adrenergic pathways in nonfailing and failing human ventricular myocardium. *Circulation* 1990;82(Suppl I):I12.

106. Schaer GL, Fink MP, Parrillo JE. Norepinephrine alone versus norepinephrine plus low-dose dopamine: enhanced renal blood flow with combination pressor therapy. *Crit Care Med* 1985;13:492.

107. Mueller HS, Evans R, Ayres SM. Effect of dopamine on hemodynamics and myocardial metabolism in shock following acute myocardial infarction in man. *Circulation* 1978;57:361.

108. Prielipp RC, Zaloga GP. Calcium action and general anesthesia. *Adv Anesth* 1991;8:241.

109. Zaloga GP, Willey S, Malcolm D, Chernow B, Holaday JW. Hypercalcemia attenuates the blood pressure response to epinephrine. *J Pharmacol Exp Ther* 1988;247:949.

110. Prielipp RC, Butterworth JF IV, Roberts PR, Black KW, Zaloga GP. Magnesium antagonizes the actions of lysophosphatidyl choline (LPC) in myocardial cells: a possible mechanism for its antiarrhythmic effects. *Anesth Analg [in press].*

111. Ginsburg R, Bristow MR, Billingham ME, Stinson EB, Schroeder JS, Harrison DC. Study of the normal and failing isolated human heart: decreased response of failing heart to isoproterenol. *Am Heart J* 1983; 106:535.

112. Goldberg LI. Dopamine and new dopamine analogs: receptors and clinical applications. *J Clin Anesth* 1988;1:66.

113. Breckenridge A, Orme M, Dollery CT. The effect of dopamine on renal blood flow in man. *Eur J Clin Pharmacol* 1971;3:131.

114. Hilberman M, Maseda J, Stinson EB, et al. The diuretic properties of dopamine in patients after open-heart operation. *Anesthesiology* 1984;61:489.

115. Costa P, Ottino GM, Matani A, et al. Low-dose dopamine during cardiopulmonary bypass in patients with renal dysfunction. *J Cardiothorac Anesth* 1990;4:469.

116. Duke GJ, Briedis JH, Weaver RA. Renal support in critically ill patients: low-dose dopamine or low-dose dobutamine? *Crit Care Med* 1994;22:1919.

117. Lass N, Goldberg LI, Lubbers N, Glock D. Cardiac and renal vascular effects of the selective DA₁ agonist, fenoldopam, alone and combined with dobutamine. *Clin Res* 1986;34:638A.

118. DiSesa VJ, Brown E, Mudge GH Jr, Collins JJ Jr, Cohn LH. Hemodynamic comparison of dopamine and dobutamine in the postoperative volume-loaded, pressure-loaded, and normal ventricle. *J Thorac Cardiovasc Surg* 1982;83:256.

119. Van Trigt P, Spray TL, Pasque MK, Peyton RB, Pellom GL, Wechsler AS. The comparative effects of dopamine and dobutamine on

120. Brown RA, Dixon J, Farmer JB, et al. Dopexamine: a novel agonist at peripheral dopamine receptors and beta₂-adrenoreceptors. *Br J Pharmacol* 1985;85:599.

121. Ghosh S, Gray B, Oduro A, Latimer RD. Dopexamine hydrochloride: pharmacology and use in low cardiac output states. *J Cardiothorac Vasc Anesth* 1991;5:382.

122. Mitchell PD, Smith GW, Wells E, West PA. Inhibition of uptake-1 by dopexamine hydrochloride *in vitro.* *Br J Pharmacol* 1987;92:265.

123. Lokhandwala MF. Renal actions of dopexamine hydrochloride. *Clin Intens Care* 1990;1:163.

124. Santman FW. Prolonged infusion of varied doses of dopexamine hydrochloride for low cardiac output after cardiac surgery. *J Cardiothorac Vasc Anesth* 1992;6:568.

125. Hunter DN, Gray H, Mudaliar Y, Morgan C, Evans TW. The effects of dopexamine hydrochloride on cardiopulmonary haemodynamics following cardiopulmonary bypass surgery. *Int J Cardiol* 1989;23: 365.

126. MacGregor DA, Butterworth JF IV, Zaloga GP, Prielipp RC, James R, Royster RL. Hemodynamic and renal effects of dopexamine and dobutamine in patients with reduced cardiac output following coronary artery bypass grafting. *Chest* 1994;106:385.

127. Cain SM, Curtis SE. Systemic and regional oxygen uptake and delivery and lactate flux in endotoxic dogs infused with dopexamine. *Crit Care Med* 1991;19:1552.

128. Boyd O, Grounds M, Bennett ED. A randomized clinical trial of the effect of deliberate perioperative increase of oxygen delivery on mortality in high-risk surgical patients. *JAMA* 1993;270:2699.

129. Leenen FH, Chan YK, Smith DL, Reeves RA. Epinephrine and left ventricular function in humans: effects of beta-1 vs nonselective beta-blockade. *Clin Pharmacol Ther* 1988;43:519.

130. Sata Y, Matsuzawa H, Eguchi S. Comparative study of effects of adrenaline, dobutamine, and dopamine on systemic hemodynamics and renal blood flow in patients following open heart surgery. *Jpn Circ J* 1982;46:1059.

131. Bollaert PE, Bauer P, Audibert G, Lambert H, Larcan A. Effects of epinephrine on hemodynamics and oxygen metabolism in dopamine-resistant septic shock. *Chest* 1990;98:949.

132. Sung BH, Robinson C, Thadani U, Lee R, Wilson MF. Effects of l-epinephrine on hemodynamics and cardiac function in coronary disease: dose-response studies. *Clin Pharmacol Ther* 1988;43:308.

133. Bersten AD, Rutten AJ, Summersides G, Ilsey AH. Epinephrine infusion in sheep: systemic and renal hemodynamic effects. *Crit Care Med* 1994;22:994.

134. Binkley PF, Murray KD, Watson KM, Myerowitz PD, Leier CV. Dobutamine increases cardiac output of the total artificial heart. Implications for vascular contribution of inotropic agents to augmented ventricular function. *Circulation* 1991;84:1210.

135. Ruffolo RR Jr. The pharmacology of dobutamine. *Am J Med Sci* 1987;294:244.

136. Kraft-Hunter F, Hinds JE. Cardiac dynamic effects of increasing myocardial contractility without changing heart rate, mean aortic pressure and end diastolic volume in conscious instrumented dogs. *Fed Proc* 1973;32:710(abst).

137. Akhtar N, Mikulic E, Cohn JN, Chaudhury MH. Hemodynamic effect of dobutamine in patients with severe heart failure. *Am J Cardiol* 1975;36:202.

138. Butterworth JF IV, Prielipp RC, Royster RL, et al. Dobutamine increases heart rate more than epinephrine in patients recovering from aortocoronary bypass surgery. *J Cardiothorac Vasc Anesth* 1992;6: 535.

139. Reyes G, Schwartz PH, Newth CJ, Eldadah MK. The pharmacokinetics of isoproterenol in critically ill pediatric patients. *J Clin Pharmacol* 1993;33:29.

140. Prielipp RC, Rosenthal MH, Pearl RG. Hemodynamic profiles of prostaglandin E₁, isoproterenol, prostacyclin, and nifedipine in vasoconstrictor pulmonary hypertension in sheep. *Anesth Analg* 1988;67: 722.

141. Molloy WD, Lee KY, Girling L, Schick U, Prewitt RM. Treatment of shock in a canine model of pulmonary embolism. *Am Rev Respir Dis* 1984;130:870.

142. Chilian WM. Functional distribution of alpha₁- and alpha₂-adrenergic receptors in the coronary microcirculation. *Circulation* 1991;84:2108.

ventricular mechanics after coronary artery bypass grafting: a pressure-dimension analysis. *Circulation* 1984;70(Suppl I):I1112.

143. Landzberg JS, Parker JD, Gauthier DF, Colucci WS. Effects of myocardial alpha$_1$-adrenergic receptor stimulation and blockade on contractility in humans. *Circulation* 1991;84:1608.

144. Bohm M, Diet F, Feiler G, Kemkes B, Erdmann E. α-Adrenoreceptors and α-adrenoreceptor-mediated positive inotropic effects in failing human myocardium. *J Cardiovasc Pharmacol* 1988;12:357.

145. Schwinn DA, McIntyre RW, Hawkins ED, Kates RA, Reves JG. Alpha$_1$-adrenergic responsiveness during coronary artery bypass surgery: effect of preoperative ejection fraction. *Anesthesiology* 1988;69:206.

146. Carcillo JA, Litten RZ, Suba EA, Roth BL. Alterations in rat aortic alpha$_1$-adrenoceptors and alpha$_1$-adrenergic stimulated phosphoinositide hydrolysis in intraperitoneal sepsis. *Circ Shock* 1988;26:331.

147. Ghosh S, Liu MS. Changes in α-adrenergic receptors in dog livers during endotoxic shock. *J Surg Res* 1983;34:239.

148. Crystal GJ, Kim SJ, Salem MM, Abdel-Latif M. Myocardial oxygen supply/demand relations during phenylephrine infusions in dogs. *Anesth Analg* 1991;73:283.

149. Feigl EO. The paradox of adrenergic coronary vasoconstriction. *Circulation* 1987;76:737.

150. Gregory JS, Bonfiglio MF, Dasta JF, Reilley TE, Townsend MC, Flancbaum L. Experience with phenylephrine as a component of the pharmacologic support of septic shock. *Crit Care Med* 1991;19:1395.

151. Meadows D, Edwards JD, Wilkins RG, Nightingale P. Reversal of intractable septic shock with norepinephrine therapy. *Crit Care Med* 1988;16:663.

152. Desjars P, Pinaud M, Bugnon D, Tasseau F. Norepinephrine therapy has no deleterious renal effects in human septic shock. *Crit Care Med* 1989;17:426.

153. Fukuoka T, Nishimura M, Imanaka H, Taenaka N, Yoshiya I, Takezawa J. Effects of norepinephrine on renal function in septic patients with normal and elevated serum lactate levels. *Crit Care Med* 1989;17:1104.

154. Chow MS. Assessing the treatment of congestive heart failure; diuretics, vasodilators, and angiotensin-converting enzyme inhibitors. *Pharmacotherapy* 1993;13:82S.

155. Cohn JN. Efficacy of vasodilators in the treatment of heart failure. *J Am Coll Cardiol* 1993;22:135A.

156. Cohn JN. The Vasodilator-Heart Failure Trials (V-HeFT). Mechanistic data from the VA Cooperative Studies. Introduction. *Circulation* 1993;87:VII.

157. Greenberg B. Role of vasodilator therapy in congestive heart failure. Effects on mortality. *Cardiol Clin* 1994;12:87.

158. Cohn JN. Treatment of infarct related heart failure: vasodilators other than ACE inhibitors. *Cardiovasc Drugs Ther* 1994;8:119.

159. Lee JM, Masuyama T, Nagano R, et al. Effects of vasodilators on pulmonary venous and mitral flow velocity patterns in patients with congestive heart failure. *Jpn Circ J* 1993;57:935.

160. Cohn JN. Nitrates versus angiotensin-converting enzyme inhibitors for congestive heart failure. *Am J Cardiol* 1993;72:21C.

161. Maxwell LP, Jain A. Therapy for congestive heart failure in the late 20th century. *West Virg Med J* 1993;89:148.

162. Stevenson LW, Fonarow G. Vasodilators. A re-evaluation of their role in heart failure. *Drugs* 1992;43:15.

163. Cavero PG, De Marco T, Kwasman M, Lau D, Liu M, Chatterjee K. Flosequinan, a new vasodilator: systemic and coronary hemodynamics and neuroendocrine effects in congestive heart failure. *J Am Coll Cardiol* 1992;20:1542.

164. Goldstein MM, Butterworth J. New role for magnesium. *Curr Opin Anaesthesiol* 1994;7:98–108.

165. Prielipp RC, Zaloga GP, Butterworth JF IV, et al. Magnesium inhibits the hypertensive but not the cardiotonic actions of low-dose epinephrine. *Anesthesiology* 1991;74:973.

166. Friederich JA, Butterworth JF IV. Sodium nitroprusside: Twenty years and counting. *Anesth Analg* 1995;81:152–162.

167. Friederich JA, Butterworth JF IV. Sodium nitroprusside: twenty years and counting—a review. *Anesth Analg [in press]*.

168. Hall VA, Guest JM. Sodium nitroprusside-induced cyanide intoxication and prevention with sodium thiosulfate prophylaxis. *Am J Crit Care* 1992;1:19.

169. Uretsky BF, Hua J. Combined intravenous pharmacotherapy in the treatment of patients with decompensated congestive heart failure. *Am Heart J* 1991;121:1879.

170. Guiha NH, Cohn JN, Mikulic E, Franciosa JA, Limas CJ. Treatment of refractory heart failure with infusion of nitroprusside. *N Engl J Med* 1974;291:587.

171. David D, Dubois C, Loria Y. Comparison of nicardipine and sodium nitroprusside in the treatment of paroxysmal hypertension following aortocoronary bypass surgery. *J Cardiothorac Vasc Anesth* 1991;5:357.

172. Roberts AJ, Niarchos AP, Subramanian VA, et al. Systemic hypertension associated with coronary artery bypass surgery. Predisposing factors, hemodynamic characteristics, humoral profile, and treatment. *J Thorac Cardiovasc Surg* 1977;74:846.

173. Williams EF, Lake CL. Nitrates. *Baillieres Clin Anaesthesiol* 1994;8(1):87.

174. Chiariello M, Gold HK, Leinbach RC, Davis MA, Maroko PR. Comparison between the effects of nitroprusside and nitroglycerin on ischaemic injury during acute myocardial infarction. *Circulation* 1976;54:766.

175. Gerson JI, Allen FB, Seltzer JL, Parker FB Jr, Markowitz AH. Arterial and venous dilation by nitroprussdie and nitroglycerin—is there a difference? *Anesth Analg* 1982;61:256.

176. Jugdutt BI, Warnica JW. Intravenous nitroglycerin therapy to limit myocardial infarct size, expansion, and complications. Effect of timing, dosage, and infarct location. *Circulation* 1988;78:906.

177. Yusuf S, Collins R, MacMahon S, Peto R. Effect of intravenous nitrates on mortality in acute myocardial infarction: an overview of the randomized trials. *Lancet* 1988;1:1088.

178. Kaplan JA, Dunbar RW, Jones EL. Nitroglycerin infusion during coronary artery surgery. *Anesthesiology* 1976;45:14.

179. Thomson IR, Mutch WAC, Culligan JD. Failure of intravenous nitroglycerin to prevent intraoperative myocardial ischemia during fentanyl-pancuronium anesthesia. *Anesthesiology* 1984;61:385.

180. Pennington DG, LaCroix JT, Shell WE, Williams MJ. Coronary vascular response to nitroglycerin following aorta-coronary saphenous vein grafting in dogs. *J Thorac Cardiovasc Surg* 1976;72:885.

181. Bauer JA, Fung HL. Pharmacodynamic models of nitroglycerin-induced hemodynamic tolerance in experimental heart failure. *Pharm Res* 1994;11:816.

182. Haber HL, Simek CL, Bergin JD, et al. Bolus intravenous nitroglycerin predominantly reduces afterload in patients with excessive arterial elastance. *J Am Coll Cardiol* 1993;22:251.

183. Imai Y, Ito H, Minatoguchi S, et al. The effects of phentolamine and nitroglycerin on right-sided hemodynamics in cardiac patients can be explained by a shift of the systemic venous return curve and right-ventricular output curve. *Jpn Circ J* 1992;56:801.

184. Rezakovic DE Jr, Popadic M, Popovic G, Pavicic L, Stalec J. Hemodynamic mechanisms of the effect of nitroglycerin in patients with acute myocardial infarction. *Cardiology* 1991;79(Suppl 2):70.

185. Met B, Miller ED. Angiotensin and angiotensin-converting enzyme inhibitors. *Baillieres Clin Anaesthesiol* 1994;8(1):151.

186. David D, Dubois C, Loria Y. Comparison of nicardipine and sodium nitroprusside in the treatment of paroxysmal hypertension following aortocoronary bypass surgery. *J Cardiothorac Vasc Anesthesiol* 1991;5:357.

187. Turlapaty P, Vary R, Kaplan JA. Nicardipine, a new intravenous calcium antagonist: a review of its pharmacology, pharmacokinetics, and perioperative applications. *J Cardiothorac Vasc Anesth* 1989;3:344.

188. Pahor M, Guralnik JM, Furberg CD, Carbonin P, Havlik RJ. Risk of gastrointestinal haemorrhage with calcium antagonists in hypertensive persons over 67 years old. *Lancet* 1996;347:1061–1065.

189. Anand KJ, Hickey PR. Halothane-morphine compared with high-dose sufentanil for anesthesia and postoperative analgesia in neonatal cardiac surgery. *N Engl J Med* 1992;326:1.

190. Cummins RO. *Textbook of advanced cardiac life support.* Dallas: American Heart Association; 1994.

191. Berne RM, Levy MN. *Physiology.* 2nd ed. St Louis: CV Mosby; 1988.

192. Rossi AF, Steinberg LG, Kipel G, Golinko RJ, Griepp RB. Use of adenosine in the management of perioperative arrhythmias in the pediatric cardiac intensive care unit. *Crit Care Med* 1992;20:1107.

193. Khan MG, ed. *Arrhythmias.* Philadelphia: Lee & Febiger; 1993:244.

194. Ellenbogen KA, Dias VC, Plumb VJ, Heywood JT, Mirvis DM. A placebo-controlled trial of continuous intravenous diltiazem infusion for 24-hour heart rate control during atrial fibrillation and atrial flutter: a multicenter study. *J Am Coll Cardiol* 1991;18:891.

195. Seitelberger R, Hannes W, Gleichauf M, Keilich M, Christoph M, Fasol R. Effects of diltiazem on perioperative ischemia, arrhythmias,

and myocardial function in patients undergoing elective coronary bypass grafting. *J Thorac Cardiovasc Surg* 1994;107:811.

196. Hannes W, Fasol R, Zajonc H, et al. Diltiazem provides anti-ischemic and anti-arrhythmic protection in patients undergoing coronary bypass grafting. *Eur J Cardio-thorac Surg* 1993;7:239.

197. Rabkin SW. The calcium antagonist diltiazem has antiarrhythmic effect which are mediated in the brain through endogenous opiods. *Neuropharmacology* 1992;31:487.

198. Clair WK, Wilkinson WE, McCarthy EA, Pritchett EL. Treatment of paroxysmal supraventricular tachycardia with oral diltiazem. *Clin Pharm Ther* 1992;51:562.

199. Buckley MM, Grant SM, Goa KL, McTavish D, Sorkin EM. Diltiazem. A reappraisal of its pharmacological properties and therapeutic use. *Drugs* 1990;39:757.

200. Hoffman BB, Lefkowitz RJ. Adrenergic receptor antagonists. In: Gilman AG, Rall TW, Nies AS, Taylor P, eds. *Goodman and Gilman's The pharmacological basis of therapeutics.* 8th ed. New York: Pergamon; 1990:221.

201. Gold EH, Chang W, Cohen M, et al. Synthesis and comparison of some cardiovascular properties of the stereoisomers of labetalol. *J Med Chem* 1982;25:1363.

202. Baum T, Watkins RW, Sybertz EJ, et al. Antihypertensive and hemodynamic actions of SCH 19927, the R,R-isomer and labetalol. *J Pharmacol Exp Ther* 1981;218:444.

203. Thorne AC, Bedford RF. Esmolol for perioperative management of thyrotoxic goiter. *Anesthesiology* 1989;71:291.

204. Gold MR, Dec GW, Cocca-Spofford D, Thompson BT. Esmolol and ventilatory function in cardiac patients with COPD. *Chest* 1991;100:1215.

205. Shettigar UR, Toole JG, Appunn DO. Combined use of esmolol and digoxin in the acute treatment of atrial fibrillation or flutter. *Am Heart J* 1993;126:368.

206. Molinoff PB, Ruddon RW. *Goodman & Gilman's The pharmacological basis of therapeutics.* 9th ed. New York: McGraw-Hill; 1996.

207. *Physicians desk reference.* Oradell, NJ: Medical Economics Company; 1995.

*The Critically Ill Cardiac Patient,*
edited by V. Kvetan and D. R. Dantzker,
Lippincott - Raven Publishers, Philadelphia © 1996.

CHAPTER 13

# Hematologic and Coagulation Considerations in Patients With Cardiac Disease

Richard C. Becker

Hematologic and coagulation abnormalities are common among critically ill patients with cardiac disease. Their assessment and management can challenge even the most astute clinicians and critical care specialists for the following reasons: In some instances, they represent a desired and controlled response to intervention (systemic anticoagulation in a patient with active thromboembolic disease). While in other circumstances the abnormality reflects an acquired condition [disseminated intravascular coagulation (DIC) in a patient with cardiogenic shock] or a complication of treatment (retroperitoneal hemorrhage following emergency coronary angioplasty). Further, it is not unusual for preexisting and acquired conditions to coexist.

Clinicians involved in the care of critically ill patients must have a solid understanding of basic hematologic principals and coagulation processes to provide a high level of care. This chapter outlines these two important areas, stressing pathobiology, differential diagnosis, and management. Each section is structured and presented with the practicing clinician specifically in mind.

## HEMATOLOGIC CONSIDERATIONS

### Anemia

Anemia is defined as a reduction of either the volume of red blood cells (hematocrit) or the concentration of hemoglobin in a sample of peripheral venous blood when compared with a reference population. By convention, the normal range is defined as including 95% of the reference population. A general classification of anemias is presented in Table 1.

R. C. Becker: Department of Medicine, University of Massachusetts Medical School, Worcester, Massachusetts 01655

### Physiologic Effects and Compensatory Mechanisms

The signs, symptoms, and physiologic effects of anemia are directly proportional to the rate of development. This point is particularly important among critically ill patients. An abrupt loss of 20% to 30% of the circulating blood volume from acute gastrointestinal hemorrhage will cause systemic hypotension, a fall in cardiac output, and unless supportive measures are provided immediately, circulatory collapse. Patients with underlying coronary artery disease may experience acute myocardial ischemia or infarction.

The response to chronic anemia is quite different. In most cases, circulating blood volume is maintained as is systemic blood pressure. Cardiac output is increased, allowing the passage of fewer red blood cells through tissues and vital organs more frequently. A reduced affinity of hemoglobin for oxygen (shift of oxyhemoglobin dissociation curve to the right) coupled with an increased cellular 2,3-diphosphoglycerate concentration increases oxygen delivery at the tissue level by nearly 30%. These latter two compensatory mechanisms are particularly important in patients with compromised left ventricular performance, in whom cardiac output may not increase significantly. In contrast, severe long-standing anemia (hematocrit < 20%) may be responsible for high-output congestive heart failure.

### Clinical Approach

With acute blood loss, blood pressure support through volume expansion and, if necessary, vasopressor administration should receive the highest priority. A prompt and thorough assessment to identify the source (or sources) should be undertaken. The coagulation status and platelet count should also be determined; although subacute and chronic anemias often carry less clinical

**TABLE 1.** *Classification of anemias*

I. Hypoproliferative anemias
  a. Myelophthisic (neoplastic, inflammatory)
  b. Marrow aplasia
  c. Chronic disease states
  d. Organ failure
    1. Renal
    2. Hepatic
    3. Hypothyroidism
    4. Hypopituitarism
II. Hyperproliferative anemias
  a. Hemorrhage (acute blood loss)
  b. Hemolytic
    1. Primary membrane defects
    2. Hemoglobinopathies
    3. Immune hemolysis
    4. Toxic hemolysis
    5. Traumatic (microangiopathic) hemolysis
    6. Hypersplenism
III. Maturation defects
  a. Hypochromic anemia
  b. Megaloblastic anemia
  c. Myelodysplastic anemia
IV. Dilutional anemia
  a. Pregnancy
  b. Aggressive fluid resuscitation
  c. Massive splenomegaly

urgency, they nonetheless are frequently of considerable importance.

Patients being evaluated for anemia should have a complete blood count, reticulocyte count, and review of the peripheral smear. The erythrocyte mean corpuscular volume (MCV) is a readily available and useful means to divide anemias into groups: microcytic ($<80$ $\mu m^3$), normocytic (80 to 100 $\mu m^3$), and macrocytic ($>100$ $\mu m^3$). Several challenges confront the clinician evaluating hospitalized patients. First, many anemias are normocytic, necessitating further testing and, second, multiple etiologies, particularly acute on chronic anemia, are common (Table 2).

A reticulocyte is a young red blood cell newly released from the bone marrow. The normal reticulocyte circulates for 24 hours before maturing. Because normal red blood cells survive on average for 120 days, the reticulocyte count is typically 1%. As anemia increases the relative concentration of reticulocytes in peripheral blood, the count should always be corrected to a normal hematocrit (45%):

Corrected reticulocyte count

$$= \text{calculated reticulocyte count} \times \frac{\text{(patient's hematocrit)}}{45}$$

A marked decrease in reticulocytes ($<0.5\%$) implies primary suppression of the bone marrow. A severe reduction (0.1%) suggests marrow aplasia. Reticulocytosis ($>5.0\%$) is the hallmark of hemolytic anemia.

Information vital to assessing patients with anemia can be obtained from a review of the peripheral blood smear (Table 3). A bone marrow examination may be necessary in challenging clinical situations, particularly when a primary blood dyscrasia or infiltrative process (tumor, infection) is a strong consideration.

### Special Considerations in the Intensive Care Unit

Blood loss from vigorous phlebotomy and invasive procedures considered collectively is the most common cause of anemia in hospitalized patients. Both should be considered and thoroughly assessed before other potential etiologies are explored. However, it is important to acknowledge two broad categories of acquired anemia: aplastic anemia and hemolytic anemia. Either can develop swiftly and have a profound impact on overall clinical status.

### Aplastic Anemia

The term *aplasia* refers to a condition of bone marrow characterized by a severe reduction or absence of

**TABLE 2.** *Diagnosing anemias on the basis of mean corpuscular volume (MCV)*

| Microcytic (MCV < 80 $\mu m^3$) | Macrocytic (MCV > 100 $\mu m^3$) |
|---|---|
| Iron deficiency | Megaloblastic anemias |
| Thalassemia | Chemotherapeutic agents[a] |
| Anemia of chronic disease[a] | Reticulocytosis |
| Sideroblastic anemia | Aplastic anemias |
| Erythrocyte fragmentation | Myelodysplastic syndromes |
| Burns[a] | Aplastic anemias[a] |
| Hereditary pyropoikilocytosis | Hypothyroidism[a] |

[a]MCV may be within normal range.

**TABLE 3.** *Peripheral blood smear: red blood cell morphologic characteristics and associated anemia*

| Red blood cell morphology | Anemia or associated condition |
|---|---|
| I. Hypoproliferative anemia | |
|   Normal | Anemia of chronic disease, aplastic anemia |
|   Rouleaux formation | Myeloma |
|   Blast cells | Blood dyscrasias |
|   Nucleated cells | Myelophthisic anemias |
|   Burr cells | Renal failure |
|   Marked poikilocytosis | Myelodysplastic syndrome |
| II. Hyperproliferative anemia | |
|   Polychromasia | Hemolysis |
|   Sickle cells | Sickle cell disease |
|   Microspherocytes | Hereditary spherocytosis, autoimmune hemolysis |
|   Bite cells | Oxidant hemolysis |
|   Schistocytes | Microangiopathic hemolysis |
| III. Maturation defects | |
|   Microcytes, hypochromia | Iron deficiency |
|   Target cells | Thalassemias |
|   Oval macrocytes | Vitamin $B_{12}$ or folate deficiency |

hematopoietic stem cells. In the majority of cases, anemia is accompanied by leukopenia and thrombocytopenia; however, pure red blood cell aplasia does occur. A general classification of aplastic anemia is presented in Table 4. Nearly half of all cases of aplastic anemia are considered idiopathic in origin. The remaining cases are associated with a diverse array of drugs, chemicals, toxins, and infectious agents (Table 5). In general, it is the acquired aplastic anemias that clinicals working in the critical care setting must be familiar with.

### Acquired Hemolytic Disorders

Hemolytic anemia is characterized by the premature destruction of essentially normal red blood cells from immunologic, physical, or chemical injury (Table 6).

In disorders of immune-mediated hemolyses, red blood cell destruction is caused by the binding of antibodies, complement components, or both to the surface membrane. This phenomenon is typically the result of autoimmunization, alloimmunization, or drug exposure.

Immunogloblulin M (IgM) antibodies are agglutinating, component fixing, and active in cold temperatures. In contrast, most IgG red blood cell antibodies are fully active at 37°C, have minimal agglutinating potential, and have variable complement-fixing activity. The synthesis of polyclonal cold agglutinins increases in response to infections, including mycoplasma, viruses (Ebstein-Barr, cytomegalovirus), and protozoa, as well as lymphoproliferative disorders. Nearly 50% of patients with IgG-mediated autoimmune hemolytic anemia have an underlying neoplastic, lymphoproliferative, collagen vascular (systemic lupus erythematosus most common), or inflammatory condition.

Alloantibodies capable of destroying transfused (but not autologous) red blood cells are most commonly products of immunologic responses to (a) colonizing bacteria of the large intestine or (b) imperfectly matched transferred red blood cells.

Drug-induced hemolysis should be considered in hospitalized patients with a rapidly decreasing hematocrit and no obvious source of blood loss. Several distinct mechanisms have been described:

1. *Drug–red blood cell binding.* In this situation, a drug-specific antibody (typically IgG) is produced and attacks the erythrocyte membrane at sites occupied by the offending drug. The cell is then sequestered in the spleen and destroyed by Fc-receptor-bearing macrophages (e.g., penicillin).

2. *Innocent bystander.* Drugs bound by plasma proteins stimulate the production of drug-specific, complement-giving antibodies. In turn, C3b generated by these complexes covalently binds to red blood cells, activating the terminal C5–C9 attack complex and causing intravascular hemolysis (e.g., quinidine, sulfonamides, and phenothiazine).

3. *Antierythrocyte antibody.* A pure, drug-induced antierythrocyte IgG antibody is rare but can occur (e.g., methyldopa).

To detect immunoproteins present on the red blood cell membrane, a direct antiglobulin (Coomb's) test is most frequently used. Almost all patients with immune hemolytic anemia exhibit a positive direct Coomb's test. An indirect antiglobulin test (indirect Coomb's) detects circulating antibodies capable of attaching to a normal red blood cell. Overall, the direct Coomb's test is more specific for autoimmune processes.

**TABLE 5.** *Drugs, chemicals, and toxins associated with aplastic anemia/pancytopenia*

| | |
|---|---|
| I. Antimibrobial agents | Penicillin, sulfonamides, cephalosporins, tetracycline derivatives, amphotericin B, chloramphenicol, streptomycin, methicillin |
| II. Antineoplastic agents | Antimetabolites, alkylating agents, antimitotic agents, radiation |
| III. Anticonvulsants | Phenytoin, carbamazepine (Tegretol) |
| IV. Antidiabetic agents | Chlorpropamide, tolbutamide |
| V. Antithyroid drugs | Carbimazole, propylthiouracil |
| VI. Sedatives and tranquilizers | Meprobamate, chlordiazepoxide |
| VII. Antiarrhythmic agents | Procainamide, quinidine |
| VIII. Other drugs | Furosemide, acetazolamide, heparin, captopril |
| IX. Infections | Hepatitis, parvovirus |
| X. Toxic chemicals | Solvents (benzene, glue, toluene, carbon tetrachloride), bismuth, mercury, arsenic, alcohol |

**TABLE 4.** *General classification of aplastic anemias*

| | |
|---|---|
| I. Acquired | |
| Idiopathic | Infectious |
| Autoimmune | Radiation |
| Drug-related | Pregnancy |
| Toxins | Paroxysmal nocturnal hemoglobinuria |

II. Other: familial, Fanconi's anemia, dyskeratosis congenita

**TABLE 6.** *Classification of acquired hemolytic anemias*

I. Immune
  a. Autoimmune
  b. Alloimmune
  c. Drug induced
II. Paroxysmal nocturnal hemoglobinuria
III. Toxins/metabolic abnormalities
IV. Red cell trauma (microangiopathic)
V. Red cell parasites
VI. Sequestrational hemolysis (hypersplenism)

When circulating red blood cells are subjected to excessive mechanical stress, hemolysis can occur. Abnormalities involving the left side of the heart, particularly those characterized by high pressures and shearing stress, are the most common. These include aortic stenosis, aortic insufficiency, and ruptured sinus of Valsalva. Significant red blood cell fragmentation may also occur as a result of traumatic atrioventricular (AV) fistulas or aortofemoral bypass procedures. Hemolysis secondary to mechanical prosthetic heart valves is less common today with the development of low-profile prosthetics; however, paravalvular leaks and malfunctioning valves may predispose to hemolysis.

Excessive shearing forces generated in the microvasculature can cause intravascular hemolysis. In a majority of cases, the vessels are either partially occluded by platelet-fibrin thrombi (e.g., DIC) or the vessel wall itself is abnormal (e.g., malignant hypertension and vasculitis). Occasionally a combination of the two coexists (e.g., thrombotic thrombocytopenia purpura and hemolytic uremic syndrome).

A diagnosis of traumatic hemolysis is supported by the presence of fragmented red blood cells (schistocytes) in the peripheral smear. Reticulocytosis (>5.0%), increased serum lactate dehydrogenase (LHD), and decreased haptoglobin are also common. In DIC, thrombocytopenia, prolonged clotting tests, and evidence of thrombin generation (prothrombin fragment 1.2) or fibrin formation (fibrinopeptide A) may also be present.

### Polycythemia

*Polycythemia* is characterized by an increased red blood cell count as measured by the hematocrit, hemoglobin, and absolute erythrocyte mass. A distinction between absolute and relative polycythemia should be made when evaluating patients with elevated counts. The former refers to conditions in which there is an absolute increase in red blood cell mass. Absolute polycythemia can also be subcategorized as primary or secondary, depending on whether the elevation in red blood cell mass is autonomous (primary polycythemia) or under hormonal (erythropoietin) control (secondary polycythemia) (Table 7).

The normal red blood cell mass averages $30 \pm 3$ mL/kg body weight in men and $27 \pm 3$ mL/kg in women. Generally, as the hematocrit nears 50%, the proportion of patients with an absolute increase in red blood cell mass increases but does not achieve complete specificity until the hematocrit exceeds 60%.

#### *Clinical Approach*

Regardless of the underlying etiology, all disorders characterized by absolute erythrocytosis share common clinical manifestations caused by expanded blood volume and increased blood viscosity. The expanded blood vol-

**TABLE 7.** *General classification or polycythemias*

I. Absolute polycythemia
  a. Primary: polycythemia rubra vera
  b. Secondary: (decreased $O_2$ transport, appropriate erythropoietin stimulation)
    1. Cyanotic congenital heart disease (R-to-L shunts)
    2. Pulmonary arteriovenous fistula
    3. High altitude
    4. Impaired ventilation (chronic lung disease)
    5. Impaired hemoglobin function
  c. Inappropriate erythropoietin stimulation
    1. Malignancy (lung, kidney, adrenal, liver)
    2. Benign tumors (Cushing's syndrome, pheochromocytoma, cerebellar)
    3. Renal: cysts, hydronephrosis
II. Relative polycythemia
  a. Dehydration
  b. Burns
  c. Adrenal insufficiency
  d. Stress (Gaisböck's syndrome)

ume leads to generalized vascular expansion and venous engorgement, while increased viscosity decreases vascular flow rate. The combination greatly increases the risk of thromboembolic events (discussed in the section on coagulation in this chapter) and may also result in both a decreased cardiac output and impaired tissue oxygenation.

In general, a hematocrit greater than 60% is rarely physiologic, and consideration should be given to therapeutic phlebotomy (target hematocrit 50%) as a means of minimizing the risk of thrombosis and tissue hypoperfusion.

### Thrombocytopenia

Under normal conditions, platelets circulate in a concentration between 150,000 and 300,000 cells/mm$^3$ for $7 \pm 2$ days. The splenic pool compromises nearly one-third of the blood platelets and is in dynamic equilibrium with the general circulation. Platelets themselves are manufactured in the bone marrow from percussor megakaryocytes; each megakaryocyte produces between 1,000 and 1,500 platelets in response to existing physiologic requirements.

*Thrombocytopenia* is defined as a reduction in the circulating platelet count to below 150,000 per mm$^3$. The most common mechanisms include (a) disorders of production, (b) disorders of distribution or dilution, and (c) platelet destruction. On occasion, a combination of abnormalities may coexist. This is particularly true in critically ill patients.

Disorders of platelet production include decreased megakaryocyte synthesis and ineffective platelet production (Table 8). A decrease in the number of megakaryocytes is characteristic of some congenital disorders, marrow damage, or bone marrow replacement. Isolated megakaryocyte hypoplasia has been observed following exposure to (a) drugs (e.g., thiazides), (b) chemicals (e.g., alcohol), and (c) toxins (e.g., solvents, glues, insecticides). It has also occurred following infections (viral, bacterial) and in association with collagen vascular disease, particularly systemic lupus erythematosus. As with many cases of aplastic anemia, megakaryocyte hypoplasia is most often idiopathic in origin. Ineffective platelet production is characterized by an increase in bone marrow megakaryocyte mass and a concomitant decrease in circulating platelets. Only a bone marrow examination can distinguish ineffective platelet production from disorders of peripheral destruction.

Drug-induced thrombocytopenia is particularly important in the intensive care unit setting. A partial list of causes is provided in Table 9, including both immune-mediated and bone marrow (megakaryocyte) abnormalities.

Disorders of platelet distribution and dilution can also be difficult to diagnose with certainty. They include splenic pooling, usually associated with moderate to marked splenomegaly (congestive, infectious, inflammatory, neoplastic), hypothermia (platelet pooling in hepatic sinusoids), and massive blood transfusions, particularly of stored blood (containing nonviable platelets).

In disorders of platelet destruction and consumption, the degree of thrombocytopenia is directly correlated with the bone marrow's ability to compensate by producing and releasing new platelets (Table 10).

### Clinical Approach

A careful history must be taken to identify the time of onset, course, past hemorrhagic complications, a family history of abnormal bleeding tendency, and associated medical illnesses. The hallmark of thrombocytopenia is petechia, most commonly involving the skin and mucous membranes (easily traumatized areas). The stool should be tested for blood and evidence of adenopathy or splenomegaly should be sought.

Several laboratory tests should be ordered, including a complete blood count with differential and review of the peripheral smear. Spurious thrombocytopenia can occur

**TABLE 8.** *Thrombocytopenia: disorders of platelet production*

I. Decreased megakaryocytes
  a. Congenital (Fanconi's anemia, intrauterine infections)
  b. Acquired hypoplasia (chemicals, drugs, infection, alcohol, radiation, collagen vascular disease, idiopathic)
  c. Marrow replacement (metastatic malignancy, myeloma, leukemia, lymphoma, myelofibrosis)
II. Ineffective platelet production
  a. Hereditary (autosomal dominant, Wiskott-Aldrich syndrome, May-Hegglin anomaly)
  b. Vitamin $B_{12}$ or folate deficiency
  c. Preleukemia, paroxysmal nocturnal hemoglobinuria

**TABLE 9.** *Drug-induced thrombocytopenia*

I. Reduced platelet production
  a. Cytotoxic drugs (alkylating agents, antimetabolites)
  b. Thiazides
  c. Alcohol
  d. Chloramphenicol, phenylbutazone
II. Immune-mediated or combined (decreased production and destruction)
  a. Antibiotics (cephalosporins, penicillins, rifampin, sulfonamides)
  b. Cardiac medication (digoxin, quinidine, nitroglycerin, heparin, amrinone, propranolol)
  c. Neuropsychiatric drugs (desipramine, phenothiazine, diphenylhydantoin, carbamazepine)
  d. Antihypertensives/diuretics (thiazides, furosemide, methyldopa)
  e. Anti-inflammatory drugs (aspirin, acetaminophen, gold salts, phenylbutazone)
  f. Oral hypoglycemic agents (chlorpropamide, tolbutamide)
  g. Other: ranitidine

with cold agglutinins, giant platelets, in vitro clotting, and ethylenediaminetetraacetic acid (EDTA)-induced clumping. Review of the peripheral smear also permits assessment of both erythrocytes and leukocytes. A bleeding time may be a useful part of the initial assessment of thrombocytopenia; however, it is a measure of both quantitative and qualitative platelet abnormalities. In the presence of normal platelet function, bleeding time is inversely related to platelet counts between 10,000 and 100,000 per mm³. Coagulation studies, including an activated partial thromboplastin time (aPTT), prothrombin time (PT), and thrombin time (TT) may be useful when DIC is being considered. A bone marrow examination may be required to assess platelet production (as well as other cell lines). Infiltrative and infectious processes can also be diagnosed.

**TABLE 10.** *Thrombocytopenia: platelet destruction and consumption*

I. Isolated platelet consumption
  a. Thrombotic thrombocytopenia purpura
  b. Hemolytic-Uremic syndrome
  c. Vasculitis
  d. Cardiopulmonary bypass
II. Immune destruction
  a. Idiopathic
  b. Alloantibodies (posttransfusion)
  c. Drug induced
  d. Other (infection, malignancy, collagen vascular disease)
III. Consumption of coagulation factors and platelets
  a. Disseminated intravascular coagulation
  b. Snake venoms
  c. Tissue injury (necrosis, trauma, surgical)
  d. Obstetric complications
  e. Infection (viral, bacteria, rickettsial)
  f. Neoplasms (promyelocytic leukemia, hemangioma)

In disorders characterized by platelet destruction, laboratory tests can either measure antibody-platelet binding or measure immune-mediated paraphenomena (lysis, complement fixation, aggregation). As the initial event in immune thrombocytopenia is antibody or immune complex binding, the measurement of platelet-associated IgG is the most commonly used, first-line test. Available assays include (a) inhibition assays, (b) direct binding assays, and (c) immunoprecipitation assays. Unfortunately, platelet-associated IgG is found in many clinical settings manifesting thrombocytopenia and, therefore, lacks specificity for immune disorders.

Heparin-associated thrombocytopenia is not uncommon in clinical practice. The frequent use of heparin in cardiac critical care requires a solid understanding of this platelet disorder that can manifest not only as thrombocytopenia and bleeding but also as multiorgan thrombotic events. An immune basis for heparin-associated thrombocytopenia is supported by the following observations:

1. Rechallenge with heparin may cause recurrent thrombocytopenia.
2. Platelet-associated IgG is present in a majority of patients.
3. Immunoglobulin G from the plasma of patients with the disorder binds to heparin in vitro and, in the presence of platelets, causes complement fixation.
4. Plasma from patients causes platelet activation (serotonin release) and platelet aggregation.

**Disorders of Platelet Function**

Platelets are required for primary hemostasis and also to maintain vascular integrity (these areas are outlined in greater detail in the coagulation section). Qualitative defects in platelet function can be caused by (a) decreased adhesion, (b) decreased aggregation, (c) reduced thromboxane synthesis, (d) impaired secretion of platelet granule contents, or (e) an inadequate contribution of platelets to blood coagulation. Disorders of platelet function can be classified broadly as congenital and acquired (Tables 11 and 12).

Drug-induced abnormalities in platelet function should be considered strongly in critically ill patients with bleeding complications despite a normal platelet count. The most common offending agents include (a) aspirin and other nonsteroidal anti-inflammatory agents, (b) antihistamines, (c) phenothiazines, (d) dextran, (e) heparin, (f) antimicrobial agents (penicillins, cephalosporins), (g) ethanol, and (h) radiographic contrast agents.

*Clinical Approach*

The hallmark of qualitative platelet disorders is a prolonged bleeding time in the presence of a normal platelet count. A history of easy bruising, hemorrhage following

**TABLE 11.** *Congenital disorders of platelet function*

I. Defects in plasma membrane
  a. Bernard-Soulier syndrome
  b. von Willebrand's disease
  c. Glanzmann's thrombasthenia
  d. Primary platelet coagulant defect (platelet factor 3)
II. Defects in storage organelles
  a. Dense body deficiency
  b. Idiopathic storage pool disease
  c. Wiskott-Aldrich syndrome
  d. Chediak-Higashi syndrome
  e. Thrombocytopenia with absent radii
  f. Alpha-granule deficiency
III. Thromboxane deficiency
  a. Cyclooxygenase deficiency
  b. Thromboxane synthase deficiency
IV. Other
  a. Ehlers-Danlo's syndrome
  b. Marfan's syndrome
  c. Osteogenesis imperfecta

minor trauma, spontaneous bleeding from mucosal surfaces, and a family history of bleeding (particularly important in congenital disorders). A series of platelet function tests can be performed, including aggregation response to adenosine diphosphate (ADP), collagen, ristocetin, and arachidonic acid. More complex tests are available in experienced laboratories, including assessment of membrane glycoproteins using monoclonal antibodies and flow cytometry, uptake and secretion of serotonin, content and secretion of adenine nucleotides, and structural assessment with electron microscopy.

**Thrombocytosis**

*Thrombocytosis* refers to an elevation in the platelet count beyond 400,000 per mm$^3$. Three forms have been recognized: (a) physiologic, (b) reactive (also known as secondary thrombocytosis) and, (c) primary.

Physiologic thrombocytosis can occur after vigorous physical exertion or stress. Epinephrine administration

**TABLE 12.** *Acquired disorders of platelet function*

  a. Uremia
  b. Myeloproliferative diseases
  c. Acute leukemia
  d. Preleukemia states
  e. Dysproteinemias
  f. Liver disease
  g. Circulating fibrin(ogen) degradation products
  h. Drug induced
  i. Acquired storage pool deficiency
    1. Autoimmune disorders
    2. Severe burns
    3. Cardiopulmonary bypass
    4. Disseminated intravascular coagulation
    5. Valvular heart disease

can elevate the platelet count by 20% to 30%. In most instances, physiologic thrombocytosis is caused by increased mobilization of platelets rather than increased production. In contrast, reactive thrombocytosis is characterized by accelerated platelet production in response to acute/subacute hemorrhage, acute/chronic inflammatory disorders, hemolysis, malignancy, iron deficiency, splenectomy, or moderate to severe thrombocytopenia (rebound phenomenon). It is rare for platelet counts to exceed 1 million per $mm^3$. Despite the observed elevations, thrombotic (and hemorrhagic) complications are rare; therefore, treatment should focus on the underlying condition or disorder rather than on the platelet count.

Essential (primary) thrombocythemia is a myeloproliferative disorder characterized by a persistent and marked elevation in platelet count to levels beyond 1 million per $mm^3$. At times, the platelet count may increase to as high as 2 million per $mm^3$. In essential thrombocythemia, increased platelet production occurs independently from normal regulatory processes; however, other cell lines are unaffected, distinguishing it from polycythemia rubra vera and other myeloproliferative disorders.

### Clinical Approach

Thrombocytosis can give rise to spurious laboratory values. The most common include psuedohyperkalemia, increased LDH, and falsely elevated acid phosphatase. These abnormalities quickly correct when cell-free plasma is used to run the tests.

Reactive and secondary forms of thrombocytosis rarely cause hemorrhagic or thrombotic complications. In contrast, essential thrombocythemia is associated with hemorrhage (related to accompanying platelet dysfunction) and thrombosis. The latter can involve both small and large vessels, causing stroke, myocardial infarction, and damage to other major viscera. Overall, thrombotic events are among the leading causes of death in patients with essential thrombocythemia. As the thrombotic diathesis reflects excessive platelet activation, prophylaxis with antiplatelet drugs (aspirin, dipyridamole) may be beneficial. Platelet phoresis and cytoreduction therapy are indicated in the acute and chronic stages, respectively, if thrombotic events occur in the presence of platelet counts greater than 1 million per $mm^3$. The target goal for maintenance should be 600,000 per $mm^3$.

### Leukopenia

Under normal circumstances, *leukopenia* refers to a condition during which the peripheral white blood cell count ranges from 5,000 to 10,000 per $mm^3$ and includes neutrophils, lymphocytes, monocytes, eosinophils, and basophils. A differential count allows abnormalities of individual components to be determined.

Neutropenia is defined as a peripheral neutrophil count below 2,000 per $mm^3$. Counts greater than 1,000 per $mm^3$ under most circumstances provide adequate host defenses; however, counts below 500 neutrophils per $mm^3$ substantially increase the risk of serious infection. A listing of conditions and disorders associated with neutropenia is presented in Table 13.

### Clinical Approach

Neutropenia occurs in a wide variety of illnesses which may dominate the clinical picture. As previously mentioned, counts below 1,000 per $mm^3$ are associated with an increased risk of infection. The organs most commonly affected include the lungs, genitourinary tract, and skin. It is important to realize that many of the signs and symptoms of infection (fever, erythema, infiltrates) may be absent. Therefore, with heightened suspicion immediate treatment should be started. In addition to broad-spec-

**TABLE 13.** *Recognized causes for neutropenia*

I. Abnormalities of bone marrow
  a. Injury
    1. Drugs
      (a) Antiarrhythmics: procainamide, quinidine, propranolol
      (b) Antibiotics: penicillins, sulfonamides, trimethoprim-sulfa, vancomycin
      (c) Phenothiazine: chlorpromazine, prochlorperazine
      (d) Antithyroid agents: methimazole, propylthiouracil
      (e) Antihypertensives: captopril, methyldopa
      (f) Antihistamines: cimetidine, ranitidine
      (g) Anticonvulsants: phenytoin, carbamazepine
      (h) Diuretics: hydrochlorothiazide, acetazolamide
      (i) Cytotoxic agents: hydroxyurea, alkylating agents, antimetabolites
      (j) Other: alcohol, allopurinol, alpha-interferon
    2. Chemicals (arsenic, bismuth, nitrous oxide, benzene)
    3. Radiation
    4. Congenital/hereditary neutropenia
    5. Infection (viral, bacterial)
    6. Infiltrative diseases (metastatic malignancy, fibrosis, CML[a])
  b. Maturation defects
    1. Neoplastic (myelodysplastic syndromes, acute non-lymphocytic leukemia)
    2. Acquired (folic acid/$B_{12}$ deficiency)
II. Abnormalities in peripheral blood
  a. Shift from circulating to marginated pool
    1. Hereditary pseudoneutropenia
    2. Protein calorie malnutrition
    3. Severe bacterial infections
  b. Sequestration
    1. Hypersplenism
    2. Leukoagglutination (complement mediated)
II. Abnormalities in extravascular compartment
  a. Destruction (antibody mediated)
  b. Increased utilization (infection, anaphylaxis)

[a]CML, Chronic Myelogenous Leukemia

trum antibiotics, some benefit may be derived from the administration granulocyte colony-stimulating factor.

A careful evaluation of blood counts and the peripheral smear is required in patients with neutropenia. A bone marrow examination may also provide insights through assessment of (a) cellularity and (b) cellular differentiation.

Lymphopenia often represents a response to an underlying disease. Several mechanisms can be involved: (a) suppressed bone marrow production (malnutrition, radiation, viral infection), (b) peripheral destruction (viral infections, autoantibodies), and (c) changes in lymphocyte mobilization (trauma, corticosteroids).

## Leukocytosis

During *leukocytosis* peripheral white blood cell counts above 11,000 per mm$^3$ are common in critically ill patients. Counts in excess of 25,000 per mm$^3$ are considered a leukomold reaction. Most often, the excess involves neutrophils (neutrophilia); however lymphocytosis, monocytosis, basophilia, and eosinophilia can also occur.

Neutrophilia (>7,500 per mm$^3$) occurs as a result of changes in the bone marrow, peripheral blood, or extravascular space. Infection and inflammatory states are the most common causes, but many other etiologies exist (Table 14).

Lymphocytosis (>5,000 per mm$^3$) is associated with a variety of infectious (viral, Brucellosis, tuberculosis, toxoplasmosis, typhoid fever), malignant (solid tumors, Hodgkin's lymphoma, chronic lymphocytic leukemia, acute lymphocytic leukemia), and endocrine (thyrotoxicosis) diseases.

Monocytosis (>500 per mm$^3$) is observed in the following circumstances: infection (Brucellosis, tuberculosis, syphilis, bacterial endocarditis, protozoal, fungal), neoplastic disease (Hodgkin's lymphoma, myelomonocytic leukemias), gastrointestinal illness (cirrhosis, ulcerative colitis), drug reactions, and recovery from bone marrow suppression. Eosinophilia (>400 per mm$^3$) is associated with a wide variety of infectious, allergic, connective tissue, cutaneous, and inflammatory disorders.

Basophilia (>150 per mm$^3$) is relatively uncommon but specific for an underlying abnormality such as (a) myeloproliferative disorders or (b) paraneoplastic syndromes.

## COAGULATION CONSIDERATIONS

Blood normally circulates through endothelium-lined vessels without appreciable coagulation or hemorrhage taking place. Vascular injury triggers the hemostatic process, typically beginning with platelet adherence to damaged or dysfunctional endothelium or exposed subendothelium. Concomitantly, plasma proteins react with the subendothelium, initiating the coagulation

**TABLE 14.** *Common causes of neutrophilia*

I. Infection
  a. Bacteria
  b. Viruses
  c. Parasites
  d. Fungi
II. Neoplastic disorders
  a. Pancreas, lung, renal
  b. Metastatic disease to bone marrow
  c. Chronic myeloproliferative disorders
  d. Hodgkin's disease
  e. Acute leukemia
III. Autoimmune disorders
  a. Vasculitis
  b. Ulcerative colitis
  c. Collagen vascular diseases
IV. Hematologic disorders
  a. Acute hemolysis
  b. Transfusion reactions
  c. Postsplenectomy
V. Drugs
  a. Corticosteroids
  b. Lithium chloride
  c. Epinephrine
  d. Chemicals
    1. Venoms (reptiles, insects)
    2. Ethylene glycol
VI. Trauma
  a. Thermal injury
  b. Crush injuries
  c. electrical shock
VII. Endocrine disorders
  a. Ketoacidosis
  b. Thyrotoxicosis
  c. Lactic acidosis
VIII. Systemic inflammatory reactions

cascade (Figs. 1 and 2). In pathologic conditions, platelet–vessel wall (or plaque) interactions initiate local thrombus formation, either causing an immediate impedance to physiologic blood flow or serving as a nidus for subsequent vascular events.

## Anatomy and Vascular Biology

### Vascular Endothelium

The vascular endothelium is structurally simple but functionally complex. Its integrity is essential for normal vessel responsiveness and thromboresistance. Until recently the vascular endothelium was thought to represent no more than a protective barrier, separating platelets and the contact-activated coagulation factors from thrombogenic subendothelial connective tissues. It is now known that the endothelial lining is, in fact, a multifunctional organ system composed of metabolically active and physiologically responsive component cells. Moreover, we now appreciate that vascular endothelial

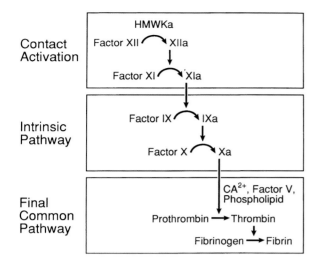

**FIG. 1.** Intrinsic coagulation cascade (pathway) is initiated by contact activation through a series of enzymatic steps involving the activation of coagulation proteins; fibrinogen is converted to fibrin in the final common pathway (HMWKA, high molecular weight kininogen).

cells are susceptible to injury (biochemical or mechanical), which may be relevant to certain disease processes such as coronary atherosclerosis.

*Structural Anatomy*

In most vertebrates vascular endothelial cells form a single layer of simple squamous lining cells (0.1 to .5μm in thickness, and elongated in the long axis of the vessel, thus orienting the cellular longitudinal dimension in the direction of blood flow).

The endothelial cell has three surfaces; nonthrombogenic (luminal), adhesive (subluminal), and cohesive.

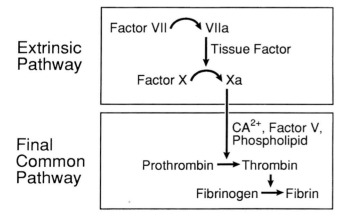

**FIG. 2.** Extrinsic coagulation cascade (pathway) is initiated by tissue factor expression, which combined with factor VIIa activates the final common pathway and fibrin generation.

The luminal surface is nonthrombogenic and devoid of any electron-dense connective tissue. It does, however, possess an exterior coat, or glycocalyx, that consists primarily of starches and proteins secreted by the endothelial cells: oligosaccharides, glycoproteins, glycolipids, and sialoconjugates. Plasma proteins, including lipoprotein lipase, $\alpha_2$-macroglobulin, antithrombin III, heparin cofactor II, albumin, and small amounts of fibrinogen and fibrin are adsorbed to the luminal surface. The luminal membrane itself adds significantly to the thromboresistant properties, carrying a negative charge that repels similarly charged circulating blood cells.

The subluminal (or abluminal) surface adheres to the connective tissue of the subendothelial zone. Small processes penetrate throughout a series of internal layers to form myoendothelial junctions with subjacent smooth muscle cells.

The third surface of the vascular endothelium is cohesive, joining endothelial cells to one another by cell junctions of two basic types: occluding (tight) junctions and communicating (gap) junctions. Occluding junctions represent a physical link between two adjoining cells, sealing the intercellular space. The communicating junctions provide the structural substrate for direct two-way communication between cells. They are instrumental in the electronic coupling and intracellular exchange of ions and small metabolites.

*Normal Function*

As an active site of protein synthesis, the vascular endothelium may be considered the largest and most productive organ system in the human body. Endothelial cells synthesize, secrete, modify, and regulate connective tissue components, vasodilators, and vasoconstrictors, anticoagulants, procoagulants, fibrinolytic compounds, and prostanoids, each contributing to the maintenance of normal vasomotion, thromboresistance, and physiologic hemostasis (Figs. 3 and 4A,B).

*Prostacyclin*

Prostacyclin (PGI$_2$) is a potent vasodilating substance released locally in response to biochemical and mechanical mediators, including thromboxane A$_2$, thrombin, bradykinin, histamine, high-density lipoprotein, platelet-derived growth factor, tissue hypoxia, and hemodynamic stress (1). By increasing intracellular cyclic adenosine monophosphate (cAMP), PGI$_2$ also inhibits platelet aggregation. Furthermore, there is evidence that PGI$_2$ increases the rate of smooth muscle cell cholesterol ester metabolism, suppresses lipid metabolism within macrophages, and inhibits the release of growth factors, which mediate proliferative responses to intravascular shear stress (2).

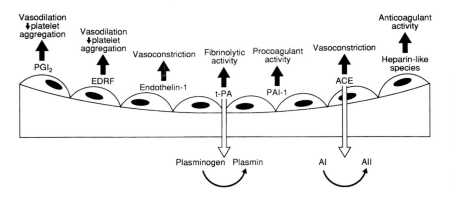

**FIG. 3.** Vascular endothelium is one of this body's most active organs, synthesizing and secreting proteins that determine thromboresistance and vasoreactivity (PGI₂, prostacyclin; EDRF, endothelium-derived relaxing factor; t-PA, tissue plasminogen activator; PAI₁, plasminogen activator inhibitor-1; ACE, angiotensin-converting anzyme; AI, angiotensin 1; AII, angiotensin 2).

### Endothelium-Derived Relaxing Factor

Utilizing strips of arteries in organ baths (isolated system), Furchgott and Zawadski (3) discovered that acetylcholine-mediated vasodilation requires an intact vascular endothelium (i.e., it is endothelium dependent) (Table 15). Endothelium-derived relaxing factor (EDRF), recently identified as nitric oxide (4), is an L-arginine derivative that relaxes smooth muscles by increasing intracellular cyclic guanosine monophosphate (cAMP). It is released locally in response to a number of mediators, including thrombin, bradykinin, thromboxane A₂, histamine, adenine nucleotides, and aggregating platelets. In addition to vasoactive properties, EDRF is also a potent inhibitor of platelet adhesion (5) and aggregation (6). Moreover, EDRF and PGI₂ appear to have synergistic antiaggregatory properties.

### Angiotensin II

Studied extensively over the past two decades, angiotensin II is a potent vasoconstrictor that exerts an important effect on vascular tone (7). Although the systemic properties of angiotensin II have been known for some time, local synthesis, release, and vascular activity have just recently been appreciated. Angiotensin-con-

verting enzyme (ACE), required for the conversion of angiotensin I to the active peptide angiotensin II, has been isolated from mammalian arteries and veins. While there has been some debate, most studies suggest that ACE is synthesized within vascular endothelial cells. Moreover, there is mounting evidence that endothelial cells are also capable of producing enzymes other than or in addition to ACE capable of angiotensin II generation (8).

### Endothelin

The vascular endothelium, in addition to synthesizing vasodilating substances such as PGI₂ and EDRF, also produces vasoconstrictors essential for maintaining vessel tone and responsiveness. Endothelin, a small peptide, has vasoconstricting properties ten times those of angiotensin II (9). Although three structurally and pharmacologically distinct isopeptides have been isolated and characterized, only endothelin-1 is synthesized by vascular endothelial cells (10). While a majority of vasoactive mediators are released in surges following local mechanical or biochemical stimulation, endothelin-1 is released slowly and, via specific receptor-mediated mechanisms, activates intracellular protein kinase C (11), leading to smooth muscle contraction (vessel constriction).

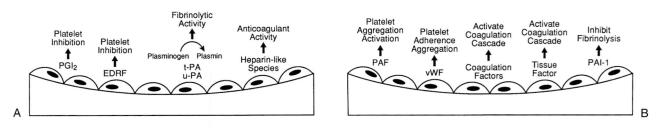

**FIG. 4. A:** Vascular endothelium normally prevents or limits thrombus formation through the synthesis and secretion of thromboresistant proteins (PGI₂, prostacyclin; U-PA, urokinase-like plasminogen activator). **B:** Damaged pr dysfunctional/endothelial cells may promote thrombus formation through platelet activation, coagulation, and impaired fibrinolytic activity (PAF, platelet activating factor; vWF, von Willebrand factor; PAI-1, plasminogen activator inhibitor-1).

**TABLE 15.** *Endothelium-independent and endothelium-dependent vasodilators*

| Independent vasodilators | Dependent vasodilators |
|---|---|
| PGE$_1$, PGE$_2$, PGI$_2$ | Acetylcholine |
| Adenosine | Histamine |
| Bradykinin | Serotonin |
| Nitroglycerin | Thrombin |
| Atrial natriuretic polypeptide | Arachidonic acid |
| Sodium nitroprusside | Substance P |
| Nitric oxide | Leukotrienes (LTC$_4$, LTD$_4$) |
| Insulin | Epinephrine, norepinephrine |
| Glucagon | |

PGE$_1$, prostaglandin E$_1$; PGE$_2$; PGI$_2$, prostacyclin.

## Plasminogen Activators

Vascular endothelial cells synthesize and release activators that are capable of converting plasminogen to the serine protease plasmin, an enzyme that proteolytically degrades fibrin (and fibrinogen). Tissue plasminogen activator and urokinase-type plasminogen activator generate plasmin locally; therefore, fibrinolysis is limited to the immediate local environment. Stimuli for the release of vascular plasminogen activators include epinephrine, thrombin, heparin, interleukin-1, venous occlusion, aggregating platelets, and desamino-8-D-arginine vasopressin (DDAVP).

## Heparin-Like Species

In the past, mast cells were thought to be the only cells capable of synthesizing anticoagulant-active heparin. Investigations performed by Teien et al. (12), Thomas et al. (13), and Rosenberg (14) have shown, however, that endothelial cells are capable of synthesizing heparin-like molecules (e.g., heparan sulfate) with anticoagulant properties. As a result, it is currently accepted that thromboresistance is mediated at least in part, through the interaction of heparin-like substances with antithrombin III and heparin cofactor II (both located on the endothelial surface), accelerating the neutralization of hemostatic (procoagulant) proteins.

## Platelet-Activating Factor

A lipid capable of inducing platelet aggregation and secretion in a concentration-dependent fashion, platelet-activating factor (PAF) mobilizes platelet surface membrane arachidonic acid, which stimulates thromboxane A$_2$ synthesis.

## Tissue Factor

Tissue factor, also known as tissue thromboplastin, is a lipoprotein present in large quantities in a number of organ systems, including the brain and lung parenchyma. Although tissue factor is, under normal conditions, produced by endothelial cells in small amounts, synthesis can be increased markedly after mechanical or biochemical stimulation, accelerating the activation of factor X by factor VIIa (15, 16).

## Von Willebrand Factor

Circulating in plasma as a series of self-aggregated structures composed of a single glycoprotein subunit, von Willebrand factor is a vital component of normal hemostasis that mediates both platelet–vessel wall interactions and platelet-platelet interactions (17).

## Plasminogen Activator Inhibitor

Plasminogen activator inhibitor-1 (PAI-1) is a single-chain glycoprotein that forms stable complexes with tissue plasminogen activator and urokinase-type plasminogen activator, inhibiting their fibrinolytic activity (18). Endothelial cells are able to increase PAI-1 production and do so following administration of exogenous tissue plasminogen activator (t-PA) or after direct exposure to platelet lysates or compounds released from activated platelets (epidermal growth factor, transforming growth factor beta (19–21).

## Platelets

Despite being simple in appearance, platelets are complex cellular elements with complicated structural and functional characteristics.

### Structural Anatomy

1. The *peripheral zone* consists of membranes and closely associated structures that provide surfaces for the platelet itself and the tortuous channels of the open canalicular system. The peripheral zone consists of three distinct structural domains: the exterior coat, the unit membrane, and the submembrane region.

The exterior coat, or glycocalyx, is rich in glycoproteins (GPs). Recent biochemical studies have identified nine distinct glycoproteins: Ia, Ib, Ic, IIa, IIb, IIIa, IV, V, and IX. Many glycoproteins act as receptors for platelet-platelet and platelet–vessel wall interactions.

The unit membrane provides a physiochemical separation between intracellular and extracellular constituents and processes. Important components of the unit membrane include Na/K, adenosinetriphospahatase (ATPase), and other anion or cation pumps that maintain transmembrane ionic gradients.

The submembrane region contains a specialized filamentous system similar to actin microfilaments. Functionally submembrane filaments assist circumferential microtubules, maintaining platelet discoid shape, controlling pseudopod extrusion, and interacting with other elements of the platelet contractile mechanism.

2. The *sol-gel zone* is the matrix of the platelet cytoplasm. It contains several fiber systems in various states of polymerization, maintaining the discoid shape of nonstimulated platelets and providing the intricate contractile system required to initiate shape change, pseudopod extension, internal contraction, and secretion.

3. The *organelle zone* consists of granules, electron-dense bodies, peroxisomes, lysosomes, and mitochondria randomly dispersed in the platelet cytoplasm. It is centrally involved with metabolic processes and also acts as a storage site for enzymes, adenine nucleotides, serotonin, calcium, and a variety of protein constituents.

## Membrane Systems

The platelet membrane systems include a surface-connected canalicular system, which provides access for plasma-borne substances to the platelet interior and an exit route for products of the release reaction, and a dense tubular system, which acts as a site for calcium sequestration and for storing prostaglandin precursors.

## Normal Platelet Physiology

### Platelet Adhesion

Platelet surface membrane receptors are essential for adhesion. Glycoprotein Ia (GPIa) binds with collagen at low shear rates and may also contribute to platelet adherence in areas of vascular damage. Glycoprotein Ib (GPIb) serves as a binding site for von Willebrand factor, particularly at high shear rates. Glycoprotein IIb/IIIa (GPIIb/IIIa) may also participate in platelet adhesion within areas of high shear rate.

### Platelet Aggregation

Activated platelets undergo a progressive change in shape and release calcium from the dense tubular system. Adenosine diphosphate (ADP), serotonin, and thromboxane $A_2$ are subsequently released, exposing platelet receptors for fibrinogen, the molecular "glue" for platelet aggregation.

### Platelet–Coagulation Protein Interactions

Beyond their ability to provide coagulation proteins, including factors II, V, VII, IX, X, XI, and XIII, high-molecular-weight kininogen, and fibrinogen, platelets contain specific receptors for a number of circulating hemostatic proteases and can also trigger contact-activated coagulation. Moreover, platelets provide a protective nidus for activated clotting factors from circulating plasma inhibitors (22).

### Platelet-Lipid Interactions

Hypercholesterolemia has been shown to influence platelet activity. Increased adhesion, aggregation, and serotonin release have been reported (23), as have increased circulating levels or the potent platelet agonist thromboxane $A_2$ (24) and decreased sensitivity to the platelet-inhibiting properties of $PGI_2$ (25). Cholesterol feeding is associated with increased platelet activatability (26, 27); however, a reduction of cholesterol through either dietary or pharmacologic means returns platelet activity to its normal state (28).

Although the mechanism(s) underlying the relation between serum cholesterol concentration and platelet activity are not fully understood, it has been shown that changes in the cholesterol content of the platelet surface membrane profoundly affect overall membrane fluidity. In turn, fluidity, or the cells' lipid-water interface, influences lipase activity. Therefore, it has been proposed that hypercholesterolemia-mediated increases in the cholesterol content of the platelet surface membrane enhance diglyceride lipase or phospholipase $A_2$ activity (or both), which increases the release of arachidonic acid, the substrate for thromboxane $A_2$ synthesis (29, 30).

Hypercholesterolemia and atherosclerosis impair endothelium-dependent relaxation of major epicardial coronary arteries. Although marked intimal atherosclerosis is frequently observed in these vessels, the endothelium is morphologically intact; however, it fails to release EDRF, a potent vasodilator and inhibitor of platelet aggregation (31, 32). It is widely believed, therefore, that hypercholesterolemia in and of itself may directly impair vascular endothelial cell function and enhance platelet–vessel wall interactions prior to the development of overt atherosclerosis (33–35).

## Acquired Disorders of Coagulation

Acquired disorders of coagulation develop in patients without a prior history of bleeding from a new condition, disease process, or medication. The coagulation disorder may be due to defective synthesis, increased loss, or the presence of substances (including therapeutic agents) that interfere with the normal function of one or more vital hemostatic components.

### Liver Disease

Fibrinogen synthesis is impaired in both acute and chronic liver disease. In addition, the fibrinogen molecule itself is frequently dysfunctional, displaying defective polymerization (36). The liver is also a primary source of prothrombin and coagulation factors VII, IX, and X. Vitamin-K-dependent carboxylation, a process occurring in hepatic microsomes, is defective in liver disease, preventing the synthesis of functionally normal coagulation proteins (acarboxy forms of factors II, VII, IX, and X cannot bind calcium and therefore cannot participate in normal hemostasis). Interestingly, defective carboxylation is one of the earliest signs of liver dysfunction. Factor V is partially synthesized by hepatocytes and partially in hepatic reticuloendothelial cells. As a result, low levels of factor V are found in acute liver failure. Plasminogen and antithrombin III levels are also decreased in liver disease. Under normal circumstances the liver metabolizes activated coagulation factors from circulating blood (37). In addition, it effectively clears both fibrin(ogen) degradation products (FDP) and plasminogen activators. Accordinly, the biochemical environment observed in patients with liver disease is both procoagulant and anticoagulant. However, this unique situation commonly favors anticoagulation. Platelet abnormalities, both qualitative and quantitative, add to the increased bleeding tendency.

## Clinical Approach

Thrombotic episodes are relatively uncommon among patients with liver disease, despite reductions in antithrombin III, plasminogen, and plasminogen activator levels. Instead, hemorrhagic complications predominate the clinical picture. The most common sites of bleeding include the nasopharynx, esophagus, stomach, small intestine, and retroperitoneum.

In acute liver disease, coagulation abnormalities parallel other signs of hepatic damage; in fact, prolongation of standard coagulation tests (PT, aPTT, TT) has prognostic value.

A major challenge confronting the clinician is treatment. Replacement of coagulation factors through fresh frozen plasma transfusion and vitamin K replacement may reduce the incidence of life-threatening hemorrhage; however, complete correlation of the coagulopathy is usually not possible in acute liver failure. Platelet transfusions should also be considered in patients with platelet counts less than 30,000 per mm$^3$.

With either acute or chronic liver disease complicated by moderate to severe bleeding, other treatment measures, including endoscopic and surgical, should be considered early given the inherent difficulty in correcting the coagulopathy.

## Renal Disease

Thrombocytopenia is common in renal disease and reflects a combination of reduced production and periph-

eral consumption. Platelet dysfunction also occurs and is thought to represent a defect in the platelet release reaction (38). An imbalance between vascular prostacyclin synthesis and platelet thromboxane synthesis may also contribute (39).

Despite increased fibrinogen and factor VIII levels in patients with renal disease, prolongation of the PT and PTT is commonly observed, probably from reduced levels of factors V, VII, and X. Low-grade DIC may also cause reduction in clotting factors through consumption. This may explain, at least in some patients, the elevations in FDP so commonly seen in renal failure. Alternatively, impaired hepatic and renal clearance may be responsible.

Antithrombin III is reduced in patients with renal disease complicated by nephrotic syndrome (40).

## Clinical Approach

Hemorrhage is not an uncommon event among patients with renal disease. In a majority of cases, the skin, mucous membranes, and gastrointestinal tract are the sites of involvement. Occasionally, life-threatening bleeding may occur, particularly in those with both platelet and coagulation abnormalities.

In contrast, serious thrombotic (arterial or venous) events have been described in patients with nephrotic syndrome (40). As a result, these individuals must be approached somewhat differently.

The general approach to bleeding problems includes the correction of underlying metabolic abnormalities. The institution of dialysis in a uremic patient may have an important impact on hemostasis. If the standard coagulation tests (PT, aPTT) are prolonged, vitamin K replacement should be provided, followed by fresh frozen plasma if the clinical setting so warrants.

Platelet transfusions and intravenous DDAVP should also be considered for moderate to severe bleeding complications.

### Disseminated Intravascular Coagulation

Disseminated intravascular coagulation is not a specific disease entity but a complex event characterized by abnormal bleeding, small-vessel obstruction, tissue necrosis, and end-organ damage. The clinical picture and natural history are extremely variable, making diagnosis and treatment difficult. The initial event in DIC is activation of the coagulation cascade. Three major mechanisms may be involved: (a) endothelial injury with activation of the intrinsic pathway, (b) tissue injury with activation of the extrinsic pathway, and (c) direct proteolytic cleavage of factor X and activation of the prothrombinase complex. Following activation of the coagulation cascades, fibrin is generated. Although it would seem that thrombosis would be the next step, this is not always the case. For reasons that are unclear, the formation of soluble fibrin results in both consumption of coagulation factors (bleeding tendency) *and* impaired fibrinolysis (thrombotic tendency).

*Clinical Approach*

The keys to management are diagnosing and treating the underlying disorder (Table 16). Antibiotics, volume replacement, inotropic/vasopressor support, and surgical intervention should be applied as indicated without delay. Several laboratory tests should be obtained, including a complete blood count, platelet count, fibrinogen and FDP concentrations, and standard coagulation measurements (PT, aPTT, TT). Other tests such as Bβ1-42 (D-dimer), antithrombin III, prothrombin fragment 1.2 (F1.2), and Fibrino-peptide A concentrations, while helpful at times, lack specificity, are expensive, and are not readily available through nonspecialized laboratories (Table 17).

The specific treatment of DIC is limited but can be broken down into three categories; (a) restoration of hemostasis, (b) thrombosis prevention, and (c) thrombus removal. Transfusion of blood and fresh frozen plasma may be required to restore blood volume and replace consumed coagulation factors. Cryoprecipitate and platelet transfusions can be used in the presence of severe bleeding; however, the theoretical risk of "fueling the fire" does exist. Low-dose heparin (300 to 400 units/hr) has been used to prevent microthrombosis in animal models of DIC. It can be used cautiously in clinical situations where the risk of bleeding is relatively minor compared with the probability of thrombosis. It also should be considered when a thrombotic event (e.g., pulmonary embolism) is the precipitating cause for DIC. In this case, standard heparin doses may be used if clinical bleeding is not evident. However, when bleeding does occur, thrombectomy (surgical, extraction catheter) may be necessary.

**TABLE 16.** *Conditions and disorders associated with disseminated intravascular coagulation*

I. Acute
   a. Shock (cardiogenic, septic, neurogenic, hypovolemic)
   b. Pulmonary embolism
   c. Cardiac arrest
   d. Major trauma
   e. Burns
   f. Hyperthermia
   g. Amnionic fluid embolism
II. Subacute
   a. Metastatic malignancy
   b. Pancreatic, gastrointestinal, ovarian cancer
   c. Promyelocytic leukemia
III. Chronic
   a. Liver disease
   b. Collagen vascular diseases
   c. Solid tumors
   d. Renal disease
   e. Liver disease

**TABLE 17.** *Standard coagulation measurements and laboratory tests in disseminated intravascular coagulation*

| Measurement | Acute | Subacute | Chronic |
|---|---|---|---|
| Prothrombin time | ↑↑ | ↑ | Normal, ↓, or ↑ |
| Partial thromboplastin time | ↑↑ | ↑ | Normal, ↓, or ↑ |
| Thrombin time | ↑↑ | ↑ | Normal, ↓, or ↑ |
| Fibrinogen level | ↓↓ | ↓ or normal | Normal, ↓, or ↑ |
| FDP[a] level | ↑↑ | ↑↑ | Normal, ↓, or ↑ |
| Platelet count | ↓ | Variable | Variable |

[a]Fibrin(ogen) degradation products.

### Cardiopulmonary Bypass

The cardiopulmonary bypass circuit consists of nearly 12 m$^2$ of synthetic surfaces, including polyvinyl chloride, silicone rubber, polyurethane (flexible tubing), and polystyrene (rigid connectors). In the roller pump, flexible tubing undergoes considerable deformation and the blood is exposed to high shear rates, turbulence, and hydraulic stresses. Additional shear stress is imposed by the heat exchanger, which contains a surface of uncoated or pyrolytic carbon-coated stainless steel. The gas exchange devices, gas interface, and membrane oxygenators impose damaging effects of high shearing stress at both the gas-blood and blood—synthetic membrane interfaces (41).

Blood coming into direct contact with synthetic surfaces is the proposed mechanism for hemostatic abnormalities observed following cardiopulmonary bypass. Quantitative and qualitative platelet abnormalities occur following platelet activation and release of intracellular granules (acquired storage pool deficiency) (42, 43). The reduced platelet count commonly seen is the result of both consumption and hemodilution (44). Contact activation of the intrinsic coagulation cascade can lead to fibrin formation and consumption of circulating coagulation proteins. Plasmin is generated as well, increasing fibrinolytic potential. For these reasons, adequate systemic anticoagulation is vital during cardiopulmonary bypass (45).

*Clinical Approach*

Bleeding complications following cardiopulmonary bypass require immediate attention. Once the source of bleeding has been identified and local measures have been undertaken, efforts must address the defective hemostatic mechanism. It is important to keep in mind that abnormalities in platelet function, coagulation, and fibrinolysis almost always coexist. The extent and severity of the acquired coagulopathy may also be augmented by preoperative medical treatment, which for many unstable cardiac patients with coronary artery disease includes heparin, aspirin, and at times, thrombolytic agents (Fig. 5).

**Guidelines For The Management of Post-operative Bleeding**

? Normal hemostatic parameters pre-op
? Adequate heparinization during cardiopulmonary bypass
? Adequate heparin neutralization with protamine sulfate

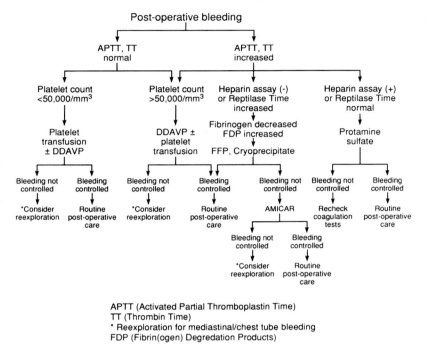

APTT (Activated Partial Thromboplastin Time)
TT (Thrombin Time)
* Reexploration for mediastinal/chest tube bleeding
FDP (Fibrin(ogen) Degredation Products)

**FIG. 5.** General approach to bleeding complications following coronary bypass grafting. High-risk patients may benefit from routine aprotinin administration in the perioperative period.

## Disorders of Hemostasis Associated with Medical Treatment

Over 50% of bleeding complications occurring in patients with cardiac disease are the result of medical treatment and invasive procedures. As many patients with advanced cardiac disease treated with antithrombotic agents and invasive procedures (central line placement, cardiac catheterization, circulatory assist device insertion, and coronary angioplasty) are commonplace, the mechanism of action, pharmacology, biology, monitoring, and treatment of commonly used drugs should be well known to practicing clinicians.

### Platelet-Inhibiting Agents

The participation of platelets in the thrombotic process depends on their ability to adhere to an abnormal surface, aggregate to form an initial platelet plug, and activate, thus stimulating further aggregation and triggering the coagulation cascade. Therefore, pharmacologic strategies designed to inhibit platelet activity have focused on these three fundamental mechanisms of action. In addition, the recognition that growth factors released from platelets may influence cellular proliferation and atheroma forma-

tion has provided yet another potential target for newer agents (46, 47) (Table 18).

### Agents That Inhibit Platelet Adhesion

In areas of severe coronary arterial narrowing caused by underlying atheroma, plaque rupture, or hemorrhage, platelet adhesion and aggregation are mediated by von Willebrand factor and the platelet receptors GPIb and GPIIb/IIIa. Monoclonal antibodies to von Willebrand factor (48) and aurintricarboxylic acid (49), a triphenylmethyl dye compound, inhibit platelets in regions of high shear stress through their binding to von Willebrand factor, preventing its interaction with platelet receptors and damaged or dysfunctional vessel walls. These agents may be useful for short-term therapy. Long-term therapy, however, may be associated with a significant risk of bleeding.

### Agents That Inhibit Platelet Aggregation

#### Aspirin

Following oral ingestion, aspirin is rapidly absorbed in the stomach and the duodenum, achieving peak serum levels within 20 to 30 minutes. Enteric-coated prepara-

**TABLE 18.** *Platelet-inhibiting agents in clinical use or development*

I. Inhibit platelet adhesion
   a. Aurintricarboxylic acid
   b. von Willebrand factor monoclonal antibody
II. Inhibit platelet aggregation
   a. Aspirin
   b. Glycoprotein IIb/IIIa receptor antagonists
      1. Monoclonal antibodies
      2. RGD-peptides
      3. Non-peptides
   c. Ticlopidine
   d. Thromboxane synthetase inhibitors
   e. Thromboxane/endoperoxide receptor inhibitors
   f. Dextran
   g. Nitrate preparations
III. Inhibit platelet activation
   a. Dipyridamole
   b. Prostaglandin $E_1$
   c. Prostacyclin
   d. Calcium channel blockers
IV. Inhibit platelet growth factors
   a. Trapidil

tions are less well absorbed (unless they are chewed), resulting in a delay in peak serum levels to approximately 60 minutes.

Aspirin irreversibly acetylates cyclooxygenase, impairing prostaglandin metabolism and thromboxane $A_2$ synthesis. As a result, platelet aggregation in response to collagen, ADP, and thrombin (in low concentrations) is inhibited (50). Adherence and platelet release, however, are not affected. Because, unlike vascular endothelial cells, platelets lack the synthetic capacity to regenerate cyclooxygenase, aspirin's inhibitory effect persists for the life span of the platelet (7 ± 2 days). The antithrombotic effect of aspirin can be achieved with doses ranging from 160 to 325 mg/day (and possibly lower); therefore, the toxic side effects seen with higher doses can be avoided (51).

Although nonsteroidal anti-inflammatory drugs also inhibit platelet cyclooxygenase, they do so in a reversible manner. In addition, these compounds have not been adequately tested in large randomized clinical trials. Therefore, their use in the prevention or treatment of cardiovascular disease cannot be recommended at this time (52).

### GPIIb/IIIa Receptor Blockers

The platelet GPIIB/IIIa receptor is unique in two ways. First, normal platelets have a large number of receptors (~50,000) on their surface. Second, platelet activation exposes the GPIIb/IIIa receptor, leading to platelet aggregation. In essence, all physiologic platelet agonists act by exposing the GPIIb/IIIa receptor.

Monoclonal antibodies to the GPIIb/IIIa receptor have been developed recently. The F(AB)$_2$ fragment of this antibody can completely block in vitro platelet aggregation induced by agonists thought to function in vivo, even in high concentrations or in combinations (53).

The ability of GPIIb/IIIa to bind a number of naturally occurring substances has been explained, at least in part by the fact that it contains a binding site for the tripeptide arginine-glycine-aspartic acid (Arg-Gly-Asp). All substances that bind to the GPIIb/IIIa receptor contain this amino acid sequence; therefore, synthetic compounds containing the sequence can inhibit the binding of fibrinogen to GPIIb/IIIa. The RGD (Arg-Gly-Asp), RGDS (Arg-Gly-Asp-Ser), and RGDF (Arg-Gly-Asp-Phe) peptides represent a new class of proteins that inhibit platelet aggregation (54).

### Ticlopidine

Ticlopidine is structurally distinct from all other antiplatelet agents. It is a potent inhibitor of platelet aggregation induced by ADP and variably inhibits aggregation provoked by collagen, epinephrine, arachidonic acid, thrombin, and platelet-activating factor. Ticlopidine also inhibits the platelet release action and may impair platelet adhesion as well (55). Structurally similar analogues are under clinical investigation.

### Thromboxane Synthetase Inhibitors

Thromboxane synthetase inhibitors (Dazoxiben, pirmagrel) have been developed to suppress platelet thromboxane $A_2$ synthesis, thereby preventing platelet aggregation (56, 57). Despite their potential beneficial effects, currently available agents have been limited by two factors: incomplete thromboxane $A_2$ inhibition and the aggregating potential of endoperoxide intermediates.

### Inhibitors of Thromboxane and Endoperoxide Receptors

The potential limitations of thromboxane synthetase inhibitors can, at least theoretically, be managed by inhibiting the receptors for both thromboxane $A_2$ and the active endoperoxide intermediates. In addition to inhibiting platelet aggregation, the vasoactive effects of thromboxane $A_2$ can also be blocked (58).

### Dextran

Dextran is a polysaccharide that ranges in molecular weight from 65,000 to 80,000 daltons. It has been shown to prolong bleeding time in humans; however, its mechanism of action is unclear. There is evidence suggesting that dextran binds to the platelet surface, altering membrane receptor function and inhibiting platelet aggregation (59). Decreased levels of the factor VIII:vWF (von Willebrand factor) complex have also been reported (60).

## Agents That Inhibit Platelet Activation

Cyclic adenosine monophosphate (cAMP) is a major modulator of platelet activation and release. The platelet response to stimulation is inhibited when intracellular cAMP levels are elevated by agents that activate adenylate cyclase (the enzyme that converts ATP to cAMP) or that inhibit phosphodiesterase (the enzyme responsible for cAMP degradation).

### Dipyridamole

Dipyridamole (Persantine) is a pyrimidopyrimidine derivative first used as an antianginal agent because of its vasodilating properties. It was subsequently known to inhibit platelet activation and has been postulated to do so through one or more mechanisms, including inhibition of phosphodiesterase, stimulation and release of endothelial prostacyclin, or inhibiting cellular uptake and metabolism of adenosine, which increases in concentration at the platelet-vessel interface (61). High concentrations of dipyridamole are required to influence platelet aggregation in vitro. It is not surprising, therefore, that the observed effects in vivo have been both modest and inconsistent.

### Prostaglandin $E_1$

Prostaglandin $E_1$ ($PGE_1$) inhibits platelet activation and aggregation primarily by increasing intracellular cAMP. It may also have the capacity to deaggregate aggregated platelets (62). The clinical usefulness of $PGE_1$ is limited by the extensive first-pass metabolism, which takes place in the lungs. Indeed, 70% of the activated compound is eliminated, resulting in extremely low plasma levels. Therefore, direct intravascular infusions are required to achieve therapeutic concentrations (63).

### Prostacyclin

Prostacyclin ($PGI_2$) is a potent, naturally occurring platelet inhibitor. Its role in the treatment of cardiovascular disease has been limited by its instability in plasma and its propensity to cause systemic hypotension when given in doses required to inhibit platelet activation (64). In contrast, the prostacyclin analogues Iloprost and ciprostene are chemically stable compounds. Because they are both platelet inhibitors, further investigation is in progress (65).

### Calcium Channel Antagonists

Because calcium plays a vital role in platelet activation and aggregation, the potential platelet-inhibiting properties of the calcium channel antagonists nifedipine, diltiazem, and verapamil have been investigated. Indeed, each has been shown to inhibit platelet release and aggregation (66–68). In addition, diltiazem appears to potentiate the inhibitory effects of aspirin (69) and prevent platelet-activating factor binding (70).

## Agent That Inhibits Growth Factors

Platelet-derived growth factor (PDGF) is a potent mitogen and chemoattractant capable of stimulating proliferation of smooth muscle cells and fibroblasts in tissue culture (71). The in vitro and in vivo stimulatory effect of PDGF is significantly reduced by Trapidil, a triazolopyrimidine derivative that also has vasodilatory and cholesterol-lowering properties (72). Trapidil is currently undergoing clinical evaluation.

## Clinical Approach

Bleeding events associated with disorders of primary hemostasis most often involve the skin and mucous membranes; however, the gastrointestinal and genitourinary tracts may occasionally be involved. The severity of bleeding is directly related to the degree of platelet dysfunction, integrity of the vasculature, and status of the intrinsic/extrinsic coagulation pathways. In general, an isolated platelet defect is rarely the cause of life-threatening hemorrhage.

The template bleeding time can be measured to provide a general estimate of platelet dysfunction; however, it is nonspecific and vulnerable to error from variable technique. Platelet aggregation studies can also be performed if time allows.

The treatment of bleeding for the most part is nonspecific. As with all hemorrhage, the source should be identified, the offending agent discontinued, and local measures (manual pressure, suturing) explored first. Thereafter, treatment is dictated by the severity of the event. Platelet transfusions either with or without DDAVP should be given for serious or life-threatening bleeding.

## Anticoagulants

### Heparin

The most widely used anticoagulant, heparin, is a heterogenous mucoplysacchoride that accelerates the inhibitory interaction between antithrombin II and several hemostatic proteins, most notably thrombin and factor X. Following intravenous administration, approximately one-third of circulating heparin molecules bind to antithrombin III. The remaining two-thirds have minimal anticoagulant activity A (73, 74).

Heparin is cleared from the circulation through a combination of a rapid saturable mechanism (binding) and a much slower first-order mechanism (renal) (75, 76). After its intravenous administration, heparin binds to vascular endothelial cells, macrophages, and plasma proteins (including von Willebrand factor). The latter phenomenon is responsible for the "heparin resistance" observed in some patients with acute thromboembolic events and subsequent release of acute phase reactant proteins into the circulation (77). Because of these complex kinetics, the anticoagulant effect of heparin at therapeutic doses is not linear, although usually both intensity and duration increase as the dose increases. Therefore, the biological half-life of heparin increases from 30 minutes following an intravenous bolus of 25 units/kg to 60 minutes after a dose of 100 units/kg and 150 minutes with a bolus of 400 units/kg (78).

The anticoagulant effects of heparin are usually monitored with the aPTT, a test sensitive to the inhibitory effects of heparin on thrombin and factor X. Prior clinical studies have shown convincingly that a therapeutic state of systemic anticoagulation (1.5 to 2.5 times control) is a prerequisite for patient benefit when heparin is used in the treatment of venous and arterial thromboembolic disorders (79–81). Because the pharmacokinetics and pharmacodynamics of heparin are complex, frequent monitoring during the course of treatment is required. Unfortunately, the different commercial aPTT reagents vary considerably in their responsiveness to heparin and excessive time delays in the laboratory prevent clinicians from providing optimal care. A recent study by our group suggested that bedside coagulation monitoring could reduce the time needed to achieve a therapeutic state of anticoagulation in heparinized patients admitted to the coronary care unit with unstable angina, acute myocardial infarction, or pulmonary embolism (82).

The most common side effect of heparin is hemorrhage. Other complications include thrombocytopenia (with or without thrombosis), skin necrosis, alopecia, hypersensitivity reaction, and hypoaldosteronism. The risk of bleeding increases with heparin dose (and anticoagulant effect), age, decreasing body weight, trauma, recent surgery, invasive procedures, and the concomitant use of aspirin.

Mild to moderate bleeding complication can be addressed by reducing the heparin dose (particularly if the aPTT is excessively prolonged) or discontinuing the infusion for a brief period of time (30 minutes). More severe hemorrhage may require complete discontinuation or, with serious life-threatening hemorrhage, neutralization with protamine sulfate (1 mg for each 100 units of heparin administered in the preceding 4 hours). However, in patients with active coronary heart disease, a careful risk-benefit assessment must be undertaken, considering the risks of coronary thrombosis versus those of bleeding. It may be in the patient's best interest to continue systemic anticoagulation, particularly if the bleeding is not serious/life threatening and can be adequately controlled with local measures (e.g., manual pressure over a site of vascular trauma).

### Warfarin

Like heparin, warfarin is a frequently used anticoagulant in clinical practice, particularly among patients with cardiac disease. It is rapidly absorbed from the gastrointestinal tract following oral administration, reaches maximal plasma concentration in 90 minutes, and has a circulating half-life of 36 to 42 hours. It circulates bound to plasma proteins. The dose-response profile of warfarin differs between individuals and is influenced by both pharmacokinetic and pharmacodynamic factors. Conditions that affect the availability of vitamin K also influence warfarin response (Table 19).

The PT is the method most commonly used for monitoring warfarin therapy. The PT increases in response to depression of three of the four vitamin-K-dependent

**TABLE 19.** *Drugs, disorders, and the conditions that influence the action of warfarin*

I. Decreased effect
  a. Impaired absorption of warfarin
    1. Cholestyramine
  b. Increase metabolic clearance of warfarin
    1. Ethanol
    2. Rifampin
    3. Barbiturates
    4. Carbamazepine
    5. Hypothyroidism
  c. Increase vitamin K intake (leafy green vegetables, nutritional supplements)
II. Increased effect
  a. Inhibit metabolic clearance of warfarin
    1. Disulfiram
    2. Metronidazole
    3. Amiodarone
    4. Cimetidine
    5. Sulfa derivatives
  b. Increase response (direct pharmacodynamic effect)
    1. Second- and third-generation cephalosporins
    2. Heparin
    3. Clofibrate
  c. Unknown mechanisms
    1. Anabolic steroids
    2. Isoniazid
    3. Ketoconazole
    4. Fluconazole
    5. Tamoxifen
    6. Quinidine
    7. Phenytoin
    8. Propafenone
  d. Potentiate effect of warfarin
    1. Low vitamin K intake
    2. Reduced vitamin K absorption
    3. Hyperthyroidism
    4. Liver disease
    5. Malnutrition (decreased serum albumin)

coagulation proteins—factors II, VII, and X. At the beginning of warfarin administration, prolongation of the PT primarily reflects factor VII depression (shortest half-life). During maintenance therapy, the test is sensitive to depressions in factors II and X as well.

Thromboplastins vary considerably in their responsiveness to depletion of vitamin-K-dependent clotting factors. As a result, PTs determined using different reagents are not interchangeable (83–85). For this reason, a calibration system known as the International Normalized Ratio (INR) was adopted by the World Health Organization in 1982 and is currently used to standardize the reporting of prothrombin times.

Bleeding is the main complication of warfarin therapy. Other complications include skin necrosis and thrombosis in protein-C-deficient patients. The risk of bleeding is directly influenced by the intensity of anticoagulant therapy, age, renal insufficiency, and occult disease of the gastrointestinal and genitourinary tracts.

The anticoagulant effect of warfarin can be reduced or entirely reversed by lowering the dose, discontinuing treatment, administering vitamin K, or replacing the defective coagulation factors with fresh frozen plasma. The severity of bleeding and inherent risks of reduced anticoagulation should dictate the course of action.

### Other Anticoagulants

Several potent and direct thrombin antagonists that can be given either subcutaneously or intravenously are currently undergoing clinical testing. Hirudin and Hirulog, both derivatives of the medicinal leech, have shown promise in animal studies and phase 2 clinical trials. Their safety and efficacy profiles will be more firmly established after the results of large-scale trials are available.

### Thrombolytic Agents

The available thrombolytic agents, including t-PA, streptokinase (SK), anisoylated plasminogen-streptokinase activator complex (APSAC), and urokinase each convert the inactive proenzyme plasminogen to the active enzyme plasmin, which then is responsible for thrombolysis. The lytic state is characterized by plasmin-mediated degradation of coagulation proteins (factors V and VIII) and fibrinogen. Fibrin and fibrinogen degradation causes the release of FDPs, which are capable of inhibiting thrombin, fibrin monomer polymerization, and platelet aggregation (86–89).

Bleeding complications of a serious nature occur in approximately 5% of patients treated with thrombolytic agents. The most feared and devastating complication, intracerebral hemorrhage, occurs in approximately 0.5% to 0.7% of treated patients. Careful patient screening can minimize the likelihood of hemorrhage (Table 20). At the present time, a majority of patients also receive adjuvant treatment with antiplatelet agents (aspirin) and anticoagulants (heparin). This practice probably increases the risk of bleeding, particularly if careful monitoring is not carried out in the first 24 to 48 hours. The challenge facing clinicians is a virtual absence of guidelines for administering and monitoring antithrombotic therapy in patients treated with thrombotics. Fortunately, serious efforts are underway to correct this deficiency (90, 91).

Even with careful patient selection and acceptable monitoring hemorrhagic events do occur. Routine management includes volume and blood pressure support as well as a prompt and thorough search for the site of bleeding. Abdominopelvic or head computed tomography may be useful in the diagnosis and management of major hemorrhagic events. Life-threatening hemorrhage warrants prompt intervention. Heparin should be discontinued and neutralized with protamine sulfate. Fresh frozen plasma is an excellent source of factors V and VIII, $\alpha_2$-antiplasmin, and plasminogen activator inhibitor. Cryoprecipitate (8 to 10 units) is the preferred source of fibrinogen (200 to 250 mg/10 to 15 cc) and factor VIII (80 units/10 to 15cc). If the platelet count is low (<80,000 per mm$^3$), platelets (10 units random donor) should be given. If indicated, DDAVP (0.3 mg/kg IV over 20 minutes) can be used to correct qualitative platelet abnormalities. Persistent and potentially life-threatening hemorrhage unresponsive to standard measures (outlined above) may require antifibrinolytic therapy. This intervention should be used with caution since serious thrombotic complications may be precipitated. Alpha-aminocaproic acid (AMICAR) and tranexamic acid are the most frequently used agents.

### Screening Tests for Hemostasis

Bleeding in critically ill patients may involve an abnormality of blood vessels, platelets, coagulation, or excessive fibrinolysis. If the bleeding diathesis is inherited, usually only one of these components is involved, whereas

---

**TABLE 20.** *Identifying patients at risk for serious hemorrhage following thrombolytic therapy*

I. Patient characteristic/conditions
  a. Bleeding diathesis (congenital or acquired)
  b. Active bleeding (current or within prior 2 months)
  c. Significant trauma (<2 months)
  d. History of cerebrovascular accident, intracranial neoplasm, arteriovenous malformation, or aneurysm
  e. Recent major surgery (<4 weeks)
  f. Recent puncture of noncompressible vessel or organ biopsy (<7 days)
  g. Pregnancy
  h. Hypertension (>180/110 mm Hg) acute or poorly controlled

acquired hemostatic disorders may involve several or all components. This is particularly true in the critically ill cardiac patient. The following are commonly used tests to assess integrity of the hemostatic mechanism.

### Bleeding Time

The bleeding time has been available for several decades, measuring platelet–vessel wall interactions and formation of a primary hemostatic plug. A prolonged bleeding time, defined as the time between the infliction of a small cut on the forearm to the moment that bleeding stops, occurs when the level of circulating platelets is decreased, the platelets function abnormally, or platelet–vessel wall interactions are abnormal. Although the test provides important information as a screening tool for the early stages of hemostasis, it has been among the most difficult tests to standardize. Indeed, the test is affected by the depth, length, site and, direction of the incision. Automated devices give the most reliable and reproducible results and therefore are used in clinical practice. A normal bleeding time is between 3 and 8 minutes.

### Partial Thromboplastin Time

The partial thromboplastin time (PTT) measures the intrinsic coagulation cascade. A partial thromboplastin (e.g., cephalin and inosithin) has an activity equivalent to platelet factor 3. They are added to citrated plasma, and the time required to form a clot is measured at 37°C after the addition of calcium. The variability of contact activation of the intrinsic cascade is standardized by the addition of an activator (e.g., Kaolin, celite, powdered glass) and referred to as the activated partial thromboplastin time (aPTT).

The aPTT is prolonged if there is decreased coagulation factor activity or if there is a circulating inhibitor or anticoagulant. Mixing the patient's plasma with normal plasma and repeating the test allows these two mechanisms to be distinguished. If the correction pattern indicates a coagulation factor deficiency, mixing tests can then be performed with artificially depleted plasmas or with patient's plasmas known to be deficient in specific coagulation proteins. The aPTT is the test used most commonly to monitor heparin. The normal range varies between reagents and automated devices; however, it typically is in the range of 25 to 35 seconds.

### Thrombin Time

The thrombin time measures the terminal portion of the common coagulation pathway and is determined by adding a solution of thrombin to anticoagulated plasma and performing a clotting time. The thrombin time is particularly sensitive to heparin as well as to low fibrinogen levels, dysfunctional fibrinogen, and the presence of FDPs. If the thrombin time is prolonged and the contribution of heparin is unknown, a reptilase time can be performed. Reptilase (derived from pit viper venom) clots fibrinogen in the presence of heparin. Therefore, the reptilase time will be normal if heparin is responsible for a prolonged thrombin time (or aPTT). In contrast, deficient or dysfunctional fibrinogen or impaired fibrin monomer polymerization (caused by circulating FDP) will prolong the reptilase time and thrombin time (and occasionally the aPTT as well).

A normal thrombin time is between 20 and 30 seconds.

### Prothrombin Time

The prothrombin time (PT) is a measure of clotting initiated by the extrinsic coagulation pathway. The test is performed by adding a thromboplastin (complete)—the equivalent of tissue thromboplastin—to citrated blood and performing a clotting time after the addition of calcium. Like the aPTT, the PT is affected by deficiencies of factors II, V, and X and fibrinogen. However, unlike the aPTT, it is also sensitive to deficiencies of factor VII (the deficiency may be absolute or relative, as is the case with circulating factor VII inhibitors).

The PT varies with the thromboplastin used. As discussed previously, this limitation has been addressed through the adoption of a standardized system (the INR). However, poor quality thromboplastins (International Sensitivity Index > 1.8) tend to limit the potential benefits of the INR system. A normal INR is between 1.0 and 1.3.

The aPTT, thrombin time, and PT can be used together in clinical practice to investigate the source or sources of bleeding complications (Table 21).

### Activated Clotting Time

The activated clotting, or coagulation, time (ACT) is a derivative of the whole blood clotting time used initially in the 1950s to assess coagulation and heparin response. Two commercially available systems are in clinical use—the medtronic Hemotec ACT (Medtronic Hemotec, Inc., Englewood, CO) and the Hemochron (International Technidyne Corporation, Edison, NJ). The Hemotec device uses a mechanical plunger that is dipped in and out of Kaolin-activated whole blood samples in cartridges. The device optically senses the time required for the plunger to move through the blood samples. Both high- and low-range cartridges are available. The high-range cartridges provide an average response of 100 seconds for each unit of heparin per milliliter of blood. The low-range cartridges provide an average response of 250 seconds for each unit of heparin per milliliter of blood. The Hemochron device uses a magnet inside prewarmed

**TABLE 21.** *Evaluation of bleeding complications and hemostatic abnormalities*

| Abnormality | aPTT | Thrombin time | PT |
|---|---|---|---|
| Intrinsic pathway | Prolonged | Normal or mildly prolonged | Normal |
| Extrinsic pathway | Normal | Normal | Prolonged |
| Common pathway | Prolonged | Normal or mildly prolonged[a] | Prolonged |
| Fibrinogen (depletion/dysfunction) | Normal[b] | Prolonged | Normal[b] |

[a]Determined by deficient component; thrombin time more sensitive to terminal portion of common pathway, particularly fibrinogen.
[b]With severe fibrinogen depletion, aPTT and PT may be prolonged.
aPTT, activated partial thromboplastin time; PT, prothrombin time.

glass specimen tubes that contain various activators (diatomaceous earth or glass beads). After whole blood is placed in the tube, they are rotated inside the device. As blood clots, a magnet is displaced, activating a proximity switch. The clotting time is derived from the time required to move the magnet a preset distance. High- and low-range cartridges are also available for use with the Hemochron device.

The ACT is used often during coronary angioplasty or bypass surgery for heparin monitoring.

## Transfusions

Blood transfusions are indicated when one or more essential components are deficient and require immediate replacement. The assumption is made that more specific and potentially safer therapy (e.g., iron supplementation) has been considered but precluded because of time and urgency. When blood transfusions are indicated, only the deficient component should be administered.

A standard unit of blood consists of 450 mL of blood mixed with 50 to 60 mL of a solution containing citrate, glucose, phosphate, and adenine for optimal preservation of red blood cell viability. A majority of anemic patients can be treated with red blood cells supplemented by an electrolyte solution (normal saline, Ringer's lactate) for blood pressure support. Whole blood replacement is typically reserved for massive hemorrhage complicated by shock.

A variety of red blood cell preparations are available through most hospital blood banks:

*Red blood cells* (*packed red blood cells*) are the primary treatment for most acute and chronic anemias. Enough plasma is maintained from the original unit to facilitate rapid transfusion when necessary.
*Leukocyte-poor red blood cells* are available for patients with prior transfusion-related febrile reactions (a majority are caused by alloantibodies reacting to donor leukocytes). Removal of 80% 90% of leukocytes is adequate. It is important to realize that the process of removing leukocytes (washing, centrifugation, filtering) also removes some red blood cells, lowering the final hematocrit of the donor unit.

*Washed red blood cells* are reserved for patients with severe febrile reactions to transfused cells.
*Frozen red blood cells* can also be used in this setting; however, the primary reason to freeze red blood cells is for the purpose of storing (up to 3 years) rare blood types.

### Blood Compatibility

The surface membrane of all blood cells (and plasma proteins) contain a large number of genetically programmed antigens. Fortunately, many of these antigens are poor immunogens, and therefore, antibody production is minimal. The red blood cell antigens are divided into blood groups, the ABO group being the most important with two antigens: A and B. The second important red blood cell group is Rh [important because one of the antigenic determinants in this group (D) is a very potent antigen]. The term Rh-positive indicates the presence of D; Rh-negative indicates its absence (approximately 15% of the population lacks the D antigen).

When a blood transfusion is clinically indicated, the blood bank must type the red blood cells of the patient (recipient) for A, B, and D and confirm the typing on the donor. Further, tests are performed on the recipient's blood for unexpected antibodies (other than the expected anti-A or anti-B). Cross-matching tests the recipient's serum with red blood cells for the intended donor unit.

Under normal circumstances, transfused cells are the same ABO type as those of the recipient. In urgent situations, incompatible cells may be transfused (type O cells can be given to a recipient of any ABO type; type AB recipients can receive cells of any ABO type). In these situations, only packed red blood cells should be used. A special effort should be made to avoid transfusing Rh-positive cells into Rh-negative female recipients of childbearing potential. Subsequent immunization to the D antigen may cause hemolytic disease of the newborn.

### Complications of Blood Transfusions

Blood transfusions have the potential for a wide variety of complications and side effects. Therefore, it is important in all clinical scenarios to carefully consider the risks and benefits of transfusion (Table 22).

## Procoagulant Disorders

The concept of hypercoagulability and its impact in medicine is commonly attributed to the celebrated pathologist Rudoth Virchow (92), who proposed that alterations in circulating blood components, changes in blood flow, and abnormalities in the blood vessel wall (Virchow's triad) were key contributors to the initiation, progression, and manifestations of intravascular thrombosis (venous and arterial). Procoagulant states or disorders, as generally defined, cause a shift in the hemostatic balance toward inappropriate or excessive thrombus formation. This definition includes conditions that favor thrombosis yet require specific physical or biologic substrate to do so (prethrombotic states) and those where the intrinsic thrombotic stimulus is so profound that thrombosis can occur even in a relatively nonthrombotic environment (hypercoagulable state).

In cardiovascular medicine, procoagulant disorders are encountered commonly (Table 23). The pathobiology and potential clinical impact of those most frequently confronting clinicians are discussed.

### Atherosclerotic Coronary Artery Disease

There is considerable evidence that most acute cardiovascular events are thrombotic in origin. However, beyond its ability to increase thrombotic tendency, the atherosclerotic process itself may be influenced directly by abnormalities in platelet activation, coagulation, and fibrinolysis, each contributing to fibrin deposition and, ultimately, plaque growth.

**TABLE 22.** *Potential hazards of blood transfusions*

a. Hemolytic reactions (ABO mismatch)
b. Febrile reactions
c. Contaminated blood
　1. Gram-negative bacillae
d. Noncardiogenic pulmonary edema
e. Posttransfusion thrombocytopenia
f. Disease transmission
　1. Hepatitis B
　2. Hepatitis non-A non-B
　3. Acquired immunodeficiency syndrome
　4. Cytomegalovirus
　5. Malaria
　6. Syphilis
g. Allergic reactions
　1. Anaphylactic shock
　2. Urticaria
h. Air embolism
i. Congestive heart failure (circulatory overload)
j. Graft-versus-host disease

**TABLE 23.** *Procoagulant disorders*

a. Atherosclerotic coronary artery disease
b. Hyperlipidemias
c. Dysplasminogenemias
d. Abnormal plasminogen activation
e. Antiphospholipid antibody syndrome
f. Antithrombin III deficiency
　1. Quantitative
　2. Qualitative
g. Protein C deficiency/protein C resistance
h. Protein S deficiency
i. Malignancy
j. Myeloproliferative disease
k. Paroxysmal nocturnal hemoglobinuria
l. Homocystinuria
m. Vasculitis

The ubiquitous fatty streak is the earliest lesion of atherosclerosis and the pathologic precursor of more advanced disease. Grossly flat, the fatty streak consists of macrophages and smooth muscle cells. Over time, each becomes lipid laden, contributing to further growth and development (93, 94). As that fatty streak grows, which depends primarily on an ample supply of lipid substrate, endothelial cell separation and retraction can occur, exposing underlying lipid-laden macrophages, smooth muscle cells, and connective tissue to the circulation. This provides an opportunity for platelet adherence and activation. In addition to serving as a template for coagulation processes, activated platelets release a number of potent chemotactic and mitogenic substances, including epidermal growth factor, platelet-derived growth factor, and transforming growth factor beta. Smooth muscle cell migration and proliferation are stimulated, as is monocyte and fibroblast migration (95–97). Even in the absence of overt denudation, functional endothelial cell abnormalities may promote monocyte adherence and subendothelial transport, platelet activation, smooth muscle cell proliferation, and paradoxical vasoconstriction (98–100).

The incrustation theory of Rokitansky (101) suggests that vascular intimal thickening results from fibrin deposition, with subsequent organization from fibroblasts and secondary lipid accumulation. Pathologic analysis of patients dying of atherosclerotic coronary artery disease has frequently revealed a morphologic appearance consistent with healed plaque fissures containing various stages of thrombus organization (102–104). Further evidence for the role of thrombosis in atherosclerotic plaque growth has been provided by the works of Woolf and Crawford (105), Bini et al. (106), and Smith et al. (107), demonstrating fibrin-related products within intimal, neointimal, and deeper medial layers of advanced atherosclerotic plaques. The presence of thrombus in general and thrombin in particular can also promote the uptake of lipid by macrophages (108) and increase smooth muscle cell proliferation, either directly or indirectly through activated platelet growth factor release (109, 110).

Atheromatous plaque rupture, associated with either partial or complete thrombotic arterial occlusion, is fundamental to the development of ischemic coronary syndromes, particularly myocardial infarction (111, 112). Rupture of small plaques, with subsequent mural thrombosis and fibrotic organization, may not cause a significant reduction in either coronary blood flow or myocardial perfusion. However, it may contribute to plaque growth. Indeed, nonocclusive thrombi developing within areas of plaque rupture may be "sealed off" by proliferating smooth muscle cells, fibroblasts, and small blood vessels (neovascularization). The residual thrombus may then act as a scaffold for additional plaque growth, progressively decreasing the cross-sectional diameter of the arterial lumen (113).

## Hyperlipidemia

Platelets obtained from individuals with type II hyperlipoproteinemia exhibit increased aggregability in response to stimulation with epinephrine, collagen, and adenosine diphosphate (114). In vitro studies varying the platelet membrane cholesterol concentration have shown that increased levels consistently cause increased aggregability (115, 116). The observed state of heightened platelet aggregation in the presence of hypercholesterolemia may be the result of changes in membrane fluidity, leading to an increased exposure of thrombin receptors on the platelet surface. In addition to its effects on platelet behavior, hypercholesterolemia, even in the absence of atherosclerosis, can impair endothelium-dependent vascular relaxation, increasing focal shear stress and thrombotic tendency.

## Dysplasminogenemias

The fibrinolytic system is a proteolytic enzyme system with a diversity of physiologic functions, of which degradation of fibrin deposits in the cardiovascular system is the most well known and widely investigated. Plasminogen variants have been identified in patients with thromboembolic disease, including deep venous thrombosis, pulmonary embolism, mesenteric vein thrombosis, cerebral vein thrombosis, and less commonly, stroke, and myocardial infarction (MI). To date, 12 reported variants have been described (117–119). Congenital dysplasminogenemias are characterized by decreased plasminogen functional activity. In contrast, familial hypoplasminogenemia exhibits a proportional decrease in both antigenic and functional activity.

## Abnormal Plasminogen Activation

Large epidemiologic studies including middle-aged men and other patient populations at risk for atherosclerotic coronary artery disease have failed to demonstrate a clear relationship between deficient fibrinolytic activity and cardiovascular events (120, 121). However, in patients with typical angina pectoris, or those with a previous MI, a number of cross-sectional studies have identified an association between impaired fibrinolytic potential and major cardiac events, including recurrent infarction and death (122–124). Fibrinolytic impairment secondary to either decreased vascular tissue plasminogen activator release or increased circulating plasminogen activator inhibitor (PAI-1) concentrations has been observed commonly, particularly in young survivors of MI (125). Prospective studies will be required, however, to define more clearly the role of impaired fibrinolysis in predicting cardiac events.

## Antiphospholipid Antibody Syndrome

Antiphospholipid antibodies are autoantibodies of either the IgG or IgM variety that can be detected in either plasma or serum using a solid-phase immunoassay in which negatively charged phospholipids serve as an antigen. Antiphospholipid antibodies commonly cross-react with cardiolipin, phosphatidylserine, phosphatidylinositol, phosphatidylethanolamine, and phosphatidylcholine, as well as endothelial cell and platelet surface membranes (126).

Antiphospholipid antibodies are typically identified in individuals with autoimmune disorders, particularly systemic lupus erythematosus. However, they may occur in other disorders as well, including acute and chronic viral infections and malignancy. Occasionally, they develop in individuals without an underlying systemic disorder (primary antiphospholipid antibody syndrome) or following ingestion of one of several drugs, such as chlorpromazine, procainamide, hydralazine, phenytoin, or quinidine.

Antiphospholipid antibodies have been associated with the development of transient ischemic attacks, cerebrovascular accidents, spontaneous abortion, livedo reticularis, and thromboembolic events. Arterial thrombosis has been documented in the retinal, intracranial, mesenteric, peripheral, and coronary arteries. Venous thrombosis occurs as well, involving the renal, hepatic, mesenteric, cerebral, retinal, and superficial and deep veins of the lower extremities (127).

The potential mechanisms for pathologic thrombosis in patients with circulating antiphospholipid antibodies are currently under investigation. Cross-reactivity with phospholipids in endothelial cell and platelet surface membranes may be directly involved, preventing prostacyclin release (128, 129) and increasing platelet aggregability, respectively (130). Increased von Willebrand factor activity and decreased fibrinolytic potential, resulting from prekallikrein inhibition and decreased plasminogen activator release, have also been described (131). More recently, however, a number of interesting observations have been made. The binding of antiphospholipid antibodies occurs only in plasma or serum, suggesting that a cofactor is required. Indeed, the cofactor $\beta_2$-glycoprotein ($\beta_2$-GPI), a single-chain polypeptide of 50,000 kDa, has recently been described (132, 133). Interestingly, $\beta_2$-GPI binds and neutralizes negatively charged macromolecules which may activate either platelets or the intrinsic coagulation pathway. Therefore, if $\beta_2$-GPI serves as an antigenic cofactor for antiphospholipid antibody binding, its own neutralization may explain, at lease in part, the observed thrombotic tendency.

Although variable, several investigators have identified the presence of antiphospholipid antibodies in patients with coronary heart disease (134). They have also been reported in patients at risk for saphenous vein occlusion following coronary bypass surgery (135) and among young survivors of MI in whom their presence predicts an increased likelihood of recurrent cardiac events (136). While in these settings the presence of circulating antiphospholipid antibodies may reflect a secondary immune response to either an acute or chronic inflammatory state rather than a primary disorder, their presence may nonetheless serve as a useful prognostic marker.

### Antithrombin III (ATIII) Deficiency

Antithrombin III is a 67,000-kDa glycoprotein which accounts for 75% of the total antithrombin activity of plasma. A naturally occurring accelerator of heparin-like species inhibitory interactions on the vascular endothelial surface, ATIII is essential for physiologic thromboresistance. In typical cases, ATIII deficiency is inherited in an autosomal dominant fashion with proportionately decreased ATIII antigenic and functional activities of 25% to 60% of normal. However, qualitative deficiencies may occur as well. Acquired ATIII deficiency has been described in patients with the nephrotic syndrome, advanced liver disease, and DIC and following high-dose intravenous nitroglycerin administration (137).

The most frequently observed clinical symptoms are recurrent deep venous thrombosis and pulmonary embolism, occurring for the first time in the second or third decades of life. Other sites may be involved as well, including the renal, mesenteric, hepatic, retinal, and cerebral veins. In contrast, arterial thrombosis is much less common, with relatively few cases of MI appearing in the medical literature (138, 139).

### Protein C Deficiency

Protein C, a 62,000-kDa glycoprotein precursor of activated protein C, participates in vascular thromboresistance by proteolytically inactivating coagulation factors Va and VIIIa in the presence of thrombomodulin. Activated protein C also has fibrinolytic generating properties. An insufficient amount of protein C would, therefore, be expected to increase local thrombus formation. Indeed, protein C deficiency, a codominantly inherited disorder, is associated with thromboembolic events, coming to clinical attention during the second and third decades of life (140). The clinical spectrum typically includes recurrent deep venous thrombosis and pulmonary embolism; however, involvement of other venous sites, albeit less common, can occur as well. As with ATIII deficiency, arterial thrombosis, including MI, is rarely encountered (141).

Activated protein C resistance may be responsible for a significant number of venous thrombotic events and requires careful consideration.

### Protein S Deficiency

Protein S, like protein C, is a vitamin-K-dependent protein which serves as a cofactor for the anticoagulant and fibrinolytic effects of activated protein C. Protein S exists in two forms within plasma, either as a free protein (40%) or complexed with C4b-binding protein, an inhibitor of the complement system. Only free protein S is functionally active. A majority of patients with inherited protein S deficiency have increased plasma levels, but most of the molecules are bound to C4b-binding protein, rendering them functionally inactive. Acquired protein S deficiency has been described in pregnancy, oral contraceptive use, DIC, advanced liver disease, nephrotic syndrome, and type I diabetes mellitus (142–144).

As with ATIII and protein C deficiency states, patients with protein S deficiency can experience recurrent thromboembolic events, most commonly deep venous thrombosis and pulmonary embolism. Arterial thrombosis has been described (145).

### Diabetes Mellitus

There is a well-established association of diabetes mellitus with the development of atherosclerosis, microvascular disorders, and thromboembolic complications. Since platelets are known to contribute directly to physiologic and pathologic coagulative processes, their involvement in the accelerated vascular disease and in thrombotic events seen in patients with diabetes mellitus has been investigated.

Studies performed in experimental animal models, coupled with those in humans, suggest that diabetes mellitus is associated with a number of platelet abnormalities, including (a) increased adhesion, (b) increased aggregation, (c) increased activation and release, and (e) increased thromboxane $A_2$ synthetic capacity. More recently, additional platelet abnormalities have been identified which include enhanced platelet responsiveness to serotonin and adenosine diphosphate and increased von Willebrand factor release. The mechanism responses for these abnormalities are currently under investigation. However, the available evidence suggests that hyperglycemia itself, associated hyperlipidemic states, and chronic endothelial cell injury (146, 147) may each contribute.

Beyond the observed abnormalities in platelet activity, diabetes mellitus has been associated with impaired fibrinolysis and enhanced coagulation, resulting from decreased tissue plasminogen activator release, increased PAI concentrations, elevated plasma fibrinogen levels, and enhanced thrombin generation (148).

## Malignancy

An association between malignancy and thromboembolic events was recognized by Armand Trousseau more than a century ago. Currently, a large body of clinical evidence suggests that coagulation abnormalities may represent an epiphenomenon of disseminated malignancy or exist as a primary abnormality with profound clinical implications.

A wide variety of thrombotic disorders have been described, including recurrent superficial and deep venous thrombosis, pulmonary embolism, MI and other arterial thrombosis, and nonbacterial (marantic) endocarditis with peripheral embolism. These events are particularly common in patients with pancreatic carcinoma, adenocarcinoma of the gastrointestinal tract, and bronchogenic carcinoma (149).

An extensive amount of information has been gathered on patients with malignancy experiencing thromboembolic events. From this experience, a number of abnormalities have been defined and potential mechanisms generated. Some investigators have proposed that chronic DIC with platelet activation and fibrin deposition is the primary abnormality. Although this entity may certainly contribute in some patients, the thrombotic tendency is likely a multifactorial phenomenon. The long list of potential contributors includes increased platelet activatability, elevated fibrinogen concentrations, and increased coagulation factor Va and VIII and decreased ATIII levels. Increased thrombin generation is supported by an observed increase in fibrinopeptide A, thrombin-antithrombin complexes, and prothrombin fragment 1.2 concentrations (150, 151).

There is increasing evidence that procoagulant activity can be expressed by tumor cells directly or by shed membrane-bound vesicles. Indeed, both have been shown to express tissue factor activity and to activate both factor X and the prothrombinase complex leading to fibrin generation and thrombus formation.

## Myeloproliferative Disorders

The myeloproliferative disorders include polycythemia vera, essential thrombocythemia, myelofibrosis, chronic myelogenous leukemia, and myeloid metaplasia. Hemorrhagic and thrombotic events occur, the latter typified by recurrent venous thrombosis, pulmonary embolism, stroke, MI, and microvascular thrombi. Although increased plasma and/or whole blood viscosity may be a contributing feature, particularly in polycythemia vera and essential thrombocythemia, qualitative platelet abnormalities with increased adhesion, aggregation, and activation are centrally involved in the observed thrombotic tendency (152, 153).

## Paroxysmal Nocturnal Hemoglobinuria

Paroxysmal nocturnal hemoglobinuria is an acquired hemolytic disorder characterized by the proliferation of an abnormal clone of stem cells which are susceptible to complement-mediated cellular membrane damage. Microcirculatory thrombosis is common, as is recurrent venous thrombosis involving the hepatic, splenic, portal, cerebral, and deep peripheral veins. Arterial thrombosis occurs rarely.

## Homocystinuria

Homocystinuria is an inborn error of metabolism with variable expression caused by a deficiency of cystathionine β-synthetase. In its homozygous form, accumulation of homocysteine in the tissues and vasculature is responsible for typical symptoms and physical findings which include premature vascular occlusive events. In addition, however, heterozygous homocystinuria may also be a cause of premature peripheral occlusive and ischemic cerebrovascular disease. Fatal MI has been described as well, reflecting thrombus formation at a site of endothelial injury (154, 155).

## Vasculitis

The vasculitides are characterized by various stages of inflammation, involving small-, medium-, or large-caliber vessels (depending on the disorder). Inflammation with accompanying structural and functional endothelial abnormalities and shear stress, increasing as a result of changes in luminal dimension, foster platelet adherence, activation, and fibrin deposition. Although some systemic disorders may be associated with circulating procoagulant factors (e.g., antiphospholipid antibodies), the majority exhibit a thrombotic tendency, primarily on the basis of focal abnormalities involving the vessel wall. Active vasculitis can cause arterial thrombosis, including MI. In addition, however, healed vasculitis involving the coronary arteries can cause accelerated atherosclerosis, itself a procoagulant state. Overall, the vasculitic disorders most commonly causing arterial thrombosis are polyarthritis nodosa and giant cell arthritis (156, 157).

## REFERENCES

1. Piper P, Vane JR. The release of prostaglandins from the vascular endothelium and other tissues. *Ann NY Acad Sci* 1971;180:363.
2. Willis AL, Smith DL, Vigo C, Kluge AF. Effects of prostacyclin and orally active stable mimetic agent RS-93427-007 on bovine mechanisms of atherogenesis. *Lancet* 1986;2:682.
3. Furchgott RF, Zawasdski JV. The obligatory role of endothelial cells in the relaxation of arterial smooth muscle cells by acetylcholine. *Nature* 1980;288:373.
4. Palmer RMJ, Ferige AG, Moncada S. Nitric oxide release accounts for the biologic activity of endothelium-derived relaxing factor. *Nature* 1987;327:524.
5. Radomski MW, Palmer RM, Moncada S. Endogenous nitric oxide inhibits human platelet adhesion to vascular endothelium. *Lancet* 1987;1:1057.
6. Radomski MW, Palmer RM, Moncada S. The antiaggregatory properties of vascular endothelium: interactions between prostacyclin and nitric oxide. *Br J Pharmacol* 1987;92:639.
7. Heeg E, Meng K. Die wirkung des bradykinins, angiotensis und vasopressins auf verhof appillarmusckel, und isoliert durstromte herzpraprate des meerschweinchens. *Navnyn schiedebergs. Arch Pharmacol* 1965;250:35.
8. Unger TH, Gohlke P, Ganten D, Lang RE. Converting enzyme inhibitors and their effects on the renin-angiotensin system of the blood vessel wall. *J Cardiovasc Pharmacol* 1988;13(Suppl 3):S8.
9. Simonson MS, Wann S, Mene P, et al. Endothelin-1 activates the phosphoinositide cascade in cultured glomerular mesangial cells. *J Cardiovasc Pharmacol* 1989;13(Suppl 5):S80.
10. Yanagisawa M, Kurihara H, Kimsura S, et al. A novel potent vasoconstrictor peptide produced by vascular endothelial cells. *Nature* 1988;332:411.
11. Miyanchi T, Tomobe Y, Shiba R, et al. Involvement of endothelin in the regulation of human vascular tonus: potent vasoconstrictor effect and existence in endothelial cells. *Circulation* 1990;81:1874.
12. Teien AN, Abildgaard U, Hook M, Lindahl U. The anticoagulant effect of heparin sulfate and dermatan sulfate. *Thromb Res* 1977;11:107.
13. Thomas DP, Merton RE, Barrowcliffe TW, et al. Antifactor Xa activity of heparin sulfate and dermatan sulfate. *Thromb Res* 1979;14:501.
14. Marcum JA, Rosenberg RD. Heparin-like molecules with anticoagulant activity are synthesized by cultured endothelial cells. *Biochem Biophys Res Commun* 1985;126:365.
15. Maynard JR, Dreyer BE, Stererman MB, Pitlick FA. Tissue factor coagulant activity of cultured human endothelial and smooth muscle cells and fibroblasts. *Blood* 1977;50:387.
16. Stern OM, Bank I, Naworth PP, et al. Self regulation of procoagulant events on the endothelial cells surface. *J Exp Med* 1985;162:1223.
17. Giddings JC, von Willebrand factor-physiology. In: Gimbrone MA Jr, ed. *Vascular endothelium in hemostasis and thrombosis.* New York: Churchill-Livingstone; 1986:142.
18. Erickson LA, Ginsberg MH, Loskutoff DJ. Detection and partial characterization of an inhibitor of plasminogen activator in human platelets. *J Clin Invest* 1984;74:1465.
19. Lucore CL, Sobel BE. Interactions of tissue type plasminogen activator with plasma inhibitors and their pharmacologic implications. *Circulation* 1988;77:660.
20. Loskutoff DJ. Type 1 plasminogen activator inhibitor and its potential influence on thrombolytic therapy. *Semin Thromb Hem* 1988;14:100-109.
21. Fujii S, Sobel BE. Induction of plasminogen activator inhibitor by products released from platelets. *Circulation* 1990;82:1485.
22. Chakrabarti R, Hocking ED. Fibrinolytic activity and coronary heart disease. *Lancet* 1968;1:987.
23. Zahavi J, Bitteridge JD, Jones NAG, et al. Enhanced in vivo platelet-release reaction and malondialdenyde formation in patients with hyperlipidemia. *Am J Med* 1981;70:59.
24. Joist JH, Baker RK, Schonfeld G. Increased in vivo and in vitro platelet function in type II and type IV hyperlipoproteinemia. *Thromb Res* 1974;15:95.
25. Strano A, Davi G, Averna M, et al. Platelet sensitivity to prostacyclin and thromboxane production in hyperlipidemic patients. *Thromb Haemost* 1982;48:18.
26. Joist JH, Dolezel G, Kinlough-Rathbone RL, Mustard JF. Effect of diet-induced hyperlipidemia on in vitro function of rabbit platelets. *Thromb Res* 1976;9:435.
27. Tremoli E, Folco G, Agradi E, Gall C. Platelet thromboxanes and serum cholesterol. *Lancet* 1979;1:107.
28. Harker LA, Hazzare W. Platelet kinetic studies in patients with hyperlipoproteinemia: effect of clofibrate therapy. *Circulation* 1979;60:492.
29. Worner P, Patscheke H. Hyperreactivity by an enhancement of the arachidonate pathway of platelets treated with cholesterol-rich phospholipid-dispersions. *Thromb Res* 1980;18:439.
30. Shattil SJ, Cooper RA. Role of membrane lipid composition organization and fluidity in human platelet function. *Prog Hemost Thromb* 1978;4:59.
31. Nabel EG, Ganz P, Selwyn AP. Atherosclerosis impairs flow-mediated dilation in human coronary arteries. *Circulation* 1988;78(Suppl II):II-474.
32. Jayakody L, Sernaratne M, Thompson A, Kapagoda T. Endothelium-dependent relaxation in experimental atherosclerosis in the rabbit. *Circ Res* 1987;60:251.
33. Cohen RA, Zitnay KM, Haudenschild CC, Cunningham LD. Loss of selective endothelial cell vasoactive functions caused by hypercholesterolemia in pig coronary arteries. *Circ Res* 1988;63:903.
34. Yasue H, Matsuyama K, Matsuyama K, et al. Responses of angiographically normal human coronary arteries to intracoronary injection of acetylcholine by age and segment. *Circulation* 1990;81:482.
35. Vita HA, Treasure CB, Nabel EG, et al. Coronary vasomotor response to acetylcholine relates to risk factors for coronary artery disease. *Circulation* 1990;81:491.
36. Mills D, Karpatkin S. The non-plasmin proteolytic origin of human fibrinogen heterogenicity. *Biochem Biophys Acta* 1977;251:121.
37. Spaet TH, Horowitz HI, Franklin DZ, Cintron J, Biezensi JJ. Reticuloendothelial clearance of blood thromboplastin by rats. *Blood* 1961;17:196.
38. Rabiner S. Uremic bleeding. In: Spaet TH, ed. *Progress in thrombosis and hemostasis,* vol 1. New York: Grune & Stratton;1972:233.
39. Remuzzi G, Marches D, Livio M, et al. Altered platelet and vascular prostaglandin-generation in patients with renal failure and prolonged bleeding time. *Thromb Res* 1978;13:1007.
40. Thompson AR. Factor XII and other hemostatic abnormalities in nephrotic syndrome patients. *Thromb Haemost* 1982;48:27.
41. Shea MA, Indeglia RA, Dorman FD. The biologic response to pumping blood. *Trans Am Soc Artif Intern Organs* 1967;13:116.
42. Salzman EW. Blood platelets and extracorporeal circulation. *Transfusion* 1963;3:274.
43. Friedenberg WR, Myers WO, Plotka ED. Platelet dysfunction associated with cardiopulmonary bypass. *Ann Thorac Surg* 1978;25:298.
44. Hope AF, DuPhens A, Lotter MG. Kinetics and sites of sequestration of indium 111-labeled human platelets during cardiopulmonary bypass. *J Thorac Cardiovasc Surg* 1981;81:880.
45. Boyd AD, Engelman RM, Beadet RL, Lackner H. Disseminated intravascular coagulation following extracorporeal circulation. *J Thorac Cardiovasc Surg* 1972;64:685.
46. Libby P, Warner SJC, Salomon RN, Birinyi LK. Production of platelet-derived growth factor-like mitogen by smooth-muscle cells from human atheroma. *N Engl J Med* 1988;318:1493.
47. Williams LT. Signal transduction by the platelet-derived growth factor receptor. *Science* 1989;243:1564.
48. Badimon L, Badimon JJ, Chesebro JH, Fuster V. Inhibition of thrombus formation: blockage of adhesive glycoprotein mechanisms versus blockage of the cyclooxygenase pathway. *J Am Coll Cardiol* 1988;11 (Suppl A):30A(abst).
49. Strony J, Phillips M, Brands D, et al. Aurintricarboxylic acid in canine model of coronary artery thrombosis. *Circulation* 1990;81:1106.
50. Cattaneo M, Chahil A, Somers D, et al. Effect of aspirin and sodium salicylate on thrombosis, fibrinolysis, prothrombin time, and platelet survival in rabbits with indwelling aortic catheters. *Blood* 1983;61:353.
51. Hirsh J. Progress review: the relationship between dose of aspirin, side effects and antithrombotic effectiveness. *Stroke* 1985;16:1.
52. Neri Serneri GG, Casellani S. Platelet and vascular prostaglandins:

pharmacological and clinical implications. In: Born GVR, Neri Serneri GG, eds. *Antiplatelet therapy: twenty years experience. Proceedings of a European conference.* Amsterdam: Elsevier Excerpta Medica; 1987:37.

53. Yasuda T, Gold HK, Leinback RC, et al. Lysis of plasminogen activator-resistant platelet rich coronary artery thrombus with combined bolus injection of recombinant tissue-type plasminogen activator and antiplatelet GPIIb/IIIa antibody. *J Am Coll Cardiol* 1990;16:1728.

54. Musial J, Niewiarowski S, Rucinski B, et al. Inhibition of platelet adhesion to surfaces of extracorporeal circuits by disintegrins. RGD-containing peptides from viper venoms. *Circulation* 1990;82:261.

55. Saltiel R, Ward A. Ticlopidine: a review of its pharmacodynamics and pharmacokinetic properties and therapeutic efficacy in platelet-dependent disease states. *Drugs* 1987;34:222.

56. Fitsgerald GA, Reilly LA, Pederson Ak. The biochemical pharmacology of thromboxane synthase inhibition in man. *Circulation* 1985;72:1194.

57. Mullane KM, Fionabaio D. Thromboxane synthetase inhibitors reduce infarct size by a platelet dependent, aspirin-sensitive mechanism. *Circ Res* 1988;62:668.

58. Saussy DL Jr, Mais DE, Knapp DR, Halushka PV. Thromboxane A$_2$ and prostaglandin endoperoxide receptors in platelets and vascular smooth muscle. *Circulation* 1985;72:1202.

59. Evans RJ, Gordon JD. Mechanisms of the antithrombotic actions of dextran. *N Engl J Med* 1974;290:748.

60. Weiss HJ. The effect of clinical dextran on platelet aggregation, adhesion, and ADP release in man: in vivo and in vitro studies. *J Lab Clin Med* 1967;69:37.

61. Fitzgerald GA. Dipyridamole. *N Engl J Med* 1987;316:1247.

62. Emmons RP, Hampton JR, Harrison MJG, et al. Effect of prostaglandin E$_1$, on platelet behavior in vitro and in vivo. *Br Med J* 1967;2:468.

63. Treers W, Beythein C, Kupper W, Bleifeld W. Effects of aspirin and prostaglandin E$_1$ on in vitro thrombolysis and urokinase. *Circulation* 1989;79:1309.

64. Weksler BB. Prostaglandins and vascular function. *Circulation* 1984;70(Suppl III):III-63.

65. Fisher CA, Kappa JR, Sinha AK, et al. Comparison of equimolar concentrations of iloprost, prostacyclin, and prostaglandin E$_1$ on human platelet function. *J Lab Clin Med* 1987;109:184.

66. Kiyomoto A, Sasaki Y, Odawara A, Morita T. Inhibition of platelet aggregation by diltiazem. Comparison with verapamil and nifedipine and inhibitory potencies of diltiazem metabolites. *Circ Res* 1983;52 (Suppl I):115.

67. Mehta P, Mehta J, Ostrowski N, Brigmon L. Inhibitory effects of diltiazem on platelet activation caused by ionophore A23187 plus ADP of epinephrine in subthreshold concentrations. *J Lab Clin Med* 1983;102:332.

68. Addonizio VP, Fisher CA, Strauss JF, et al. Effects of verapamil and diltiazem on human platelet function. *Am J Physiol* 1986;250:H366.

69. Wade PJ, Lunt DO, Lad N, et al. Effect of calcium and calcium antagonists on [$^3$H]-PAF-Acether binding to washed human platelets. *Thromb Res* 1986;41:251.

70. Altman R, Scazziota A, Dujovne C. Diltiazem potentiates the inhibitory effect of aspirin on platelet aggregation. *Clin Pharmacol Ther* 1988;44:320.

71. Fischer-Dzoga K, Kuo YF, Wissler RW. The proliferative effect of platelets and hyperlipidemic serum on stationary primary cultures. *Atherosclerosis* 1983;47:35.

72. Tiell ML, Sussman II, Gordon PB. Suppression of fibroblast proliferation in vitro and of myointimal hyperplasia in vivo by the triazolopyrimadine, trapidil. *Artery* 1983;12:33.

73. Lam LH, Silbert JE, Rosenberg RD. The separation of active and inactive forms of heparin. *Biochem Biophys Res Commun* 1976;69:570.

74. Andersson LO, Barrowcliffe TW, Holmer E, Johnson EA, Sims GE. Anticoagulant properties of heparin fractionated by affinity chromatography on matrix-bound antithrombin III and by gel filtration. *Thromb Res* 1976;9:575.

75. de Swart CA, Nijmeyer B, Roelofs JM, Sixma JJ. Kinetics of intravenously administered heparin in normal humans. *Blood* 1982;60:1251.

76. Olsson P, Lagergren H, Ek S. The elimination from plasma of intravenous heparin: an experimental study on dogs and humans. *Acta Med Scand* 1963;173:619.

77. Young E, Prins M, Levine MN, Hirsh J. Heparin binding to plasma proteins, an important mechanism for heparin resistance. *Thromb Haemost* 1992;67:639.

78. Bjornsson TD, Wolfram KM, Kitchell BB. Heparin kinetics determined by three assay methods. *Clin Pharmacol Ther* 1982;31:104.

79. Hsia J, Hamilton WP, Kleiman N, et al. A comparison between heparin and low dose aspirin as adjunctive therapy with tissue plasminogen activator for acute myocardial infarction. *N Engl J Med* 1990;323:1433.

80. de Bono DP, Simoons ML, Tijssen J, et al. Effect of early intravenous heparin on coronary patency, infarct size and bleeding complications after alteplase thrombolysis: results of a randomized double blind European Cooperative Study Group trial. *Br Heart J* 1992;67:122.

81. Hull RD, Raskob GE, Hirsh J, et al. Continuous intravenous heparin compared with intermittent subcutaneous heparin in the initial treatment of proximal-vein thrombosis. *N Engl J Med* 1986;315:1109.

82. Becker RC, Cyr J, Corrao JM, Ball SP. Bedside coagulation monitoring in heparinized patients with active thromboembolic disease: a coronary care unit experience. *Am Heart J.* 1994;128:719.

83. Poller L. Progress in standardisation in anticoagulant control. *Hematol Rev* 1987;1:225.

84. Poller L, Taberner DA. Dosage and control of oral anticoagulants: an international collaborative survey. *Br J Haematol* 1982;51:479.

85. Bussey HI, Force RW, Bianco TM, Leonard AD. Reliance on prothrombin time ratios causes significant errors in anticoagulation therapy. *Arch Intern Med* 1992;152;278.

86. Wate R, Savidge GF. Rapid thrombolysis and preservation of valvular function in high deep venous thrombosis. *Acta Med Scand* 1979;205:293.

87. Stricker RB, Wond D, Shin DT, et al. Activation of plasminogen by tPA in normal and thromboasthenic platelets: effect of surface proteins and platelet aggregation. *Blood* 1986;68:275.

88. Loscalzo J, Vaughan DE. Tissue plasminogen activator promotes platelet disaggregation in plasma. *J Clin Invest* 1987;79:1749.

89. Schafer AL, Adelman B. Plasmin inhibition of platelet function and of arachidonic acid metabolism. *J Clin Invest* 1985;75:456.

90. Bovill E, Tracy R, Granger C, Hardin N. Monitoring anticoagulant therapy in the setting of thrombolytic therapy. In: Becker RC. ed. *The modern era of coronary thrombolysis.* Norwell, MA: Klumer Academic; 1994.

91. Becker RC. Toward establishing universal guidelines for antithrombotic therapy. *J Thromb Thrombol* 1995;1:225.

92. Virchow R. Ein vortrag uber die Thrombose vom Jahre 1845. In: *Gesammelte Abhandlungen zur wissenschaftlichen Medizin.* Frankfurt: Meidinger; 1856:478.

93. Faggiotto A, Ross R, Harker L. Studies of hypercholesterolemia in the nonhuman primate. I. Changes that lead to fatty streak formation. *Arteriosclerosis* 1984;4:323.

94. Faggiotto A, Ross R. Studies of hypercholesterolemia in the nonhuman primate. II. Fatty streak conversion to fibrous plaque. *Arteriosclerosis* 1984;4:341.

95. Fisherman JA, Ryan GB, Karnovsky MJ. Endothelial regeneration in the rat carotid artery and the significance of endothelial denudation in the pathogenesis of myointimal thickening. *Lab Invest* 1977;32:339.

96. Castellot JJ Jr, Addonizio ML, Rosenberg R, et al. Cultured endothelial cells produce a heparin-like inhibitor of smooth muscle cell growth. *J Cell Biol* 1981;90:372.

97. Richardson M, Ihnatowycz I, Moore S. Glycosaminoglycan distribution in rabbit aortic wall following balloon catheter endothelialiation: an ultrastructural study. *Lab Invest* 1980;43:509.

98. Gajdusek CM, DeCorleto P, Ross R, et al. An endothelial cell-derived growth factor. *J Cell Biol* 1980;85:467.

99. DiCorleto PE, Gajdusek CM, Schwartz SM, et al. Biochemical properties of the endothelium-derived growth factor. Comparison to other growth factors. *J Cell Physiol* 1983;114:339.

100. DiCorleto PE, Bowen-Pope DF. Cultured endothelial cells produce a platelet-derived growth factor like protein. *Proc Natl Acad Sci USA* 1983;80:1919.

101. Rokitansky C. *Annual of pathological anatomy*, vol 4. London: Sydenham Society; 1852:261.

102. Davies MJ. Thrombosis and coronary atherosclerosis. In: Julian D, Kubler WS, Norris RM, et al., eds. *Thrombolysis in cardiovascular disease.* New York: Dekker; 1989:25.

103. Davies MJ, Thomas AC. Thrombosis and acute coronary artery lesions in sudden cardiac death. *N Engl J Med* 1984;310:1137.

104. Davies MJ, Thomas AC. Plaque fissuring: the cause of acute myocardial infarction, sudden ischemic death and crescendo angina. *Br Heart J* 1985;53:363.

105. Woolf N, Crawford T. Fatty streaks in the aortic intima. Studies by an immune-histochemical technique. *J Pathol Bacterial* 1960;80:405.

106. Bini A, Genoglia JJ, Mesa-Tejada R, et al. Identification and distribution of fibrinogen, fibrin and fibrin degradation products in atherosclerosis: use of monoclonal antibody. *Atherosclerosis* 1989;1:109.

107. Smith EB, Kean A, Grant A, et al. Fate of fibrinogen in human arterial intima. *Arteriosclerosis* 1990;10:265.

108. Schwartz CJ, Valente AJ, Kelly JL, et al. Thrombosis and the development of atherosclerosis: Rokitanksy revisited. *Semin Thromb Hemost* 1988;14:189.

109. Cunningham DD, Farrel DH. Thrombin interactions in cultured fibroblasts: relationship to mitogenic stimulation. *Ann NY Acad Sci* 1986;485:240.

110. Shuman MA. Thrombin-cellular interactions. *Ann NY Acad Sci* 1986; 485:288.

111. Davies MJ, Thomas AC. Plaque fissuring: the cause of acute myocardial angina. *Br Heart J* 1985;53:363.

112. Falk E. Plaque rupture with severe pre-existing stenosis precipitating coronary thrombosis. Characteristics of coronary atherosclerotic plaques underlying fatal occlusive thrombi. *Br Heart J* 1983;50:127.

113. Davies MJ. A macro and micro view of coronary vascular insult in ischemic heart disease. *Circulation* 1990;82(Suppl II):38.

114. Carvalho A, Colmon E, Lees R. Platelet function in hyperlipoproteinemia. *N Engl J Med* 1987;240:434.

115. Shattil SJ, Anaya-Galindo R, Bennett J, et al. Platelet hypersensitivity induced by cholesterol incorporation. *J Clin Invest* 1975;55:636.

116. Tandon N, Harman J, Robbard D, et al. Thrombin receptors define responsiveness of cholesterol modified platelets. *J Biochem* 1983; 184:11840.

117. Aoki N, Moroi M, Sakata Y, et al. Abnormal plasminogen. A hereditary molecular abnormality found in a patient with recurrent thrombosis. *J Clin Invest* 1978;61:1186.

118. Wohl RC, Summaria L, Robbins KC. Physiologic activation of the human fibrinolytic system. Isolation and the characterization of human plasminogen variants. Chicago I and Chicago II. *J Biol Chem* 1979;254:9063.

119. Liu Y, Lyons RM, McDonah J. Plasminogen San Antonio: an abnormal plasminogen with a more cathodic migration, decreased activation and associated thrombosis. *Thromb Haemost* 1988;59:49.

120. Meade TW, North WRS. Chakrabarti RR, et al. Hemostatic function and cardiovascular death: early results of a prospective study. *Lancet* 1980;i:1050.

121. Wilhelmsen L, Svardsudd K, Korsan-Bengsten K, et al. Fibrinogen as a risk factor for stroke and myocardial infarction. *N Engl J Med* 1984; 311:501.

122. Johnson O, Mellbring G, Nilsson T. Defective fibrinolysis in survivors of myocardial infarction. *Int J Cardiol* 1984;6:380.

123. Paramo JA, Colucci M, Collen D, et al. Plasminogen activator inhibitor in the blood of patients with coronary artery disease. *Br Med J* 1985;291:573.

124. Hamsten A, Blomback M, Wiman B, et al. Hemostatic function in myocardial infarction. *Thromb Haemost* 1986;55:58.

125. Hamsten A, Wiman B, de Faire U, et al. Increased plasma levels of a rapid inhibitor of tissue plasminogen activator in young survivors of myocardial infarction. *N Engl J Med* 1985;313:1557.

126. Hasselaar P, Derksen RHWM, Blokzijil L, et al. Crossreactivity of antibodies directed against cardiolipin DNA, endothelial cells and blood platelets. *Thromb Haemost* 1990;63:169.

127. Asherson RA, Khamashta MA, Gil A, et al. Cerebrovascular disease and antiphospholipid antibodies in systemic lupus erythematosus, lupus like disease, and the primary antiphospholipid syndrome. *Am J Med* 1989;86:391.

128. Carreras LO, Defreyn G, Machin SJ, et al. Arterial thrombosis, intrauterine death and lupus anticoagulant. Detection of immunoglobulin interfering with prostacyclin formation. *Lancet* 1981;i:244.

129. De Castellaranau C, Vila L, Sancho MJ, et al. Lupus anticoagulant recurrent abortion and prostacyclin production by cultured smooth muscle cells. *Lancet* 1983;ii:1137.

130. Recker DP, Leff Rl. The broach clinical reach of antiphospholipid antibodies. *Comtemp Intern Med* 1989;Nov/Dec:30.

131. Sanfelippo MJ, Drayna J. Prekallikrein inhibition associated with the lupus anticoagulant. A mechanism of thrombosis. *Am J Clin Pathol* 1982;77:275.

132. McNeil HP, Simpson RJ, Chesterman CN, et al. Antiphospholipid antibodies are directed against a complex antigen that includes a lipid binding inhibitor of coagulation: $\beta_2$-glycoprotein I (apolipoprotein H). *Proc Natl Acad Sci USA* 1990;87:4120.

133. Galli M, Comfurius P, Maassen C, et al. Anticardiolipin antibodies (ACA) directed not to cardiolipin but to a plasma protein cofactor. *Lancet* 1990;335:1544.

134. Klemp P, Rosemary C, Cooper FJ, et al. Anticardiolipin antibodies in ischaemic heart disease. *Clin Exp Immunol* 1988;74;254.

135. Morton KE, Gavaghan TP, Krilis TP, et al. Coronary artery bypass graft failure: an autoimmune phenomenon. *Lancet* 1986;ii:1353.

136. Hamsten A, Bjorkholm M, Norberg R, et al. Antibodies to cardiolipin in young survivors of acute myocardial infarction: an association with recurrent cardiovascular events. *Lancet* 1986;i:113.

137. Becker RC, Corrao JM, Bovill EG, et al. Intravenous nitroglycerin-induced heparin resistance: a qualitative antithrombin III abnormality. *Am Heart J* 1990;119:1254.

138. Innerfield I, Goldfischer JD, Reicher-Reiss H, et al. Serum antithrombin in coronary artery disease. *Am J Clin Pathol* 1976;65:64.

139. Shapiro ME, Rodvein R, Bauer KA, et al. Acute aortic thrombosis in antithrombin III deficiency. *JAMA* 1981;254:1759.

140. Bovill EG, Bauer KA, Dickerman JD, et al. The clinical spectrum of heterozygous protein C deficiency in large New England kindred. *Blood* 1989;73:712.

141. Hacker SM, Williamson BD, Lisco S, et al. Protein C deficiency and acute myocardial infarction in the third decade. *Am J Cardiol* 1991; 68:137.

142. D'Angelo A, Vigano-D'Angelo S, Esmon CT, et al. Acquired deficiencies of protein S. Protein S activity during oral anticoagulation, in liver disease and in disseminated intravascular coagulation. *J Clin Invest* 1988;81;1445.

143. Vigano-D'Angelo S, D'Angelo A, Kaufman J, et al. Protein S deficiency occurs in the nephrotic syndrome. *Ann Intern Med* 1987;107: 42.

144. Schwarz HP, Schernthaner G, Griffin JH. Decreased plasma levels of protein S in well-controlled type I diabetes mellitus (letter). *Thromb Haemost* 1987;57:240.

145. Coller BS, Owen J, Jesty J, et al. Deficiency of plasma protein S, protein C, or antithrombin II and arterial thrombosis. *Arteriosclerosis* 1987;7:456.

146. Lepapte A, Gutman N, Guitton JD, et al. Nonenzymatic glycosylation increases platelet aggregation potency of collagen from placenta of diabetic human beings. *Biochem Biophys Res Commun* 1983;111: 602.

147. Silberhaur K, Schernthaner G, Sinzinger H, et al. Decreased vascular prostacyclin in juvenile-onset diabetes. *N Engl J Med* 1979;300:366.

148. McLaren M, Jennings PE, Alexander W, et al. Responses to venous occlusion in non-insulin dependent diabetic and its relationship to blood glucose. *Thromb Haemost* 1991;65:987(abst).

149. Weick JK. Intravascular coagulation in cancer. *Semin Oncol* 1978;5: 203.

150. Yoda Y, Abe T. Fibrinopeptide A (FPA) level in fibrinogen kinetics in patients with malignant disease. *Thromb Haemost* 1981;46:706.

151. Rickles FR, Edwards RL, Barb C, et al. Abnormalities of blood coagulation in patients with cancer. Fibrinopeptide A generation and tumor growth. *Cancer* 1983;51:301.

152. Murphy S. Thrombocytosis and thrombocythemia. *Clin Haematol* 1983;12:89.

153. Maldonado JE, Pinaido T, Pherre RV. Dysplastic platelets and circulating megakaryocytes in chronic myeloproliferative disease. 1. The platelets: ultrastructure and peroxidase reaction. *Blood* 1974;43:797.

154. Newman G, Mitchell JRA. Homocystinuria presenting as multiple arterial occlusions. *Q J Med* 1984;210:251.

155. Boers GHJ, Smals AGH, Trigbels FJM, et al. Heterozygosity for homocystinuria in premature peripheral and cerebral occlusive arterial disease. *N Engl J Med* 1985;313:709.

156. Fauci AS, Haynes BF, Katz P. The spectrum of vasculitis: clinical, pathologic, immunologic and therapeutic considerations. *Ann Intern Med* 1978;89:660.

157. Angels-Cano E, Sultan Y, Clauvel JP. Predisposing factors to thrombosis in systemic lupus erythematosus: possible relation to endothelial cell damage. *J Lab Clin Med* 1979;94:312.

*The Critically Ill Cardiac Patient,*
edited by V. Kvetan and D. R. Dantzker,
Lippincott - Raven Publishers, Philadelphia © 1996.

CHAPTER 14

# Cardiac Trauma

Panagiotis N. Symbas and Alexander G. Justicz

Traumatic heart disease has been known since antiquity as is evident in Homer's *Iliad* (1): "He fell with a crash and the lance fixed in his heart that was still beating."

Through the centuries thereafter, wounds of the heart were considered untreatable and universally lethal (2), until 1897, when Rehn (3) performed the first successful cardiography in humans. Since then traumatic heart disease has been considered predominately a surgical disease. However, with the advancement of technology, the participation of internists and cardiologists in the diagnosis and management of these diseases is increasing.

Traumatic heart disease is commonly caused from penetrating and blunt trauma, although with the increase of the scope and frequency of invasive procedures, the incidence of traumatic heart disease caused by them is becoming more prevalent (4–6). Cardiac injury from ionizing radiation or electric current also rarely occurs (7, 8).

Trauma is a leading cause of morbidity, mortality, and loss of work force in the industrialized nations. During 1985, 59 million people were injured in the United States, 143,000 deceased, and 2.3 million were hospitalized (9). Injury to the heart is responsible for a portion of these fatalities. It has been estimated that about 10% of the victims of penetrating trauma to the chest have injury to the heart, and 60% to 80% of them develop lethal cardiac tamponade or exsanguinate (10). Also, autopsies of unselected deaths from automobile accidents have shown a 15% to 17% incidence of cardiac contusion (11).

## PENETRATING TRAUMA TO THE HEART

Penetrating cardiac injuries usually are due to knife or missile wounds. They frequently involve only the free cardiac wall, but injury to other structures of the heart—cardiac valves, chordae tendineae, papillary muscles, atrial or ventricular septa, coronary arteries, and conduction system—may occur (12). The cardiac wounds may be single or multiple; the latter are more commonly caused by missiles (13) (Table 1).

The clinical manifestations of penetrating injuries to the heart depend upon the size and site of the wound, the mode of injury, and especially the state of the pericardial wound. When the pericardial wound remains open, the bleeding occurs freely into the pleural space. The cardiac wound then presents with signs and symptoms of hemothorax and loss of blood volume (Fig. 1A). When the pericardial wound is sealed, the bleeding is confined in the pericardial space, manifesting with a clinical picture of cardiac tamponade (14) (Fig. 1B). When either of these two clinical entities or a combination of both is present, the diagnosis of cardiac injury is strongly suspected and is confirmed at the time of exploratory thoracotomy. Occasionally neither cardiac tamponade nor significant bleeding is present; rather the patients only have a precordial wound. In the past these patients presented a considerable diagnostic and therapeutic dilemma, as to whether they had a heart wound or not. The management of such patients has heretofore been either close observation with the accompanying risk of sudden hemodynamic deterioration and even death or exploration of the heart through a subxyphoid approach. Currently the use of echocardiography has greatly facilitated the management of these patients. The demonstration of presence or absence of fluid in the pericardial cavity usually correlates with the presence or absence of a cardiac wound. The timely use of echocardiography renders the management of this group of patients safer, avoids unnecessary surgery, and reduces the cost of their care. The treatment of acute penetrating wounds of the heart is immediate open drainage of the pericardial space and repair of the cardiac wound. During the waiting period for thoracotomy the patient's circulating blood volume is expanded by autotransfusing the blood drained from the pleural space and

P. N. Symbas: Department of Cardiothoracic Surgery, Grady Memorial Hospital, Emory University School of Medicine, Atlanta, Georgia 30309.

A. G. Justicz: Department of Thoracic and Cardiovascular Surgery, Piedmont Hospital, Atlanta, Georgia 30309.

**TABLE 1.** *Sites of cardiac wounds*

| Site | Number |
| --- | --- |
| RV | 48 |
| LV | 22 |
| RA | 8 |
| LA | 4 |
| PA | 6 |
| RV, LV | 5 |
| RV, LA | 3 |
| LV, RA | 1 |
| RV, MV, LA | 1 |
| LV, RV, LA, BA | 1 |
| LV, LA | 2 |
| LV, LAD | 5 |
| LV, diagonal | 1 |
| RV, RCA | 1 |
| LV coronary vein | 3 |

From Symbas PN. *Cardiothoracic trauma: current problems in surgery.* St Louis, MO: Mosby Year-Book; 1991:752, with permission.
Data from patients treated at Grady Memorial Hospital, 1975–1985. LV, left ventricle; RV, right ventricle; LA, left atrium; RA, right atrium; PA, pulmonary artery; LAD, anterior descending coronary artery; RCA, right coronary artery; MV, mitral valve.

by the rapid intravenous administration of fluids, and pericardiocentesis may be done (Fig. 2).

Once a wound of the free cardiac wall is successfully closed, many trauma victims do not recover their preinjury cardiac status. Rather, they have a variety of residual or delayed sequelae: ventricular or atrial septal defect; injury of the valve cusps, leaflets, or chordae tendineae; aortocardiac, aortopulmonary, coronary artery to coronary vein or to cardiac chamber communication; ventricular aneurysm; posttraumatic or postoperative pericarditis (Table 2). In addition, they may have a host of electrocardiographic abnormalities (12, 13) (Table 3). Echocardiography before the patient's discharge excludes the presence of most of these sequelae. After discharge they should be followed for clinical manifestations of any posttraumatic cardiac sequelae. When a patient develops symptoms and signs of a structural defect, appropriate diagnostic studies including echocardiography and/or cardiac catheterization should be performed to define the lesion and its hemodynamic significance and to determine the proper mode of therapy. The therapy for posttraumatic sequelae is the same as for other similar acquired cardiac lesions, except for retained missiles in the heart (14).

Frequently the question arises as to whether they should be removed or not. Retention of a projectile in the heart may result from a direct injury to the heart or an injury to a systemic vein with subsequent migration of the missile to the heart. The missile may cause a variety of complications; it may embolize into the systemic or pulmonary arteries, bacterial endocarditis may also occur if the projectile is not completely embedded in the myocardium and occasional patients develop cardiac neurosis (15–19). In most patients, however, the retained missile in the heart results in no ill effects over a long period of observation (20, 21). A review of our own experience as well as that of other investigators concerning the management and outcome of retained missiles in the heart indicated that their treatment should be individualized according to the patient's clinical course and the site, size, and shape of the missile (20, 21). All symptomatic missiles and large missiles with irregular margins should be removed. Similarly, missiles free or partially protruding into a left cardiac chamber should be removed, because they may embolize into the systemic arterial system and cause serious complications. Missiles in a right chamber may be removed or may be left to embolize in the pulmonary vascular bed,

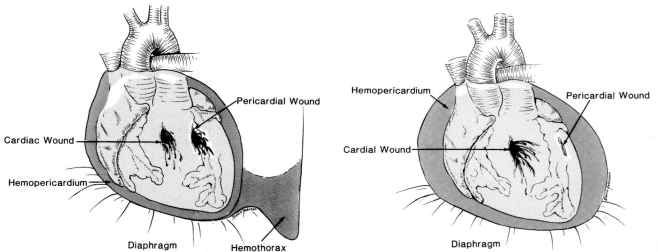

**FIG. 1.** Penetrating wounds of the heart. With **(A)** open and **(B)** sealed pericardial wound. From Symbas PN. *Cardiothoracic trauma.* Philadelphia: WB Saunders; 1989:31, with permission.

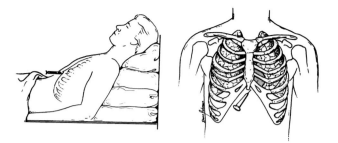

**FIG. 2.** Pericardiocentesis through the left paraxiphoid route. From Symbas PN. *Cardiothoracic trauma.* Philadelphia: WB Saunders; 1989:23, with permission.

**TABLE 3.** *Recorded postoperative ECG findings*

| | |
|---|---|
| Nonspecific ST-T wave changes | 8 |
| Right bundle branch block | 1 |
| Atrial fibrillation | 1 |
| One degree block with ischemic changes | 3 |
| Normal electrocardiogram | 12 |
| Ischemic/injury changes | 18 |
| Q waves | 5 |
| T-wave inversion | 3 |

From Symbas PN. Cardiothoracic trauma: current problems in surgery. St Louis, MO: Mosby Year-Book; 1991:752, with permission.
Data from 113 patients with penetrating cardiac wounds treated at Grady Memorial Hospital, 1975–1985.

from which they can be easily retrieved (15). Bullets or pellets in the myocardium or intrapericardial are tolerated well, and they can be left in place.

## BLUNT INJURIES

The vast majority of the blunt trauma to the heart is due to vehicular accidents, although other forms of trauma, even from various sports, may also cause such injuries. The spectrum of blunt cardiac injuries extends from concussion to various structural lesions of the heart. Concussion is a functional cardiac injury caused by a sharp precordial blunt trauma. It results in a dysrhythmia causing sudden hemodynamic collapse and even death without associated structural cardiac damage (22). Its treatment consists of immediate cardiopulmonary resuscitation, precordial thump, assisted ventilation, and defibrillation, as indicated by electrocardiographic monitoring. The structural traumatic lesions include rupture of pericardium, free cardiac wall, ventricular septum and valves, and myocardial contusion. Each lesion, except for cardiac contusion, can be diagnosed and managed similarly to those from penetrating trauma. Appropriate tests include echocardiography and/or cardiac catheterization. As far as cardiac contusion is concerned, considerable controversy exists in the literature, particularly concerning its diagnosis.

**TABLE 2.** *Residual sequelae in 113 patients with penetrating cardiac wounds treated during 1975 to 1985*

| | |
|---|---|
| VSD[a] | 4 |
| VSD with mitral regurgitation | 1 |
| Mitral valve prolapse | 2 |
| Abnormal septal motion | 2 |
| Retained missiles | 2 |
| Ventricular aneurysm | 1 |
| Murmur | 2 |

From Symbas PN. *Cardiothoracic trauma: current problems in surgery.* St Louis, MO: Mosby Year-Book; 1991:752, with permission.
[a]Ventricular septal defect.

Cardiac contusion is the blunt injury which results in identifiable histopathologic changes of the myocardium. These lesions may vary considerably in extent and character, ranging from small areas of petechiae or ecchymosis to contusion of the full thickness of the myocardial wall (14). As a result, the clinical manifestation of cardiac contusions varies. Patients with contusion of the heart are usually asymptomatic. Rarely they may complain of angina, such as chest pain (23) which is unresponsive to nitroglycerin and commonly is transient unless there is concomitant coronary artery injury. In patients with severe contusion of the heart, congestive heart failure may be present.

The diagnosis of cardiac contusion should be suspected in all patients who have sustained significant trauma to the chest. Although the agreement is universal that a high index of suspicion is of paramount importance in the diagnosis of contusion, there is very little agreement as to the relative diagnostic value of each of the available tests. This is because, other than by pathologic examination of the heart, there is no gold standard test against which to measure the sensitivity and specificity of the currently available diagnostic tests. As a result, the diagnostic accuracy of each of these tests has been derived by comparing one test with another unproven one. Electrocardiography, creatine phosphokinase and its cardiac enzyme (CPK-MB) cardiac radioisotope scanning, radionuclide ventriculography, and echocardiography have been the usual tests for diagnosing cardiac contusion. Numerous studies on the specificity and sensitivity of each of these diagnostic methods have been performed, yielding conflicting results. These differences are difficult to resolve. In addition, each of the available tests has additional individual limitations.

Electrocardiography is the most widely used test. The electrocardiographic abnormalities which may accompany cardiac contusion include various tachycardias, premature contractions, conduction abnormalities, and QRS and ST- and T-wave changes. However, in traumatized patients many of these abnormalities are nonspecific since they may be due to hypotension, hypoxia, stress, electrolyte abnormalities (especially hyperkalemia), or head trauma (24, 27). Interestingly, occasional trauma victims with no electrocardiographic abnormalities have demonstrated myocardial contusion at autopsy (28). As a result, the electrocardiogram has generally been considered to lack both specificity and sensitivity for the diagnosis of myocardial contusion.

The use of CPK-MB has been extended from diagnosing acute myocardial infarction to diagnosing cardiac contusion. Although some studies have shown improved overall sensitivity in detecting contusion when compared with the admission electrocardiogram, others have demonstrated no elevation of the CPK-MB in patients with and abnormal two-dimensional echocardiogram and radionuclide ventriculogram (29—33). Moreover, other conditions (33), such as tachyarrhythmias, gas gangrene, muscular dystrophies, Reye's syndrome, Rocky Mountain spotted fever, and major crush injuries to the skeletal muscle with CPK values greater than 20,000 IU/L as well as trauma to the tongue, have been shown to be accompanied by an increase in CPK-MB. Additionally, the CPK-MB activity has been shown to be negligible in endomyocardial biopsy specimens of normal ventricles (34). As a result, young healthy trauma victims may have negligible elevations of serum CPK-MB. Therefore this test also has been considered to lack specificity and sensitivity in the diagnosis of myocardial contusion.

Myocardial radioisotope scanning with $_{99}$Tc pyrophosphate in dogs with experimentally produced full-thickness contusion of the heart has readily identified areas of injury. However, in the animals with contusion limited to subepicardial ecchymosis, the scanning showed no abnormality (35). Similarly, in electrocardiographically proven myocardial contusion the diagnostic accuracy of radionuclide imaging was disappointing (36).

Radionuclide ventriculography has shown promise in evaluation of patients with cardiac trauma. Some investigators have shown improved sensitivity of this diagnostic test compared with electrocardiography or CPK-MB determinations. Others were unable to demonstrate prognostic value of radionuclide ventriculography in victims from blunt trauma (32, 37, 38). In addition the technical complexity, the cost, and the lack of easy availability at the bedside are currently its disadvantages.

Transthoracic echocardiography has been found to be a valuable diagnostic test for contusion of the heart, particularly when performed early and interpreted by a highly skilled physician (39, 40). A variety of echocardiographic abnormalities have been considered indicative of cardiac contusion, but the real specificity of some of these abnormalities is not known (31). While some investigators have shown poor correlation with other diagnostic tests and failure of echocardiography to provide prognostic information in trauma victims, others have demonstrated significant sensitivity in predicting cardiac complications, particularly arrhythmias (32, 41). Not uncommonly, bedside two-dimensional transthoracic echocardiography in a patient with a traumatized chest may be difficult, and the quality of the study may not be satisfactory. Therefore the routine screening of trauma victims with this technique does not appear to be warranted. The diagnostic value of transesophageal echocardiography in blunt cardiac trauma has not been evaluated extensively. It is a test that can be easily done in critically ill patients, and its potential appears to be promising.

Considering the sensitivity, specificity, accessibility, and cost of all the currently available tests, it appears that the appropriate use and interpretation of electrocardiography, CPK-MB isoenzyme determination, and in selected patients echocardiography will provide acceptable accuracy in the diagnosis of cardiac contusion (30, 32, 41–47). A 12-lead electrocardiogram should be obtained in all patients with history of blunt trauma even when there are no external stigmata of injury. Another electrocardiogram should be done at 24 and 48 hours to determine whether the electrocardiographic abnormality persists or, if the initial electrocardiogram was normal, to see whether any evolutionary changes have occurred. As mentioned earlier, abnormal electrocardiographic findings following blunt trauma from causes other than cardiac injury usually disappear after the stabilization of the acute situation. Therefore, with the exception of sinus tachycardia, new and persistent electrocardiographic changes and particularly the presence of Q waves can be considered with relative safety, indicative of the presence of myocardial contusion. Elevation of serum CPK-MB in the absence of other causes also should be considered indicative of the presence of contusion of the heart. Echocardiography should be obtained in all symptomatic patients and in patients with signs and symptoms of other structural cardiac injury. New echocardiographic abnormalities should be considered indicative of cardiac contusion. Thus, until better tests are found, the prudent use and interpretation of a combination of electrocardiography, serum levels of CPK-MB, and echocardiography appears to be an accurate and cost-effective algorithm for detecting cardiac contusions of clinical significance.

The treatment of myocardial contusion is expectant and directed toward symptoms. The regimen includes administration of antiarrhythmic drugs and digitalis as needed. When angina such as chest pain is present, it is controlled with either analgesics or narcotics, since coronary vasodilators have virtually no effect on it. Anticoagulants are contraindicated during the early postinjury days because they may precipitate intrapericardial hemorrhage.

Patients with cardiac contusion who require early surgical intervention under general anesthesia for other organ injuries, as with patients with acute myocardial infarction, should be considered a high operative risk. However, several studies now have shown that the required surgical procedure can be done safely (32, 46) under close electrocardiographic and hemodynamic monitoring during the intraoperative and perioperative periods.

When congestive heart failure is present during the acute postinjury period, appropriate treatment with digitalis, diuretics, and other inotropic agents should be initiated. Also, the patients should be studied to determine whether the failure is due to the contusion only, which is a rare occurrence, or to additional structural injury, such as rupture of the ventricular septum or of a valve. Echocardiography and/or cardiac catheterization will reveal the diagnosis, determine its relative contribution to the cardiac failure, and indicate the mode of treatment. Patients with decompensation due only to the contusion who cannot be controlled with routine supportive measures should be maintained with intra-aortic balloon counterpulsation or other ventricular-assist devices (48) while the myocardium recovers.

The prognosis for patients with cardiac contusion who recover from the acute insult is usually good. These injuries, whether superficial or full thickness, heal without any significant residual lesion. Occasionally, delayed sequelae such as ventricular aneurysm, traumatic pericarditis, and coronary artery fistula may appear weeks or months later. For this reason patients who sustain cardiac contusion should be followed, and the appropriate studies should be done when cardiac symptoms persist or new ones appear.

# REFERENCES

1. Homer. *The Iliad*. Pope A (trans). New York: Heritage Press; 1934: 314.
2. Paget S. *The surgery of the chest*. London: John Wright and Sons; 1896:121.
3. Rehn L. Ueber penetrirende Herzwunden und Herznaht. *Arch Klin Chir* 1897;55:315.
4. Bredlau CE, Roubin GS, Leimgruber PP, Douglas JS Jr, King SB Jd, Gruentzig AR. In-hospital morbidity and mortality in patients undergoing elective coronary angioplasty. *Circulation* 1985;72:52.
5. Safian RD, Berman AD, Diver DJ, et al. Balloon aortic valvuloplasty in 170 consecutive patients. *N Engl J Med* 1988;319:125.
6. Shah KB, Rao TL, Laughlin S, El Etr AA. A review of pulmonary artery catheterization in 6,245 patients. *Anesthesiology* 1984;61:271.
7. Morton DL, Glancy DL, Joseph WL, Adkins PC. Management of patients with radiation-induced pericarditis with effusions: a note on the development of aortic regurgitation in two of them. *Chest* 1973;64:291.
8. Jackson SH, Parry DJ. Lightning and the heart. *Br Heart J* 1980;43: 454.
9. Rice DP, MacKenzie EJ and Associates. Cost of injury in the United States. A report to congress. San Francisco, CA: Institute for Health and Aging, University of California and Injury Prevention Center, The Johns Hopkins University; 1989:2.
10. Sugg WL, Rea WJ, Ecker RR, et al. Penetrating wounds of the heart: an analysis of 459 cases. *J Thorac Cardiovasc Surg* 1968;56:531.
11. Schulz E, Maghsudi AA. Herzverletzungen und ihre beziehungen zu anderen organverletzungen bei verkehrsunfallen. *Dtsch Z Ges Gerichtl Med* 1969;65:65.
12. Symbas PN, DiOrio DA, Tyras DH, et al. Penetrating cardiac wounds: significant residual and delayed sequelae. *J Thorac Cardiovasc Surg* 1973; 66:526.
13. Symbas PN. *Traumatic heart disease current problems in cardiology*. St Louis, MO: Mosby; 1991:544.
14. Symbas PN. *Cardiothoracic trauma*. Philadelphia: WB Saunders; 1989:1159.
15. Symbas PN, Hatcher CR Jr, Mansour KA. Projectile embolus of the lung. *J Thor Cardiovasc Surg* 1968;56:97.
16. Symbas PN, Harlaftis N. Bullet emboli in the pulmonary and systemic arteries. *Ann Surg* 1977;185:318.
17. Decker HR. Foreign bodies in the heart and pericardium should they be removed? *J Thorac Surg* 1939;9:62.
18. Harken DE. Experiments in intracardiac surgery. I. Bacterial endocarditis. *J Thorac Surg* 1942;11:656.
19. Turner GG. Bullets in the heart for 23 years. *Surgery* 1942;9:832.
20. Symbas PN, Picone AL, Hatcher CR Jr, Vlasis SE. Cardiac missiles: a review of the literature and personal experience. *Ann Surg* 1990; 211:639.
21. Symbas PN, Vlasis SE, Picone AL, Hatcher CR Jr. Missiles in the heart. *Ann Thorac Surg* 1989;48:192.
22. Abrunzo TJ. Commotio cordis, the single, most common cause of traumatic death in youth baseball. *Am J Dis Child* 1991;145:1279.
23. Kissane RW. Traumatic heart diseases, especially myocardial contusion. *Postgrad Med* 1954;15:114.
24. Bayer MJ, Burdick D. Diagnosis of myocardial contusion in blunt chest trauma. *JACEP* 1977;6:238–242.
25. Hoffman B. The genesis of cardiac arrhythmias. *Prog Cardiovasc Dis* 1966;8:319.
26. Marriott HY. Physiologic stimuli simulating ischemic heart disease. *JAMA* 1967;200:715.
27. Tindall GT, Kinjiro I. Cardiorespiratory changes associated with intracranial pressure waves: evaluation of these changes in 27 patients with head injuries. *South Med J* 1975;68:407.
28. Blair E, Topuzlu C, Davis JH. Delayed or missed diagnosis of cardiac damage in blunt chest trauma. *J Trauma* 1971;11:129.
29. Keller KD, Shatney CH. Creatine phosphokinase-MB assays in patients with suspected myocardial contusion: diagnostic test or test of diagnosis? *J Trauma* 1988;28:58.
30. Helling TS, Duke P, Beggs CW, Crouse LJ. A prospective evaluation of 68 patients suffering blunt chest trauma for evidence of cardiac injury. *J Trauma* 1989;29:961.
31. Potkin RT, Werner JA, Trobaugh GB, et al. Evaluation of noninvasive tests of cardiac damage in suspected cardiac contusion. *Circulation* 1982;66:625.
32. Fabian TC, Mangiante EC, Patterson CR, et al. Myocardial contusion in blunt trauma: clinical characteristics, means of diagnosis, and implications for patient management. *J Trauma* 1988;28:50.
33. Marmor A, Alpin G. Specificity of creatine kinase MBV isoenzymes for myocardial injury. *Clin Chem* 1978;24:2206.
34. Ingwall JS, Kramer MF, Fifer MA, et al. The creatine kinase system in normal and diseased human myocardium. *N Engl J Med* 1985;313: 1050.
35. Gonzalez AC, Harlaftis N, Gravanis M, Symbas PN. Imaging of experimental myocardial contusion. Observations and pathologic correlations. *Am J Roentgenol* 1977;128:1039.
36. Rodriguez A, Shatney C. The value of technetium pyrophosphate scanning in the diagnosis of myocardial contusion. *Am Surg* 1982;48:472.
37. Harley DP, Mena I, Miranda R, et al. Myocardial dysfunction following blunt chest trauma. *Arch Surg* 1983;118:1384.
38. Harley DP, Mena I, Narahara KA, et al. Traumatic myocardial dysfunction. *J Thorac Cardiovasc Surg* 1984;87:386.
39. Miller FA Jr, Seward JB, Gersh BJ, et al. Two-dimensional echocardiographic findings in cardiac trauma. *Am J Cardiol* 1982;50:1022.
40. King RM, Mucha P Jr, Seward JB, et al. Cardiac contusion: a new diagnostic approach utilizing two-dimension echocardiography. *J Trauma* 1983;23:610.
41. Reif J, Justice JL, Olsen WR, Prager RL. Selective monitoring of patients with suspected blunt cardiac injury. *Ann Thorac Surg* 1990; 50:5303.
42. Baxter BT, Moore EE, Moore FA, McCrosky BL, Ammons LA. A plea for sensible management of myocardial contusion. *Am J Surg* 1989;158:557.
43. Wisner DH, Reed WH, Riddick RS. Suspected myocardial contusion. Triage and indications for monitoring. *Ann Surg* 1990;212(1):82–86.
44. Miller FB, Shumate CR, Richardson JD. Myocardial contusion. When can the diagnosis be eliminated? *Arch Surg* 1989:124:8058.
45. Foil MB, Mackersie RC, Furst SR, et al. The asymptomatic patient with suspected myocardial contusion. *Am J Surg* 1990;160:638.
46. Norton MJ, Stanford GG, Weigelt JA. Early detection of myocardial contusion and its complications in patients with blunt trauma. *Am J Surg* 1990:160:577.
47. Healey MA, Brown R, Fleiszer D. Blunt cardiac injury: Is this diagnosis necessary? *J Trauma* 1990;30(2):137.
48. Snow N, Lucas AE, Richard JD. Intraaortic balloon counterpulsation for cardiogenic shock from cardiac contusion. *J Trauma* 1982;22:426.

*The Critically Ill Cardiac Patient,*
edited by V. Kvetan and D. R. Dantzker,
Lippincott-Raven Publishers, Philadelphia © 1996.

CHAPTER 15

# Cardiovascular Complications of Organ Transplantation

Sunil Mankad, Adelaida M. Miro, G. Daniel Martich, and Ake Grenvik

Organ transplantation has come of age. Individual patients have now lived more than 35 years after such impressive procedures as kidney, liver, or heart transplantations which were pioneered 30 to 40 years ago. By January 1, 1995, approximately 500,000 transplantations have been performed worldwide, and this figure is expected to double by the year 2000. Current 1-year survival after heart or liver transplantation approximates 90%. For kidney recipients, this figure is above 95%. The results of pancreas and lung transplantation are also improving rapidly. Any physician is likely to encounter patients with a transplanted organ even if not personally involved in such a program. Patients who have undergone organ transplantation are usually admitted to an intensive care unit (ICU) postoperatively but may also develop complications later in the post-transplantation period which may necessitate admission to an ICU. Their complications frequently involve the cardiovascular system. Therefore, it is important for cardiologists to be familiar with these problems commonly experienced by transplanted patients.

S. Mankad: Department of Medicine, University of Pittsburgh, School of Medicine, Pittsburgh, Pennsylvania 15213.

A. M. Miro: Department of Anesthesiology/CCM and Medicine, University of Pittsburgh, School of Medicine, Pittsburgh, Pennsylvania 15213.

G. D. Martich: Department of Anesthesiology/CCM and Medicine, University of Pittsburgh, School of Medicine, Pittsburgh, Pennsylvania 15213.

A. Grenvik: Department of Anesthesiology, Medicine and Surgery, University of Pittsburgh, School of Medicine, Pittsburgh, Pennsylvania 15213.

## THORACIC ORGAN TRANSPLANTATION

### Heart Transplantation

#### *Right Ventricular Dysfunction*

Right ventricular (RV) failure early in the postoperative period is a common complication after orthotopic heart transplantation (OHTX). Its diagnosis should be suspected when systemic hypotension, elevated central venous pressure, low to normal pulmonary capillary wedge pressure despite an elevated pulmonary arterial pressure, and low cardiac index are observed. Right ventricular dilatation and hypokinesis can be confirmed with echocardiography. Elevated pulmonary vascular resistance (usually defined as more than 4 to 5 Wood units despite maximum pulmonary vasodilation) is the most important factor responsible for acute RV failure following OHTX (1). The newly transplanted heart usually has not had to work against high RV afterload and, therefore, is quite prone to developing acute RV failure when significant pulmonary hypertension exists. Although every effort is made at screening recipients for pulmonary hypertension, acute RV failure secondary to this problem remains a significant cause of early mortality in OHTX (2–4). Multiple other factors also contribute to transient RV dysfunction after OHTX, including suboptimal donor quality, prolonged donor organ ischemic time, and inadequate cardiac preservation technique (5).

Once acute RV failure occurs, treatment is aimed simultaneously at two specific goals. First, inotropic agents are infused in an attempt to improve RV contractility. Dobutamine, isoproterenol, or amrinone are preferred since they possess pulmonary vasodilatory properties, but dopamine or epinephrine may certainly be substituted. Often, a combination of these various agents brings about the highest degree of improvement in RV contractility.

Intravenous sodium nitroprusside or nitroglycerin is concurrently utilized to reduce pulmonary vascular resistance. Should these standard agents prove ineffective at lowering pulmonary vascular resistance, intravenous infusion of prostaglandin $E_1$ can be successfully utilized to treat acute RV failure in this setting (6–9). Norepinephrine, which provides some beta-adrenergic effects in addition to excellent alpha-adrenergic action, is occasionally required to maintain systemic vascular resistance when these pulmonary vasodilating agents are used. Severe RV failure, refractory to the above treatment modalities, may warrant insertion of a RV assist device (RVAD). An RVAD may provide the failing right ventricle sufficient time for recovery and has been used with limited success for this purpose (10–12). Such heroic support may, however, carry an increased risk of infection and subsequent morbidity in the immunosuppressed patient (13). Fortunately, rapid resolution of posttransplant pulmonary hypertension is normally observed (14). Therefore, prolonged aggressive treatment usually is not required. Furthermore, the use of moderately "oversized" donor hearts in recipients with elevated pulmonary vascular resistance has also been effective in limiting the early postoperative incidence of right-sided heart failure (13).

Heterotopic heart transplantation is another modality utilized to protect against RV dysfunction in the setting of pulmonary hypertension. In this situation, the native heart is not removed and the transplanted heart is inserted parallel to the native heart (Fig. 1). The native right ventricle, which is adapted to a high afterload, protects the transplanted heart against this sudden burden, thus facilitating support of the native left ventricle by the transplanted heart.

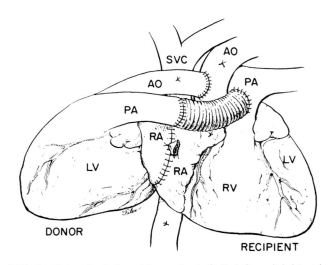

**FIG. 1.** Heterotopic heart transplant. Both left and right atria are anastamosed side to side in a parallel fashion. End-to-side anastamoses are used for the aorta and pulmonary arteries. An interposition graft may be needed to connect the pulmonary arteries.

## Rejection

Although immunosuppression strategies have improved greatly over the past decade, rejection is still one of the leading causes of death in the first year after OHTX (15–17). Historically, cardiac rejection was functionally classified as hyperacute, acute, or chronic, depending on temporal appearance. A clinically more meaningful classification has emerged based on immunologic mechanisms, and cardiac rejection is now classified as either (a) cell mediated (humoral) or (b) antibody mediated (vascular).

Hyperacute rejection is a form of humoral rejection and is both rare and difficult to diagnose. This complication may manifest immediately after reperfusion of the graft in the operating room, or it may follow a more insidious course marked by a progressive rise in central venous pressure with concomitant decline in cardiac index unresponsive to pharmacotherapy (13). It carries a grave prognosis and appears to occur as a result of preformed recipient antibodies directed against the donor heart. These antibodies may be the result of a previous exposure to human antigens such as might occur with pregnancy or blood transfusions (2, 18). Hyperacute rejection occurred in 19 of our first 450 patients at the University of Pittsburgh, and only one of these patients survived following heroic support with a Jarvik-7 total artificial heart, plasmapheresis, and subsequent retransplantation (13, 19, 20). Fortunately, this complication is exceedingly rare today, because of improved donor-recipient antigen screening.

Acute rejection occurs with a frequency of approximately $1.3 \pm 0.7$ episodes per patient within the first year of OHTX based on information from the Transplant Cardiologists Research Database (TCRD) (21). The TCRD data indicate that 37% of patients had no rejection episode, 40% had one episode, and 23% had more than one episode in the first year after transplantation. The acute rejection episodes (most often cell mediated) were asymptomatic in the majority of these patients and, thus, were found only on endomyocardial biopsy. The clinical spectrum of acute rejection ranges from asymptomatic patients to those with acute myocardial decompensation with congestive heart failure, hypotension, elevated cardiac filling pressures, and a low cardiac index. Arrhythmias, both supraventricular and ventricular, can occur and recur until the rejection episode is brought under control. When the clinical presentation is severe, urgent endomyocardial biopsy is performed, but aggressive antirejection treatment is often empirically initiated. Despite advances in treatment, death from acute rejection represented 17% of all lethal cases in the TCRD series (21).

Allograft coronary artery disease has been described as a form of chronic rejection, although some authorities now discourage that description and believe that this form of vasculopathy is not truly a form of rejection. A better term to describe this disorder is allograft arteriopathy. Immunologic factors certainly have a significant role in its development, but other processes such as viral infection, hypertension, and hyperlipidemia have also been implicated (22). This topic will be discussed in greater detail later in this chapter.

Factors implicated in augmenting the risk of rejection following OHTX include female gender in the donor or recipient (21, 23), human leukocyte antigen (HLA) mismatch (18), young age (24), non-O blood types (25), panel-reactive antibody (PRA) screen above 10% (26, 27), positive donor-specific crossmatch (25), OKT3 murine monoclonal antibody sensitization (27), and the presence of HLA antibodies (28). Although there are continued attempts at identifying noninvasive means of diagnosing rejection, endomyocardial biopsy remains the gold standard. The International Society of Heart and Lung Transplantation has published a grading scale to quantify the degree of rejection present on endomyocardial biopsy (29) (Table 1). This provides objective means of describing how much rejection exists and also assists in quantifying the success of antirejection therapy.

There are a variety of treatment strategies for acute rejection. The particular strategy utilized depends on multiple factors, including (a) the histologic grade of rejection, (b) the severity of clinical symptoms and hemodynamic compromise, (c) the experience of the clinician, (d) the previous antirejection therapy rendered and its success or failure, and (e) the time course after transplantation. A detailed discussion of immunosuppressive therapy is beyond the scope of this chapter but is summarized elsewhere (30). In general, mild rejection is not usually treated but rather is followed closely as it usually progresses to greater rejection in only a minority of cases (31, 32). Moderate or severe rejection, on the other hand, is almost invariably treated with increased immunosuppression. The usual initial therapy is 0.5 to 1 gram of methylprednisolone intravenously daily over 3 days (33). Rejection episodes that are inadequately controlled with a single treatment course of corticosteroids are often treated with a second course. Should that second course fail or the clinical presentation be extremely severe, monoclonal antibody (usually OKT3) (34, 35), antithymocyte globulin (36, 37), or cyclophosphamide therapy is often added. The likelihood of rejection is greatest within 6 to 9 months of OHTX. The incidence of rejection markedly decreases after this time has elapsed.

### Cardiac Allograft Arteriopathy

An unusual type of post-OHTX coronary artery disease, cardiac allograft arteriopathy, is both the leading cause of death after the first posttransplant year and the most common indication for retransplantation (2, 22, 38–43). The angiographic prevalence of this allograft arteriopathy is between 2% and 28% one year posttransplant and increases around 10% per year to between 30% and 70% five years after transplantation (44–48). This proliferative vascular disease of the coronary arteries is pathophysiologically similar to the *vanishing bile duct syndrome* seen in liver transplants, the *obliterative bronchiolitis* in lung transplants, and the *chronic rejection* of renal allografts (49). In contrast to the proximal, focal stenoses seen in native coronary artery disease, this disorder is primarily diffuse and involves the coronary arteries at more distal locations and often without collaterals (48). The lesions may be further described as having longitudinal concentric narrowing with pruning or complete obstruction of the most distal segments. Routine posttransplant coronary arteriograms are necessary for diagnosis since the denervation of the cardiac allograft makes angina distinctly unusual, although it has been reported (50).

The etiology of allograft arteriopathy involves two primary interrelated conditions: (a) immune-mediated or infection-related endothelial injury and (b) environmental factors such as hyperlipidemia, hypertension, nicotine abuse, and obesity (22, 42, 51, 52). The environmental factors that play so critical a role in the development of native coronary artery disease probably take on a more limited role in the development of allograft arteriopathy. Evidence is accumulating in favor of an immune-mediated process of endothelial injury, subsequent nonspecific response to that injury being the primary inciting factor for the development of allograft arteriopathy (2, 42, 53–55). It should be borne in mind that the allograft vascular endothelium is the site at which the recipient initially and continuously meets the transplanted organ. However, data as to whether the incidence of cellular rejection correlates with the subsequent development of allograft arteriopathy are mixed (56–58).

Cytomegalovirus infection–related endothelial injury has also been implicated as a possible etiologic factor in the development of allograft arteriopathy (59–62). This

**TABLE 1.** *International Society of Heart and Lung Transplantation standardized cardiac biopsy grading scale*

| Grade | Definition |
| --- | --- |
| 0 | No rejection |
| 1 | Focal (perivascular or interstitial) infiltrate without myocardial necrosis |
| 1B | Diffuse but sparse infiltrate without myocardial necrosis |
| 2 | One focus only with aggressive infiltration and/or focal myocyte damage |
| 3A | Multifocal aggressive infiltrates and/or myocyte damage |
| 3B | Diffuse inflammatory process with myocardial necrosis |
| 4 | Diffuse aggressive polymorphous ± infiltrate, ± hemorrhage ± vasculitis, with myocardial necrosis |

idea has not yet been proven, however, and it has been argued that the presence of cytomegalovirus infection itself is more likely to occur should aggressive antirejection treatment have been needed. A reasonable hypothesis is that endothelial injury, regardless of whether it was primarily immune mediated or infection related, initiates a cascade of events that eventually lead to allograft arteriopathy. Environmental factors may then influence the rapidity with which this process develops.

Coronary allograft arteriopathy occurs with equal frequency in patients transplanted for ischemic cardiomyopathy and those transplanted for other reasons. Most patients have silent ischemia up until the time they present with arrhythmias (63), progressive congestive heart failure, or decompensated acute myocardial infarction. Thus, the symptoms at the time of their presentation might include dyspnea, palpitations, profound weakness, or sudden death (64). The electrocardiogram is often difficult to interpret secondary to the diffuse and atypical pattern of infarction (64) . Since this disease usually is asymptomatic and may progress rapidly to catastrophic events, surveillance coronary arteriography is the current standard. Noninvasive methods for the detection of ischemia have proven ineffective so far, probably related to the diffuse nature of the vasculopathy (65, 66). Coronary arteriography also underdiagnoses this disease (45), but quantitative angiography and intracoronary Doppler measurement of blood flow may increase its sensitivity (39, 67, 68).

The therapy of allograft arteriopathy has not been very effective at changing the clinical course of the disease (2). Medical treatment that has been tried includes exercise, smoking cessation, meticulous blood pressure control, lipid-lowering measures, antiplatelet and anticoagulant drugs, calcium channel blockers, and vasodilators (2, 42, 69–72). Angioplasty has been performed on more proximal lesions with good initial results but unknown long-term success rates (73). Typically, however, the diffuse and distal nature of allograft arteriopathy precludes the use of angioplasty. Coronary artery bypass grafting has been successfully performed in a few patients (74, 75) but is also not usually possible because of diffuse lesions and poor distal target vessels. Ultimately, retransplantation is the only definitive treatment for allograft arteriopathy, but the success rate in this setting is significantly lower than for a first transplant with only 55% and 25% survival at 1 and 2 years, respectively (76).

### Arrhythmias

A variety of both bradyarrhythmias and tachyarrhythmias occur following heart transplantation. Supraventricular, junctional, and ventricular arrhythmias all can be seen. The diagnosis of these various arrhythmias can be complicated in heart transplant recipients since their elec-

trocardiograms often demonstrate two distinct P waves. One atrial signal originates from both the transplanted heart and the other from the residual cuff of the native right atrium. The native atrial depolarization may be affected by alterations in parasympathetic and sympathetic tone, but the denervated donor heart atrial activity is not. Electrocardiographic interpretation may be even more difficult in the setting of heterotopic heart transplantation as both native and donor electrocardiographic (EKG) complexes may be seen independently (Fig. 2). As the denervated transplanted heart usually lacks physiologic responses to both sympathetic and parasympathetic mediated stimuli, unique treatment of arrhythmias in this setting is sometimes required.

As a result of exposure to hypothermia in combination with possible preservation, ischemic, and reperfusion injury, the intrinsic rate of the denervated heart may be quite slow (1, 13, 77). Sinus bradycardia or low-grade atrioventricular nodal block is the most frequent rhythm disturbance in the early postoperative period (1). Heart rate must be supported with either pacing or chronotropic agents (usually to a rate of at least 90 beats/min) since both myocardial and systemic oxygen delivery appear to be heart rate dependent during this period (78). Dobutamine (usually at doses of 5 to 10 mcg/kg/min) or isoproterenol (usually at doses of 0.01 to 0.05 mcg/kg/min) are utilized for chronotropy when bradycardia exists early in the posttransplant period. These drugs are slowly tapered over the following weeks. Ventricular pacing is incorporated if the agents are ineffective, although atrioventricular synchrony is lost in this setting. It should be noted that atropine has no effect on the denervated transplanted heart. Terbutaline (79) or aminophylline has been successfully utilized as a more chronic treatment for persistent bradycardia after cardiac transplantation. Fewer than 10% of patients require implantation of a permanent pacemaker prior to hospital discharge (1, 80).

Supraventricular arrhythmias occurring following cardiac transplantation also require unorthodox treatment strategies, again relating to the denervation of the transplanted heart. Vagal maneuvers have an extremely limited role in management of the denervated transplanted heart. Similarly, digoxin, which acutely decreases atrioventricular conduction by indirectly increasing vagal tone, has no effect in acutely slowing atrial tachyarrhythmias in the transplanted heart. It may still, however, have a role in long-term control of ventricular rates in cardiac transplant patients with atrial tachyarrhythmias (81). Because of their potential anti-inotropic activity, calcium channel blockers and beta-blockers are seldom used to control arrhythmias in transplanted hearts. Type IA antiarrhythmics are utilized in the treatment of supraventricular arrhythmias in transplanted hearts in much the same fashion as they are normally utilized. The vagolytic effects of these drugs do not exist in transplanted hearts, but their numerous other side effects still do. There is limited infor-

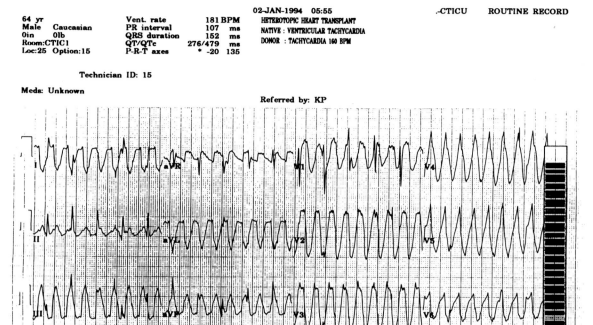

64 yr
Male    Caucasian
0in    0lb
Room:CTIC1
Loc:25 Option:15

Vent. rate        181 BPM
PR interval       107  ms
QRS duration      152  ms
QT/QTc       276/479  ms
P-R-T axes    *  -20  135

02-JAN-1994  05:55
HETEROTOPIC HEART TRANSPLANT
NATIVE : VENTRICULAR TACHYCARDIA
DONOR : TACHYCARDIA 160 BPM

.-CTICU    ROUTINE RECORD

Technician ID: 15

Meds: Unknown

Referred by: KP

25mm/s    10mm/mV    100Hz    ?A-001-002A    128L 110    CID: 2        EID:    8  EDT: 21:07 03-JAN-1994  ORDER:

**FIG. 2.** Electrocardiogram of a heterotopic heart transplant recipient in which the native heart is in ventricular tachycardia and the donor heart is in sinus rhythm.

mation on the use of adenosine in transplanted hearts, but it likely will have a significant role in the treatment of supraventricular arrhythmias in this setting. Adenosine may, however, have an exaggerated magnitude and duration of effect in transplanted hearts. Therefore, smaller initial doses (1.5 to 2.0 mg) should be used, and backup pacemaker function should be checked prior to its use. The clinical significance and relationship to rejection of supraventricular arrhythmias is much debated (77, 82, 83). Atrial flutter, in particular, does appear to be closely associated with rejection and may be regarded as an indication for endomyocardial biopsy (77).

Ventricular ectopic beats occur commonly in transplanted hearts, but unless complex ventricular depolarizations are demonstrated, they are usually not clinically important (82). Treatment of complex ventricular arrhythmias occurring in cardiac transplant recipients is much the same as in any other population. Therapy aimed at correction of electrolyte disturbances, evaluation of ischemia, and reduction of inotropic support is initiated. The use of lidocaine, phenytoin, quinidine, and procainamide in cardiac transplant recipients is not much different than in normal populations. Bretylium is rarely

used in cardiac transplant recipients, as its antiarrhythmic properties are poorly understood and may depend on intact autonomic innervation (1) (Table 2).

### Inotropic Dependence, Hypertension, and Other Complications

The transplanted heart invariably requires inotropic support secondary to the impairment of ventricular contractility resulting from hypothermic cardioplegic preservation and possible ischemic injury (1). Inotropic support is used, usually with dobutamine or isoproterenol, since these drugs also possess pulmonary vasodilating properties, to maintain a cardiac index of at least 2.5 L/min/m$^2$. Close observation of both hemodynamic and other physiologic variables is important. The duration of this support is often related to the quality of the transplanted heart, the length of donor organ ischemic time, and the underlying medical condition of the transplant recipient.

Hypertension is extremely common in cardiac transplant recipients and occurs in between 50% and 90% (2) of cases (40, 84). Cyclosporine is clearly implicated as an

**TABLE 2.** *Efficacy of antiarrhythmic agents after cardiac transplantation*

| | |
|---|---|
| Class IA antiarrhythmics | Yes |
| Class IB antiarrhythmics | Yes |
| Class IC antiarrhythmics | ? |
| Class II antiarrhythmics | Yes[a] |
| Class III antiarrhytmics | ? |
| Class IV antiarrhytmics | Yes[a] |
| Digoxin | No[b] |
| Atropine | No |
| Adenosine | Yes |

[a]Use limited by anti-inotropic activity.
[b]May have role in chronic treatment.

etiologic factor in the development of this transplant hypertension (84–89), but corticosteroids play an important role as well (84, 90). Although increased sympathetic tone and resultant loss of the nocturnal decline in blood pressure is associated with cyclosporine-induced hypertension (87, 89), multiple other etiologies have been suggested as well. These include cyclosporine nephrotoxicity, increased renal tubular reabsorption of sodium in conjunction with volume expansion, alteration of intracellular calcium regulation, and vasoconstriction secondary to excessive production of prostaglandins (2, 40, 87—89, 91). The efficacy of various agents in the treatment of transplant hypertension has not been tested in prospective randomized trials. Calcium antagonists and ace inhibitors are the most commonly employed antihypertensive drugs in this setting (40), but alpha-blockers, hydralazine, beta-blockers, and diuretics have all been prescribed with varying success. These drugs may be used alone or in combination and exert their typical adverse side effects.

Atrial septal defects (ASDs) may rarely occur following heart transplantation. This is a result of the increased wall tension created along the intra-atrial septum by the surgical procedure itself or may be the result of a patent foramen ovale or ASD present in the donor heart which was not appreciated at the time of procurement or implantation (1, 13). An ASD may increase RV strain, and if elevation of right atrial pressure were to occur, significant right-to-left shunting may be seen with resultant systemic embolic risk and hypoxia. Therefore, the presence of either a patent foramen ovale or an ASD are carefully evaluated and surgically repaired, if found.

Precise orientation between new and native vascular structures in both pulmonary and cardiac transplantation can be difficult. Although extremely rare, pulmonary artery torsion and obstruction may be seen as a result of rotational misalignment (13). This entity is usually recognized immediately after separation from cardiopulmonary bypass, but delayed diagnosis has been reported (92). Should such an event occur, severe hemodynamic and pulmonary embarrassment is usually the case. Treatment requires surgical correction involving cardiopul-

monary bypass. Because the recipient's pulmonary veins are anastomosed to the donor left atrium via the recipient left atrium cuffs, true stenosis of these veins is not a common complication of OHTx, but kinking or twisting of the pulmonary veins may occur with resultant increase in PVR (pulmonary vascular resistance). This also causes RV strain and possibly failure necessitating surgical correction when diagnosed.

**Lung Transplantation**

Cardiovascular complications of lung transplantation are rare. The two most frequent complications can be divided according to the underlying pathology which necessitated transplantation initially.

Patients with chronic obstructive pulmonary disease from any etiology who undergo single-lung transplant (SLT) are managed in the early postoperative period with a double-lumen endotracheal tube and differential lung ventilation (DLV). Typically, over the next 24 to 48 hours these patients will be converted to a single-lumen endotracheal tube, weaned from mechanical ventilation, and extubated without difficulty (93). However, should the patient develop primary failure of the pulmonary allograft either from an ischemic or reperfusion injury, the time course can be markedly prolonged with continued need for DLV. In this scenario, there is an increased requirement for oxygenation and ventilation placed on the native lung. Because of this increased need with higher than usual tidal volumes and respiratory rates used on the native lung, auto–positive emd-expiratory pressure (PEEP) can develop and cause the native lung to hyperinflate. Hyperinflation of the native lung can then cause a thoracic tamponade effect with hemodynamic compromise. To treat this condition, the patient is removed from positive pressure on the native lung by disconnecting that side from the ventilator.

The other major cardiovascular complication of lung transplantation involves the need for cardiopulmonary bypass (CPB) during the procedure. Cardiopulmonary bypass is required for nearly all patients undergoing double-lung transplantation or SLT for pulmonary hypertension (94). The cardiovascular consequence of CPB principally is depression of ventricular function for 8 to 10 hours after surgery (95). The need for total heparinization during CPB increases the amount of bleeding both intra- and postoperatively. To avoid these CPB consequences, double-lung transplant can be performed as sequential SLTs with lung function, first by the remaining native lung, then by the first SLT while the second lung is being implanted. However, pulmonary failure during this procedure may still necessitate conversion to CPB.

There is continued controversy over the best surgical approach to the patient with end-stage lung disease and pulmonary hypertension. Many centers exclusively use heart-lung transplantation as the treatment of choice.

However, because of the shortage of acceptable heart-lung donor *blocs*, several centers have successfully performed SLT also in this group of patients (96). The hemodynamic consequences of SLT in patients with severe pulmonary hypertension merit discussion in this section. Although ventricular failure has been reported in a patient undergoing SLT for pulmonary hypertension, in general, there is an improvement in the patient's cardio-vascular status after the operation (97, 98). Despite systemic or suprasystemic pulmonary artery pressures prior to transplantation, these patients can have a significant decrement in pulmonary artery pressures following SLT. Patients with severe pulmonary hypertension may have RV dilatation and dysfunction prior to transplant; however, RV failure is unlikely following SLT (98).

Right ventricular dysfunction may also be seen following single- or double-lung transplantation. Significant PEEP is employed on newly transplanted lungs. In general, PEEP adversely affects RV function. The practice of restricting the administration of fluids following lung transplantation in order to avoid the development of pulmonary edema is also commonly utilized and brings about a situation in which left ventricular (LV) function may be preload dependent. Thus, the high levels of PEEP often utilized in lung transplantation can significantly increase RV afterload which may compromise RV function. This, in turn, can bring about a decrease in LV preload and subsequent fall in cardiac output.

Pulmonary venous obstruction following lung transplantation may result secondary to kinking of the pulmonary veins or a narrow venous anastomosis with or without thrombosis (99, 100). The diagnosis should be entertained whenever pulmonary edema develops in the transplanted lung. Diagnosis is best achieved with transesophageal echocardiography, pulmonary angiography, or radionucleotide evaluation. Surgical treatment is usually needed, although anticoagulation may be of help if partial thrombosis has occurred.

## ABDOMINAL ORGAN TRANSPLANTATION

There are several organs in the abdominal cavity that may be transplanted following irreversible end-stage disease. These organs include the kidneys, liver, pancreas, islet cells, small bowel, and different combinations of multivisceral allografts. With the many diseases that lead to end-stage organ failure, there may be concurrent cardiac involvement predisposing to perioperative cardiovascular complications either in the operating room or afterward in the ICU. Cardiac disease may even be associated with the primary disease process necessitating the organ transplant. Because these patients have multiple problems, physicians must have a logical and systematic approach to the evaluation and medical optimization prior to transplant surgery.

### Kidney Transplantation

With the current advance in surgical technique and immunosuppression, all patients with end-stage renal disease, regardless of age, should be considered eligible for kidney transplantion in the absence of a contraindication to the procedure.

Patients with end-stage renal failure from diabetic nephropathy represent a large proportion of kidney transplant candidates and the group most extensively studied with respect to cardiac complications. In the diabetic patient population, there is an extremely high incidence of concurrent ischemic heart disease, which is a major determinant of outcome following the transplant procedure (101–104). Because of autonomic neuropathy, many patients with diabetic nephropathy may have significant coronary artery disease with relatively little or no symptomatology (101). In a study by Braun and colleagues where coronary arteriography was performed in patients who were active renal transplant candidates, 40% of diabetic patients with significant coronary artery disease (>70% occlusion in one or more vessels) were completely asymptomatic and without any ischemic EKG changes compared to only 26% of asymptomatic nondiabetic patients. Furthermore, the diabetic patients who ultimately progressed to myocardial infarction were significantly younger than their nondiabetic counterparts (average age 36 vs. 54 years). Among transplant and nontransplant renal failure patients with a positive angiogram, fatal coronary artery events were the leading cause of death within the first year (105). Thus, an extremely thorough preoperative cardiac evaluation is mandatory in both symptomatic and asymptomatic patients with diabetes who are candidates for kidney transplantion.

Several diagnostic strategies have been evaluated in order to identify cardiac risk patients considered for kidney transplantation. Thallium stress testing, which is useful in nondiabetic and nonuremic populations, was no better in predicting subsequent cardiovascular events (angina, myocardial infarction, arrhythmia, stroke, pulmonary embolism) than a positive history and abnormal electrocardiogram in renal transplant candidates (106). The limited exercise capacity of diabetic patients with renal failure may have explained the low sensitivity and poor predictive value of the exercise stress test. However, a subsequent study with thallium stress testing as the initial diagnostic test used stricter criteria for interpretation of negative results (107). In this study, the stress test was reported as negative only if patients were able to attain 85% or greater of the age-predicted maximal heart rate without any symptoms (chest pain, EKG changes, or perfusion defects). In this group, there were no cardiac complications or deaths in the 6 to 34 months of follow-up. However, only 12 of 60 patients subjected to the exercise stress testing were able to achieve greater than 85% of their age-predicted maximal heart rate. Patients who had an indeterminate or positive stress thallium test were further evaluated by a coronary angiogram. If patients had normal coronary arteries (<50% stenosis) and/or LV ejection fraction (EF) between 30% and 50%, no cardiovascular death occurred after renal transplantation. In patients with one- or two-vessel disease and normal or mild LV impairment, 25% of patients (two of eight) died of cardiovascular causes within approximately 1 year after transplantation. Patients with severe LV dysfunction (EF < 30%) and three-vessel disease, including left main coronary artery disease, were not considered candidates for renal transplantation. There was no mortality and only 1 case of a significant hematoma among the 53 patients who underwent cardiac catheterization.

Transthoracic two-dimensional and M-mode echocardiography has also been evaluated as a noninvasive screening tool to asses the preoperative cardiac risk factors among diabetic renal transplant patients. Of multiple echo-derived estimates of systolic function that were studied, an increase in end-systolic diameter and a decreased velocity of circumferential shortening were most predictive of a poor survival after surgery (104).

If operable coronary artery disease is detected among renal transplant candidates, one needs to consider the optimal timing of a coronary artery bypass grafting (CABG) operation. In a study by Swift et al., open-heart surgery was associated with a higher incidence of bleeding requiring reoperation in the early postoperative period (108). Among nine patients who underwent

CABG after renal transplantation, there was an increased incidence of infectious complications, two of which were fatal, yielding a 22% mortality. However, there was a reasonably good 71% overall combined survival (43- to 52-month follow-up), indicating that although these patients represent a high risk for perioperative complications, open-heart surgery in patients with end-stage renal disease, both before and after kidney transplantation, should remain a viable therapeutic option. It appears that such heart surgery is best performed before transplantation and subsequent immunosuppression.

In summary, uremic patients who are considered for kidney transplantion as a minimum should have a thorough medical history analysis, physical examination, and electrocardiogram to screen for any evidence of underlying coronary artery disease that would increase perioperative risk and reduce survival. Any positive risk factors should be further investigated, first, with noninvasive tests such as stress thallium or by echocardiography. Any positive findings on these tests should be followed by a coronary angiogram. If operable lesions are detected, CABG may be undertaken with reasonable safety, although these uremic patients are at an increased risk for perioperative bleeding and subsequent infection. In patients with diabetes, the high incidence of asymptomatic significant coronary artery disease warrants a more aggressive diagnostic intervention. An algorithmic approach to the preoperative cardiac evaluation is depicted in Fig. 3.

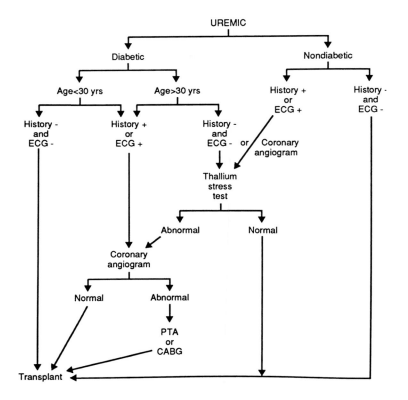

**FIG. 3.** Preoperative cardiac evaluation strategy for potential renal transplant candidates.

## Liver Transplantation

In general, patients with end-stage liver disease requiring transplantation are at risk for a variety of cardiac complications. Certain complications are similar to those seen with any extensive surgical procedure. Others are specifically associated with the etiology of the liver disease and the transplantation procedure.

### PreTransplant Considerations

Patients with end-stage liver disease and clinical risk factors associated with heart disease are described in Table 3. Our cardiac approach to liver transplant candidates at the University of Pittsburgh Medical Center is summarized in Table 4.

One particular group of patients with cirrhosis that requires a more aggressive diagnostic cardiac intervention is comprised of patients with alcoholic liver disease. Chronic alcoholism can lead to the development of a dilated congestive cardiomyopathy (109–112). Even acute alcoholic binging can have direct toxic effect on the myocardium. The etiology of alcoholic cardiomyopathy is not clear, but there is definitely a spectrum of diseases ranging from mild to severe cardiac contractile dysfunction. Even asymptomatic individuals without clinical evidence of heart disease may demonstrate contractile dysfunction on noninvasive imaging such as echocardiography (110, 113, 114). Information regarding the cardiac status of a liver transplant candidate is extremely important to the anesthesiologist for intraoperative hemodynamic management and also the liver transplant intensivist, who must manage the postoperative cardiovascular conditions in liver transplant recipients.

It also appears that alcohol-induced cardiomyopathy may be partially or completely reversible after cessation of alcohol abuse (115, 116). Therefore, it is mandatory that liver transplant candidates demonstrate a minimum of 6 months of abstinence before being considered eligible for transplantation. Optimization of cardiac function would be expected to have a favorable impact on perioperative morbidity including hypotension, renal failure, and venous congestion of the allograft. Therefore, a documented sobriety is essential from a hepatic, cardiac, and psychosocial standpoint for achieving successful liver transplantation.

**TABLE 3.** *High cardiac risk in patients with liver failure*

Age > 60 years
Preexisting heart disease
Abnormal electrocardiogram
Alcoholic liver disease
Diabetes
Hemochromatosis
Smoking history

**TABLE 4.** *Cardiac evaluation for liver transplant candidates*

Asymptomatic
  <40 years, electrocardiogram only
  40–60 years, MUGA[a] scan
  >60 years, echocardiography
Symptomatic (myocardial infarction, angina, dyspnea)
  Echocardiography
  Cardiac evaluation (stress thallium/adenosine thallium test, cardiac catheterization, and coronary angiography)
  Cardiac diseases with liver failure
  Alcoholic cardiomyopathy
  Wilson's disease
  Hemochromatosis

[a]MUGA, Multiple Gated Acquisition images.

Other patients with end-stage liver disease associated with a concurrent cardiomyopathy include those with iron storage diseases, specifically hemochromatosis. Primary or idiopathic hemochromatosis is a genetic disorder with an increase in the absorption of dietary iron, which ultimately is deposited in various organs throughout the body. Whether iron deposits in the liver cause cirrhosis or iron deposition is simply superimposed on an already cirrhotic liver is not known. It is also not clear whether the primary defect is in the liver or at some other site. There is a report of a patient with iron overload disease for up to 4 years following transplantation after inadvertently receiving a donor liver from a patient with subclinical primary hemochromatosis. This would implicate the liver as the primary site for the metabolic impairment (117). However, another report failed to demonstrate any problems of iron overload in a liver transplant recipient who also inadvertently received an organ from a donor with hereditary hemochromatosis (118).

It is controversial whether myocardial iron deposits of themselves lead to congestive cardiac failure (119, 120). Cardiac arrhythmias occur frequently in patients presumably due to iron deposition within the cardiac conduction system or myocardial muscle (121). The most frequent types of arrhythmias are supraventricular tachycardia and abnormal atrioventricular conduction. Ventricular arrhythmias are much less common (119, 122). Therefore, patients who are candidates for liver transplantation secondary to cirrhosis from iron storage diseases should have an extremely thorough preoperative cardiac work-up to evaluate the possibility of poor cardiac pump function or significant arrhythmias that would increase the perioperative cardiac risks. Interestingly, it appears that successful liver transplantation may not reverse the hemochromatosis cardiomyopathy, as was seen in one patient who had progressive cardiac failure after liver transplantation and ultimately required heart transplantation (123).

Finally, an extremely important group that requires preoperative cardiac evaluation is comprised of patients with cirrhosis associated with pulmonary hypertension (124–127). Pulmonary hypertension may be seen in patients with autoimmune liver disease such as systemic sclerosis (125). However, pulmonary hypertension has also been found in patients with a variety of liver diseases both with and without cirrhosis. The predisposing factor appears to be the presence of portal hypertension rather than cirrhosis (124, 127). The etiology of increased pulmonary vascular pressures is not known but is presumed to be from possible vasoactive substances secreted by the damaged liver or perhaps a circulating factor that is not metabolized by the liver and gains access to the pulmonary circulation through portosystemic or portopulmonary shunts. Proposed pathophysiologic mechanisms are indicated in Fig. 4.

The associated pulmonary hypertension ranges from mild to severe. When the pulmonary hypertension is long standing, there is evidence of progressive cor pulmonale with manifestations of right-sided heart failure such as elevated central venous pressure and low cardiac output. Using a specialized type of pulmonary artery catheter which can measure RV ejection fraction, we have shown that those patients who are candidates for liver transplantation may have significant impairment of RV contractility (128, 129). Furthermore, when pulmonary vasodilators such as nifedipine, nitroglycerin, or prostaglandin $E_1$ are administered, there is no reduction in pulmonary artery pressure, indicating that there is no reversible or reactive component (128). We are planning to evaluate

whether inhalation of nitric oxide, an extremely potent and selective pulmonary vasodilator, will reduce pulmonary artery pressure in these patients (130).

There are important clinical implications of the presence of pulmonary hypertension in patients considered for liver transplantation. In our early experience, the presence of pulmonary hypertension was often detected in the operating room after insertion of a pulmonary artery catheter when the liver transplant procedure was initiated. Most patients had not been evaluated preoperatively from a cardiac standpoint. Under these circumstances, a decision was made by the anesthesiology and surgical team whether to proceed with the transplantion. If it was decided to proceed, it was often extremely difficult to maintain stable cardiovascular support during the operation, since there was almost invariably some right-sided heart contractile dysfunction. In our early experience, these cases did poorly, with many early deaths from intractable right-sided heart failure after such transplant surgery (128, 131). If there are any suspicious clinical signs or symptoms or electrocardiographic abnormalities such as indications of right atrial enlargement, RV hypertrophy, or right bundle branch block, these patients currently are referred for transthoracic echocardiography, with special attention to estimation of pulmonary artery pressure and presence and quantification of the degree of tricuspid regurgitation. If the echocardiogram suggests, further investigations are performed to determine the etiology. Secondary pulmonary hypertension is investigated

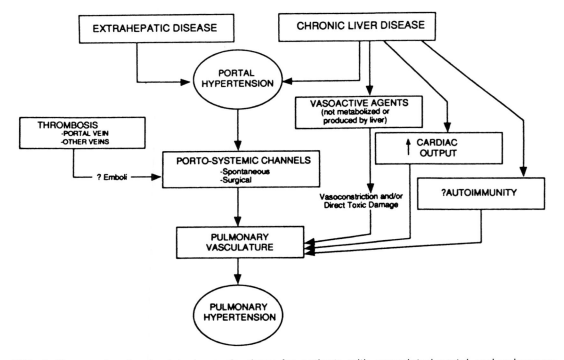

**FIG. 4.** Proposed pathophysiologic mechanisms for patients with associated portal and pulmonary hypertension.

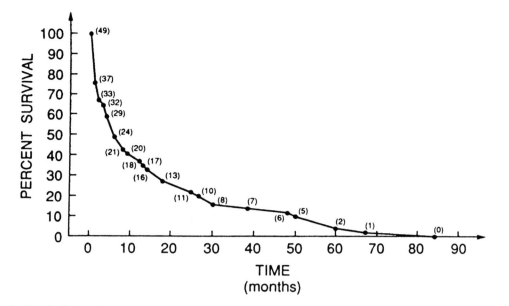

**FIG. 5.** Survival time in 49 patients with coexistent pulmonary and portal hypertension. Numbers in parentheses represent total survivors at any given time.

by obtaining an arterial blood gas to exclude chronic hypoxemia. A ventilation-perfusion scan and lower extremity Doppler studies are also performed to exclude venous thrombosis and chronic pulmonary embolism. A right-sided heart catheterization with the RV ejection fraction (RVEF) catheter is performed to exclude evidence of left-sided heart failure. A trial of pulmonary vasodilators is undertaken to assess the degree of reversibility. If there is significant RV contractility depression (RVEF < 30%) and severe pulmonary hypertension (systolic pressure > 60 mm Hg), patients are not considered for liver transplantation. However, this step should not be taken lightly since the prognosis for patients with coexistent pulmonary and portal hypertension is extremely poor, as depicted in Fig. 5 (127).

It is important to keep in mind that if a patient's right-sided heart function can be supported in the intra- and postoperative period, there is the possibility that the pulmonary hypertension may regress and pulmonary artery pressures normalize with successful transplantation. Future considerations for this multiple-organ failure may be the role of multivisceral transplantation such as heart and liver together (132). Another possibility may be more aggressive support of RV function with mechanical assist devices during the critical early postoperative period.

### Intraoperative Cardiac Complications

There are several different causes of cardiovascular instability in the intraoperative setting, as depicted in Table 5. All patients who are undergoing liver transplantation have invasive hemodynamic monitoring with pul-

monary and systemic arterial catheters. Complications are usually related to the events occurring in the operative field and tend to be seen during certain surgical phases of the transplant procedure. Specifically, profound hemodynamic alterations are seen during the native hepatectomy, the anhepatic and reperfusion stages. Familiarity of the anesthesiologist with these complications and their timing can prevent serious perioperative sequelae.

### Decreased Cardiac Preload

Significant intraoperative blood loss is the hallmark of the native hepatectomy stage in the transplant procedure. This will reduce LV preload, decrease cardiac output, and cause hypotension. Patients with liver failure usually have a coagulopathy, which when associated with serious portal hypertension can make the recipient hepatectomy arduous. It is during the recipient hepatectomy phase that the majority of the blood loss occurs. To adequately maintain circulating blood volume, all patients have at least two large-bore (8.5 Fr) intravenous catheters

**TABLE 5.** *Causes of hemodynamic instability during liver transplantation*

| Surgical stage | Mechanism of hemodynamic instability |
|---|---|
| Native hepatectomy | Blood loss, portal vein and inferior vena cava occlusion |
| Anhepatic stage | Hypocalcemia, myocardial depressants (?) |
| Reperfusion | Hyperkalemic cardiac arrest, myocardial depressants (?) |

inserted prior to the procedure. These catheters are connected to the rapid infusion system (RIS; Haemonetics, Braintree, MA) (133), which is capable of delivering up to 2,000 mL/min of diluted blood and coagulation components. Furthermore, two arterial catheters are placed with no interruption in arterial pressure monitoring during blood aspiration for blood gas or other hematologic determinations. With the RIS, adequate intravascular fluid resuscitation can be accomplished even in extremes of surgical hemorrhages.

During the operations in the early 1980s, patients often became hemodynamically unstable in the anhepatic phase, since both the portal vein and the inferior vena cava were cross clamped, thereby severely reducing systemic venous return to the heart. Furthermore, the obstructed venous beds lead to blood stagnation within the involved organs. Once the portal and vena cava clamps were removed, stagnant blood rich in potassium would return to the systemic circulation and often lead to a hyperkalemic cardiac arrest (134). To circumvent this problem, a venovenous bypass for both portal and systemic venous circulation was developed, with blood from these two venous systems directed to the left axillary vein, thereby returning this blood to the systemic circulation and maintaining cardiac preload (Fig. 6) (133). In Pittsburgh, venovenous bypass is currently employed in almost all liver transplant procedures and is maintained throughout the hepatectomy and donor liver implantation phase until the portal and inferior vena cava anastomoses are completed and circulation reestablished. However, this technique prolongs the duration of the procedure, and if the shunt flow is low, there is risk for clotting and potentially lethal pulmonary embolism.

### Decreased Myocardial Contractility

During the transplant procedure, blood loss is replaced by variable amounts of citrated bank blood. Since citrate is metabolized by the liver, in patients with liver dysfunction, there can be up to a 20-fold increase in serum citrate concentrations during the transplant procedure (135). These increases in serum citrate can then avidly bind to calcium, resulting in significant decreases in ionized serum calcium concentration. Citrate-induced hypocalcemia results in cardiovascular depression manifested by decreases in cardiac index, stroke index, and LV stroke work index. Such hypocalcemic-induced cardiovascular deterioration can be reversed by administration of calcium chloride, restoring normal ionized calcium levels. This phenomenon is most frequently seen during the anhepatic stage of the surgical procedure. Ionized calcium levels need to be monitored closely, not only intra- but also postoperatively, especially if additional blood transfusions are administered and if there is ischemic damage to the transplanted liver, decreasing its ability to regain normal citrate metabolism.

Other significant hemodynamic changes have been documented during the anhepatic and reperfusion stages through the use of pulmonary artery catheters and transesophageal echocardiography (TEE) intraoperative monitoring. Using a RVEF catheter (Baxter-Edwards), De Wolf and colleagues showed depression of RV function during the anhepatic stage which may be secondary to circulating cardiodepressants such as endotoxin (136). During the remainder of the transplant procedure, RV function was preserved. However, other studies have reported TEE evidence of acute right-sided heart failure such as "paradoxical" motion of the interventricular and/or intera-

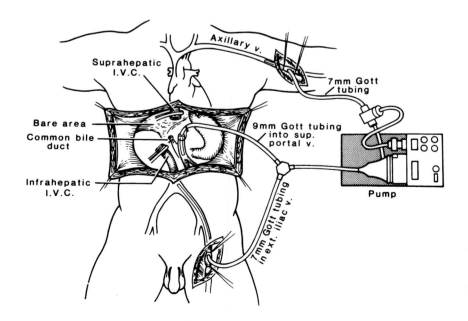

**FIG. 6.** Pump-driven venovenous bypass which allows decompression of the splanchnic and systemic venous beds without the need for heparinization. Redrawn from Griffith BP, et al. *Surg Gynecol Obstet* 1985; 160:270.

trial septum (137, 138). These right-sided heart abnormalities were thought to be related to factors such as pulmonary thromboemboli with low flow (<1 L/min) of non-heparinized venovenous bypass or air embolism during reperfusion (136). Interestingly, both of these studies documented an uncoupling of the pulmonary capillary wedge pressure and central venous pressure (CVP) to the echocardiographic left and right end-diastolic ventricular volumes, respectively, indicating that filling pressure may not accurately estimate preload during the liver transplant procedure. This observation underscores the important role of continuous intraoperative TEE monitoring of patients undergoing liver transplantation.

Finally, during reperfusion of the transplanted liver, it is common to have an increase in the serum potassium concentration which may be mild to very dramatic. The rise of serum potassium is probably caused by a combination of high potassium levels in the preservation solution of the allograft, ischemic injury, and blood stagnation in the recipient, especially if venovenous bypass is not used. Reperfusion cardiac arrest is not an uncommon intraoperative phenomenon but is usually self-limited. However, it requires several minutes of CPR and rapid correction of hyperkalemia with administration of calcium, sodium bicarbonate, glucose, and insulin.

### Postoperative Cardiac Complications

#### Fluid Management

In the immediate postoperative setting, it is extremely important to closely monitor intravascular fluid status. On arrival in the ICU, these patients are usually hypothermic and vasoconstricted. As they rewarm, they will manifest signs of intravascular hypovolemia indicated by tachycardia, fall in arterial blood pressure, oliguria, decreased pulmonary capillary occlusion, and CVP. Under these circumstances, patients usually require additional fluid administration titrated against the above-mentioned clinical indicators of intravascular volume. It is important to avoid both hypo- and hypervolemia. Any hypotension caused by hypovolemia can lead to ischemic injury of the newly transplanted liver and also acute tubular necrosis in the kidney, resulting in a possible need for posttransplant dialysis. Conversely, fluid overload or hypervolemia may prolong the need for mechanical ventilation, and an elevated CVP can decrease venous return from the liver, resulting in hepatic congestion and dysfunction.

It is always critical to maintain a high degree of suspicion for specific causes of hypovolemia such as postoperative bleeding. Intra-abdominal bleeding is monitored by inspection of the abdominal drains that are routinely placed during surgery. If the drainage is hemorrhagic in appearance, a hematocrit of the drainage fluid should be obtained. If this hematocrit is elevated (>5), it is indicative of postoperative bleeding. Under these circumstances, the next step is to determine whether this is a "medical" bleeding amenable to replacement of clotting components or a "surgical" bleeding necessitating reexploration. In general, if the patient is hemodynamically stable and a coagulopathy is present, management of the postoperative bleeding is first attempted through the transfusion of blood components (fresh frozen plasma, cryoprecipitate, and/or platelets), as indicated by thromboelastography (133). However, if the bleeding persists or significantly increases, surgical exploration is warranted. Close collaboration between the medical and surgical ICU team members is crucial in regards to the management and timing of indicated reoperation.

Finally, patients with postoperative liver dysfunction or other complications may have significant third spacing of fluid that can lead to peripheral edema and ascites with low circulating intravascular volume. Under these circumstance, the main emphasis should be on determining the cause of capillary leakage such as sepsis, rejection, pancreatitis, portal vein thrombosis, or hypoalbuminemia. Treatment should be directed to the underlying cause and to maintaining adequate circulating blood volume.

#### Hypotension

The causes of postoperative hypotension are diverse. As mentioned above, in the immediate postoperative setting, factors such as rewarming, hemorrhage, capillary leakage, and other causes all need to be considered.

If a patient has postoperative fever and hypotension anytime after the fifth postoperative day, there are two principal diagnoses that need to be entertained. The first is the possibility of infection. During the postoperative period, sepsis may be caused by a technical complication such as a biliary leak or hepatic artery thrombosis. Therefore, it is imperative that these possibilities be investigated by the appropriate means. Other more general causes of infection such as catheter sepsis, nosocomial pneumonia, and urinary infection should also be considered. The second cause of a septiclike picture in the post-transplant setting is acute cellular rejection. Patients with rejection often present in a manner that is clinically indistinguishable from sepsis. In both cases one can see fever, rise in liver enzymes, and hypotension with a hyperdynamic circulation. It is difficult or even impossible to distinguish sepsis from rejection by clinical parameters alone. In the case of sepsis, one would reduce the degree of immunosuppression to allow the normal host defense to combat the infection. With rejection, the treatment would be an increase in immunosuppression to prevent further graft dysfunction or loss. Thus, the treatment of these two clinically similar presentations is completely opposite. This dilemma is usually resolved by performing a liver biopsy, which can distinguish infection from rejection on the basis of the cellular type and location of the inflammatory infiltrates (139).

*Hypertension*

Elevated blood pressure in the postoperative setting is common. If there is preexisting hypertension, the antihypertensive medications can be resumed once the patient is able to tolerate oral intake. It may be necessary to utilize parenteral drug administration such as sublingual nifedipine or intravenous agents until the patient can use the gastrointestinal route. The combination of tachycardia and hypertension should raise the suspicion of inadequate analgesia, especially in patients who remain intubated and have limited ability to communicate adequately. Finally, if one is employing a cyclosporine-based regimen of immunosuppression, cyclosporine-induced hypertension is seen with relatively high frequency and is usually best managed with angiotensin-converting enzyme inhibitors (140, 141). At the University of Pittsburgh Medical Center, we have been using the new immunosuppressive agent tacrolimus (FK506) for approximately 5 years and have not commonly seen the secondary hypertension that is associated with cyclosporine.

## Pancreas Transplantation

The most common indication for pancreatic transplantation is in conjunction with a kidney transplant in patients with insulin-dependent diabetes mellitus. However, with current improvements in surgical technique and more efficient immunosuppression, there is renewed interest in performing pancreatic transplant alone for diabetic patients before the onset of renal failure. The perioperative management of these patients is identical to that previously discussed for diabetic candidates for renal transplantation. The major emphasis to decrease perioperative cardiovascular morbidity is strict attention to the preoperative evaluation and assessment of cardiac risk factors.

The transplantation of pancreatic islets for glucose control is currently evolving and may be preferable to whole-organ transplantation in that it can be carried out in an ICU with patients fully conscious during catheterization of the portal vein and administration of the islet-containing suspension. In the past, patients developed hypotension after the intraportal infusion of islet cells, which was probably due to the presence of vasoactive substances in the crudely purified tissue suspension (142). However, with recent advances in islet cell isolation and purification, this complication is much more infrequent (143).

## Multivisceral and Intestinal Transplantation

Transplantation of multiple abdominal viscera is an innovative solution to previously untreatable forms of many different types of abdominal diseases (144). The primary indications for multivisceral and intestinal trans-

**TABLE 6.** *Indications for intestinal and multivisceral transplantion*

| |
|---|
| Malignancies |
|   Hepatoma ± direct metastases |
|   Bile duct tumors ± direct metastases |
|   Endocrine tumor with liver metastasis |
|   Short gut syndromes with total parenteral nutrition–induced cirrhosis |
| Short gut syndromes after massive bowel resection for: |
|   Congenital disorders |
|   Malrotation |
|   Inflammatory bowel disease |
|   Radiation enteritis |
|   Mesenteric vascular disease |
|   Abdominal trauma |

plantation are summarized in Table 6. In general, the cardiac complications in this group of patients should be approached similarly to that described for liver transplant recipients. Perioperative management focuses on adequate fluid resuscitation without volume overloading. Distinguishing infection from rejection is challenging with clinically similar clinical presentations that require allograft biopsy to make the distinction. It should be noted that graft versus host disease (GVHD), commonly seen in in bone marrow transplant patients, also occurs with a significant frequency in small-bowel transplant recipients, due to the ample presence of lymphatic tissue in these allografts.

## ACKNOWLEDGMENT

The authors thank Shawna Leech for her secretarial assistance in the preparation of this manuscript.

## REFERENCES

1. Stein KL, Darby JM, Armitage J, Grenvik A. Intensive care of the cardiac transplant recipient. In: Rippe J, ed. *Intensive care medicine.* 2nd ed. Boston: Little, Brown; 1991.
2. Miller LW, Schlant RC, Kobashigawa J, Kubo S, Renlund DG. Task Force 5: complications (of cardiac transplantation). *J Am Coll Cardiol* 1993;22(1):41.
3. Murali S, Uretsky BF, Armitage JM, et al. Utility of prostaglandin E₁ in the pretransplantation evaluation of heart failure patients with significant pulmonary hypertension. *J Heart Lung Transplant* 1992;11:716.
4. Kirklin JK, Naftel DC, McGiffin DC, McVay RF, Blackstone EH, Karp RB. Analysis of morbid events and risk factors for death after cardiac transplantation. *J Am Coll Cardiol* 1988;11:917.
5. McGregor CG. Cardiac transplantation: surgical considerations and early post operative management. *Mayo Clin Proc* 1992;67:577.
6. Vincent JL, Carlier E, Pinsky MR, et al. Prostaglandin E₁ infusion for right ventricular failure after cardiac transplantation. *J Thorac Cardiovasc Surg* 1992;103:33.
7. Armitage JM, Hardesty RL, Griffith BP. Prostaglandin E₁: an effective treatment of right heart failure after orthotopic heart transplantation. *J Heart Transplant* 1987;6:348.
8. D'Ambra MN, LaRaia PJ, Philbin DM, Watkins WD, Hilgenberg AD, Buckley MJ. Prostaglandin E₁: a new therapy for refractory right

heart failure and pulmonary hypertension after mitral valve replacement. *J Thorac Cardiovasc Surg* 1985;89:567.

9. Dewhirst WE. Prostaglandin E$_1$ for refractory right heart failure after coronary artery grafting. *J Cardiothorac Anesth* 1988;2:56.

10. Odom NJ, Richens D, Glenville BE, Kirk AJ, Hilton CJ, Dark JH. Successful use of mechanical assist device for right ventricular failure after orthotopic heart transplantation. *J Heart Transplant* 1990;9:652.

11. Zumbro GL, Kithens WR, Shearer G, Harville G, Bailey L, Galloway RF. Mechanical assistance for cardiogenic shock following cardiac surgery, myocardial infarction, and cardiac transplantation. *Ann Thorac Surg* 1987;44:11.

12. Hetzer R, Hennig E, Schiessler A, Friedel N, Warnecke H, Adt M. Mechanical circulatory support and heart transplantation. *J Heart Lung Transplant* 1992;11:S175.

13. Stein KL, Armitage J, Martich GD, Hardesty RL, Kormos RL, Griffith BP. Intensive care of the cardiac transplant recipient. In: Shoemaker W, Ayres S, Grenvik A, Holbrook P, eds. *Textbook of critical care.* 3rd ed. WB Saunders, Philadelphia. *[in press].*

14. Bhatia SJS, Kirshenbaum JM, Shermin RJ, et al. Time course of resolution of pulmonary hypertension and right ventricular remodeling after orthotopic cardiac transplantation. *Circulation* 1987;76:819.

15. Kirklin JK, Naftel DC, McGiffin DC, McVay RF, Blackstone EH, Karp RB. Analysis of morbid events and risk factors for death after cardiac transplantation. *J Am Coll Cardiol* 1988;11:917.

16. Kriett JM, Kaye MP. The registry of the International Society for Heart Transplantation: seventh official report 1990. *J Heart Transplant* 1990;9:323.

17. O'Connell JB, Renlund DG. Diagnosis and treatment of cardiac allograft rejection. *Cardiovasc Clin* 1990;20:147.

18. Costanzo-Nordin MR. Cardiac allograft vasculopathy: relationship with acute cellular rejection and histocompatibility. *J Heart Lung Transplant* 1992;11:S90.

19. Jacquet L, Stein K, Kormos R, et al. Hyperacute rejection following heart transplantation: clinical hemodynamic evolution. *Chest* 1989;96:233S.

20. Griffith BP, Hardesty RL, Kormos RL, et al. Temporary use of the Jarvik-7 total artificial heart before transplantation. *N Engl J Med* 1987;316:130.

21. Kobashigawa JA, Naftel DC, Bourge RC, et al. Pre-transplant risk factors for acute rejection after cardiac transplantation: a multi-institutional study. *J Heart Lung Transplant* 1993;12:355.

22. Young BY. Cardiac allograft arteriopathy: an ischemic burden of a different sort. *Am J Cardiol* 1992;70:9F.

23. Crandall BG, Renlund DG, O'Connell JB, et al. Increased cardiac allograft rejection in female heart transplant recipients. *J Heart Transplant* 1988;7:419.

24. Renlund DG, Gilbert EM, O'Connell JB, et al. Age associated decline in cardiac allograft rejection. *Am J Med* 1987;83:391.

25. Lavee J, Kormos RL, Duquesnoy RJ, et al. Influence of panel-reactive antibody and lymphocytotoxic crossmatch on survival after heart transplantation. *J Heart Lung Transplant* 1991;10:921.

26. Kormos RL, Colson YL, Hardesty RL, et al. Immunologic and blood group compatibility in cardiac transplantation. *Transplant Proc* 1988;20:741.

27. Hammond EH, Wittwer CT, Greeenwood J, et al. Relationship of OKT3 sensitization and vascular rejection in cardiac patients receiving OKT3 rejection prophylaxis. *Transplantation* 1990;50:776.

28. Suciu-Foca N, Reed E, Marboe C, et al. Role of anti-HLA antibodies in heart transplantation. *Transplantation* 1991;10:674.

29. Billingham ME, Cary NR, Hammond ME, et al. A working formulation for the standardization of nomenclature in the diagnosis of heart and lung rejection: Heart Rejection Study Group. *J Heart Transplant* 1990;9:587.

30. Council on Scientific Affairs. Introduction to the management of immunosuppression. *JAMA* 1987;257:1781.

31. Laufer G, Laczkovics A, Wollenek G, et al. The progression of mild acute cardiac rejection evaluated by risk factor analysis. *Transplantation* 1991;51:184.

32. LLoveras JJ, Escourrou G, Delisle MG, et al. Evolution of untreated mild rejection in heart transplant recipients. *J Heart Lung Transplant* 1992;11:751.

33. Miller LW. Treatment of cardiac allograft rejection with intravenous corticosteroids. *J Heart Transplant* 1990;9:283.

34. O'Connell JB, Renlund DG, Gay WA, et al. Efficacy of OKT3

35. Gilbert EM, Dewitt CW, Eiswirth CC, et al. Treatment of refractory cardiac allograft rejection with OKT3 monoclonal antibody. *Am J Med* 1987;82:202.

36. Renlund DG, O'Connell JB, Gilbert EM, et al. A prospective comparison of murine monoclonal CD-3 (OKT) antibody based and equine antithymocyte globulin-based rejection prophylaxis in cardiac transplantation. *Transplantation* 1989;47:599.

37. Costanzo-Nordin MR, O'Sullivan EJ, Johnson MR, et al. Prospective randomized trial of OKT3 vs. horse antithymocyte globulin based immunosuppressive prophylaxis in heart transplantation. *J Heart Transplant* 1990;9:306.

38. Johnson DE, Alderman EL, Schroeder JS, et al. Transplant coronary artery disease: histopathologic correlations with angiographic morphology. *J Am Coll Cardiol* 1991;17:449.

39. Scott CD, Dark JH. Coronary artery disease after heart transplantation: clinical aspects. *Br Heart J* 1992;68(3):255.

40. Olson LJ, Rodeheffer RJ. Management of patients after cardiac transplantation. *Mayo Clin Proc* 1992;67:775.

41. Billingham ME. Graft coronary disease: the lesions and the patients. *Transplant Proc* 1989;21:3665.

42. Miller LW. Long-term complications of cardiac transplantation. *Prog Cardiovasc Dis* 1991;33:229.

43. Kriett JM, Kaye MP. The Registry of the International Society for Heart and Lung Transplantation: eighth official report. *J Heart Lung Transplant* 1991;10:491.

44. O'Neill BJ, Pflugfelder PW, Singh NR, Menkis AH, McKenzie FN, Kostuk WJ. Frequency of angiographic detection and quantitative assessment of coronary arterial disease one and three years after cardiac transplantation. *Am J Cardiol* 1989;63:1221.

45. Gao SZ, Schroeder JS, Alderman EL, et al. Prevalence of accelerated coronary artery disease in heart transplant survivors. *Circulation* 1989;80(5,Pt 2):III100.

46. Olivari MT, Homans DC, Wilson RF, Kubo SH, Ring WS. Coronary artery disease in cardiac transplant patients receiving triple drug immunosuppressive therapy. *Circulation* 1989;80(5,Pt 2):III111.

47. Billingham ME. Cardiac transplant atherosclerosis. *Transplant Proc* 1987;19(Suppl 5):19.

48. Gao SZ, Alderman EL, Schroeder JS, Silverman JF, Hunt SA. Accelerated coronary vascular disease in the heart transplant patient: coronary arteriographic findings. *J Am Coll Cardiol* 1988;12(2):334.

49. Miller LW. Allograft vascular disease: a disease not limited to hearts. *J Heart Lung Transplant* 1992;11:S32.

50. Schroeder JS, Hunt SA. Chest pain in heart transplant patients. *N Engl J Med* 1991;324:1805.

51. Farmer JA, Ballantyne CM, Frazier OH, et al. Lipoprotein(a) apolipoprotein changes after cardiac transplantation. *J Am Coll Cardiol* 1991;18:926.

52. Winters GL, Kendall TJ, Radio SJ, et al. Posttransplant obesity and hyperlipidemia: major predictors of severity of coronary arteriopathy in failed human heart allografts. *J Heart Transplant* 1990;9:364.

53. Pollack MS, Ballantyne CM, Payton-Ross C, et al. HLA match and other immunological parameters in relation to survival, rejection, severity and accelerated coronary artery disease after heart transplant. *Clin Transplant* 1990;4:269.

54. Rose EA, Smith CR, Petrossian GA, Barr ML, Reemtsma K. Humoral immune responses after cardiac transplantation: correlation with fatal rejection and graft atherosclerosis. *Surgery* 1989;106:203.

55. Young JB, Lloyd KS, Windsor NT, et al. Elevated soluble interleukin-2 receptor levels early after heart transplantation and long-term survival and development of coronary arteriopathy. *J Heart Lung Transplant* 1991;10:243.

56. Uretsky BF, Murali S, Reddy, PS, et al. Development of coronary artery disease in cardiac transplant patients receiving immunosuppression therapy with cyclosporine and prednisone. *Circulation* 1987;76:827.

57. Costanzo-Nordin MR. Cardiac allograft vasculopathy: relationship with acute cellular rejection and histocompatibility. *J Heart Lung Transplant* 1992;11:S90.

58. Zerbe T, Uretsky B, Kormos R, et al. Graft atherosclerosis: effects of cellular rejection and human lymphocyte antigen. *J Heart Lung Transplant* 1992;11:S104.

59. Virella G, Lopes-Virella MF. Infections and atherosclerosis. *Transplant Proc* 1987;19(Suppl 5):26.
60. Everett JP, Hershberger RE, Norman DJ, et al. Prolonged cytomegalovirus infection with viremia is associated with development of cardiac allograft vasculopathy. *J Heart Lung Transplant* 1992;11:S133.
61. Grattan MT, Moreno-Cabral CE, Starnes VA, Oyer PE, Stinson EB. Cytomegalovirus infection is associated with cardiac allograft rejection and atherosclerosis. *JAMA* 1989;261:3561.
62. McDonald K, Rector TS, Braulin EA, Kubo SH, Olivari MT. Association of coronary artery disease in cardiac transplant recipients with cytomegalovirus infection. *Am J Cardiol* 1989;64:359.
63. Romhilt DW, Doyle M, Sagar KB, et al. Prevalence and significance of arrythmias in long-term survivors of cardiac transplantation. *Circulation* 1982;66:I219.
64. Gao SZ, Schroeder JS, Hunt SA, Billingham ME, Valantine HA, Stinson EB. Acute myocardial infarction in cardiac transplant recipients. *Am J Cardiol* 1989;64:1093.
65. Mckillop JH, Goris ML. Thallium-201 myocardial imaging in patients with previous cardiac transplantation. *Clin Radiol* 1981;32:447.
66. Smart FW, Ballantyne CM, Cocanougher B, et al. Insensitivity of noninvasive tests to detect coronary artery vasculopathy after heart transplant. *Am J Cardiol* 1991;67:243.
67. Gao SZ, Alderman EL, Schroeder JS, Hunt SA, Widerhold V, Stinson EB. Progressive coronary luminal narrowing after cardiac transplantation. *Circulation* 1990;82:IV269.
68. St. Goar FG, Pinto FJ, Alderman EL, et al. Intracoronary ultrasound in cardiac transplant recipients. In vivo evidence of angiographically silent intimal thickening. *Circulation* 1992;85:979.
69. Gibbons GH. Preventitive treatment of graft coronary vascular disease: the potential role of vasodilator therapy. *J Heart Lung Transplant* 1992;11:S22.
70. deLorgeril M, Boissonnat P, Dureau G. Low dose aspirin and accelerated coronary disease in heart transplant recipients. *J Heart Transplant* 1990;9:449.
71. Sarris GE, Mitchell RS, Billingham ME, Glasson JR, Cahill PD, Miller DC. Inhibition of accelerated cardiac allograft arteriosclerosis by fish oil. *J Thorac Cardiovasc Surg* 1989;97:841.
72. Schroeder JS, Gao SZ, Alderman EA, et al. A preliminary study of diltiazem in the prevention of coronary artery disease in heart transplant recipients. *N Engl J Med* 1993;328:164.
73. Halle AA, Wilson RF, Vetrovec GW for the Cardiac Transplant Angioplasty Study Group. Multicenter evaluation of percutaneous transluminal coronary angioplasty in heart transplant recipients. *J Heart Lung Transplant* 1992;11:S138.
74. Frazier OH, Vega JD, Duncan JM, et al. Coronary artery bypass two years after orthotopic heart transplantation: a case report. *J Heart Lung Transplant* 1991;10:1036.
75. Copeland JG, Butman SM, Sethi G. Successful coronary artery bypass grafting for high-risk left main coronary artery atherosclerosis after cardiac transplantation. *Ann Thorac Surg* 1990;49:106.
76. Gao SZ, Schroeder JS, Hunt S, et al. Retransplantation for severe accelerated coronary artery disease in heart transplant recipients. *Am J Cardiol* 1988;62:876.
77. Scott CD, Dark JH, McComb JM. Arrhythmias after cardiac transplantation. *Am J Cardiol* 1992;70:1061.
78. Stinson EB, Caves PK, Griepp RB, Oyer PE, Rider AK, Shumway NE. Hemodynamic observations in the period after human heart transplantation. *J Thorac Cardiovasc Surg* 1975;69:264.
79. Cook LS, Will KR, Moran J. Treatment of junctional rhythm after heart transplantation with terbutaline. *J Heart Transplant* 1989;8(4):342.
80. Scott CD, Omar I, McComb JM, Dark JH, Bexton RS. Long-term pacing in heart transplant recipients is usually unecessary. *PACE Pacing Clin Electrophysiol* 1991;14:1792.
81. Ricci DR, Orlick AE, Reitz BA, Mason JW, Stinson EB, Harrison DC. Depressant effect of digoxin on atrioventricular conduction in man. *Circulation* 1978;57:898.
82. Romhilt DW, Doyle M, Sagar KB, et al. Prevalence and significance of arrhythmias in long-term survivors of cardiac transplantation. *Circulation* 1992;66:I219.
83. Little RE, Kay N, Epstein AE, et al. Arrhythmias after orthotopic cardiac transplantation—prevalence and determinants during initial hospitalization and late follow-up. *Circulation* 1989;80(Suppl III):III140.
84. Greenberg ML, Uretsky BF, Reddy PS, et al. Long term hemodynamic follow-up of cardiac transplant patients treated with cyclosporin and prednisone. *Circulation* 1985;71:487.
85. Starling RC, Cody RJ. Cardiac transplant hypertension. *Am J Cardiol* 1990;65:106.
86. Oliveri MT, Antolick A, Ring WS. Arterial hypertension in heart transplant recipients treated with triple drug immunosuppressive therapy. *J Heart Transplant* 1989;8:34.
87. Scherrer U, Vissing SF, Morgan BJ, et al. Cyclosporin induced sympathetic activation and hypertension after heart transplantation. *N Engl J Med* 1990;323:693.
88. Porter GA, Bennet WM, Sheps SG. Cyclosporin-associated hypertension. *Arch Intern Med* 1990;150:280.
89. Mark AL. Cyclosporine, sympathetic activity, and hypertension. *N Engl J Med* 1990;323:748.
90. Renlund DG, O'Connell JB, Gilbert EM, Watson FS, Bristow MR. Feasibility of discontinuation of corticosteroid maintenance therapy in heart transplantation. *J Heart Transplant* 1987;6:71.
91. Yang Z, Richard V, Von Segesser L, et al. Threshold concentrations of endothelin-1 potentiate contractions to norepinephrine and serotonin in human arteries: a new mechanism of vasospasm? *Circulation* 1990;82:188.
92. Demarchena E, Futterman L, Wozniak P, et al. Pulmonary artery torsion: a potentially lethal complication after orthotopic cardiac transplantation. *Heart Transplant* 1989;8:499.
93. Bierman MI, Stein KL, Dauber J, Hardesty RL, Griffith BP. Lung transplantation: thirty years of progress. In: Shoemaker W, Ayres S, Grenvik A, Holbrook P, eds. *Textbook of critical care.* 3rd ed. WB Saunders, Philadelphia. *[in press].*
94. Girard C, Mornex JF, Gamondes JP, Griffith N, Clerc J. Single lung transplantation for primary pulmonary hypertension without cardiopulmonary bypass. *Chest* 1992;102(3):967.
95. Breisblatt WM, Stein KL, Wolfe CJ, et al. Acute myocardial dysfunction and recovery: a common occurrence after coronary bypass surgery. *J Am Coll Cardiol* 1990;15:1261.
96. Hosenpud JD, Novick RJ, Breen TJ, Daily OP. The Registry of the International Society for Heart and Lung Transplantation: eleventh official report—1994. *J Heart Lung Transplant* 1994;13:561.
97. Chapelier A, Vouhe P, Macchiarini P, et al. Comparative outcome of heart-lung and lung transplantation for pulmonary hypertension. *J Thorac Cardiovasc Surg* 1993;106:299.
98. Levine SM, Gibbons WJ, Bryan CL, et al. Single lung transplantation for primary pulmonary hypertension. *Chest* 1990;98:1107.
99. Haydock DA, Trulock EP, Kaiser LR. Management of dysfunction in the transplanted lung: experience with seven clinical cases. Washington University Lung Transplant Group. *Ann Thorac Surg* 1992;53:635.
100. Malden ES, Kaiser LR, Gutierrez FR. Pulmonary vein obstruction following single lung transplantation. *Chest* 1992;102(2):645.
101. Braun WE, Phillips D, Vidt DG, et al. Coronary arteriography and coronary artery disease in 99 diabetic and nondiabetic patients on chronic hemodialysis or renal transplantation programs. *Transplant Proc* 1981;13:128.
102. Weinrauch LA, D'Elia JA, Healy RW, et al. Asymptomatic coronary artery disease: angiography in diabetic patients before renal transplantation. *Ann Intern Med* 1978;88:436.
103. Bennet WM, Kloster F, Rosch J, Barry J, Porter GA. Natural history of asymptomatic coronary arteriographic lesions in diabetic patients with end-stage renal disease. *Am J Med* 1978;65:779.
104. Weinrauch LA, D'Elia JA, Monaco AP, et al. Preoperative evaluation for diabetic renal transplantation: impact of clinical, laboratory, and echocardiographic parameters on patient and allograft survival. *Am J Med* 1992;93:19.
105. Khauli RB, Novick AC, Braun WE, Steinmuller D, Buszta C, Goormastic M. Improved results of cadaver renal transplantation in the diabetic patient. *J Urol* 1983;130:867.
106. Morrow CE, Schwartz JS, Sutherland DER, et al. Predictive value of thallium stress testing for coronary and cardiovascular events in uremic diabetic patients before renal transplantation. *Am J Surg* 1983;146:331.
107. Philipson JD, Carpenter BJ, Itzkoff J, et al. Evaluation of cardiovascular risk for renal transplantation in diabetic patients. *Am J Med* 1986;81:630.
108. Swift C, Steinmuller DR, Novick AC, et al. Open-heart surgery in patients undergoing renal transplantation: comparison of surgery pre- vs post-transplantation. *Transplant Proc* 1989;21:2137.

109. Ferrans VJ. Alcoholic cardiomyopathy. *Am J Med Sci* 1966;252:89.
110. Mathews E, Gardin JM, Henry WL, et al. Echocardiographic abnormalities in chronic alcoholics with and without overt congestive heart failure. *Am J Cardiol* 1981;47:570.
111. Piano MR, Schwertz DW. Alcoholic heart disease: a review. *Heart Lung* 1994;23:3.
112. Teragaki M, Takeuchi K, Takeda T. Clinical and histologic features of alcohol drinkers with congestive heart failure. *Am Heart J* 1993;125:808.
113. Spodick DH, Pigott VM, Chirife R. Preclinical cardiac malfunction in chronic alcoholism. *N Engl J Med* 1972;287:677.
114. Zambrano SS, Mazzotta JF, Sherman D, Spodick DH. Cardiac dysfunction in unselected chronic alcoholic patients: noninvasive screening by systolic time intervals. *Am Heart J* 1974;87:318.
115. Jacob AJ, McLaren KM, Boon NA. Effects of abstinence on alcoholic heart muscle disease. *Am J Cardiol* 1991;68:805.
116. Hicks RJ, Low RD, Arkles LB. Marked improvement in left ventricular systolic function 3 months after cessation of excess alcohol intake. *Clin Nucl Med* 1993;18:101.
117. Koskinas J, Portmann B, Lombard M, Smith T, Williams R. Persistent iron overload 4 years after inadvertent transplantation of a haemochromatotic liver in a patient with primary biliary cirrhosis. *J Hepatol* 1992;16:351.
118. Adams PC, Ghent CN, Grant DR, Frei JV, Wall WJ. Transplantation of a donor liver with haemochromatosis: evidence against an inherited intrahepatic defect. *Gut* 1991;32:1082.
119. Finch SC, Finch CA. Idiopathic hemochromatosis, an iron storage disease. *Medicine (Baltimore)* 1955;34:381
120. MacDonald RA, Mallory GK. Hemochromatosis and hemosiderosis: study of 211 autopsied cases. *Arch Intern Med* 1960;105:686.
121. Buja LM, Roberts WC. Iron in the heart: etiology and clinical significance. *Am J Med* 1971;51:209.
122. Engle MA, Erlandson M, Smith CH. Late cardiac complications of chronic severe, refractory anemia with hemochromatosis. *Circulation* 1964;30:698.
123. Westra WH, Hruban RH, Baughman KL, et al. Progressive homochromatotic cardiomyopathy despite reversal of iron deposition after liver transplantation. *Am J Clin Pathol* 1993;99:39.
124. Edwards BS, Weir EK, Edwards WD, Ludwig J, Dykoski RK, Edwards JE. Coexistent pulmonary and portal hypertension: morphologic and clinical features. *J Am Coll Cardiol* 1987;10:1233.
125. Morrison EB, Gaffney FA, Eigenbrodt EH, Reynolds RC, Buja LM. Severe pulmonary hypertension associated with macronodular (postnecrotic) cirrhosis and autoimmune phenomena. *Am J Med* 1980;69:513.
126. McDonnell PJ, Toye PA, Hutchins GM. Primary pulmonary hypertension and cirrhosis: are they related? *Am Rev Respir Dis* 1983;127:437.
127. Robalino BD, Moodie DS. Association between primary pulmonary hypertension and portal hypertension: analysis of its pathophysiology and clinical, laboratory and hemodynamic manifestations. *J Am Coll Cardiol* 1991;17:492.
128. De Wolf AM, Scott VL, Gasior T, Kang Y. Pulmonary hypertension and liver transplantation. *Anesthesiology* 1993;78:213.
129. Scott V, DeWolf A, Kang Y, et al. Reversibility of pulmonary hypertension after liver transplantation: a case report. *Transplant Proc* 1993;25:1789.
130. Rossaint R, Falke KJ, Lopez F, Slama K, Pison U, Zapol WM. Inhaled nitric oxide for the adult respiratory distress syndrome. *N Engl J Med* 1993;328:399.
131. De Wolf AM, Gasior T, Kang Y. Pulmonary hypertension in a patient undergoing liver transplantation. *Transplant Proc* 1991;23:2000.
132. Wallwork J, Williams R, Calne RY. Transplantation of liver, heart, and lungs for primary biliary cirrhosis and primary pulmonary hypertension. *Lancet* 1987;2:182.
133. Kang YG, Martin DJ, Marquez J, et al. Intraoperative changes in blood coagulation and thromboelastographic monitoring in liver transplantation. *Anesth Analg* 1985;64:888.
134. Shaw BW, Martin DJ, Marquez JM, et al. Venous bypass in clinical liver transplantation. *Ann Surg* 1984;200:524.
135. Marquez J, Martin D, Virji MA, et al. Cardiovascular depression secondary to ionic hypocalcemia during hepatic transplantation in humans. *Anesthesiology* 1986;65(5):457.
136. De Wolf AM, Begliomini B, Gasior TA, Kang Y, Pinsky MR. Right ventricular function during orthotopic liver transplantation. *Anesth Analg* 1993;76:562.
137. Ellis JE, Lichtor JL, Feinstein SB, et al. Right heart dysfunction, pulmonary embolism, and paradoxical embolization during liver transplantation. *Anesth Analg* 1989;68:777.
138. Lichtor JL. Ventricular dysfunction does occur during liver transplantation. *Tranplant Proc* 1991;23:1924.
139. Demetris AJ, Jaffe R, Starzl TE. A review of adults and pediatric post-transplant liver pathology. *Pathol Annu* 1987;22:347.
140. Curtis JJ, Luke RG, Jones P, Diethelm AG. Hypertension in cyclosporine-treated renal transplant recipients is sodium dependent. *Am J Med* 1988;85:134.
141. Bennett WM. Porter GA. Cyclosporine-associated hypertension [Editorial]. *Am J Med* 1988;85:131.
142. Torres LE, Traverso LW, Sohn YZ. Intraoperative hemodynamic changes in patients undergoing mixed-cell intraportal autotransplantation of pancreatic tissue. *Anesthesiology* 1980;53:427.
143. Ricordi C, Lacy PE, Finke EH, Olack BJ, Scharp DW. Automated method for isolation of human pancreatic islets. *Diabetes* 1988;37:413.
144. Starzl TE, Rowe MI, Todo, et al. Transplantation of multiple abdominal viscera. *JAMA* 1989;261:1449.
145. Copeland JG, Icenogle TB, Williams RJ, et al. Rabbit antithymocyte globulin. A 10-year experience in cardiac transplantation. *J Thorac Cardiovasc Surg* 1990;99:852.
146. O'Connell JB, Bristow MR, Hammond EH, et al. Antimurine antibody to OKT3 in cardiac transplantation: implications for prophylaxis and retreatment of rejection. *Transplant Proc* 1991;23:1157.
147. Liem LB, Dibiase A, Schroeder JS. Arrhythmias and clinical electrophysiology of the transplanted human heart. *Semin Thorac Cardiovasc Surg* 1990;2(3):271.
148. Schellhammer PF, Engle MA, Hagstrom JWC. Histochemical studies of the myocardium and conduction system in acquired iron-storage disease. *Circulation* 1967;35:631.

*The Critically Ill Cardiac Patient,*
edited by V. Kvetan and D. R. Dantzker,
Lippincott-Raven Publishers, Philadelphia © 1996.

CHAPTER 16

# Obstetric Emergencies in the Patient With Cardiac Disease

Janice E. Whitty and David B. Cotton

When pregnancy is complicated by cardiac disease, a unique challenge is presented to the management team. The normal cardiorespiratory changes in pregnancy, which are easily tolerated by the patient without underlying disease, can stress the cardiovascular system of the patient with cardiac disease, leading to the death of her fetus and even herself. It is understandable, therefore, that the obstetric emergencies that can occur antepartum, intrapartum, and postpartum (including severe preeclampsia or eclampsia, amniotic fluid embolus, obstetric hemorrhage during any trimester, respiratory failure, preterm labor, or fetal compromise necessitating emergency cesarean section) will quickly cause the pregnant patient with cardiac disease to succumb. Such patients should be managed by a multidisciplinary team that includes the maternal-fetal medicine specialist, the cardiologist, the obstetric anesthesiologist, and a neonatologist with liberal consultation with other subspecialists as needed. The purpose of this chapter is to familiarize the cardiologist with the normal cardiorespiratory changes that occur during pregnancy. In addition, we will discuss some of the obstetric emergencies that can occur during gestation and the implications of such emergencies for the patient who has underlying cardiac disease. The management of these patients will require thoughtful integration of this information to achieve the optimal outcome for mother and fetus.

## CARDIORESPIRATORY CHANGES IN NORMAL PREGNANCY

The hemodynamic changes that take place in pregnancy include alterations in blood volume, heart rate,

blood pressure, stroke volume, cardiac output, and systemic vascular resistance. An understanding of these changes and their clinical significance is necessary when managing the patient who has cardiac disease. It is imperative that the cardiologist understand not only the significance of these cardiorespiratory changes in normal pregnancy but also the particular challenge that these normally well tolerated changes can present to the patient who has underlying cardiac disease.

### Blood Volume

Maternal blood volume increases by 11% as early as the seventh week of gestation (1). Plasma volume continues to increase, reaching a plateau at 32 weeks, and remains stable until delivery (2). Plasma volume at term averages 45% to 50% above nonpregnant values. Two popular theories exist regarding the mechanism underlying the increase in maternal plasma volume. It has been postulated that the low-resistance uteroplacental circulation acts as a functional arteriovenous shunt, which causes maternal plasma volume expansion. Similar volume increases have been noted in nonpregnant patients with arteriovenous fistulas (3, 4). The other proposed mechanism is related to the hormonal changes that occur during pregnancy. Estrogen stimulates hepatic production of angiotensinogen, angiotensin, and serum aldosterone (5). This secondary hyperaldosteronism results in an accumulation of about 500 to 900 mEq of sodium and 6 to 8 L of total body water (6). In addition to the increase in plasma volume, there is an increase in red cell mass secondary to placental production of chorionic somatomammotropin, progesterone, and possibly prolactin, all of which stimulates maternal erythropoiesis (7). The resultant increase in red cell mass is 20% less than the increase in plasma volume, accounting for the

J.E. Whitty: Maternal Special Care Unit, Hutzel Hospital, Wayne State University, Detroit, Michigan 48201.

D.B. Cotton: Department of Obstetrics and Gynecology, Hutzel Hospital, Wayne State University, Detroit, Michigan 48201.

physiologic anemia observed in pregnancy. This hemodilution may have a beneficial effect on the uteroplacental circulation by decreasing blood viscosity and intervillous thrombotic events. The maternal hypervolemia also serves to protect the gravida if excessive peripartum blood loss occurs.

The pregnant patient whose cardiac output is limited by intrinsic myocardial dysfunction, valvular lesions, or ischemic heart disease will poorly tolerate this normal volume increase. These patients may rapidly develop congestive failure or worsening ischemia. Patients with an anatomic predisposition such as Marfan syndrome may have aneurysm formation or dissection secondary to increased shearing forces accompanying this volume expansion.

## Heart Rate

Maternal heart rate increases early in pregnancy and is about 20% greater than postpartum levels at term (8). The etiology of this maternal tachycardia is not well understood. Hemodynamic adjustments such as an increased heart rate and size could occur in response to the temporary volume overload state that exists during pregnancy (9). These hemodynamic changes have been observed with cardiac decompensation and volume overload in the nonpregnant state (9). This normal increase in heart rate during pregnancy may be poorly tolerated by the patient with severe cardiac disease, who is particularly dependent upon ventricular filling time to maintain cardiac output. The pregnant patient with underlying ischemic heart disease may suffer worsening ischemia secondary to this tachycardia and attendant decreased coronary perfusion.

## Blood Pressure

Blood pressure decreases during pregnancy, reaching a nadir at 28 weeks gestation (8). This decrease is observed in both systolic and diastolic blood pressure and is greatest with the patient in the left lateral recumbent position (Fig. 1). This decrease is most likely related to hormonally induced cardiovascular changes in pregnancy. Phippard and colleagues (10) studied blood pressure changes in pregnant baboons. Peripheral vasodilation and cardiac

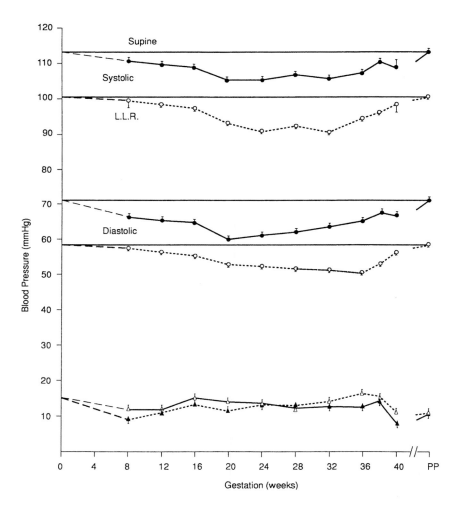

**FIG. 1.** Sequential changes in blood pressure throughout pregnancy with research subjects in supine and left lateral recumbent (LRR) positions [±SE (standard error of the mean), *n* = 69]. The change in systolic *(open triangles)* and diastolic *(closed triangles)* blood pressure produced by movement from the left lateral recumbent to the supine position is illustrated below. From Wilson M, et al. *Am J Med* 1980;68: 97, with permission.

output augmentation were found to precede gestational hypervolemia. In addition, they noted that the increased cardiac output did not compensate completely for the decreased afterload, providing an explanation for mean arterial blood pressure decreases. After the nadir in blood pressure is reached at 28 weeks, there is a gradual rise to prepregnancy values by term (see Fig. 1). If hypertension rather than vasodilation occurs during pregnancy, significantly increased fetal and maternal morbidity and mortality from intrauterine growth retardation, premature delivery, placental abruption, and superimposed preeclampsia may result (11, 12). Hypertension in pregnancy is defined by the American College of Obstetricians and Gynecologists as a blood pressure of 140/90 mm Hg, a rise in the systolic pressure of 30 mm Hg, or a rise in the diastolic pressure of 15 mm Hg from baseline. These blood pressure readings must be obtained on at least two occasions 6 or more hours apart.

## Cardiac Output

Hamilton (13) used the direct Fick principle to calculate cardiac output in 24 nonpregnant and 68 normal pregnant women. Cardiac output in the nonpregnant women averaged 4.51 L/min, compared to 5.73 L/min at 26 to 29 weeks gestational age. The increase in cardiac output begins at about 10 to 13 weeks gestation and peaks by the later part of the second trimester at 30% to 50% over nonpregnant values. This increase is sustained for the remainder of the pregnancy. Evaluation of cardiac output by Laird-Meeter (14) with M-mode echocardiography in normal pregnancy suggested that the increase in cardiac output that occurred before 20 weeks gestation was attributable to maternal tachycardia, whereas subsequent increases were secondary to significant increases in stroke volume. Robson (15) evaluated 13 women twice before conception and monthly during gestation with Doppler ultrasound measurement of transvalvular flow and estimations of valve area with real-time ultrasound. Cardiac chamber size and ventricular function were evaluated with M-mode ultrasound. Heart rate increased significantly (17%) by 32 weeks gestation and stroke volume increased 48% between 8 and 32 weeks gestation.

Clark (16) evaluated normal pregnant patients in the third trimester of pregnancy and reported about equal contributions of heart rate and stroke volume to the increased cardiac output in late pregnancy. In that study, the mean cardiac output obtained by thermodilution in the third trimester of pregnancy was 6.2 ± 1.0 L/min. This increase in cardiac output is necessary in order to meet the circulatory requirements of the fetal placental unit. The patient with cardiac disease may be unable to normally augment cardiac output and therefore may not deliver sufficient oxygen to maternal and fetal tissues.

This may result in maternal cardiac ischemia and failure and/or intrauterine growth retardation.

## Systemic Vascular Resistance

Systemic vascular resistance is decreased in pregnancy, falling from prepregnancy values of 1,240 to 980 dyn/sec/cm$^{-5}$ by the middle of pregnancy and then returning to normal by term (17). Possible explanations for this phenomenon include hormonal effects of estrogen, progesterone, and local prostaglandins, causing peripheral vasodilation (18, 19). Another theory is that the uteroplacental circulation is a major low-resistance circuit that reduces cardiac afterload (4, 20). Clark (16) found that the systemic vascular resistance in late pregnancy (1,210 ± 266 dyn/s/cm$^{-5}$) was significantly (−21%) different from that found in the nonpregnant woman (1,530 ± 520 dyn/s/cm$^{-5}$). It should be recognized that this decrease in systemic vascular resistance is of clinical importance in patients who have the potential for right-to-left shunts. These shunts will invariably be increased by the falling systemic vascular resistance seen during normal pregnancy. Changes in afterload can also compromise patients with certain types of valvular disease.

## Effect of Maternal Posture on Hemodynamics During Pregnancy

Consideration of the effect of maternal posture on hemodynamic status during pregnancy is of profound importance, particularly in the patient with cardiac disease. Uterine blood flow increases from approximately 50 to 500 mL/min at term. This represents over 10% of systemic cardiac output. Vorys and colleagues (21) first described a reduction in cardiac output due to mechanical venocaval obstruction by the gravid uterus during late pregnancy. Ueland and colleagues (22) reported their experiences with maternal postural effects on heart rate, stroke volume, and cardiac output throughout pregnancy (Fig. 2). Eleven women were serially studied with a dye dilution technique at four different periods in gestation: 20 to 24 weeks, 28 to 32 weeks, 38 to 42 weeks, and 6 to 8 weeks postpartum. Measurements were taken from the sitting supine and left lateral positions. Maternal heart rate was maximal (+13% to 20%) by 28 to 32 weeks gestation, with the highest values observed in the sitting position. Stroke volume was maximal by 20 to 24 weeks gestation and progressively declined toward term. Patients were generally able to maintain cardiac output values beyond 20 to 24 weeks through augmentation of maternal heart rate, despite a progressive decrease in stroke volume toward term. These investigators noted that the assumption of the supine position at term led to stroke volume and cardiac output values that were even

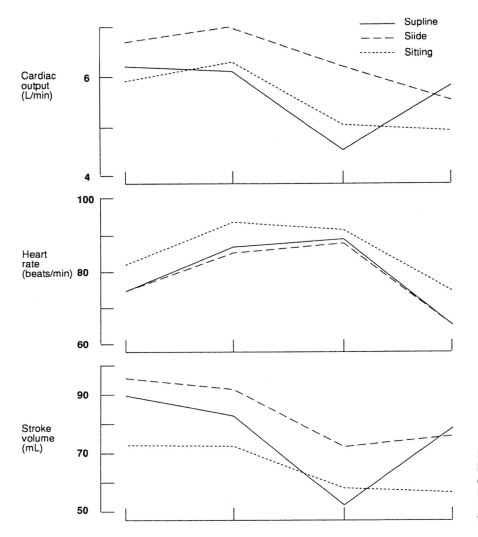

FIG. 2. Effect of posture on maternal hemodynamics. From Ueland K, Metcalfe J. *Clin Obstet Gynecol* 1975;18:41. Modified from Ueland K, et al. *Am J Obstet Gynecol* 1969;104:856. Used with permission.

lower than the corresponding measurements in the postpartum period.

It should be kept in mind, therefore, that the patient with cardiac disease may be severely compromised by the assumption of the supine position with subsequent decrease in stroke volume and cardiac output. This decrease in cardiac output can rapidly lead to fetal compromise because of decreased oxygen delivery to the gravid uterus, as well as maternal compromise, secondary to cardiac ischemia.

### Central Hemodynamic Values in Pregnancy

Right-sided heart catheterization studies by Bader and colleagues (23) failed to demonstrate significant differences for right ventricular (RV) and pulmonary artery pressures throughout pregnancy. Clark and colleagues (16, 24) examined 10 primiparous women during late pregnancy (35 to 38 weeks) and again postpartum (11 to

13 weeks) in order to establish normaive values for central maternal hemodynamics. They noted that, when compared with the postpartum state, late pregnancy was characterized by significant increases in heart rate (+17%), stroke volume (+23%), and cardiac output (+43%), confirming data presented previously. Pulmonary capillary wedge pressure, central venous pressure, and mean arterial blood pressure were not altered. In addition, they documented significant decreases in systemic vascular resistance (–21%), pulmonary vascular resistance (–34%), serum colloid osmotic pressure (–14%), and colloid osmotic pressure—pulmonary capillary wedge pressure gradient (–28%), confirming evidence presented by other investigators.

### Oxygen Delivery and Consumption in Pregnancy

The physiologic anemia of pregnancy results in a reduction in the hemoglobin concentration and arterial oxygen content. Oxygen delivery ($DO_2$) is maintained at or above normal in spite of this because of the 50% increase that occurs in cardiac output. It is important to remember, therefore, that the pregnant woman is more dependent on cardiac output for maintenance of oxygen delivery than is the nonpregnant patient (25). Oxygen consumption increases steadily throughout pregnancy and is greatest at term, reaching an average of 331 mL/min at rest and 1,167 mL/min with exercise (26). During labor, oxygen consumption increases by 40% to 60% and cardiac output increases by about 22% (27, 28). Because oxygen delivery normally far exceeds consumption, the normal pregnant patient is usually able to maintain adequate delivery of oxygen to herself and her fetus even during labor. When a pregnant patient has a low oxygen delivery, however, she can very quickly reach the "critical $DO_2$" during labor, compromising both herself and her fetus (29). Therefore, every attempt should be made to optimize oxygen delivery in the pregnant patient with cardiac disease or other conditions compromising $DO_2$ prior to allowing labor to begin. This can be accomplished by increasing cardiac output and/or oxygen-carrying capacity. Hemodynamic manipulation may be guided by the use of a flow-directed pulmonary artery catheter prior to the initiation of labor.

## MATERNAL-FETAL PHYSIOLOGIC INTERACTIONS

Information regarding the respiratory exchange of the placental-fetal unit has been derived predominately from experimental data obtained from animal models. This work has been extrapolated to the human fetus; however, the results are limited by the use of anesthesia in the operative procedure, which places an acute stress on mother and fetus that can alter baseline observations. An additional consideration is that placental structure differs markedly among various mammals.

### Fetal Oxygen Transport

Maternal red cells enter the intervillous spaces of the placenta. In the intervillous spaces, oxygen diffuses from the maternal blood into the fetal red blood cells. This oxygenated blood then flows from the placenta to the fetus, where it supplies fetal tissues. Each of these steps results in a progressive decrease in the partial pressure of oxygen ($PO_2$) (see Table 1) (30). The Fick principle has been used to calculate oxygen uptake from a chronically catheterized sheep model (31). The uterus has a higher oxygen uptake (42 mL/min) than does the fetus (28 mL/min). This phenomenon is explained by the metabolic activity of the placenta, with its relatively high uptake of oxygen. Using the diffusion equilibrium principle, it is also evident that the fetus consumes a large quantity of oxygen even with a low $PO_2$ in the umbilical

**TABLE 1.** *Stepwise decrement of $po_2$ from inspired air to fetal tissue*

| Site | $po_2$ (mm Hg) |
| --- | --- |
| Inspired air | 120 |
| Alveolar air | 90 |
| Maternal artery | 80 |
| Uterine vein | 48 |
| Umbilical vein | 30 |
| Umbilical artery | 20 |

From Thorp JM Jr, Cefale RC. *Critical care obstetrics.* 2nd ed. Blackwell Scientific Publications, 1991;6:103.
This table demonstrates the stepwise decrement of $PO_2$ as oxygen is transported from the atmosphere to the fetus.

circulation. If fetal oxygen uptake is calculated using the Fick principle and divided by total body weight, the oxygen uptake per unit body weight by the fetus far exceeds that of the adult (32).

The major reason the umbilical venous blood has such a low $PO_2$ is that the ovine placenta and, quite possibly, the human placenta functions as a venous equilibrator (31). This system of concurrent blood flow is depicted in Fig. 3. Maternal blood and fetal blood runs through two channels in the same direction. Exchange of oxygen occurs across the semipermeable membrane of the placenta. As the two blood streams move toward the end of their channels, the $PO_2$ in the uterine venous circulation is higher than the umbilical system. The $PO_2$ in the umbilical vein rises until the $PO_2$ is equal to that in the uterine venous system. The umbilical venous stream cannot exit with a higher $PO_2$ than the uterine venous stream. The system attempts to equilibrate the $PO_2$ of fetal blood in the maternal circulation. In reality, the ovine placenta and probably the human placenta cannot reach the goal of equilibration. Reasons for the lack of complete equilibration include the shunting of uterine blood flow away from the placenta to the myometrium, the uneven perfusion of various cotyledons, and possible limitations in the diffusion capacity of the placenta (30). From the concept of venous equilibration, it is obvious that the uterine venous $PO_2$ is the major determinant of the umbilical venous $PO_2$. If uterine venous $PO_2$ is elevated, there is an increase in umbilical venous $PO_2$. Likewise, a reduction in uterine venous $PO_2$ will result in a similar fall in umbilical venous $PO_2$. The oxygen saturation of uterine venous blood is affected by three major variables: (a) the oxygen saturation of maternal arterial blood, (b) The oxygen-carrying capacity of maternal blood, and (c) the uterine blood flow. A decrease in the $PO_2$ of maternal blood, anemia, or reduced cardiac output will reduce uterine venous $PO_2$ and ultimately reduce umbilical venous $PO_2$.

### Fetal Adaptation to Low $PO_2$

Fetal $PO_2$ is low; however, fetal blood delivers large amounts of oxygen to fetal tissues to enable normal

## MODEL OF CONCURRENT EXCHANGE

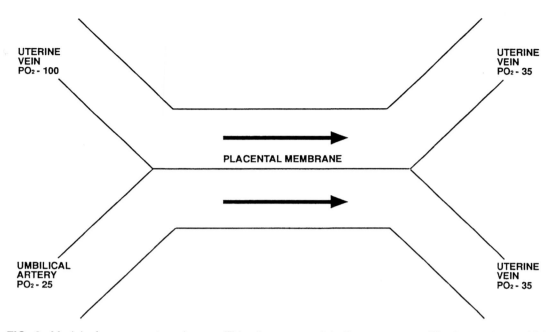

**FIG. 3.** Model of concurrent exchange. This diagram models the venous equilibrator system, which explains why umbilical vein $po_2$ cannot exceed the uterine vein $po_2$. From Thorp JM Jr, Cefalo RC. *Critical Care Obstetrics* 1991;6:105.

growth and development. This oxygen delivery to fetal tissues is accomplished by two mechanisms: the high affinity of fetal hemoglobin for oxygen and the high rate of perfusion of fetal vital organs (30). If one examines the oxyhemoglobin saturation curves of maternal and fetal hemoglobin, it is obvious that at the same $PO_2$ fetal hemoglobin has a higher affinity for oxygen than does maternal hemoglobin. This high oxygen affinity of fetal hemoglobin assures that each fetal red cell that travels through the placenta returns to the fetus almost fully saturated with oxygen. The fetus also has an increased heart rate and stroke volume which results in increased cardiac output. A comparison of the perfusion rates of adult and fetal brain has shown that the fetal brain receives 2.5 times more blood per milliliter of oxygen consumed than does the adult organ (33). The fetus accomplishes this by-passing fetal lungs via the ductus arteriosus and having a biventricular cardiac output supplying the systemic circulation.

### Uterine Perfusion

Two adaptations occur in the mother that enable her to provide adequate blood flow to the fetus and placenta. The first is the previously mentioned increase in maternal blood volume that occurs early in pregnancy and results in blood volume up to 50% greater than normal by the third trimester. The second is that uterine blood flow increases tremendously, rising to 20 times above the normal nonpregnant levels at term. These changes serve to maximize blood flow and oxygen delivery to the placenta. The development of the uteroplacental circulation is analogous to grafting a low-resistance vascular bed in parallel with the maternal circulation. The end result is a tenfold decrease in uterine vascular resistance. The diameters of uterine arteries and veins increase dramatically during gestation.

Blood flow to the uterus is dependent on systemic blood pressure. Autoregulation has not been clearly demonstrated in the uteroplacental circulation of either acute or chronic animal preparation. Thus, changes in maternal $PO_2$ do not seem to exert direct control on the placental circulation. It is important, therefore, to keep in mind that the uterus is maximally perfused at all times and that any fall in cardiac output or oxygen delivery to the uterus cannot be compensated for by autoregulation.

Uterine contractions result in a decrease in uterine blood flow that is proportional to the magnitude and the duration of the contraction. This decrease is caused by an increased vascular resistance within the uterus rather than by a change in the perfusion pressure. The increased resistance is a local phenomenon resulting from increased intrauterine pressure and is not due to central changes. As the intrauterine pressure rises, the intervillous blood flow slows and ultimately ceases.

## Fetal Response to Diminished Oxygen

As umbilical venous oxygen is reduced, the fetus goes through three major stages of acute hypoxemia (34). In the first stage, the oxygen content of fetal blood may be reduced up to 50% without the development of acidosis. The fetus initially compensates for this hypoxemia by redirecting cardiac output to the heart and brain. In the second stage, the fetus uses anaerobic metabolism, ultimately resulting in a base deficit and metabolic acidosis. There is an outpouring of catecholamines within the fetus that diminishes blood flow to every organ but the brain, heart, and placenta. If the uterus begins to contract during this second stage of hypoxemia, uterine blood will slow, further impairing fetal oxygenation. The fetal brainstem and heart will respond to this insult with brief episodes of bradycardia. The third stage of hypoxemia occurs when oxygen content is reduced by over 75%. Under these conditions, perfusion of the brain cannot be adequately maintained and central nervous system damage or even death may ensue if this stage persists.

## Interventions to Improve Fetal Oxygenation

In clinical situations where the fetus appears hypoxemic or has the potential for its development, the clinician must assess the mother and determine how to maximize fetal oxygenation. In some situations, delivery will be the optimum management for both mother and fetus. However, in other situations, particularly involving critically ill pregnant women, the maternal condition precludes operative intervention. Likewise, prematurity may place the fetus at greater risk of harm outside of the uterus than in. In these particular situations, the physician must maximize oxygen delivery and achieve in utero fetal resuscitation if possible. Particular attention should be paid to maternal cardiac output, oxygen-carrying capacity, and uterine blood flow, as these will be the determinants of fetal oxygenation in utero.

An additional consideration is maternal acidosis and fever which will shift the hemoglobin saturation curve to the right and lower oxygen-carrying capacity. Even in mothers with normal arterial $PO_2$, increasing the partial pressure of oxygen of inspired air can have favorable effects on the fetus (35). Giving oxygen to the mother causes a marked increase in maternal arterial $PO_2$ and oxygen content. The uterine venous $PO_2$ will rise by an amount much less than that of the uterine artery. However, increasing uterine venous $PO_2$ is followed by an identical increase in umbilical venous $PO_2$. This shifts the umbilical venous $O_2$ content upward. The umbilical artery $O_2$ content will move upward in the same fashion,

ultimately resulting in an increased umbilical artery $PO_2$. Small changes in fetal $PO_2$ result in proportionately larger changes in $O_2$ content because the fetus is operating on the steep portion of the oxygen dissociation curve (35).

In a similar fashion, decreases in arterial $PO_2$ below 60 mL Hg result in an even more dramatic decline in fetal oxygen content. In addition to arterial oxygen content, oxygenation will depend on uterine blood flow, and this should be maximized in the critically ill gravida to ensure adequate fetal oxygenation. Avoidance of the supine position with its potential to occlude the maternal vena cava and diminish preload and lower cardiac output is essential in maintaining uterine blood flow. Additional attention must be given to volume status, peripheral vascular resistance, and ventricular performance. In some instances this will require pulmonary artery catheterization to assess and optimize cardiac function.

## Effects of Labor and Delivery on Maternal Hemodynamics

Maternal cardiovascular response is influenced by uterine contractions, pain, labor and analgesia, surgery, and peripartum blood loss. During uterine contractions, approximately 300 to 500 mL of blood is expressed from the uterus, resulting in "autotransfusion" (36, 37). This infusion of blood into the maternal circulation increases venous return and can influence stroke volume by the Frank-Starling mechanism. Kjeldsen (38) reported cardiac output increases during latent, acceleration, and deceleration phases of labor. Similar cardiac output increases over prelabor values between contractions were described by Ueland and Hansen (39). The increase in cardiac output was not as pronounced in patients under the influence of caudal labor analgesia when compared with parturients who received only local agents. Ueland (40) observed that when the pregnant woman was in the left lateral position, the increase in stroke volume and cardiac output was maintained between contractions and changes during contractions were minimized (Fig. 4).

Robson and colleagues (41) performed noninvasive Doppler studies during labor that have provided insight as to why the changes in cardiac output occur. They documented a 13% increase in cardiac output by 8 cm of cervical dilatation that was primarily related to stroke volume augmentation. Uterine contractions led to additional cardiac output increases due to augmentation of both heart rate and stroke volume. The magnitude of these additional cardiac output changes increased with progression of labor: 3 cm or less, +17%; 4 to 7 cm, +23%; 8 cm or more, +34%. Maternal pain and anxiety may result in increased sympathetic stimulation with a rise in blood pressure and heart rate during advancing stages of labor.

Lee (42) examined the magnitude of cardiac output augmentation during contractions and found they were less in women laboring under epidural analgesia. Labor-

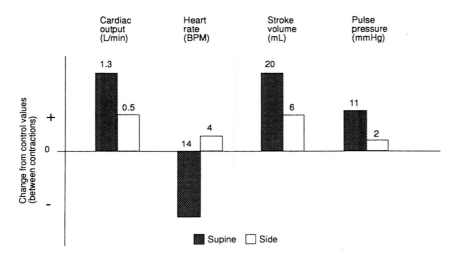

**FIG. 4.** Effect of posture on the maternal hemodynamic response to uterine contractions in early labor. From Ueland K, Metcalfe J. *Clin Obstet Gynecol* 1975;18:41. Modified from Ueland K, Hansen JM. *Am J Obstet Gynecol* 1969;103:8. Used with permission.

ing in the left lateral decubitus position with epidural analgesia for pain control is particularly important in the patient with cardiac disease who will benefit from minimal hemodynamic fluctuations during labor.

Women with cardiovascular compromise can usually deliver vaginally, and cesarean section should be reserved for obstetric indications. Ueland (40) studied the influence of anesthesia analgesia on maternal cardiac output (Fig. 5). Patients who delivered vaginally exhibited the greatest cardiac output changes with local anesthesia. The greatest perioperative changes were related to subarachnoid anesthesia. Epidural anesthesia with epinephrine led to a 29% decrease in cardiac output prior to surgery but was associated with a significant number of women requiring further therapy to treat iatrogenic hypotension. However, the patients developing postepidural hypotension may not have received adequate fluid preload prior to activation of regional anesthesia. Epidural anesthesia reduces maternal pain and anxiety, thereby avoiding the rise in blood pressure, heart rate, and cardiac output seen during the second stage of labor. In addition, due to its vasodilator action, epidural anesthesia results in reduced systemic vascular resistance, reflecting its peripheral vasodilator affects. The latter appears to be a benefit in conditions such as congestive heart failure and mitral and aortic regurgitation. However, in conditions in which a decrease in systemic vascular resistance is not tolerated, such as pulmonary hypertension, obstructive cardiomyopathy, and aortic stenosis, epidural anesthesia may be both harmful and dangerous.

There has been a decline in cardiovascular complications associated with cesarean section over the past decade because of improved surgical techniques, more knowledgeable manipulation of cardiac loading conditions, and the use of flow-directed pulmonary artery catheters to guide hemodynamic manipulations. Cesarean section can be safely performed with either lumbar epidural or general anesthesia provided the anesthesiolo-

gist is armed with the necessary hemodynamic information and a thorough understanding of the effect of a given anesthetic agent on the patient's specific cardiac lesion. Spinal anesthesia is generally associated with considerable hemodynamic imbalance and should therefore be avoided in pregnant patients with severe cardiac disease. Inhalation agents with negative inotropic effects may be beneficial in conditions such as obstructive cardiomyopathy, coarctation of the aorta, or Marfan's syndrome. In contrast, these agents may be dangerous in patients with severe dilated cardiomyopathies, aortic stenosis, and hemodynamically important mitral or aortic regurgitation.

## POSTPARTUM HEMODYNAMICS

Maternal cardiac output increases by 20% to 30% above prelabor values during the first 24 hours after delivery (38). This postpartum stroke volume augmentation probably results from increased venous return to the

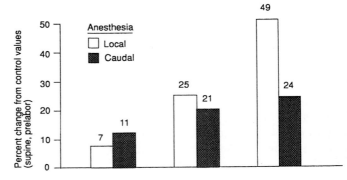

**FIG. 5.** Changes in cardiac output during local and caudal anesthesia. From Ueland K, Metcalfe J. *Clin Obstet Gynecol* 1975;18:41. Modified from Ueland K, Hansen JM. *Am J Obstet Gynecol* 1969;103:8. Used with permission.

heart from autotransfusion of uteroplacental blood back into the maternal circulation, release of venocaval compression, and mobilization of extravascular fluid back into the intravascular space. The increase in stroke volume is such that cardiac output remains elevated for at least 48 hours after normal delivery, in spite of a decrease in maternal pulse rate (−10 beats/min) (43).

Robson (43) serially characterized puerperal hemodynamics from 15 normal pregnant women by Doppler and M-mode echocardiography. Measurements were taken before delivery, at 38 weeks gestation, and then again at 2, 6, 12, and 24 weeks after delivery. A 33% decrease in cardiac output was observed by 2 weeks after delivery due to a reduction in both heart rate and stroke volume. Left ventricular (LV) contractility in the postnatal group was slightly less than age-matched nongravid control subjects by 24 weeks after delivery. These findings suggested that the reduced postnatal LV function may place women at higher risk for developing postpartum cardiomyopathy.

The hemodynamic changes characterized above, which include an increase in venous return and stroke volume and a decrease in cardiac contractility, dictate that the patient with cardiac disease should continue to be closely monitored during the postpartum period, particularly the initial 48 hours. The increase in stroke volume and decrease in contractility can lead to overt failure in these patients, and invasive monitoring in patients who have New York Heart Association (NYHA) functional classifications III and IV would be prudent.

## Respiratory System

Minute ventilation is increased in the first trimester and is elevated by 48% at term (44). Because there is no increase in respiratory rate, the increase in minute ventilation is secondary to an increase in tidal volume (44). The increase in tidal volume occurs at the expense of an 18% decrease in the functional residual capacity. This hyperventilation of pregnancy results in a respiratory alkalosis ($PCO_2 < 30$ mm Hg) and an increase in arterial oxygen tension (101 to 104 mm Hg in the third trimester) (45). The chronic respiratory alkalosis is partially compensated by increased renal bicarbonate excretion. It has been suggested that the respiratory changes of pregnancy result primarily from progesterone acting as a respiratory stimulant (46).

There is a postural effect on arterial oxygen tension at term in the pregnant patient. Work by Awe and colleagues (47) indicated that arterial oxygen tension is usually greater than 90 mm Hg when measured in the sitting position. A moderate hypoxemia ($pO_2 < 90$ mm Hg) was observed in 25% of supine gravid women. The supine position was also more likely to be associated with an abnormal alveolar oxygen tension gradient (>10 mm Hg) that significantly improved when shifted back to the sitting position. This is an additional reason why women in labor,

particularly those who have underlying cardiac disease, should be maintained in the left lateral recumbent position.

We have reviewed the cardiorespiratory changes that can be anticipated in normal pregnancy, some maternal-fetal physiologic interactions, and the hemodynamics of labor and the postpartum period. With that knowledge in hand, we will now discuss specific obstetric emergencies that might present to or require comanagement with the cardiologist.

## CARDIAC DISEASE IN PREGNANCY

We have previously discussed the alterations in maternal cardiorespiratory function during pregnancy. Patients with normal cardiac function tolerate the normal physiologic changes in pregnancy without difficulty. However, when a patient has significant cardiac disease, pregnancy can result in decompensation and even death. Death from cardiac disease in pregnancies accounts for considerable maternal mortality (48, 49). In this section we will discuss specific cardiac lesions that can be seen during gestation and their management.

Because of the high risk of maternal mortality, counseling the pregnant patient with cardiac disease is extremely important. Clark and colleagues presented a synthesis of current maternal mortality estimates for various types of cardiac disease (Table 2) (30). Counseling of the pregnant cardiac patient and general management of approaches are based on this classification. Group 1 includes conditions which, with proper management, should have negligible maternal mortality (<1%). Cardiac lesions in group

**TABLE 2.** *Mortality risk associated with pregnancy*

| Group I |
| --- |
| Atrial septal defect[a] |
| Ventricular septal defect[a] |
| Patent ductus arteriosus[a] |
| Pulmonic/tricuspid disease |
| Corrected tetralogy of Fallot |
| Porcine valve |
| Mitral stenosis, NYHA[b] classes I and II |
| Group II: mortality 5–15% |
| Mitral stenosis with atrial fibrillation |
| Artificial valve |
| Mitral stenosis, NYHA classes III and IV |
| Aortic stenosis |
| Coarctation of aorta, uncomplicated |
| Uncorrected tetralogy of Fallot |
| Previous myocardial infarction |
| Marfan's syndrome with normal aorta |
| Group III: mortality 25–50% |
| Pulmonary hypertension |
| Coarctation of aorta, complicated |
| Marfan's syndrome with aortic involvement |

[a]Uncomplicated. Data from Clark SL, et al. *Critical care obstetrics.* 2nd. ed. *Blackwell Scientific Publications* 1991;7: 115.
[b]New York Heart Association.

2 have a 5% to 15% risk of maternal mortality; in individual cases, and after appropriate counseling, this may prove acceptable to some women. Patients with cardiac lesions in group 3 are subject to a mortality risk exceeding 25%. In all but exceptional cases, this risk will prove unacceptable to the patient, and prevention or interruption of pregnancy should be recommended strongly. Up to 40% of patients developing congestive heart failure and pulmonary edema during pregnancy were to be in functional class 1 prior to pregnancy, and in one review, the majority of maternal deaths during pregnancy that occurred are initially class I or class II (Criteria Committee of the New York Heart Association, functional classes I to IV) (50). An additional consideration when counseling the pregnant cardiac patient is that recent advances in medical and surgical therapy, fetal surveillance, and neonatal care may render invalid many of the older estimates of maternal mortality and fetal wastage.

## Congenital Cardiac Disease

The relative frequency of congenital as opposed to acquired heart disease is changing (51). Rheumatic fever is less common in the United States, and more patients with congenital cardiac disease now survive to reproductive age. The ratio of rheumatic to congenital heart disease has changed from 16:1 reported in 1954 to 3:1 in 1967.

The problems encountered by the pregnant woman with cardiac disease are secondary to four principal physiologic changes seen in pregnancy (52). The 50% increase in intravascular volume seen in a normal pregnancy may lead to congestive heart failure or worsening ischemia in patients whose cardiac output is limited by intrinsic myocardial dysfunction, valvular lesions, or ischemic heart disease. In patients with conditions such as Marfan's syndrome, this volume expansion may result in increased shearing forces and aneurism or dissection. The normal decrease in systemic vascular resistance becomes especially important in patients with the potential for right-to-left shunts, which will be increased by a falling systemic vascular resistance. This decrease in cardiac afterload will also cause complications in pregnant patients with some types of valvular disease.

The hypercoagulable state associated with pregnancy can be particularly risky in patients at risk for arterial thrombosis such as patients with artificial valves and patients with atrial fibrillation. An additional consideration in these patients is the increased risk of postpartum hemorrhage in women receiving any type of therapeutic anticoagulation. The marked fluctuations in cardiac output required during normal labor and the potential for further dramatic volume shifts at the time of delivery may be poorly tolerated by a woman whose cardiac output is highly dependent on adequate preload (pulmonary hypertension) and those with a fixed cardiac output (mitral stenosis).

The antepartum management of all patients with cardiac disease should include meticulous prenatal care including serial ultrasound scans to document adequate fetal growth and the use of antepartum bed rest and close maternal surveillance. Patients with congenital cardiac abnormalities should be evaluated with fetal echocardiography in order to identify fetal cardiac abnormalities. Intrapartum management principles include laboring in the left lateral position, the use of epidural anesthesia which will minimize intrapartum fluctuations in cardiac output, the administration of oxygen and endocarditis prophylaxis when appropriate (52). Additional management recommendations may vary according to the specific lesion present. Patients with significant cardiac disease should be managed and delivered in a tertiary care center. We will now discuss specific cardiac lesions seen during pregnancy and their appropriate management.

## Atrial Septal Defect

Atrial septal defect (ASD), the most common congenital lesion seen during pregnancy, is usually asymptomatic (53). The significant potential complications seen with ASD are arrhythmias and heart failure. Atrial arrhythmias are not uncommon in patients with ASD; however, their onset generally occurs after the fourth decade of life; therefore, such arrhythmias are unlikely to be encountered in the pregnant woman. Atrial fibrillation is the most common arrythmia encountered, but superventricular tachycardia and atrial flutter may also occur (54). The hypervolemia associated with pregnancy may result in an increased left-to-right shunt through the ASD and a significant burden on the right ventricle. This additional burden is well tolerated by most patients; however, congestive heart failure and death have been reported (55, 56). Atrial septal defect is characterized by high pulmonary blood flow; however, pulmonary hypertension is unusual. The majority of patients with ASD will tolerate pregnancy, labor, and delivery without complications. During labor, it is important to avoid fluid overload, give oxygen, labor the patients in left lateral recumbent position, and obtain adequate pain relief with epidural anesthesia. Patients should also receive prophylaxis against bacterial endocarditis.

## Ventricular Septal Defect

Ventricular septal defect (VSD) may occur as an isolated lesion or in conjunction with other congenital cardiac anomalies, including tetralogy of Fallot, transposition of the great vessels, and coarctation of the aorta. The most important determinant of clinical prognosis during pregnancy is the size of the septal defect. Small defects are usually tolerated well, whereas larger defects are associated with congestive failure, arrhythmias, or the development of pulmonary hypertension (52). In addition, a large VSD is often associated with some degree of aortic regurgitation, which may add to the risk of congestive failure.

Patients with uncomplicated VSD generally tolerate pregnancy, labor, and delivery well. In a series of 141 pregnancies and 56 women with VSD the only two maternal deaths were in women whose VSD was complicated by pulmonary hypertension (56). Intrapartum management considerations for patients with uncomplicated VSD are similar to those outlined for ASD.

## Patent Ductus Arteriosus

Although patent ductus arteriosus (PDA) is one of the most common congenital cardiac anomalies, it is almost universally detected and closed in the newborn period and is an uncommon diagnosis during pregnancy (57). Most patients are asymptomatic and PDA is generally tolerated well during pregnancy, labor, and delivery. However, the high pressure/high flow left-to-right shunt associated with a large uncorrected PDA can lead to pulmonary hypertension and the associated poor prognosis (30).

## Pulmonic Stenosis

Pulmonic stenosis is a common congenital cardiac defect. Most patients tolerate pulmonic stenosis during pregnancy, labor, and delivery, but the degree of obstruction correlates with the clinical outcome. If stenosis is severe, that is, a transvalvular pressure gradient exceeding 80 mm of mercury, surgical correction should be strongly recommended. When stenosis is this severe, right-sided heart failure can occur. Nonetheless, the outcome in this group of patients is generally favorable (55, 56).

## Tetralogy of Fallot

Tetralogy of Fallot is the most frequently encountered lesion, causing right-to-left shunt. The defects include pulmonary outflow obstruction, RV hypertrophy, ventriculoseptal defect, and "overriding aorta." Most cases of tetralogy of Fallot are corrected during infancy or childhood, so this condition is rarely encountered in the pregnant population. When tetralogy of Fallot has been corrected, the outcome of pregnancy is relatively good (58). In patients with uncorrected tetralogy of Fallot, reported maternal mortality ranges from 4% to 15%, with a 30% fetal mortality, secondary to hypoxia (58). In these patients, the decline in systemic vascular resistance that accompanies pregnancy can lead to a worsening of the right-to-left shunt, and hypotension as a result of peripar-

tum blood loss can further aggravate this condition. A prepregnancy hematocrit exceeding 65%, a history of syncope or congestive failure, electrocardiographic evidence of RV strain, cardiomegaly, RV pressure exceeding 120 mm Hg, and peripheral oxygen saturation less than 80% have all been associated with a particularly poor prognosis in patients with uncorrected tetralogy of Fallot (58). In view of the combined higher maternal risk and the high incidence of fetal loss, it would be prudent to discourage pregnancy in women with uncorrected tetralogy of Fallot.

## Coarctation of the Aorta

Coarctation is diagnosed when a large difference in blood pressure is found between measurements in the upper extremities and legs. Because the constriction is often located at the origin of the left subclavian artery, there may be isolated hypertension when blood pressure is determined in the right arm. Associated anomalies of the aorta and left-sided heart including VSD and PDA are common, as are intracranial aneurysms of the circle of Willis (59).

Coarctation of the aorta is infrequently encountered in pregnant women. Although earlier studies report a maternal mortality rate as high as 17%, maternal death is now a rare complication of this lesion (56). Goodwin (60) reviewed the literature and reported a maternal mortality rate of 3.5% in pregnancies with uncorrected coarctation. Deal and Wooley (61) examined data from 185 pregnancies with uncorrected coarctation and reported no maternal deaths. In the presence of aortic or interventricular aneurysm, known aneurysm of the circle of Willis, or associated cardiac lesions, the risk of death may approach 15% and therapeutic abortion should be strongly considered. Both of these studies noted a high fetal loss rate which may have been the result of inadequate uteroplacental blood flow. Shime (58) reported that four of seven pregnancies with corrected coarctation demonstrated pregnancy-induced hypertension. One patient had severe pregnancy-induced hypertension with renal failure and neonatal death.

Left ventricular compromise may be exacerbated during pregnancy if significant aortic obstruction is present. Hypotension should be avoided during labor, and during the postpartum period, because stroke volume is fixed in these patients, and normal compensatory mechanisms such as tachycardia may not be sufficient to maintain an adequate cardiac output. There is a 2% risk that the fetus will inherit this cardiac lesion.

## Marfan's Syndrome

Marfan's syndrome is an autosomal dominant disorder of connective tissue marked by joint deformities, arachnodactyly, dislocations of the ocular lenses, and cardiac manifestations. These cardiac manifestations include weakness of the aortic root and wall, and mitral valve prolapse is found in 90% of cases. Patients with Marfan's syndrome should receive genetic counseling and be made aware of the risks of pregnancy with this condition. The cardiovascular system of each patient should be studied prior to counseling them about the dangers of pregnancy, as findings will influence the amount of risk the individual patient takes. Ultrasound can be utilized to measure the width of the aorta and may be helpful in selecting patients at greatest risk for aortic dissection. It has been suggested that dilatation of the aortic root of greater than 40 mm is a contraindication to pregnancy (62). The mortality rate of up to 50% associated with Marfan's syndrome in pregnancy reflects cases in which significant maternal cardiovascular disease existed prior to conception. Women with no abnormality of the aortic valve and an aortic root diameter less than 40 mm have a mortality less than 5% (62).

Aortic dissection occurs frequently during pregnancy and may be influenced by hypertension. Symptoms of dissection include excruciating chest pain that migrates posteriorly. Painless dissection may be accompanied by hypertension and tachycardia. Patients with progressive dissection will require emergent surgical correction. The management of patients with Marfan's syndrome includes efforts to minimize both the hypertension and the contractile force transmitted to the aortic wall. This can be accomplished with the use of beta-blockers such as propranolol. These patients generally tolerate regional anesthesia for labor and delivery very well. If general anesthesia is necessary, avoidance of agents that promote hypertension during induction is recommended.

Patients with Marfan's syndrome should be advised that in addition to the considerable potential maternal risk quoted above, offspring have a 50% risk of inheriting the disorder. Another consideration is the shortened life span (half of normal) that may prevent the woman from raising the child to adulthood.

## Acquired Cardiac Lesions

Acquired cardiac lesions are generally rheumatic in origin; however, endocarditis may occasionally be a cause, especially with right-sided heart lesions.

Although the incidence of rheumatic fever has declined in the United States, it still remains a problem throughout much of the world and is still the most common cause of severe heart disease encountered in pregnancy. The large immigrant population in the United States ensures that the cardiologist will encounter pregnant patients who have rheumatic heart disease. In this section, we will briefly discuss the types of acquired heart disease found in pregnant patients, the specific effects of pregnancy on these conditions, and their management.

During pregnancy, maternal morbidity and mortality secondary to acquired cardiac lesions usually result from congestive failure or arrhythmias. Pulmonary edema is the leading cause of death in rheumatic heart disease patients during pregnancy (49). The risk of pulmonary edema in pregnant patients with rheumatic heart disease increases with increasing maternal age and increasing duration of gestation (49). There is a higher risk of RV and LV failure (63%) when atrial fibrillation first presents during gestation compared to presentation prior to gestation (22%). In addition, the risk of systemic embolization after the onset of atrial fibrillation during pregnancy appears to exceed that associated with onset in the nonpregnant state (49).

Chesley (63) followed 134 women who had functionally severe rheumatic heart disease and who had completed pregnancy. He followed these women for up to 44 years and reported a mortality of 6.4% per year but concluded that in patients who survived pregnancy maternal life expectancy was not shortened. Pregnancy apparently has no long-term sequelae for patients with rheumatic heart disease who survive the pregnancy.

Intrapartum management of patients with valvular disease and/or pulmonary hypertension has been facilitated by the use of the pulmonary artery catheter (64). Clark has reported that patients who are NYHA functional class 1 or 2 at term usually tolerate appropriately managed labor without invasive monitoring. Patients who have been class 3 or 4 or those in whom pulmonary hypertension is present or suspected may benefit from pulmonary artery catheterization during the intrapartum and immediate postpartum periods (64, 65).

## Mitral Stenosis

Mitral stenosis is the most common rheumatic valvular lesion encountered during pregnancy and accounts for 90% of rheumatic heart disease during pregnancy (66). It can occur as an isolated lesion or in conjunction with aortic or right-sided lesions. This valvular lesion, which impedes blood flow from the left atrium to the left ventricle, presents a particularly challenging set of problems, since the increasing blood volume, cardiac output, and heart rate accompanying pregnancy increase pulmonary venous pressure and may lead to symptoms of congestive heart failure. Congestive failure is most likely to occur in the third trimester, during labor, or following delivery.

The most common symptom of mitral stenosis is dyspnea, initially on exertion and eventually at rest. The predominant symptoms of uncomplicated mitral stenosis are due to pulmonary venous hypertension and reflect the need for high left atrial (LA) to LV pressure gradients to maintain adequate transmitral blood flow. As LA and pulmonary venous pressures rise, there is usually a passive obligatory increase in mean pulmonary arterial pressure to ensure blood flow across the pulmonary vascular bed. However, in some patients with mitral stenosis, pulmonary artery pressure increases out of proportion to the rise of LA and pulmonary venous pressures. This reactive pulmonary hypertension can lead to RV dilatation and dysfunction in association with functional tricuspid regurgitation. Therefore, symptoms of right-sided heart failure may supercede those of pulmonary venous hypertension in these patients.

Due to the "normal physiologic" changes that occur during pregnancy, that is, increased cardiac output, heart rate, and blood volume, in association with reduced systemic and pulmonary vascular resistances, a seemingly well compensated patient with mitral stenosis may decompensate and suddenly experience symptoms. Symptoms may occur in as many as 25% of patients with mitral stenosis during pregnancy, and worsening of symptoms is common at the time of labor and delivery.

Nonpregnant women with symptoms or a mitral valve area less than 1.0 cm$^2$ (normal 4 to 6 cm$^2$) should receive surgical therapy prior to conception. When a pregnant patient with mitral stenosis develops pulmonary edema or hemodynamic compromise unresponsive to medical therapy, surgical therapies need to be considered. Mitral valve replacement has been reported to have a 23% fetal loss and a 2.6% maternal mortality (67). Since its introduction in 1984, percutaneous mitral commissurotomy (PMC) has steadily gained ground as an alternative to surgical commissurotomy. Iung (68) treated 13 pregnant women with PMC and reported this technique was efficacious in terms of improving maternal hemodynamics and was well tolerated by the fetus.

Cardiac output in patients with mitral stenosis is largely dependent on two factors (66). One is an adequate diastolic filling time; the other is LV preload. Although tachycardia is a clinical sign of underlying hemodynamic instability in most patients, in those with mitral stenosis the tachycardia itself, regardless of cause, may contribute significantly to hemodynamic decompensation. During labor, tachycardia may accompany the exertion of pushing or be secondary to pain or anxiety. Thus, patients with mitral stenosis in labor may exhibit a rapid and dramatic drop in cardiac output and blood pressure in response to an expected tachycardia. This drop in cardiac output will compromise maternal and fetal well-being. To avoid such tachycardia, the physician managing the patient should consider oral beta-blocker therapy for any patient with severe mitral stenosis who enters labor with a pulse exceeding 90 beats/min. In patients who are not initially tachycardic, acute control of tachycardia with an intravenous beta-blocking agent is rarely necessary (66).

Left ventricular preload is a very important consideration in patients with mitral stenosis. The presence of mitral stenosis makes the pulmonary capillary wedge pressure an inaccurate reflection of LV filling pressure. These patients often require high normal or elevated pulmonary capillary wedge pressure to maintain adequate ventricular filling pressure and cardiac output. Preload manipulation, such as diuresis, must be undertaken with extreme caution and careful attention to maintenance of cardiac output in these patients. Judicious use of epidural anesthesia may minimize potentially dangerous intrapartum fluctuations in cardiac output (69).

The immediate postpartum period is the most hazardous time for pregnant patients with mitral stenosis. Clark and colleagues (66) examined a series of patients with severe mitral stenosis and reported that a postpartum rise in wedge pressure of up to 16 mm Hg could be expected in the immediate postpartum period. This group suggested that pulmonary edema could be avoided in these patients by optimizing predelivery wedge pressures at 14 mm Hg or lower using the pulmonary artery catheter to monitor these patients and assure the maintenance of adequate cardiac output. Fluid restriction or careful diuresis may be used to achieve optimum pulmonary capillary wedge pressures.

Atrial fibrillation is frequently associated with mitral stenosis and has important hemodynamic consequences due to the resultant increased heart rate and loss of atrial contribution to LV filling. If atrial fibrillation occurs suddenly, it can lead to pulmonary congestion and pulmonary edema. In these cases, intravenous verapamil (5 to 10 mg IV) should be given or electrocardioversion should be attempted promptly. The latter has been performed successfully during pregnancy without apparent adverse fetal affects, but it is recommended that fetal heart rate (FHR) monitoring be instituted prior to attempting electrocardioversion. Chronic oral digoxin or beta blockade will usually ensure a reasonably slow ventricular response should atrial fibrillation occur. The potential for development of thrombus in the left atrium is an important consideration in the pregnant patient who is in a "hypercoagulable" state secondary to pregnancy. Thrombus in the left atrium may fragment and shed into the systemic arterial circulation. Atrial fibrillation in the presence of mitral valve disease is an indication for anticoagulation during pregnancy. An additional consideration in the management of the patient with rheumatic mitral stenosis should include both rheumatic fever and endocarditis prophylaxis.

In summary, the successful hemodynamic management of the pregnant woman with mitral stenosis requires anticipation of cardiovascular events. Elective induction of labor is prudent in order to insure the availability of the subspecialist necessary for optimal management of labor and delivery as well as neonatal problems. Evaluation of hemodynamic status and optimizing oxygen delivery prior to induction is also indicated. The patient with classes III and IV cardiac disease will require invasive hemodynamic monitoring during the intrapartum and postpartum periods. They should also be monitored with a bedside electrocardiogram in order to assess the presence of any disturbances in cardiac rhythm. In addition, effective epidural anesthesia during labor should minimize pain and anxiety and, therefore, decrease the hemodynamic burden on the heart. If the patient should become hypotensive secondary to regional anesthesia, treatment with large amounts of volume expansion can be performed cautiously with the use of the pulmonary artery catheter to monitor hemodynamic status. During delivery, blood loss should be replaced "milliliter for milliliter" and attention should be paid to cardiac output and urine output as well. A fall in urine output will result from poor renal perfusion and signals aberration in maternal hemodynamic status. Careful fetal monitoring during labor and delivery is essential and will assist in monitoring maternal hemodynamic status, as often the first sign of maternal compromise will be abnormal changes in the FHR (30).

## Mitral Regurgitation

Hemodynamically significant mitral regurgitation is usually rheumatic in origin but may have multiple etiologies. This lesion is generally well tolerated during pregnancy because of the low systemic vascular resistance, which may actually result in a decrease in the severity of valvular incompetence. In general, the symptoms of congestive heart failure due to mitral regurgitation in the pregnant patient are rare, and valve replacement is almost never indicated. Prophylaxis against bacterial endocarditis is usually recommended in patients with mitral regurgitation. Congenital mitral valve prolapse is much more common during pregnancy than is rheumatic mitral insufficiency and can occur in up to 17% of young healthy women. This condition is usually asymptomatic (70). Endocarditis prophylaxis is recommended for patients with mitral valve prolapse if associated with a click or a murmur.

## Aortic Stenosis

Aortic stenosis is usually of rheumatic origin but may occur congenitally and represents 5% of congenital cardiac lesions. In contrast to mitral valve stenosis, aortic stenosis generally does not become hemodynamically significant until the orifice has diminished to one-third or less of normal. The major problem experienced by patients with aortic stenosis is maintenance of cardiac output. Because of the relative hypervolemia associated with gestation, most patients generally tolerate pregnancy well. With severe disease, however, cardiac output will be relatively fixed and may be inadequate to maintain coronary artery or cerebral perfusion during exertion (71). This can result in angina, myocardial infarction, syncope, or sudden death. Therefore, during gestation, marked limitation of physical activity will be vital to patients with severe disease. If activity is limited and the

mitral valve is normal, pulmonary edema will rarely occur during pregnancy. Percutaneous commissurotomy has been successfully used to treat symptomatic aortic stenosis during gestation (72).

The times of greatest risk for patients with aortic stenosis are delivery and pregnancy termination (71). The maintenance of cardiac output is crucial. Any factor which leads to diminished venous return will compromise cardiac output. The literature suggests that pregnancy termination may be particularly hazardous in this regard and carries a mortality of up to 40%. Hypotension, from any cause, may result in myocardial ischemia, arrhythmias, and sudden death for the pregnant patient with aortic stenosis.

An additional consideration in patients with aortic stenosis is the frequent coexistence of ischemic heart disease. Patients with ischemic heart disease may suffer fatal myocardial infarction during gestation (71). The overall reported mortality associated with aortic stenosis in pregnancy is 17% (71). A shunt gradient greater than 100 mm Hg is associated with the greatest risk of maternal mortality. Right-sided heart catheterization may allow precise hemodynamic assessment and control during labor and delivery (73). The wedge pressure should be maintained in the range of 16 mm Hg to maintain a margin of safety against peripartum blood loss and hypotension (74). Lao (75) reported a recent experience with 25 pregnancies in 13 patients with congenital aortic stenosis. There were no maternal deaths or perinatal mortality in that group.

## Aortic Insufficiency

Aortic insufficiency is also commonly rheumatic in origin and almost always associated with mitral valve disease. Aortic insufficiency is well tolerated during pregnancy because the increased heart rate seen with advancing gestation decreases time for regurgitive flow during diastole. In a review of 28 maternal rheumatic cardiac deaths, only one was associated with aortic insufficiency in the absence of concurrent mitral stenosis (55). Patients with aortic insufficiency should receive prophylaxis for endocarditis during labor and delivery.

## Pulmonic and Tricuspid Lesions

Isolated right-sided valvular lesions of rheumatic origin are uncommon. Recently, such lesions are seen with increased frequency in intravenous drug abusers secondary to valvular endocarditis. Pregnancy-associated hypervolemia is far less likely to be symptomatic with right-sided lesions than those involving the left side of the heart. Hibbard (55) reported no deaths associated with right-sided lesions. In another report, congestive failure occurred in only 2.8% of women with pulmonic stenosis (76). Cautious fluid administration is usually all that is necessary for labor and delivery management in patients with pulmonic and tricuspid lesions.

## Peripartum Cardiomyopathy

Peripartum cardiomyopathy is cardiomyopathy developing in the last month of pregnancy or the first 6 months postpartum in a woman without previous cardiac disease and after exclusion of other causes of cardiac failure (77). It is a diagnosis of exclusion that should not be made without an effort to identify valvular, metabolic, infectious, or toxic causes of cardiomyopathy. Other peripartum complications such as severe preeclampsia, amniotic fluid embolism, corticosteroid, or sympathomimetic-induced pulmonary edema must also be considered before making the diagnosis of peripartum cardiomyopathy. Cunningham (78) reported that peripartum congestive heart failure occurs approximately once in every 4,000 deliveries and that true peripartum cardiomyopathy occurs only once in every 15,000 deliveries. In the United States, the peak incidence of peripartum cardiomyopathy occurs in the second postpartum month and there is a higher incidence among older, nulliparous, black women (79). Other risk factors include twinning and pregnancy-induced hypertension (79). Sympathomimetic agents used for tocolysis may unmask peripartum cardiomyopathy in previously asymptomatic pregnant women. A familial recurrence pattern has been reported in some cases.

Clinically, peripartum cardiomyopathy may present with a gradual onset of increasing fatigue, dyspnea, and peripheral or pulmonary edema. On physical examination, classical evidence of congestive heart failure is usually evident, including jugular venous distension, rales, and an $S_3$ gallop. On chest radiograph, cardiomegaly and pulmonary edema may be evident and the electrocardiogram is consistent with LV and LA dilation and diminished ventricular performance. Up to 50% of patients with peripartum cardiomyopathy may have evidence of pulmonary or systemic embolic phenomena. The mortality rate for pure peripartum cardiomyopathy is reportedly 57% (78).

If myocardial specimens are examined histologically, nonspecific cellular hypertrophy, degeneration, fibrosis, and increased lipid deposition are noted. Some reports have documented the presence of a diffuse myocarditis; however, it is questionable whether or not such cases represent the same syndrome (80–82). Because the clinical and pathologic nature of peripartum cardiomyopathy is nonspecific, its existence as a distinct entity has been questioned.

The existence of peripartum cardiomyopathy is supported primarily by epidemiologic evidence suggesting that 80% of cases of cardiomyopathy in women in child-bearing age occur in the peripartum period (78, 79). Another consideration is that this epidemiologic distribution may also be attributed to an exacerbation of underlying subclinical cardiac disease related to the hemodynamic changes accompanying normal pregnancy. However, the hemodynamic changes in pregnancy are maximal in the third trimester and gradually return to normal within a few weeks postpartum and therefore do not explain the peak incidence of peripartum cardiomyopathy occurring in the second month postpartum.

Therapy for peripartum cardiomyopathy includes digitalization, diuretic agents, sodium restriction, and prolonged bed rest (65). Afterload reduction with Ace inhibitors, hydralazine, or nitrates may be useful. Women with peripartum cardiomyopathy have a high frequency of systemic and pulmonary emboli. Prophylactic subcutaneous heparin should be used during the antepartum period. Warfarin can be used postpartum even in women who are breast feeding.

Peripartum cardiomyopathy has a tendency to recur in subsequent pregnancies. Several reports have suggested that the prognosis for future pregnancies is related to heart size. Patients whose cardiac size return to normal within 6 to 12 months had an 11% to 14% mortality in subsequent pregnancies. Patients with persistent cardiomegaly, however, had a 40% to 80% mortality (77). Pregnancy, therefore, is definitely contraindicated in all patients with persistent cardiomegaly. The 11% to 14% risk of mortality seen in patients with a return to normal heart size, in all but exceptional cases, would appear unacceptable as well.

## Idiopathic Hypertrophic Subaortic Stenosis

Idiopathic hypertrophic subaortic stenosis (IHSS) is an autosomal dominant condition with variable penetrance. It commonly becomes clinically manifest in the second or third decade of life and may often be first diagnosed during pregnancy. Idiopathic hypertrophic subaortic stenosis primarily involves LV hypertrophy typically involving the septum to a greater extent than the free wall. The hypertrophy results in an obstruction to LV outflow and secondary mitral regurgitation. These are the two principal hemodynamic concerns for clinical management of the patient with this condition. Increased blood volume associated with normal pregnancy should enhance LV filling and improve hemodynamic performance (73). However, the drop in arterial pressure and the venocaval obstruction that are found in late pregnancy may result in hemodynamic impairment and depressed cardiac output. Tachycardia resulting from pain or fear in labor will also diminish LV filling and aggravate the relative outflow obstruction. The Valsalva effect during pushing in the second stage of labor will have the same effect (73).

Important issues involved in successful management of the peripartum period in patients with IHSS involves avoidance of hypotension and tachycardia as well as conducting labor in the left lateral recumbent position. The use of forceps to shorten the second stage of labor has also been recommended. As with other cardiac diseases, cesarean section should be reserved for obstetric indications only.

Maternal and fetal outcome in IHSS patients is generally good. A report of 54 pregnancies in 23 patients with IHSS revealed no maternal or neonatal deaths (83). Antibiotic prophylaxis against bacterial endocarditis is recommended for patients with IHSS.

## Myocardial Infarction

Myocardial infarction during pregnancy is rare, occurring approximately once in 10,000 pregnancies. Hankins (84) reviewed 68 reported cases of myocardial infarction during pregnancy and noted a 35% mortality rate. Only 13% of patients were known to have had coronary artery disease prior to pregnancy. Two-thirds of these patients suffered myocardial infarction during the third trimester; the mortality for these women was 45%, compared with 23% for infarction in the first or second trimester. The increased hemodynamic burden imposed on the maternal cardiovascular system in late pregnancy may unmask latent coronary artery disease in some women and worsen the prognosis for patients suffering infarction. Women who survive myocardial infarction during pregnancy appear to have an increased rate of spontaneous abortion and unexplained still birth.

Diagnostic radionucleotide cardiac imaging during pregnancy results in a fetal dose no more than 0.08 Gy and does not carry the potential for teratogenesis; therefore this testing should be done when indicated (85). If cardiac catheterization is indicated, the simultaneous use of contrast echocardiography may reduce the need for cineangiography, thereby reducing radiation exposure to the fetus (86).

Antepartum care in women who suffer myocardial infarction during gestation includes bedrest to minimize myocardial oxygen demands. Delivery within 2 weeks of myocardial infarction has been associated with increased mortality. Therefore, attempts should be made to allow adequate convalescence prior to attempting delivery. If delivery is necessary, the patients should be hemodynamically stabilized, preferably with a pulmonary artery catheter in place. The patient should labor in the lateral recumbent position, optimizing venous return. Oxygen should be administered during labor in order to maximize oxygen delivery to the injured myocardium. Pain relief should be adequate and is best obtained with epidural anesthesia.

In one report, two patients were presented who suffered myocardial infarction during gestation (87). One patient had a triplet gestation. Both patients had documentation of myocardial infarction based on clinical and laboratory evidence, and both underwent coronary angiography. Both patients developed preeclampsia and were prematurely delivered of viable fetuses. One patient suffered angina during labor and was successfully treated with sublingual nitroglycerin. Neither patient received invasive hemodynamic monitoring during labor, and the mode of delivery was determined solely on obstetric indications. Neither suffered reinfarction or heart failure. These authors concluded that pregnant patients who suffered myocardial infarction during gestation did not require invasive hemodynamic monitoring as long as they had good cardiac function and reserve.

The safety of pregnancy in patients who have a history of myocardial infarction was examined by Frenkel (88). Twenty cases of pregnancy after myocardial infarction were reviewed, and in addition the management of four cases was presented. Conception occurred in these patients 9 months to 9 years after myocardial infarction. Each patient had a uneventful pregnancy with no cardiac or obstetric complications related to myocardial infarction. The mode of delivery in these patients was based on obstetric indications, and this reported experience demonstrated a good prognosis for pregnancy in patients who have a history of myocardial infarction.

## CARDIAC SURGERY DURING PREGNANCY

The pregnant patient with cardiac disease is best managed with conservative medical management during gestation (30). The majority of women with cardiac disease can be managed successfully with use of diet, bed rest, and cardiovascular drugs. However, when these conservative measures fail, cardiac surgery is an acceptable alternative. Before surgical intervention is undertaken, the potential risks and complications for the pregnant woman and her fetus should be considered. If the decision to perform surgery is made, a team approach including the cardiologist, cardiovascular surgeon, and obstetrician is required (89). With current advanced medical and surgical management, the risk of cardiac surgery in the pregnant patient is probably not increased over that of the nonpregnant patient. In addition, perinatal mortality has declined 67% in patients undergoing cardiac surgery since 1969 (89). The use of electronic FHR monitoring during bypass surgery has been the major contributing factor to this improved perinatal outcome (90). Fetal heart rate monitoring allows the team to continuously monitor the fetal condition and promptly identify and treat any evidence of fetal distress. Fetal bradycardia followed by compensatory tachycardia is often noted during bypass surgery. The basis for the FHR changes has been suggested to be diminished uteroplacental perfusion. The decline in perfusion is thought to be secondary to a lack of pulsatile flow, the opening of uterine arteriovenous shunts, uterine artery spasm, or insufficient flow rates. There appears to be a direct relationship between flow rates and FHR. Intraoperative correction of fetal bradycardia has been achieved simply by increasing flow rates. In addition, repositioning the mother to relieve possible umbilical cord compression or compression of the inferior vena cava has been suggested (91). If these measures fail and surgery is to be prolonged, cesarean delivery may be required.

Spontaneous uterine activity is increased during and immediately following bypass surgery, and this may require tocolytic therapy. Use of magnesium sulfate for tocolysis will avoid the tachycardia associated with beta-agonists. In addition to continuous electronic FHR monitoring and high-flow, high-pressure nonthermic perfusion, fetal outcome may be improved by avoiding vasopressors, correcting maternal hemorrhage with blood or component replacement, and increasing maternal oxygenation (91).

## Pregnancy After Cardiac Transplantation

Cardiac transplantation has been performed in women of childbearing age. There are reports in the literature describing pregnancy after heart transplantation in female recipients (92–96). Three of the reports describe patients who had received cardiac transplantation because of intractable peripartum cardiomyopathy. One patient was 29 years old, and she conceived 5 years after cardiac transplantation (92). She was maintained on prednisone, azothioprine, and aspirin. Her pregnancy was complicated at 34 weeks by *Listeria monocytogenes.* At 36 weeks the patient was delivered by elective cesarean section of a 3,100-gram male infant who had no gross fetal anomalies and did well. This patient died at 5 months postpartum because she stopped her immunosuppressive therapy and suffered acute rejection. Another patient who had cardiac transplantation because of previous postpartum cardiomyopathy was also treated with immunosuppressive therapy with prednisone and cyclosporine (96). Her pregnancy was uneventful; however, 1 year after birth, her infant developed cardiomyopathy. The other case reports outlined the course and management of patients who were postcardiac transplantation for other diagnosis. These patients had good perinatal outcome. Although there are only a few reports in the literature, the overall positive outcome for these patients would seem to imply that prior cardiac transplantation is not necessarily a contraindication to pregnancy.

## Artificial Valves and Anticoagulation in Pregnancy

When considering the best mode of anticoagulation in the pregnant woman with an artificial valve and/or atrial fibrillation during pregnancy, consideration must be given to the known teratogenic effects of oral anticoagulants weighed against the potential increased risk of thrombosis and thromboembolism incurred by using heparin rather than warfarin. Cases have been reported in which heparin failed to prevent thrombosis of an artificial valve during pregnancy (97–99). One should consider, however, the fact that with mechanical prosthetic valves there is a rate of approximately 2% to 4% per year of thromboembolism or valve thrombosis, even with the use of oral anticoagulants. An additional consideration is that warfarin is associated with spontaneous abortion, warfarin embryopathy, and central nervous system anomalies.

Some investigators have favored using warfarin therapy in the presence of an artificial heart valve or arterial fibrillation because of a perception that the actual fetal risks associated with warfarin appear less frequently than have been reported. Oakley (97) estimated the chance of a live born abnormal baby is less than 5% following coumarin exposure. However, the use of heparin rather than coumarin during pregnancy is still currently recommended by most experts and remains the standard of care in the United States (100). Heparin is advised for the following reasons: heparin regimens during pregnancy for treatment or prophylaxis of venous thromboembolic disease appear safe, the risk of bleeding is low, and heparin-induced thrombocytopenia and systemic osteoporosis are uncommon (101). Although experience is limited in patients with prosthetic heart valves, it appears that subcutaneous adjusted-dose heparin may be as effective as oral anticoagulants (102, 103).

The adjusted-dose regimen employs heparin given subcutaneously every 12 hours in a dose sufficient to prolong the activated partial thromboplastin time, obtained 6 hours after the dose, to 1.5 to 2 times the normal control value. This should provide plasma heparin levels of 0.2 to 0.4 units/mL if measured by the available $S_a$ assay. There is one exception to the recommendation for heparin use during gestation, and that is in the patient who has continuing gestation and is unable to tolerate heparin, for example, a patient who develops heparin-induced thrombocytopenia or a patient who accepts the risks associated with warfarin therapy during pregnancy after a full discussion of the risks as well as the medical/legal consequences. There are no reports specifically describing the use of low molecular weight heparin for anticoagulation in patients with artificial valves.

There is a small series of patients with prosthetic heart valves who have been treated during gestation with antiplatelet agents without reported maternal or neonatal complications. Biale (104) reported on 4 women with

Star-Edwards prosthetic valves treated with aspirin and dipyridamole who had no thromboembolic complications. Nunez (105) described 20 women with nonbiologic prosthetic valves treated with either 1 gram of aspirin daily or 500 mg every 48 hours. Although 13 of the women had atrial fibrillation, none had thromboembolic complications. This observation, however, does not change the need to fully anticoagulate patients in chronic atrial fibrillation (59).

The biprosthetic valves might be considered the ideal choice of prosthesis for a young woman contemplating pregnancy because anticoagulation is not required beyond 3 months after insertion. However, the valve has a rapid rate of deterioration and a need for subsequent replacement (106). One report suggests that the frequent need to surgically replace a deteriorated biprosthetic valve may pose a greater mortality risk to the patient than does the thromboembolic risk of a mechanical valve (107).

Subcutaneous minidose heparin is insufficient for anticoagulation of prosthetic valve patients during gestation. Wang (108) treated 7 women having artificial heart valves with subcutaneous heparin, 5,000 units every 12 hours. Four of the women had serious thromboembolic complications. Salzar (109) reported 1 case of cerebral embolism among 12 patients receiving minidose heparin. Therefore, if heparin is to be used in artificial valve patients, full anticoagulation is required. In one series, 6 patients were treated with a continuous subcutaneous heparin infusion pump (110). Five patients had had venous thromboembolic events and 1 patient had a prosthetic heart valve. There were no additional thrombotic complications; however, 5 of the 6 patients had major bleeding complications from treatment despite having partial thromboplastin times in the therapeutic range. Newer approaches in which anticoagulation with a heparin pump is monitored with serum heparin assays are preferable to monitoring the partial thromboplastin times alone.

### Prevention of Infective Endocarditis

Infective endocarditis is nearly always fatal if untreated and continues to cause substantial morbidity and mortality despite modern antimicrobial and surgical treatment (111). Therefore, prevention is a priority. The rationale for prophylaxis against endocarditis with antibiotics is as follows: endocarditis usually follows bacteremia; several health care procedures cause bacteremia with organisms that can cause endocarditis; these bacteria are usually sensitive to antibiotics; therefore, antibiotics should be given to patients with predisposing heart disease before procedures that may cause bacteremia (111). On this basis, prophylaxis against endocarditis has become routine in most developed countries. However, no prospective study has proved its efficacy. Transient

bacteremia is thought to occur after 1.0% to 4.9% of normal vaginal deliveries (112). The incidence of bacteremia after cesarean section is unknown. A review of infective endocarditis in obstetric and gynecologic practice revealed only 18 cases that developed postpartum and were attributable to infection at the time of delivery (112). Sixteen of these cases occurred after vaginal delivery and 2 cases developed after cesarean section. Of the 17 cases for which there was adequate information, 14 had underlying cardiac disease.

The committee on rheumatic fever and infective endocarditis of the Council on Cardiovascular Disease in The Young revised recommendations for bacterial endocarditis in 1984 (113). The common conditions for which patients are considered to be at risk for endocarditis are prosthetic valves, most congenital cardiac malformations, surgical systemic pulmonary shunts, rheumatic and other acquired valvular dysfunction, idiopathic hypertrophic subaortic stenosis, previous history of bacterial endocarditis, and mitral valve prolapse with insufficiency.

The issue of whether to utilize prophylaxis of endocarditis in patients with mitral valve prolapse occurs frequently because mitral valve prolapse is the most common valvular disease in productive age women. At least 5% of women are affected (114). Mitral valve prolapse with regurgitation requires prophylaxis (114). The patient with silent mitral valve prolapse without a regurgitant murmur or click is not at increased risk for endocarditis and therefore does not require prophylaxis.

### PREECLAMPSIA/ECLAMPSIA

*Preeclampsia* complicates approximately 5% of pregnancies in the United States (115). The Committee on Terminology of the American College of Obstetricians and Gynecologists (ACOG) (116) has determined that the diagnosis of preeclampsia is based on elevated blood pressure, proteinuria and/or edema. Blood pressure is considered elevated if prior blood pressure is unknown and readings of 140/90 mm Hg or a mean arterial pressure of 104 mm Hg is obtained. If prior blood pressures are known, and the systolic blood pressure increases by 30 mm Hg, or the diastolic blood pressure increases by 15 mm Hg, the blood pressure is considered elevated. These elevations must be present on two measurements taken 6 hours apart. Edema is diagnosed as clinically evident swelling; however, fluid retention can also be manifest as a rapid increase in weight, without evidence of edema. Proteinuria is defined as a concentration of 1 g/L or more in at least two random urine specimens collected 6 hours apart, or more than 0.3 g/L in a 24-hour urine collection.

The criteria for severe preeclampsia are as follows (116):

1. Blood pressure ≥ 160 mm Hg systolic, or ≥110 mm Hg diastolic; recorded on at least two occasions, at least 6 hours apart with the patient at bed rest
2. Proteinuria ≥ 5 g in a 24-hour urine specimen (3+ or 4+ on quantitative examination)
3. Oliguria (≤400 mL in 24 hours)
4. Epigastric pain
5. Pulmonary edema or cyanosis
6. Impaired liver function of unclear etiology
7. Thrombocytopenia

*Eclampsia* is diagnosed when tonic clonic seizures occur in a pregnant patient with preeclampsia that cannot be attributed to other causes (116). Eclampsia is most common in the last trimester and becomes increasingly more frequent as term approaches. Preeclampsia usually precedes the onset of eclamptic convulsions. Patients will often relate symptoms such as headache, visual disturbance, and epigastric or right upper quadrant pain that should make one suspicious of preeclampsia. Such symptoms should always be investigated. Eclampsia is one of the most dangerous conditions that one may face in pregnancy. The reported maternal mortality rate has ranged from less than 1% to as much as 17.5%.

The perinatal outcome in preeclampsia is dependent on gestational age at onset of preeclampsia, and at the time of delivery, the severity of the disease process, the presence of multiple gestation, and the presence of underlying hypertensive or renal disease (117). In patients with mild preeclampsia at term, the perinatal mortality rate, incidence of fetal growth retardation, and neonatal morbidity are no different than those of normotensive pregnancies. Long and colleagues (118) reported the pregnancy outcome in 2,434 singleton pregnancies with preeclampsia during a 7-year period. They noted that patients with preterm preeclampsia (<37 weeks) had a worse perinatal outcome than those with preeclampsia at 37 weeks or later. The perinatal mortality rate in the preterm group was 10.5%. The incidence of fetal growth retardation was 18.2%, and the incidence of abruptio placenta was 4.5%. For women at term with preeclampsia, the perinatal mortality rate was 0.6%, the incidence of fetal growth retardation was 5.6%, and the incidence of abruptio placenta was 0.4%. Preeclampsia tends to develop earlier in a twin gestation, and maternal disease is usually more severe than in singleton pregnancies.

Pregnancies complicated by severe preeclampsia are usually associated with high perinatal mortality and morbidity rates. Sibai and associates (117) reported the pregnancy outcome in 303 pregnancies complicated by severe preeclampsia. There were 28 stillbirths and 15 neonatal deaths, for an uncorrected perinatal mortality rate of 145 per 1,000. The corrected perinatal mortality rate was 135 per 1,000. In this series 20% of newborns were small for gestational age.

Severe preeclampsia usually results in progressive deterioration in both the maternal and fetal conditions. The management plan should seek to optimize maternal outcome first but should also give consideration to obtaining the best fetal outcome possible under the circumstances. In formulating the management plan, the gestational age at the onset of severe preeclampsia should be taken into consideration.

When severe preeclampsia develops at 34 weeks gestational age or beyond or if there is evidence of fetal lung maturity or maternal or fetal compromise, delivery should be undertaken. Antiseizure prophylaxis with magnesium sulfate is indicated, and the patient should be in a monitored setting in the left lateral recumbent position, and blood pressures should be controlled (30). Induction of labor should be undertaken with specific goals in mind; that is, safe delivery of the fetus within a reasonable time frame. During induction it is extremely important that blood pressure and urine output be monitored closely as well as the patient's hemoglobin, platelet count, liver function tests, and serum creatinine.

Close fetal surveillance is necessary, as the fetus is at risk for abruptio placenta and, in addition, may have evidence of fetal compromise because of inadequate uteroplacental perfusion. The preeclamptic patient does not increase intravascular volume compared to normal pregnant patients. Because of this, she is at increased risk of decreased uteroplacental perfusion when hypotension occurs with regional anesthesia (119, 120). Therefore, it is important to maintain intravascular volume during regional anesthesia. If evidence of fetal compromise develops, such as prolonged absence of FHR reactivity or persistent late decelerations, cesarean delivery should be undertaken once the maternal condition has been stabilized. Evidence of worsening maternal condition such as severe thrombocytopenia, continued elevation of liver function tests, or oliguria is also an indication for immediate delivery. The patient should be stabilized, transfused platelets if necessary, and cesarean delivery undertaken for maternal indications if vaginal delivery is not imminent.

The management of patients who have severe preeclampsia and are less than 34 weeks gestation is not as clearcut. Some institutions recommend delivery for all cases of severe preeclampsia, regardless of gestational age, but many others recommend prolonging pregnancy in patients who are remote from term until development of fetal or maternal jeopardy, fetal lung maturity, or a gestational age of 36 weeks or greater. If conservative management is undertaken, patients should be admitted to the labor and delivery area for intense maternal and fetal surveillance. Patients should be given intravenous magnesium sulfate for seizure prophylaxis, and when indicated, hydralazine should be administered to control blood pressures greater than 160 mm Hg systolic or 110 mm Hg diastolic.

Patients should be monitored in the left lateral recumbent position and frequent determinations of hemoglobin, arterial blood pressure, urine output, platelet count, liver function tests, and serum creatinine should be obtained. In addition, the fetus should be assessed with nonstress testing or a biophysical profile. The nonstress test (NST) is based on the fact that fetal movement typically is accompanied by transient acceleration of the FHR (121). Each time fetal movement is felt by the mother she presses a button to record the instant of movement on the same moving paper strip that the heart rate is recorded. The test is generally considered normal (reactive) when two or more fetal movements are accompanied by acceleration of the FHR of 15 beats/min for at least 15 seconds duration within a 20-minute period (121). The biophysical profile, which is performed utilizing an ultrasound examination and the NST, is defined in Table 3 (122). If the patient is 25 weeks gestational age or greater and there is evidence of fetal compromise, the maternal condition should be stabilized and operative delivery undertaken in a tertiary care center. Patients who continue to show evidence of maternal compromise, such as persistent severe hypertension, low platelets, oliguria, or pulmonary edema, should also be delivered. If possible, vaginal delivery should be undertaken and labor should be induced.

Patients with oliguria unresponsive to fluid challenge, pulmonary edema that does not resolve with diuresis, or blood pressures unresponsive to hydralazine that require intensive therapy with agents such as nitroprusside may require right-sided heart catheterization and intra-arterial blood pressure monitoring during induction of labor (123). In these circumstances the use of the pulmonary artery catheter may help to elucidate the pathophysiologic derangement. Data presented by several authors have demonstrated that central venous pressure and pulmonary capillary wedge pressure often do not correlate in severe preeclampsia (123–126). Clark and Cotton (123) have proposed that increased LV afterload accompanied by normal to high cardiac output and a well-compensated myocardium result in a higher intracavitary pressure for a given blood volume on the left side of the heart when compared with the RV system. Under these circumstances, the filling pressures of the right and left sides of the heart would not be expected to be similar. As it is impossible to predict in which patient central venous pressure and pulmonary capillary wedge pressure will correlate, central venous pressure is a clinically unacceptable measurement of preload in the patient with severe preeclampsia (123). Therefore, preeclamptic patients who require central monitoring should have a pulmonary artery catheter inserted.

When a gravida develops eclamptic seizures, the fetus is at risk for morbidity or mortality from abruptio placenta, prematurity, intrauterine growth retardation, and the hypoxia that develops during a convulsion (120, 127). Lopez-Llera and colleagues (120) reported a perinatal mortality rate of 45% in women who had eclampsia and developed abruptio placenta. Abdella and colleagues (128) reported an incidence of 23.6% of abruptio placenta in women who developed eclampsia before delivery at the University of Tennessee. In this group of patients there were three stillbirths and three neonatal deaths for a perinatal mortality rate of 460 per 1,000.

Brazy and colleagues (129) reported on 28 infants from pregnancies complicated by severe hypertension. Eight of these patients had eclampsia, 39% of patients had infants that were less than the 10th percentile, and 29% of these infants were symmetrically growth

**TABLE 3.** *Fetal biophysical profile score*

| Variable | Score 2 | Score 0 |
|---|---|---|
| Fetal breathing movements (FBM) | Presence of at least 30 s of sustained FBM in 30 min of observation | Less than 30 cc of FBM in 30 min |
| Fetal movements | Three or more gross body movements in 30 min of observation; simultaneous limb and trunk movements counted as a single movement | Two or less gross body movements in 30 min of observation |
| Fetal tone | At least one episode of motion of a limb from a position of flexion to extension and a rapid return to flexion | Fetus in a position of semi- or full-limb extension with no return to flexion with movement; absence of fetal movement counted as absent tone |
| Fetal reactivity | Presence of two or more fetal heart rate accelerations of at least 15 beats/min lasting at least 15 s and associated with fetal movement in 40 min | No acceleration or less than two accelerations of the fetal heart rate in 40 min of observation |
| Qualitative amniotic fluid volume | Pocket of amniotic fluid that measures at least 1 cm in two perpendicular planes | Largest pocket of amniotic fluid measures <1 cm in two perpendicular planes |
| Maximal score | 10 | — |
| Minimal score | — | 0 |

From Manning et al. *Am J Obstet Gynecol* 1981;140:289, with permission.

retarded. This group of patients had a high incidence of perinatal asphyxia, low Apgar scores, and hematologic abnormalities. Sibai and colleagues (130) followed 28 premature infants and 14 full-term infants of eclamptic mothers for up to 50 months. Eight of 12 infants who were small for gestational age by birth weight showed catch-up growth at an average of 20.6 months. A total of 3 infants had major neurologic deficits resulting in cerebral palsy and mental retardation on follow-up evaluation. Of the mentally retarded infants, two remained growth retarded by weight, height, and head circumference. Several premature infants required multiple hospitalizations for pulmonary or neurologic complications during the first year of life.

Paul and colleagues (131) examined the changes in FHR and uterine contraction patterns associated with eclampsia. They reported that maternal convulsions were usually associated with sustained uterine contractions and a sudden rise in maternal blood pressure. During seizure activity, which generally lasts less than 1.5 minutes, transient maternal hypoxia and uterine artery vasospasm occur and combine to produce a decline in uterine blood flow. Spontaneous uterine activity is further increased, resulting in additional compromise of uteroplacental perfusion. Fetal hypoxia develops and FHR bradycardia ensues. Fetal heart rate bradycardia may last up to 9 minutes. The normal beat-to-beat variability of the FHR is lost, and compensatory fetal tachycardia is characteristically seen. After an eclamptic seizure occurs, the obstetrician must maintain an adequate airway and administer oxygen. Anticonvulsant therapy should be instituted, and in the United States intravenous magnesium sulfate is the drug of choice, for both treatment of eclamptic seizures and prevention of seizure recurrence (132). The patient should be placed in the left lateral recumbent position in order to optimize uteroplacental perfusion. Intrauterine resuscitation with additional magnesium sulfate or a betamimetic may decrease eclampsia-induced uterine hypertonia and minimize FHR abnormalities (133, 134). Continuous electronic FHR monitoring should be utilized in order to monitor the fetal condition. Care must be taken during this time period to be sure that the gravida has been stabilized before attempting to intervene for fetal indications. One should remember that prolonged fetal bradycardia often follows eclamptic seizures and that intervention to rescue the fetus may not be necessary, as most of the time the FHR pattern will improve with therapeutic intervention.

If the fetus continues to show signs of distress, fetal acid-base status should be assessed if possible. This is done by obtaining a sample of blood from the fetal scalp. Values above 7.25 are considered normal and should be repeated, as indicated by the FHR pattern and progress in labor (135, 136). Values between 7.20 and 7.25 are considered to be suspicious or borderline and generally should be repeated in 15 to 30 minutes to detect the possibility of a downward trend in pH. A scalp blood pH of less than 7.20 is considered abnormal and generally is an indication for some type of medical or surgical intervention. If assessment confirms fetal compromise, delivery by cesarean section should be undertaken once the maternal condition has been stabilized. If the fetal assessment is reassuring and conditions are favorable, an attempt should be made to deliver the patient vaginally, as there is less maternal morbidity and mortality when delivery is by this route. When the fetal acid-base status cannot be assessed or evidence of fetal compromise persists, the fetus should be delivered by cesarean section once the maternal condition has been stabilized.

## Obstetric Hemorrhage and Hypovolemic Shock

Obstetric hemorrhage is a frequent cause of maternal death in the United States, accounting for 11% of maternal mortality in the United States between 1980 and 1985 (137). Hypovolemic shock in pregnancy is also responsible for serious nonfatal complications. The pregnant woman undergoes physiologic changes to prepare for the blood loss that will occur at parturition. By the end of the second trimester of pregnancy, maternal blood volume has increased by 1,000 to 2,000 mL (138). Cardiac output increases by 50% while total peripheral resistance decreases. Therefore, the parturient has been prepared for blood volume loss of up to 1,000 mL. The usual estimated blood loss at delivery is notoriously underestimated. Actual measurements show that the average blood loss after normal spontaneous vaginal delivery is over 600 mL (138). Following a postpartum blood loss of less than 1,000 mL, the parturient's vital signs may not reflect acute blood loss, and a first-day postpartum hematocrit is usually not altered significantly from the admission hematocrit.

Any disruption of the maternal vascular system during pregnancy has the potential for devastating blood loss. After the first trimester, obstetric hemorrhage usually results from a disruption of the placental attachment site. This could be secondary to abruptio placenta, that is, separation of a normally implanted placenta prior to delivery of the fetus or to separation of the placental attachment of a placenta previa. Uterine rupture can occur spontaneously or related to trauma.

Most obstetric hemorrhage occurs in the postpartum period. The most common cause is uterine atony following placental separation. Shortening of the myometrial fibers acts as a physiologic ligature around the arterioles of the separated placental bed. Therefore, uterine atony will result in arterial hemorrhage. Factors that can predispose the patient to uterine atony include precipitous or prolonged labor, oxytocin augmentation, magnesium sulfate infusion, chorioamnionitis, and enlarged uterus resulting from increased intrauterine contents and operative deliveries (30). Obstetric trauma is another common cause of postpartum hemorrhage. Additional causes include uterine inversion, placenta accreta, amniotic fluid embolism, retroperitoneal bleeding from birth trauma or episiotomy, and coagulopathies. Most obstetric patients will tolerate a blood loss of up to 1 liter and remain hemodynamically stable. However, patients with preeclampsia do not enhance their intravascular volume during gestation adequately as compared to normal pregnant patients. Because of the depleted intravascular volume associated with preeclampsia, even the usual blood loss associated with delivery may result in clinical instability.

Antepartum hemorrhage is most often associated with abruptio placenta or placenta previa. When antepartum hemorrhage occurs, the obstetrician must be concerned with both maternal and fetal well-being. Fetal oxygenation decreases in proportion to the decrease in maternal cardiac output. During shock, catecholamine output may preferentially increase arteriolar resistance of the spiral arterioles in the placental bed, further decreasing fetal oxygenation. Thus, the fetus may be in jeopardy even though this is a compensatory mechanism to maintain stable maternal vital signs. Even in the absence of overt hypotension, concern for the well-being of the fetus dictates that intravascular volume must be replaced in an antepartum patient who has lost blood. The FHR should be monitored closely during an antepartum bleeding event in a potentially viable fetus (≥24 weeks gestational age) because it is often possible to gauge maternal response to therapy such as blood transfusion, oxygen administration, positional change, etc., by assessing the fetal response to these resuscitative measures. If, in spite of what seems to be adequate maternal resuscitative efforts the fetus continues to show evidence of stress, one may make the assumption that maternal hemorrhage continues and that operative therapy may be indicated.

Three maternal organs are particularly susceptible to damage when perfusion pressure decreases as a result of hemorrhagic shock. These include the anterior pituitary gland, the kidneys, and the lungs. During pregnancy, the anterior pituitary enlarges in size and receives an increased blood flow. When shock ensues, blood flow is shunted away from the anterior pituitary gland which may then undergo ischemic necrosis. Sheehan and Murdoch (139) first described the syndrome of hypopituitarism secondary to postpartum hypotension as a result of hemorrhage. This condition is rare and has an incidence of 1:10,000 pregnancies. Hypovolemia from any cause leads to reduced renal perfusion which can result in acute tubular necrosis. In one series, hemorrhage and hypovolemia were precipitating factors in 75% of obstetric patients with acute renal failure (140). Lung injury resulting from hypovolemic shock can lead to the adult respiratory distress syndrome (ARDS). In one report on maternal mortality in a maternal-fetal intensive care unit, preeclampsia hemorrhage and infection were the most common initiat-ing causes of maternal death (141). In that report the terminal event in ten of the maternal deaths was ARDS.

In patients with underlying cardiac disease who are very dependent on preload in order to maintain cardiac output, acute blood loss, both in the antepartum and postpartum periods, can result in devastating maternal outcome. Therefore, one needs to anticipate potential for blood loss. Transfusion should be readily available and liberally used in patients who have underlying cardiac disease and are experiencing blood loss in the antepartum or postpartum periods. Oxygen should also be administered, and if there is any question about the adequacy of the resuscitative measure, central hemodynamic monitoring with the flow-directed pulmonary artery catheter can be used to optimize volume status and oxygen delivery to both the maternal and fetal compartments.

## AMNIOTIC FLUID EMBOLISM

Amniotic fluid embolism (AFE) is responsible for roughly 10% of all maternal deaths in the United States and is the most common cause of peripartum death. The mortality rate from AFE may be as high as 80% (142). Amniotic fluid embolism is classically characterized by hypotension, hypoxemia, and coagulopathy. However, the pathogenesis of this condition is still not completely understood. Animal studies of AFE had been conducted in various animal models including the dog, cat, rat, rabbit, sheep, calf, and monkey. The physiologic derangements obtained in these studies differ from study to study and from one species to the other (30). Studies that are often quoted are models of Reis and Attwood (143, 144).

In the sheep study by Reis (143), the intravenous injection of amniotic fluid resulted in a 90% increase in main pulmonary artery pressure, a 69% increase in central venous pressure, and a 150% increase in pulmonary vascular resistance without a rise in pulmonary capillary wedge pressure. In this study, pulmonary artery pressure rapidly returned to normal within 30 minutes in all animals, and pulmonary edema was never observed. Attwood (144) observed an almost identical response and prompt resolution in the canine model. Reliance in these animal models to the exclusion of others had led many authors to conclude that the pathophysiology of AFE in humans principally involves severe pulmonary hypertension secondary to occlusive or vasal spastic changes in the pulmonary vasculature leading to acute cor pulmonale. In the past, recommendations for therapy have been based on this assumption and have included a variety of measures directed at the release of pulmonary artery vasospasm including atropine, papaverine, aminophylline, and nonspecific "vasodilating agents" (30).

In contrast to observations in animal models, all published cases of AFE in humans involving central hemodynamic monitoring are similar and involve only mild to moderate elevations in pulmonary artery pressure, variable increases in central venous pressure, elevated pulmonary capillary wedge pressures, and most importantly, evidence of LV dysfunction or failure (145–152). Clark (146) reviewed the published data of AFE and noted that in all cases pulmonary vascular resistance was either normal or well within the range consistent with left-sided heart failure alone. He proposed that this evidence supports the contention of recent investigative publishing since 1985, that left-sided heart failure is the major physiologic aberration seen in humans with AFE. left-sided heart failure appears to be the only significant hemodynamic abnormality consistently documented in human patients. Data supporting intrinsic pulmonary artery spasm and secondary cor pulmonale are lacking. Additional animal data suggest that hypoxic injury to the left ventricle may be involved in this left-sided heart failure (153). An in vitro observation of decreased myometrial contractility in the presence of amniotic fluid also suggests the possibility of a direct depressant effect of amniotic fluid on the myocardium (154).

Clark (30) suggests that AFE is a biphasic process, apparently initiated by sudden embolism of amniotic fluid or debris of fetal origin into the maternal venous circulation. The initial transient physiologic disturbances involve profound alterations in cardiovascular hemodynamics and oxygenation, often followed by the development of consumptive coagulopathy. Patients who survive this initial phase experience a secondary phase of hemodynamic compromise which involves left-sided heart failure, a variable secondary elevation of pulmonary artery pressure, and return of normal right-sided heart function. The classic presentation is sudden dyspnea and hypotension often followed within minutes by cardiorespiratory arrest (30). In 10% to 20% of cases, these initial events may be accompanied by seizures (142). In up to 70% of patients who survive the initial hemodynamic collapse, the adult respiratory distress syndrome develops (30).

Clark (155) recently reported on 46 patients in a national registry of AFE. All patients presented with hypotension and fetal distress, 93% presented with pulmonary edema or the adult respiratory distress syndrome, 80% suffered cardiac arrest, and 83% had cyanosis and coagulopathy. Dyspnea was reported in 49%, seizure in 48%, apnea in 23%, bronchospasm in 15%, and transient hypertension in 11%. Additional symptoms were cough, headache, and chest pain.

In this series (155), 40 patients, or 87%, experienced cardiac arrest and an additional 4 patients manifested a serious dysrhythmia without frank arrest. The time interval between onset of symptoms and cardiac arrest varied from less than 1 minute to 18 hours. In 15 of the 40 patients, cardiac arrest occurred within 5 minutes from symptom onset. In this series, 28 women died, for an overall maternal mortality rate of 61%. Death occurred from 30 minutes to 2 months after the initial event. Only

7% of the 46 patients survived neurologically intact. Twelve patients with cardiac arrest were successfully resuscitated and survived; however, only 3 of the 40, or 8%, with cardiac arrest survived neurologically intact. In this series, 28 patients had AFE while the fetus was alive in utero. Of these, 22 fetuses survived (79%); however, only 11 (50%) were neurologically normal. Overall, neurologically intact survival was 39%.

Analysis of Clark's data revealed no demographic maternal risk factors predisposing to AFE. Age, race, parity, obstetric history, weight gain, and blood pressure were no different from those expected in the general obstetric population (155). The data suggested that previous descriptions of AFE occurring after long hard labors were not valid. They also observed no relation between oxytocin or antecedent hyperstimulation and amniotic embolism. In this series, 5 of 40 patients exhibited a striking temporal relationship between artificial rupture of membranes or placement of an intrauterine pressure catheter and acute cardiovascular collapse. This observation suggests that simple exposure of the maternal circulatory system to even small amounts of amniotic fluid contents may, under the right circumstances, initiate AFE syndrome (155).

Clark (155) reported a remarkable similarity of the clinical course in hemodynamic and laboratory findings between women with AFE syndrome and patients with anaphylactic or septic shock. These similarities suggest similar pathophysiologic mechanisms. In both septic and anaphylactic shock, entrance into the circulation of foreign substance, bacterial endotoxin, or specific antigens directly or indirectly result in a release of various primary and secondary indigenous mediators (156–158). It is the release of these mediators that results in the physiologic derangement characterized in these syndromes, including profound myocardial depression and decreased cardiac output, described in experimental animals and man; pulmonary hypotension demonstrated in lower primate models of anaphylaxis and disseminated intravascular coagulation also described in human anaphylactic reactions and septic shock (155). These same clinical and hemodynamic derangements are virtually identical to those seen in AFE (155).

Treatment of AFE revolves around three goals: oxygenating the patient, maintaining cardiac output and blood pressure, and combating what is usually a self-limited but severe coagulopathy (30). When sudden intrapartum hypotension and dyspnea suggest AFE, the following steps should be taken: Administer oxygen, intubate, and ventilate. Hypotension is usually on the basis of cardiogenic shock and treatment involves initial optimization of cardiac preload by rapid crystalloid administration. This should be followed by pressor administration such as dopamine or dobutamine if the patient remains hypotensive. A pulmonary artery catheter should be inserted to guide further hemodynamic management and optimize fetal and maternal oxygen delivery. Fetal heart rate should be monitored carefully if the gestational age is sufficient to consider intervention for fetal distress. After resolution of hypotension, fluid should be restricted in order to minimize pulmonary edema secondary to developing ARDS. Component therapy should be administered to treat bleeding secondary to disseminated intravascular coagulation (DIC). Clark's (155) recent report confirms that even in patients who survive very few survive neurologically intact, thus stressing the need for optimization of oxygen delivery to the maternal vital organs during this devastating syndrome.

## THROMBOEMBOLIC DISEASE

Pulmonary embolism complicates between 0.09 and 0.7 per 1,000 pregnancies and is the leading cause of maternal mortality in the United States (159). Untreated pulmonary embolus during pregnancy carries a 12.8% mortality rate, while treatment lowers this to 0.7% (160). The majority of pulmonary emboli arise from thrombophlebitis of the deep femoral and pelvic veins. The reported incidence of deep venous thrombosis during pregnancy is 0.4 per 1,000 (159).

The increased frequency of thromboembolic disease associated with pregnancy has been attributed to an increase in clotting factors VII, VIII, and X as well as increased fibrinogen level and decreased fibrinolytic activity (160). Depression in antithrombin III activity may also have a role, as evidenced by data on estrogen therapy (161). In addition, venostasis caused by uterine pressure on the inferior vena cava may also be a contributing factor. Several factors further increase the risk of thromboembolic disease during pregnancy and the puerperium (162). These risk factors include cesarean delivery, which has a ten times greater risk of fatal pulmonary embolism, when compared to vaginal delivery, increased maternal age, multiparity, obesity, prolonged bed rest, and surgical procedures during pregnancy and the early postpartum period.

Respiratory failure in pulmonary embolism may be caused by extensive occlusion of the pulmonary vasculature or by concomitant pulmonary edema. Pulmonary edema has been associated with pulmonary embolism in areas of intact blood flow (163, 164). It has been attributed to increased hydrostatic pressure in nonoccluded vessels, to vigorous crystalloid resuscitation, and to increased microvascular permeability caused by platelet-derived mediators (165). Hemodynamic findings in patients with cardiovascular compromise caused by massive pulmonary emboli include normal to low pulmonary capillary wedge pressure, moderate elevation of mean pulmonary artery pressure, and moderate elevation of right atrial pressure (166). Pulmonary vascular resistance is usually elevated, and pulmonary hypertension develops when approximately 40% to 60% of the pulmonary circuit is acutely obstructed by pulmonary emboli. When mean pulmonary artery pressures increase greater than 35 to 45 mm of Hg, RV failure ensues with consequent decreases in RV ejection fraction and cardiac index as well as an increase in right atrial pressure.

The evaluation of patients with suspected pulmonary embolism without hemodynamic compromise is usually accomplished with tests, such as impedance plethysmography, venography, and perfusion lung scanning. However, in patients with massive pulmonary embolism, pulmonary angiography frequently becomes the diagnostic procedure of choice in order to document the presence of pulmonary embolism and the extent of obstruction.

The major goals of therapy for massive pulmonary embolism are to provide adequate oxygenation, treat hypotension and organ hypoperfusion, and interrupt clot propagation by immediate anticoagulation with intravenous heparin (167). In patients without detectable blood pressure or pulse, closed-chest compression may break up large proximal pulmonary emboli, improve pulmonary perfusion, reduce RV afterload, and possibly restore adequate circulation (166). In patients with massive and submassive pulmonary emboli with no contraindications to anticoagulation, heparin is the initial drug of choice. Large studies have failed to document that thrombolytic therapy results in any significant improvement in mortality or morbidity, compared with heparinization (168). In patients with massive pulmonary embolism and significant hemodynamic compromise, despite vasopressor therapy, thrombolytic therapy is an appropriate consideration as an alternative to pulmonary endarterectomy (167). The problem that is encountered with thrombolytic therapy is that if it is unsuccessful in achieving clot lysis, subsequent endarterectomy may be impossible because of the lytic state.

Pregnancy and the immediate postpartum state are relative contraindications to thrombolytic therapy because of the risk of hemorrhage during labor, delivery, and the first several days postpartum (169). However, streptokinase has been used successfully in pregnant patients with deep venous thrombosis and pulmonary embolism (170, 171). Animal studies have suggested that minimal amounts of streptokinase, if any, cross the placenta. Thrombolytic therapy during pregnancy should be limited to the duration of therapy needed for restoration of acceptable hemodynamic function. Therapy should be discontinued at least 4 to 6 hours prior to delivery, and if a patient delivers after recent thrombolytic therapy, careful observation for uterine bleeding is necessary. Cryoprecipitate or aprotinin can be used when rapid reversal of the lytic state is needed prior to delivery (167). Administration of heparin should follow thrombolysis in all patients. Heparin therapy should be delayed until the activated thromboplastin time is less than two times the normal value.

Low molecular weight heparin (LMWH), a fraction with high bioavailability and a relatively long half-life, is produced by the enzymatic or chemical breakdown of the unfractionated heparin molecule. The use of daily LMWH is at least as effective as the traditionally prescribed unfractionated heparin in preventing thromboembolic events with fewer side effects and complications (172). Low molecular weight heparin has been used during pregnancy (173). The LMWH does not cross the placenta and has not been associated with fetal or maternal morbidity. This preparation may be the anticoagulant preparation of choice for pregnant patients who cannot be treated with unfractionated heparin because of heparin-induced thrombocytopenia. In addition, the once daily dosing of LMWH may make women more comfortable with therapy and, therefore, more compliant.

Inferior vena caval interruption should be strongly considered in any patient with cardiopulmonary compromise caused by pulmonary embolism who does not receive thrombolytic therapy and in patients who have a contraindication to heparin or have recurrent emboli despite heparin anticoagulation. The best method now available for treatment of recurrent emboli unresponsive to heparin is transvenous placement of a Greenfield vena cava filter (174). This filter can be placed during pregnancy if indicated.

## BETA-AGONIST THERAPY AND PULMONARY EDEMA

Beta-agonist therapy is instituted in order to prevent preterm delivery of the fetus. Beta-agonist tocolytic therapy is contraindicated in gravidas with known heart disease but may unmask unsuspected cardiac abnormalities in the normally asymptomatic patient. The cardiologist may also be called on to assist in the management of the patient who develops arrhythmias or pulmonary edema in response to beta-agonist tocolysis.

Pulmonary edema is the most frequently reported life-threatening complication of beta-agonist therapy and has occurred in 3% to 9% of women reported in some studies (175–178). Pulmonary edema has occurred during the antepartum, intrapartum, and postpartum periods, and its onset has also been noted to occur several hours after therapy has been discontinued (179). Pulmonary edema was a key clinical presentation in 11 of the 14 maternal deaths that have been reported in conjunction with beta-agonist tocolytic therapy (30).

Several possible mechanisms to explain beta-adrenergic tocolytic induced pulmonary edema have been proposed. These include fluid overload, myocardial toxicity, reduced colloid osmotic pressure, and increased pulmonary capillary permeability (30). Fluid overload is suggested, by the known increased release of antidiuretic hormone, which occurs 30 minutes after initiation of intravenous

betamimetic therapy (180, 181). This observation is additionally supported by the clinical evidence of a decrease in hematocrit, consistent with an increase in plasma volume shortly after administration of betamimetic therapy (30). The antidiuretic hormone (ADH) effect of beta-adrenergic therapy may also be accentuated by the large volumes of crystalloids that are often given during tocolysis.

The possibility of direct myocardial toxicity has not been supported by any pathologic correlation in patients receiving beta-adrenergic tocolytic therapy. Heart failure can occur solely on the basis of tachycardia, resulting in decreased diastolic filling and systolic ejection times. Titrating betamimetics to the heart rate, with the goal of limiting maternal tachycardia to 140 beats/min or less, has served as an excellent safeguard to prevent this mechanism of heart failure (30). Supraventricular tachycardia in conjunction with the use of betamimetic therapy and the subsequent treatment of tachycardia appears to have been etiologic in the development of pulmonary edema in one woman. In addition, rate-related myocardial ischemia occurred in three women who developed pulmonary edema, and cardiac valvular lesions were found in two women who developed pulmonary edema (176, 182).

There is no evidence that use of betamimetic therapy alone has resulted in an increase in pulmonary capillary membrane permeability (183–185). Clinically apparent infections, including pneumonias, urinary tract infection, gram-negative sepsis, chorioamnionitis, and peritonitis, have been identified in 29% of women who developed pulmonary edema in conjunction with beta-agonist therapy for premature labor (30). Infection is the leading cause of lung injury. The injury is, in a large part, due to increased pulmonary capillary permeability. Additionally, most cases of pulmonary edema have occurred in the setting of prolonged tocolysis for refractory preterm labor; a scenario that has been shown to represent silent chorioamnionitis in many instances (186–191). It is reasonable to hypothesize that seeding of the maternal blood stream with either bacteria or their by-products may result in small alterations in the permeability of these women's lungs.

Irrespective of the mechanism of pulmonary edema, initial therapy should consist of oxygen, furosemide, and discontinuation of the beta-agonist (30). The patient's clinical status can be monitored with arterial blood gas determination and arterial oxygen saturation monitoring with pulse oximetry. If the patient's clinical condition improves, no further therapy is necessary. If the patient's clinical condition does not improve or deteriorates, invasive hemodynamic monitoring should be instituted and used to guide further therapy. Pulmonary edema with betamimetic therapy can be avoided by avoiding the use of betamimetic therapy in cases where patients have active infection, avoiding volume overload by strict attention to intake and output status.

## TRAUMA IN PREGNANCY

Continuous electronic FHR monitoring should be initiated early in the course of the evaluation of the pregnant trauma patient. Late decelerations indicating uteroplacental insufficiency may be observed in a hypovolemic trauma patient. This may be relieved by volume replacement with blood or crystalloids and oxygen therapy. Uterine perfusion may also be augmented by left lateral uterine displacement with a resultant increase in venous return and cardiac output. Care should be taken not to intervene on behalf of the fetus in an unstable mother, as such intervention may lead to death of both mother and fetus. However, if fetal distress is evident in a viable fetus and hemodynamically stable mother, cesarean delivery may be appropriate. All efforts should be made to manage the situation conservatively with volume resuscitation, oxygen administration, and left lateral uterine displacement before proceeding to delivery.

One of the greatest clinical concerns in a trauma patient is abruptio placenta. Placental abruptio has been reported in 5.9% of patients involved in severe automobile collisions (192). Consequently in the patient with serious abdominal trauma, the clinician should undertake an evaluation for abruptio. The patient should be observed for abdominal or uterine tenderness, preterm labor, or vaginal bleeding. The trauma patient should have an ultrasound examination for gestational age, placental location, and viability. Ultrasound can never exclude placental abruptio. Additionally, serial evaluation of the coagulation profile is important in the management of patients who are being observed for placental abruptio. Evidence of fetal distress on FHR monitoring, heavy vaginal bleeding, and coagulopathy are indications for delivery.

Another consideration in the patient who has had abdominal trauma and is being observed for abruptio placenta is the potential for fetal/maternal hemorrhage. This can lead to fetal anemia distress and death. In addition, the Rh-negative patient may develop sensitization secondary to fetal/maternal hemorrhage and hemolytic disease of a surviving or subsequent fetus. When a severely anemic fetus is delivered following maternal trauma, a positive maternal Kleihauer-Betke test may be noted. In one prospective series, 28% of patients had evidence of fetal/maternal hemorrhage (193). A Kleihauer-Betke test should therefore be considered in all pregnant trauma patients. A positive test should be an indication for prolonged FHR monitoring. The Rh-negative patient should be treated with hyperimmune anti-D globulin (194, 195).

The duration of fetal monitoring that is necessary after blunt trauma remains controversial. Earlier reviews suggested continuous fetal monitoring for longer than 24 hours; however, recent studies support a shorter observation period, provided that the patient does not have significant uterine activity or tenderness, vaginal bleeding, an abnormal FHR tracing, or a positive Kleihauer-Betke test (194, 195).

In late pregnancy, the enlarged gravid uterus is the intraperitoneal organ most likely to be injured by penetrating wounds (196). Gunshot wounds and stabbings are the most common injuries sustained (197). All gunshot wounds to the abdomen mandate exploration. Bushbaum (198) reported a 19% incidence of injury to organs other than the uterus. When the uterus was identified, the incidence of fetal injury varied from 59% to 89%, and fetal mortality rates ranged from 41% to 71% (198). Injuries involving umbilical cord, placenta, or membranes can also contribute to fetal morbidity and mortality. With uterine injury at or near term, cesarean delivery is often indicated. However, if the fetus is less than 28 weeks gestation, repair of the uterine injury and close monitoring of the fetal condition may be more beneficial than delivery for the fetus. When the enlarged uterus interferes with affective surgical repair of other maternal injuries, cesarean delivery may be necessary.

Stab wounds are the second most frequent penetrating abdominal wounds. Mortality is generally lower with stab wounds than gunshot wounds. The extent of intraabdominal injury is less, because bowel may slide away from the knife. However, stab wounds to the upper abdomen are more likely to injure bowel because the enlarge uterus has crowded the intestine together and cephalad (30). Controversy exists as to whether all stab wounds need exploration; however, exploration is indicated when the extent of injury is in question.

In summary, the fetus may sustain considerable injury or be threatened by maternal injury or blood loss when maternal trauma is sustained. The goal of the management team is to maintain a healthy mother and fetus. However, there are times in which the intervention on behalf of a fetus in a hemodynamically unstable mother may be inappropriate. Every attempt should be made to stabilize the mother, as this alone may affect rescue of the fetus.

## CARDIAC ARREST DURING PREGNANCY

We have already discussed the hemodynamic and cardiovascular alterations that occur during gestation. These changes render the pregnant woman more susceptible and less tolerant of major cardiovascular and respiratory insults. Precipitating events for cardiac arrest during pregnancy include many of the clinical situations discussed in this chapter, such as pulmonary embolism and AFE, trauma, peripartum hemorrhage, congenital and acquired cardiac disease, and complications of tocolytic therapy. When cardiac arrest occurs during gestation, standard resuscitative measures and procedures should be taken without modification (199). If ventricular fibrillation is present, it should be treated with defibrillation according to the ventricular fibrillation algorithm.

Closed-chest compressions and supportive ventilation should be done in accord with the usual protocol. In order to minimize the effects of the gravid uterus on venous return and cardiac output, a wedge, such as a pillow, should be placed under the right abdominal flank and hip to displace the uterus to the left side of the abdomen (200). One practical proposal is for a second rescuer to form a human wedge to help relieve aortocaval compression (201). In this maneuver, the back of the victim is rolled onto the thighs of a kneeling second rescuer who can then stabilize the shoulder and pelvis of the victim. Alternatively, continuous manual displacement to the left may be used or a Cardif resuscitation wedge which tilts the patient such that the uterus is displaced to the left side may be utilized (200).

Standard pharmacologic therapy should be used without modifications. Specifically, vasopressors such as epinephrine, norepinephrine, and dopamine should not be withheld when clinically indicated (199). Although a large clinical experience with the pharmacologic agents used in advanced cardiac life support is lacking in pregnancy, theoretical problems exist. The volume of distribution and drug metabolism may vary from nonpregnant norms, and if standard doses do not produce the predicted response, one should not hesitate to give higher doses to account for the expanded plasma volume of pregnancy. Vasopressors may reduce uteroplacental perfusion; lidocaine in high doses may lead to fetal acidosis; and beta-blockers may induce fetal bradycardia (202, 203). Nevertheless, at therapeutic maternal levels no adverse fetal affects have been shown, and the agents used in advanced cardiac life support are recommended in standard doses during pregnancy (30).

Cardiopulmonary resuscitation (CPR) during pregnancy may impose complications on both mother and fetus (30). Maternal injuries may include fractures of the ribs and sternum, hemothorax, and hemopericardium; rupture of internal organs, specifically spleen and uterus; and laceration or organs, notably the liver. Potential damaging effects on the fetus include central nervous system toxicity from medications, altered uterine activity, and reduced uteroplacental perfusion with possible fetal hypoxemia and acidemia.

Perimortem cesarean section should be considered early when efforts at cardiopulmonary resuscitation are unsuccessful.

## Postmortem Cesarean Delivery

When unanticipated or sudden death is encountered in a pregnant patient, the timing of cesarean delivery is a critical issue. It has been suggested that cesarean delivery should be begun within 4 minutes, and the baby delivered within 5 minutes of maternal cardiac arrest to optimize maternal and fetal outcome (204). Delivery within that time frame permits restoration of maternal cardiac output and the greatest possibility of maternal and fetal survival. Care must be taken to continue maternal CPR, not only until birth of the fetus, but also after the delivery. On occasion, a woman has been resuscitated and has lived postcesarean (30). Fetal survival is linked closely to the interval between maternal cardiac arrest and delivery of the fetus. Although the probability of a surviving normal infant diminishes the longer the time interval from maternal death to delivery of the fetus, the potential still exists for a favorable fetal outcome at more than 20 minutes from maternal cardiac arrest. The gestational age of the fetus is an important consideration, as the probability of fetal survival is directly related to the neonatal birth weight or gestation age (205). As a general rule, intervention is prudent whenever the fetus is potentially viable or capable of existence outside the mother's womb (206). Criteria for intervention need to be established for each institution with the aid of current neonatal survival statistics and guidance from the Bioethic Committee.

In summary, the suggested approach to a perimortem event during pregnancy includes the following principles (207):

1. Attempts at delivery of a gestationally viable fetus should begin within 4 minutes after maternal cardiac arrest.
2. Cardiopulmonary resuscitation should be continued during and after the procedure in cases in which the potential for maternal survival exists.
3. Time should not be wasted preparing a sterile field.
4. Because there have been isolated reports of infant survival well beyond the 4- to 6-minute time limit, attempts at delivery usually should be undertaken at any time after maternal death if signs of fetal life are present.
5. Cesarean delivery associated with significant blood loss may further compromise maternal stability unless blood volume is replaced.
6. Cesarean section should not be performed in an unstable patient because of anticipated cardiac arrest.
7. If a patient undergoes successful CPR before an attempt is made to deliver the infant, this operative procedure should not be performed because successful in utero resuscitation is likely.

## FETAL SURVIVAL AFTER MATERNAL BRAIN DEATH

The sophistication of current artificial life support systems has made possible successful prolongation of gestation in women who have sustained massive brain injury or brain death. One report describes maternal support in the intensive care for 107 days after the diagnosis of brain death and delivery of a normal 1,550-gram male infant at 32 weeks gestation by repeat cesarean section (208).

Other pregnancies have been maintained for 1, 9, and 10 weeks (209, 210).

The goal of management of the brain-dead patient is to maintain maternal somatic survival until fetal viability is documented. To achieve this goal, a number of maternal and fetal considerations are essential. Maternal medical considerations involve the regulation of most, if not all, maternal bodily functions (210). A loss of the pneumotactic center in the pons that is responsible for cyclic respirations and the medullary center responsible for spontaneous respirations make mechanical ventilation mandatory. Ventilation is similar to the nonpregnant patient; however, maternal partial pressure of carbon dioxide should be kept between 28 and 32 mm Hg, and the partial pressure of oxygen greater than 60 mm Hg, in order to avoid deleterious effects on uteroplacental perfusion (30). If the adult respiratory distress syndrome develops, the use of positive end-expiratory pressure (PEEP) may become necessary.

Cases of brain death reported in the literature thus far consistently show a constellation of clinical problems which include pituitary insufficiency, glucose intolerance, thermovariability, and cardiovascular instability (208–210). In addition, infectious complications and thromboembolic phenomena are potential complications.

Maternal hypotension occurs frequently and is believed to be due to a combination of factors such as hypothermia, myocardial hypoxia, and panhypopituitarism. Maintenance of maternal pressure can be achieved with an infusion of low-dose dopamine and careful central hemodynamic monitoring. When panhypopituitarism occurs, the results may be a variety of hypoendocrinopathies such as diabetes insipidus, adrenal insufficiency, and hypothyroidism. Treatment of these conditions will require the use of vasopressin, corticosteroids, and thyroid replacement therapy as indicated.

When maternal brain death occurs, the thermoregulatory center located in the hypothalamus no longer functions, and hypothermia develops. Maintenance of normal maternal temperature can usually be accomplished with the use of warming blankets and the administration of warm humidified air. If maternal pyrexia develops, this suggests an infectious process and the need for the usual investigation for an infectious source. If maternal temperature remains elevated, cooling blankets and acetaminophen are indicated to avoid the deleterious effect of hyperthermia on the fetus (30).

Maternal nutritional support is necessary for maternal maintenance and also for fetal growth and development. Gastric motility is generally poor in the brain-dead patient, and therefore parenteral hyperalimentation is the preferred form of nutrition support (210). However, in one case report a patient received enteral nutrition throughout her course (208). The amount of alimentation should be in keeping with the caloric requirements of pregnancy and may need to be increase when infection or the adult respiratory distress syndrome exists.

Pregnancy is a hypercoagulable state, and bran-dead gravidas are immobile and therefore at increased risk of thromboembolism. To minimize the risk for a deep-vein thrombosis or pulmonary embolus, prophylactic heparin should be used.

The obstetric management should include frequent monitoring of fetal growth with serial ultrasounds and assessment of fetal well-being with nonstress testing and biophysical profile scoring as indicated. Corticosteroids can be administered to enhance fetal lung maturation (210). This therapy should be started at approximately 25 weeks gestational age and continued weekly until fetal lung maturity has been documented or delivery of the fetus has been accomplished.

The timing of delivery is based on either the deterioration of maternal or fetal status or the presence of fetal lung maturity. A team should be prepared to deliver the fetus at any time that evidence of maternal or fetal deterioration presents. To that end, a cesarean delivery pack and neonatal resuscitation equipment should be available at the bedside. Classical cesarean section is the preferred method of delivery and is the least traumatic procedure to the fetus (30).

When establishing a management plan for the pregnant woman with brain death, the moral and ethical issues revolving around the maintenance of pregnancy after death must be considered (211–214). Reviews of the ethics of this subject strongly support the role of the family in planning the care of the brain-dead patient and that the physician should not be required to provide all available care against the wishes of the family. The wishes of the next of kin, the physician, and the patient, if they were expressed before brain death, may hold different legal priorities state to state.

The legal responsibility for decision making is likely to hinge on the following unresolved issues and their interpretation by local courts. First, is the brain-dead mother legally alive or dead? If she is legally dead, does the maintenance of systemic integrative function for the benefit of the fetus fall under the auspices of the uniform anatomic gift act? Second, how does the state view interest of the fetus at a given point in gestation? Would it be legal at a given time in the pregnancy to discontinue maternal support and terminate the pregnancy? Does the fetus have interest that could outweigh the next of kin's decision to discontinue support? Third, how does the state view its own interests? In the absence of an identifiable next of kin or in the event of significant disagreement among the parties involved in the decision making, will the state maintain that it shares an interest in the well-being of the fetus? The answers to these questions are likely to vary among jurisdictions. Some of these questions have been explored in detail in papers reviewing the ethical issues pertinent to the management of the brain-dead patient (211–214). Another important issue when considering the maintenance of pregnancy beyond brain death is the issue of cost. In one report the hospital bills totaled over $100,000, the majority of which were paid by insurance. Maternal brain death in pregnancy is infrequent but does occur. The management of each individual case will have to be based upon the decisions made by family, physician, and the courts. With careful clinical management of these complicated patients, a favorable fetal outcome can be achieved.

In summary, we have described the normal cardiorespiratory changes in pregnancy and the potential effect of these changes on the cardiovascular status of patients with heart disease. In addition, we have reviewed several obstetric emergencies which might be encountered by the practicing cardiologist. It should be clear from these discussions that an interdisciplinary approach to the management of cardiac disease in pregnancy, which includes perinatologists, cardiologists, intensivists, and neonatalogists, should assure the best outcome for both mother and fetus.

## REFERENCES

1. Clap JF, Seaward BL, Sleamaker RH, Hiser J. Maternal physiologic adaptations to early human pregnancy. *Am J Obstet Gynecol* 1988;159:1456.
2. Scott DE. Anemia during pregnancy. *Obstet Gynecol Annu* 1972;1:219.
3. Warren JV, Elkin DC, Nicerson JL. The blood volume in patients with arteriovenous fistulas. *J Clin Invest* 1951;30:220.
4. Burwell CS. The influence of pregnancy on the course of heart disease. *South Med J* 1936;29:1194.
5. Watanabe M, Meoder C, Gray MJ, et al. Secretion rate of aldosterone in normal pregnancy. *J Clin Invest* 1963;43:1619.
6. Seitchik J. Total body water and total body density of pregnant women. *Obstet Gynecol* 1967;29:155.
7. Jepson JH. Endocrine control of maternal and fetal erythropoiesis. *Can Med Assoc J* 1968;98:844.
8. Wilson M, Morganti AA, Zervodakis I, et al. Blood pressure, The renin-aldosterone system and sex steroids throughout normal pregnancy. *Am J Med* 1980;68:97.
9. Katz R, Karliner JS, Resnik R. Effects of a natural volume overload state (pregnancy) on left ventricular performance in normal human subjects. *Circulation* 1978;58:434.
10. Phippard AF, Horvath JS, Glynn EM. Serial studies of hemodynamics, blood volume, renin and aldosterone in the baboon (Papio Hamadryas). *J Hypertens* 1986;4:773.
11. Sibai BM, Abdella TN, Anderson GD. Pregnancy outcome in 211 patients with mild chronic hypertension. *Obstet Gynecol* 1983;61:571.
12. Lin CC, Lindheimer MD, River P, Moawad AH. Fetal outcome in hypertensive disorders of pregnancy. *Am J Obstet Gynecol* 1982;142:255.
13. Hamilton HFH. The cardiac output in normal pregnancy as determined by the Cournard right heart catheterization technique. *J Obstet Gynecol Br Emp* 1949;56:548.
14. Laird-Meeter K, VandeLey G, Bom TH, et al. Cardio circulatory adjustments during pregnancy—an echo cardiographic study. *Clin Cardiol* 1979;2:328.
15. Robson SC, Hunter S, Boys RJ, Dunlop W. Serial study of factors influencing cardiac output during human pregnancy. *Am J Physiol* 1989;256:H1060.
16. Clark SL, Cotton DB, Lee W, et al. Central hemodynamic assessment of normal term pregnancy. *Am J Obstet Gynecol* 1989;161:1439.
17. Bader RA, Bader ME, Rose DJ, et al. Hemodynamics at rest and during exercise in normal pregnancy as studied by cardiac catheterization. *J Clin Invest* 1955;34:1524.
18. Walters WAW, Lim YL. Cardiovascular dynamics in women receiving oral contraceptive therapy. *Lancet* 1969;2:879.
19. Gerber JG, Payne NA, Murphy RC, Nios AS. Prostacycline produced by the pregnant uterus in the dog may act as a circulating vasodepressor substance. *J Clin Invest* 1981;67:632.
20. Burwell CS, Strayhorn WD, Flickinger D, et al. Circulation during pregnancy. *Arch Intern Med* 1938;62:979.
21. Vorys N, Ullery Jc, Hanusek GE. The cardiac output changes in various positions in pregnancy. *Am J Obstet Gynecol* 1961;82:1312.
22. Ueland K, Novy MJ, Peterson EN, Metcalfe J. Maternal cardiovascular dynamics. IV, The influence of gestational age on the maternal cardiovascular response to posture and exercise. *Am J Obstet Gynecol* 1969;104:856.
23. Bader RA, Bader ME, Rose DJ, et al. Hemodynamics at rest and during exercise in normal pregnancy as studied by cardiac catheterization. *Eur J Clin Invest* 1955;34:1524.
24. Clark SL, Cotton DB, Lee W, et al. Central hemodynamic assessment of normal third trimester pregnancy. *Am J Obstet Gynecol* 1989;161:1439.
25. Barron W, Lindheimer M. *Medical disorders during pregnancy.* 1st ed. St Louis: Mosby-Year Book; 1991:234.
26. Pernoll ML, Metcalf J, Schlenker TL, et al. Oxygen consumption at rest and during exercise in pregnancy. *Respir Physiol,* 1975;25:285.
27. Gemzell CA, Robbe H, Strom G, et al. Observations on circulatory changes and muscular work in normal labor. *Acta Obstet Gynecol Scand* 1957;36:75.
28. Ueland K, Hansen JM. Maternal cardiovascular hemodynamics. II. Posture and uterine contractions. *Am J Obstet Gynecol* 1969;103:1.
29. Shibutani K, Komatsu T, Kubal K, et al. Critical level of oxygen delivery in anesthetized man. *Crit Care Med* 1983;11:640.
30. Clark SL, Cotton DB, Hankins GDV, Phelan JP. *Critical care obstetrics.* 2nd ed. Blackwell Scientific Publications 1991.
31. Battaglia FC, Meschia G. *An introduction to fetal physiology.* New York: Academic; 1986.
32. Wilkening RB, Meschia G. Fetal oxygen uptake oxygenation, acid base balance as a function of uterine blood flow. *Am J Physiol* 1983;244:749.
33. Sheldon RE, Peters LH, Jones M, Makowski EL, Meschia G. Redistribution of cardiac output and oxygen delivery in the hypoxemic fetal lamb. *Am J Obstet Gynecol* 1979;135:1071.
34. Peeters LH, Sheldon RE, Jones MD, Makowski EL, Meschia G. Blood flow to fetal organs as a function of arterial oxygen content. *Am J Obstet Gynecol* 1979;135:637.
35. Meschia G. Transfer of oxygen across the placenta. In: Gluck L, ed. *Intrauterine asphyxia and the fetal brain.* Chicago, IL: Yearbook Medical Publishers; 1977.
36. Adams JQ, Alexander AM. Alterations in cardiovascular physiology during labor. *Obstet Gynecol* 1958;12:542.
37. Hendricks CH, Quilligan EF. Cardiac output during labor. *Am J Obstet Gynecol* 1958;76:969.
38. Kjeldsen J. Hemodynamic investigations during labor and delivery. *Acta Obstet Gynecol Scand* 1979;89(Suppl):1.
39. Ueland K, Hansen JM. Maternal cardiovascular hemodynamics. III. Labor and delivery under local and caudal anesthesia. *Am J Obstet Gynecol* 1969;103:8.
40. Ueland K, Metcalfe J. Circulatory changes in pregnancy. *Clin Obstet Gynecol* 1975;18:41.
41. Robson SC, Dunlop W, Boys RJ, Hunter S. Cardiac output during labor. *Br Med J* 1987;295:1169.
42. Lee W, Rokey R, Cotton DB, Mille JF. Maternal hemodynamic effects of uterine contractions by M-mode and pulsed-Doppler echocardiography. *Am J Obstet Gynecol* 1989;161:974.
43. Robson SC, Hunter S, Moore M, Dunlop W. Haemodynamic changes during the puerperium: a doppler and M-mode echocardiographic study. *Br J Obstet Gynaecol* 1987;94:1028.
44. Prowse CM, Gaenster EA. Respiratory and acid-base changes during pregnancy. *Anesthesiology* 1965;26:381.
45. Templeton A, Kelman GR. Maternal blood gases (PAO2-PaO2), physiologic shunt, and VD/VT in normal pregnancy. *Br J Anaesth* 1976;48:1000.
46. Skatrud JB, Dempsey JA, Kaiser DG. Ventilatory response to medroxyprogesterone acetate in normal subjects: time course and mechanism. *J Appl Physiol* 1978;44:393.
47. Awe RJ, Nicotra MB, Newsom TD, Viles R. Arterial oxygenation

and alveolar-arterial gradients in term pregnancy. *Obstet Gynecol* 1979;53:182.

48. Steinberg WM, Farine D. Maternal mortality in Ontario from 1970 to 1980. *Obstet Gynecol* 1985;66:510.

49. Szekely P, Turner R, Snaith L. Pregnancy and the changing pattern of rheumatic heart disease. *Br Heart J* 1973;35:1923.

50. The Criteria Committee of the New York Heart Association. *Nomenclature and criteria for diagnosis of diseases of the heart and great vessels.* ed 8. New York: New York Heart Association; 1979.

51. Szekely P, Turner R, Snaith L. Pregnancy and the changing pattern of rheumatic heart disease. *Br Heart J* 1973;35:1293.

52. Clark SL. Cardiac disease in pregnancy in obstetric emergencies. *Crit Care Clin* 1991;7(4):777.

53. Veran FX, Cibes-Hernandez JJ, Pelegrina I. Heart disease in pregnancy. *Obstet Gynecol* 1968;34:424.

54. Ellison CR, Sloss CJ. Electrocardiographic features of congenital heart disease in the adult. In: Roberts WC, ed. *Congenital heart disease in adults.* Philadelphia: FA Davis; 1979:119.

55. Hibbard LT. Maternal mortality due to cardiac disease. *Clin Obstet Gynecol* 1975;18:27.

56. Schaefer G, Arditi LI, Solomon HA, Ringland JE. Congenital heart disease and pregnancy. *Clin Obstet Gynecol* 1968;11:1048.

57. Szekely P, Julian DG. Heart disease and pregnancy. *Curr Probl Cardiol* 1979;4:1.

58. Shime J, Mocarski EJM, Hastings D, Webb GD, McLaughlin PR. Congenital heart disease in pregnancy: short- and long-term implications. *Am J Obstet Gynecol* 1987;156:313.

59. Stratton JR. Common causes of cardiac emboli—left ventricular thrombi and atrial fibrillation. *West J Med* 1989;151:172.

60. Goodwin JF. Pregnancy and coarctation of the aorta. *Clin Obstet Gynecol* 1961;4:645.

61. Deal K, Wooley CF. Coarctation of the aorta and pregnancy. *Ann Intern Med* 1973;78:706.

62. Pyeritz RE. Maternal and fetal complications of pregnancy in the Marfan syndrome. *Am J Med* 1984;71:784.

63. Chesley LC. Severe rheumatic cardiac disease and pregnancy: the ultimate prognosis. *Am J Obstet Gynecol* 1980;126:552.

64. Clark SL. How labor and delivery influence mitral stenosis. *Contemp OB-GYN* 1986;27:127.

65. Clark SL. Structural cardiac disease in pregnancy. In: Clark SL, Cotton DB, Hankins GD, Phelan JP, eds. *Critical care obstetrics.* 2nd ed. Cambridge, MA: Blackwell Scientific; 1991:115.

66. Clark SL, Phelan JP, Greenspoon J, Aldahl D, Horenstein J. Labor and delivery in the presence of mitral stenosis: central hemodynamic observations. *Am J Obstet Gynecol* 1985;152:984.

67. Larrea JL, Nunez L, Reque JA, et al. Pregnancy and mechanical valve prostheses: a high-risk situation for the mother and fetus. *Ann Thorac Surg* 1983;36:459.

68. Iung B, Cormier B, Elias J, et al. Usefulness of percutaneous balloon commissurotomy for mitral stenosis during pregnancy. *Am J Cardiol* 1994;73:398.

69. Ueland K, Akamatsu TJ, Eng M, Bonica JJ, Hansen JM. Maternal cardiovascular dynamics: VI: Cesarean section under epidural anesthesia without epinephrine. *Am J Obstet Gynecol* 1972;114:775.

70. Markiewicz W, Stoner J, London E, et al. Mitral valve prolapse in one hundred previously healthy young females. *Circulation* 1976;53:464.

71. Arias F, Pineda J. Aortic stenosis and pregnancy. *J Reprod Med* 1978;20:229.

72. Lao TT, Adelman AG, Sermer M, Colman JM. Balloon valvuloplasty for congenital aortic stenosis in pregnancy. *Br J Obstet Gynaecol* 1993;100:1141.

73. Clark SL. Labor and delivery in the patient with structural cardiac disease. *Clin Perinatol* 1986;13:695.

74. Easterling TR, Chadwick HS, Otto CM, Benedetti TJ. Aortic stenosis in pregnancy. *Obstet Gynecol* 1988;72:113.

75. Lao TT, Sermer M, MaGee L, Farine D, Colman JM. Congenital aortic stenosis and pregnancy—a reappraisal. *Am J Obstet Gynecol* 1993;169:540.

76. Whittmore R, Hobbins JC, Engle MA. Pregnancy and its outcome in women with and without surgical treatment of congenital heart disease. *Am J Cardiol* 1982;50:641.

77. Demakis JG, Rahimtoola SH, Sutton GC, et al. Natural course of peripartum cardiomyopathy. *Circulation* 1971;44:1053.

78. Cunningham FG, Pritchard JA, Hankins GDV, et al. Peripartum heart failure: idiopathic cardiomyopathy or compounding cardiovascular events. *Obstet Gynecol* 1986;67:157.

79. Veille JC. Peripartum cardiomyopathies: a review. *Am J Obstet Gynecol* 1984;148:805.

80. Melvin KR, Richardson PJ, Olsen EG, et al. Peripartum cardiomyopathy due to myocarditis. *N Engl J Med* 1982;307:731.

81. Huerta EM, Erice A, Espiro RF, et al. Postpartum cardiomyopathy and acute myocarditis. *Am Heart J* 1985;110:1079.

82. Sanderson JE, Olsen EG, Gatei D. Peripartum heart disease: an endomyocardial biopsy study. *Br Heart J* 1986;56:285.

83. Oakley DG, McGarry K, Limb DG, Oakley CM. Management of pregnancy in patients with hypertrophic cardiomyopathy. *Br Med J* 1979;1:1749.

84. Hankins GDV, Wendel GD, Leveno KJ, Stoneham J. Myocardial infarction during pregnancy: a review. *Obstet Gynecol* 1985;65:139.

85. Elkayam V, Gleicher N. Cardiac problems in pregnancy, I. Maternal aspects: the approach to the pregnant patient with heart disease. *JAMA* 1984;251:2838.

86. Elkayam V, Kawanishi D, Reid CL, Chandraratna PAN, Gleicher N, Rahimtoola SH. Contrast echocardiography to reduce ionizing radiation associated with cardiac catheterization during pregnancy. *Am J Cardiol* 1983;52:213.

87. Sheikh AU, Harper MA. Myocardial infarction during pregnancy: management and outcome of two pregnancies. *Am J Obstet Gynecol* 1993;169(2):279.

88. Frenkel Y, Barkai G, Reisin L, Rath S, Mashiach S, Battler A. Pregnancy after myocardial infection: are we playing safe? *Obstet Gynecol* 1991;77(6):822.

89. Bernal JM, Growdon JH. Cardiac surgery with cardiopulmonary bypass during pregnancy. *Am J Obstet Gynecol Surv* 1986;41:1.

90. Koh KS, Friesen RM, Livingstone RA, et al. Fetal monitoring during maternal cardiac surgery with cardiopulmonary bypass. *Can Med Assoc J* 1975;112:1102.

91. Werch A, Lamberg HM. Fetal monitoring and maternal open heart surgery. *South Med J* 1977;70:1024.

92. Camann W, Goldman G, Johnson M, et al. Cesarean delivery in a patient with a transplanted heart. *Anesthesiology* 1989;71:618.

93. Akin SJ. Pregnancy after heart transplantation [Review]. *Prog Cardiovasc Nurs* 1992;7(3):2.

94. Carvalho AC, Almeida D, Cohen M, et al. Successful pregnancy, delivery and puerperium in a heart transplant patient with previous peripartum cardiomyopathy. *Eur Heart J* 1992;13(11):1589.

95. Baxi LV, Rho RB. Pregnancy after cardiac transplantation. *Am J Obstet Gynecol* 1993;169(1):33.

96. Liljestrand J, Lindstrom B. Childbirth after postpartum cardiac insufficiency treated with cardiac transplant. *Acta Obstet Gynaecol Scand* 1993;72(5):406.

97. Oakley CM, Doherty P. Pregnancy in patients after heart valve replacement. *Br Heart J* 1976;38:1140.

98. Antunes MJ, Myer IG, Santos LP. Thrombosis of mitral valve prosthesis in pregnancy: management by simultaneous cesarean section and mitral valve replacement. Case report. *Br J Obstet Gynaecol* 1984;91:716.

99. Hawkins Ottman E, Gall SA. Myocardial infarction in the third trimester of pregnancy secondary to an aortic valve thrombus. *Obstet Gynecol* 1993;81(5):804.

100. Dalen E, Hirsh J (co-chairmen). American College of Chest Physicians and the National Heart, Lung, and Blood Institute National Conference on Antithrombotic Therapy. *Chest* 1986;89(Suppl 2):1S.

101. Ginsberg JS, Hirsch J. Anticoagulants during pregnancy. *Annu Rev Med* 1989;40:79.

102. Hirsh J, Levine MN. The optimal intensity of oral anticoagulant therapy. *JAMA* 1987;258:2723.

103. Hirsh J, Levine MN. Confusion over the therapeutic range for monitoring oral anticoagulant therapy in North America. Review article. *Thromb Haemost* 1988;59:129.

104. Biale Y, Cantor A, Lewenthal H, Gueron M. The course of pregnancy in patients treated with artificial heart valves treated with dipyridamole. *Int J Gynaecol Obstet* 1980;18:128.

105. Nunez L, Larrea JL, Aguado MG, Reque JA, Matorras R, Minguez JA. Pregnancy in 20 patients with bioprosthetic valve replacement. *Chest* 1983;84:26.

106. Deviri E, Levinsky L, Yechezkel M, Levy MJ. Pregnancy after valve

replacement with porcine xenograft prosthesis. *Surg Gynecol Obstet* 1985;160:437.

107. Oakley C. Valve prostheses and pregnancy [Editorial]. *Br Heart J* 1987;58:303.

108. Wang RYC, Lee PK, Chow JSF, Chen WWC. Efficacy of low-dose subcutaneously administered heparin in treatment of pregnant women with artificial heart valves. *Med J Aust* 1983;2:126.

109. Salazar E, Zajarias A, Gutierrez N, Iturbe I. The problem of cardiac valve prostheses, anticoagulants, and pregnancy. *Circulation* 1984;70 (Suppl I):I-169.

110. Baras VA, Schwartz PA, Greene MF, Phillippe M, Saltzman D, Frigoletto FD. Use of subcutaneous heparin during pregnancy. *J Reprod Med* 1985;30(12):899.

111. Durack DT, Phil D. Prevention of infective endocarditis. *N Engl J Med* 1995;332(1):38.

112. Seaworth BJ, Durack DT. Infective endocarditis in obstetric and gynecologic practice. *Am J Obstet Gynecol* 1986;154:180.

113. Shulman ST, Amren DP, Bisno AL, et al. Prevention of bacterial endocarditis: a statement for health professionals by the Committee on Rheumatic Fever and Infective Endocarditis of the Council on Cardiovascular Disease in the Young. *Circulation* 1984;70(6):1123A.

114. Jeresaty RM. Mitral valve prolapse: an update. *JAMA* 1985;254(6):793.

115. Cunningham FG, MacDonald PL, Gant NF, Leveno KG, Gilstrap III LC, eds. Hypertensive disorders in pregnancy. In: *Williams Obstetrics*. 19 ed. Norwalk, CT: Appleton-Century-Crofts; 1993:767.

116. *ACOG Technical Bulletin*. No. 91. Washington, DC: The American College of Obstetrics and Gynecology; 1986.

117. Sibai BM. Preeclampsia-eclampsia: maternal perinatal outcomes. *Contemp Obstet Gynaecol* 1979;19:203.

118. Long PA, Abell DA, Beischer NA. Parity and preeclampsia. *Aust NZ J Obstet Gynaecol* 1979;19:203.

119. Graham C, Goldstein A. Epidural analgesia and cardiac output in severe preeclamptics. *Anaesthesia* 1980;35:709.

120. Lopez-Llera M, Horta JLH. Perinatal mortality in preeclampsia. *J Reprod Med* 1972;8:281.

121. Creasy RK, Resnik R, eds. *Fetal heart rate in maternal fetal medicine. Principles and practice*. 3rd ed. Philadelphia, PA: WB Saunders; 1994;322.

122. Manning F, Baskett T, Morrison I, Lange I. Fetal biophysical profile scoring: a prospective study in 1,184 high-risk patients. *Am J Obstet Gynecol* 1981;140:289.

123. Clark SL, Cotton DB. Clinical indications for pulmonary artery catheterization in the patient with severe preeclampsia. *Am J Obstet Gynecol* 1988;158:453.

124. Benedetti TJ, Cotton DB, Read JC, et al. Hemodynamic observations in severe pre-eclampsia with a flow-directed pulmonary artery catheter. *Am J Obstet Gynecol* 1980;136:465.

125. Clark SL, Divon MY, Phelan JP. Preeclampsia/eclampsia: hemodynamic and neurologic correlations. *Obstet Gynecol* 1985;66:337.

126. Cotton DB, Gonik B, Dorman K, et al. Cardiovascular alterations in severe pregnancy induced hypertension: relationship of central venous pressure to pulmonary capillary wedge pressure. *Am J Obstet Gynecol* 1985;151:762.

127. Neutra R. Fetal death in eclampsia. I: Its relation to low gestational age, retarded fetal growth and low birthweight. *Br J Obstet Gynaecol* 1975;82:382.

128. Abdella TN, Sibai BM, Hays JM, et al. Relationship of hypertensive disease to abruptio placentae. *Obstet Gynecol* 1984;63:365.

129. Brazy JE, Grimm JK, Little VA. Neonatal manifestations of severe maternal hypertension occurring before the thirty-sixth week of pregnancy. *J Pediatr* 1982;100:165.

130. Sibai BM, Anderson GD, Abdella TN, et al. Eclampsia. III: Neonatal outcome, growth and development. *Am J Obstet Gynecol* 1983;146:307.

131. Paul RH, Koh KS, Bernstein SG. Changes in fetal heart rate: uterine contraction patterns associated with eclampsia. *Am J Obstet Gynecol* 1978;130:165.

132. Pritchard JA, Cunningham FG, Pritchard SA. The Parkland Memorial Hospital protocol for treatment of eclampsia: evaluation of 245 cases. *Am J Obstet Gynecol* 1984;148:951.

133. Barrett JM. Fetal resuscitation with terbutaline during eclampsia-induced uterine hypertonus. *Am J Obstet Gynecol* 1984;150:895.

134. Reece E, Chervenak F, Romero R, Hobbins J. Magnesium sulfate in the management of acute intrapartum fetal distress. *Am J Obstet Gynecol* 1984;148:104.

135. *ACOG Technical Bulletin*. Number 127. Assessment of fetal and newborn acid-base status. Washington, DC: The American College of Obstetrics and Gynecology; 1989.

136. Gilstrap LC, Hauth JC, Hankins GDV, et al. Secondstage fetal heart rate abnormalities and type of neonatal acidemia. *Obstet Gynecol* 1987;70(2):191.

137. Rochat RW, Koonin LM, Atrash HK, et al. Maternal mortality in the United States: report for the Maternal Mortality Collaborative. *Obstet Gynecol* 1988;72:91.

138. Pritchard JA. Changes in the blood volume during pregnancy and delivery. *Anesthesiology* 1965;26:393.

139. Sheehan HL, Murdoch R. Postpartum necrosis of the anterior pituitary: pathological and clinical aspects. *Br J Obstet Gynaecol* 1938;45:456.

140. Smith K, Browne JCM, Shackman R, et al. Renal failure of obstetric origin. *Br Med Bull* 1968;24:49.

141. Kirshon B, Hinkley CM, Cotton DB, Miller J. Maternal mortality in a maternal-fetal medicine intensive care unit. *J Reprod Med* 1990;35 (1):25.

142. Clark SL, ed. Amniotic fluid embolism. *Clin Perinatol* 1986;13:801.

143. Reis RL, Pierce WS, Behrendt DM. Hemodynamic effects of amniotic fluid embolism. *Surg Obstet Gynecol* 1965;129:45.

144. Attwood HD, Downing SE. Experimental amniotic fluid embolism. *Surg Gynecol Obstet* 1965;120:255.

145. Clark SL, Montz FJ, Phelan JP. Hemodynamic alterations associated with amniotic fluid embolism: a reappraisal. *Am J Obstet Gynecol* 1985;151:617.

146. Clark SL, Cotton DB, Gonik B, et al. Central hemodynamic alterations in amniotic fluid embosism. *Am J Obstet Gynecol* 1988;158:1124.

147. Dolynuik M, Orfei E, Vania H, et al. Rapid diagnosis of amniotic fluid embolism. *Obstet Gynecol* 1983;61:28(S).

148. Duff P, Engelsjerd B, Zingery LW, et al. Hemodynamic observations in a patient with intrapartum amniotic fluid embolism. *Am J Obstet Gynecol* 1983;146:112.

149. Girard P, Mal H, Laine JF, et al. Left heart failure in amniotic fluid embolism. *Anesthesiology* 1986;64:262.

150. Masson RG, Ruggeiri J, Siggiqui MM. Amniotic fluid embolism: definitive diagnosis in a survivor. *Am Rev Respir Dis* 1979;120:187.

151. Moore PG, James OF, Saltos N. Severe amniotic fluid embolism: case report with hemodynamic findings. *Anaesth Intens Care* 1982;10:40.

152. Schaerf RH, de Campo T, Civetta JM. Hemodynamic alterations and rapid diagnosis in a case of amniotic fluid embolus. *Anesthesiology* 1977;46:155.

153. Richards DS, Carter LS, Corke B, et al. The effect of human amniotic fluid on the isolated perfused rat heart. *Am J Obstet Gynecol* 1988;158:210.

154. Courtney LD. Amniotic fluid embolism. *Obstet Gynecol Surv* 1974;29:169.

155. Clark SL, Hankins GDV, Dudley DA, Dildy GA, Porter TF. Amniotic fluid embolism: analysis of the national registry. *Am J Obstet Gynecol* 1995;172(4):1158.

156. Raper RF, Fisher MM. Profound reversible myocardial depression after anaphylaxis. *Lancet* 1988;1:386.

157. Parrillo JE. Pathogenic mechanisms of septic shock. *N Engl J Med* 1993;328:1471.

158. Enjeti S, Bleecker ER, Smith PL, Rabson J, Permutt S, Traystman RJ. Hemodynamic mechanisms in anaphylaxis. *Circ Shock* 1983;11:297.

159. Aaro LA, Jzergans JL. Thrombophlebitis associated with pregnancy. *Am J Obstet Gynecol* 1971;109:1128.

160. Villa Santa U. Thromboembolic disease in pregnancy. *Am J Obstet Gynecol* 1965;93:142.

161. Benotti JR, Pratter MR, Dalen JE. Pulmonary embolism. *Curr Pulmonol* 1984;6:91.

162. Bonnar J. Venous thromboembolism and pregnancy. *Clin Obstet Gynecol* 1981;8:455.

163. Hyers TM, Fowler AA, Wicks AB. Focal pulmonary edema after massive pulmonary embolism. *Am Rev Respir Dis* 1981;123:232.

164. Meth RF, Tashkin DP, Hansen KS, et al. Pulmonary edema and wheezing after pulmonary embolism. *Am Rev Respir Dis* 1975;111:693.

165. Staub NC. Pulmonary edema due to increased microvascular permeability to fluid and protein. *Circ Res* 1978;43:143.

166. Benotti JR, Dalen JE. Pulmonary embolism. In: Rippe JM, Irwin RS, Alpert JS, Dalen JE, eds. *Intensive care medicine.* Boston: Little, Brown; 1985:226.

167. Hollingsworth HM, Pratter MR, Irwin RS. Acute respiratory failure in pregnancy. *J Intens Care Med* 1989;4:11.

168. Urokinase—streptokinase pulmonary embolism trials: Phase 2 results. A cooperative study. *JAMA* 1974;229:1606.

169. Moran KT, Jewell ER, Persson AV. The role of thrombolytic therapy in surgical practice. *Br J Surg* 1989;76:298.

170. Dekloss GL, Davilla F. Thrombolytic therapy for pulmonary embolism in pregnancy. *Am J Obstet Gynecol* 1986;155:375.

171. Ludwig H. Results of streptokinase therapy in deep venous thrombosis during pregnancy. *Postgrad Med J* 1973;8:65.

172. Leyvraz PF, Bachman F, Hoek J, et al. Prevention of deep vein thrombosis after hip replacement: randomized comparison between unfractionated heparin and low-molecular-weight heparin. *BMJ* 1991;303:543.

173. Fejgin MD, Lourwood DL. Low molecular weight haparins and their use in obstetrics and gynecology [Review]. *Obstet Gynecol Surv* 1994;49(6):424.

174. Hux CH, Wapner RJ, Chayen B, et al. Use of the Greeenfield filter for thromboembolic disease in pregnancy. *Am J Obstet Gynecol* 1986; 155:734.

175. Robertson PA, Herron M, Katz, M, Creasy RK. Maternal morbidity associated with isoxsuprine and terbutaline tocolysis. *Eur J Obstet Gynecol Reprod Biol* 1981;11:371.

176. Katz M, Robertson PA, Creasy RK. Cardiovascular complications associated with terbutaline treatment for preterm labor. *Am J Obstet Gynecol* 1981;139:605.

177. Hatjis CG, Swain M. Systemic tocolysis for premature labor is associated with an increased incidence of pulmonary edema in the presence of maternal infection. *Am J Obstet Gynecol* 1988;159:723.

178. Watson P, Shapiro K, Fure J, Lees E. Betamimetic-associated pulmonary edema: time and dose relationships. Society of Perinatal Obstetricians, Fifth Annual Meeting, Las Vegas, Nevada, February 1985.

179. Bloss JD, Hankins GDV, Gilstrap LC, Hauth JC. Pulmonary edema as a delayed complication of ritodrine therapy. A case report. *J Reprod Med* 1987;32:469.

180. Schrier RW, Lieberman R, Ufferman RC. Mechanism of antidiuretic effect of beta adrenergic stimulation. *J Clin Invest* 1972;51:97.

181. Grospietsch G, Fenske M, Girndt J, Uhlich E, Kuhn W. The renin-angiotensin-aldosterone system, antidiuretic hormone levels and water balance under tocolytic therapy with fenoterol and verapamil. *Int J Gynaecol Obstet* 1980;17:590.

182. Blickstein I, Zalel Y, Katz Z, Lancet M. Ritodrine-induced pulmonary edema unmasking underlying peripartum cardiomyopathy. *Am J Obstet Gynecol* 1988;159:332.

183. Hankins GDV, Hauth JC, Kuehl TJ, Brans YW, Cunningham FG, Pierson W. Ritodrine hydrochloride infusion in pregnant baboons. II. Sodium and water compartment alterations. *Am J Obstet Gynecol* 1983;147:254.

184. Hauth JC, Hankins GDV, Kuehl TJ, Pierson WP. Ritodrine hydrochloride infusion in pregnant baboons. I. Biophysical effects. *Am J Obstet Gynecol* 1983;146:916.

185. Hankins GDV, Hauth JC. A comparison of the relative toxicities of β-sympathomimetic tocolytic agents. *Am J Perinatol* 1985;2:338.

186. Romero R, Brody DT, Oyarzun E, et al. Infection and labor. III. Interleukin-1: a signal for the onset of parturition. *Am J Obstet Gynecol* 1989;160:1117.

187. Romero R, Wu YK, Brody DT, Oyarzun E, Duff GW, Durum SK. Human decidua: a source of interleukin-1. *Obstet Gynecol* 1989;73:31.

188. Bennett PR, Rose MP, Myatt L, Elder MG. Preterm labor: stimulation of arachidonic acid metabolism in human amnion cells by bacterial products. *Am J Obstet Gynecol* 1987;156:649.

189. Romero R, Hobbins JC, Mitchell MD. Endotoxin stimulates prostaglandins $E_2$ production by human amnion. *Obstet Gynecol* 1988;71:227.

190. Hameed C, Tejani N, Verma UL, Archbald F. Silent chorioamnionitis as a cause of preterm labor refractory to tocolytic therapy. *Am J Obstet Gynecol* 1984;149:726.

191. Duff P, Kopelman JN. Subclinical intra-amniotic infection in asymptomatic patients with refractory preterm labor. *Obstet Gynecol* 1987; 69:756.

192. Crosby WM, Costiloe JD. Safety of lap-belt restraint for pregnant victims of automobile collisions. *N Engl J Med* 1971;284:362.

193. Rose PG, Strohm PL, Zuspan FP. Fetomaternal hemorrhage following trauma. *Am J Obstet Gynecol* 1985;153:844.

194. Goodwin TM, Breen MT. Pregnancy outcome and fetomaternal hemorrhage after noncatastrophic trauma. *Am J Obstet Gynecol* 1990;162:665.

195. Pearlman MD, Tintinalli JE, Lorenz RP. Blunt trauma in pregnancy. *N Engl J Med* 1990;323:1609.

196. Dyer T, Barclay DL. Accidental trauma complicating pregnancy and delivery. *Am J Obstet Gynecol* 1962;83:907.

197. Lavin JP, Polsky SS. Abdominal trauma during pregnancy. *Clin Perinatol* 1983;10:423.

198. Buchsbaum HJ. Penetrating injury of the abdomen. In: Buchsbaum HJ, ed. *Trauma in pregnancy.* Philadelphia, PA: WB Saunders; 1979.

199. Cummins RO, ed. *Textbook of advanced cardiac life support.* New York: American Heart Association; 1994.

200. Rees GA, Willis BA. Resuscitation in late pregnancy. *Anaesthesia* 1988;43:347.

201. Goodwin AP, Pearce AJ. The human wedge: a manoeuvre to relieve aortocaval compression during resuscitation in late pregnancy. *Anaesthesia* 1992;47:433.

202. Briggs GG, Garite TJ. Effects on the fetus of drugs used in critical care. In: Clark Sl, Cotton DB, Hankins GDV, Phelan JP, eds. *Critical care obstetrics.* 2nd ed. Blackwell Scientific Publications 1991.

203. Rubin PC. Beta-blockers in pregnancy. *N Engl J Med* 1981;305:1323.

204. Katz VL, Dotters DJ, Droegemueller W. Perimortem cesarean delivery. *Obstet Gynecol* 1986;68:571.

205. Westgren M, Paul RH. Delivery of the low birth weight infant by cesarean section. *Clin Obstet Gynecol* 1985;28:752.

206. Roe v Wade, 410 US 113, 93 Sct 705, 35 Led 2d 147 (1973).

207. *Maternal/fetal medicine: principles and practice.* 3rd ed. Creasy RK, Resnik R, eds. Cambridge, MA: Blackwell Scientific; 1993.

208. Bernstein IM, Watson M, Simmons GM, et al. Maternal brain death and prolonged fetal survival. *Obstet Gynecol* 1989;74:434.

209. Dillon WP, Lee RV, Tronolone MJ, et al. Life support and maternal brain death during pregnancy. *JAMA* 1982;248:1089.

210. Field DR, Gates EA, Creasy RK, Jonsen AR, Laros RK. Maternal brain death during pregnancy: medical and ethical issues. *JAMA* 1988;260:816.

211. Loewy EH. The pregnant brain death and the fetus: must we always try to wrest life from death? *Am J Obstet Gynecol* 1987;157:1097.

212. Feinberg J. The mistreatment of dead bodies. *Hastings Cent Rep* 1985;15:31.

213. Veatch RM. Maternal brain death: an ethicist's thoughts. *JAMA* 1982; 248:1102.

214. Siegler WD. Brain death and live birth. *JAMA* 1982;248:1101.

*The Critically Ill Cardiac Patient,*
edited by V. Kvetan and D. R. Dantzker,
Lippincott - Raven Publishers, Philadelphia © 1996.

CHAPTER 17

# Commonly Encountered Cardiac Toxicities in the Intensive Care Unit Setting

David Rubinstein and Peter M. Buttrick

Various drugs, whether taken therapeutically, in overdose, or as environmental toxins, can have profound pathologic effects. Many of these effects are specific for the cardiovascular system and sometimes may be severe enough to require management in an intensive care unit (ICU). A number of sources provide comprehensive reviews of cardiac toxins in general (1–3). Rather than recapitulating these, this chapter will focus on issues that are relevant to the identification and management of common cardiac toxicities as they arise in the ICU. Specifically, we will review the pathophysiology, clinical manifestations, and treatment of toxicities involving cocaine, the cyclic antidepressants, methylxanthines (theophylline and aminophylline), the anthracycline chemotherapeutic agents, digitalis, calcium channel blockers, and beta-blockers. In addition, we will review the unique manifestations and treatment of torsade des pointes, an arrhythmia commonly seen in the ICU in association with a number of drug toxicities. The goals of this chapter are to provide a basis for rapid recognition of the cardiac effects of these toxins and a strategy for specific treatments where they exist.

## GENERAL MANAGEMENT

An important, if obvious, first step in managing a hemodynamically compromised patient in a unit setting is entertaining the diagnosis of bloodstream toxins. While this may seem self-evident, the presumption that hemodynamic compromise reflects the far more common diagnosis of, for example, coronary artery or valvular disease may preclude prompt and expedient therapy of toxin exposure. The first step, therefore, is maintaining a high index of suspicion. Although the majority of patients experiencing toxic ingestions fall into a younger age group, it is important to realize that older patients, often receiving treatment for arrhythmias, heart failure, clinical depression, or concurrent medical diseases such as chronic obstructive pulmonary disease might also have been exposed to toxic agents (4).

A careful history with attention to medications, a history of drug use and potential toxin exposure, and a physical examination with emphasis on abnormalities of sympathetic or parasympathetic tone are at the core of the physician's initial assessment. General management, as with any critically ill patient, requires assurance of adequate ventilatory and circulatory support. Drugs suspected of initiating the toxic episode, whether they were administered on an outpatient basis or in-hospital, should be discontinued. In general, a toxic ingestion known to have occurred within an hour or two of presentation should be treated with gastric lavage. The use of syrup of ipecac to induce emesis should be reserved for the limited circumstance of an ingestion of a substance not known to cause sudden hemodynamic or central nervous system (CNS) compromise. Generally, all ingestions should be followed by intestinal absorption of the toxin via activated charcoal combined with a cathartic such as sorbitol, with repeated doses of charcoal given in the setting of serious intoxications (3). It is routine for most emergency rooms to also administer glucose (i.e., D50), naloxone, and thiamine to any patient presenting with altered mental status.

This general treatment outline has usually been initiated before the patient presents to the ICU, either in the emergency department or during the primary evaluation of the patient in a noncritical hospital setting. However, for the patient with iatrogenic toxin exposure, the above important principles of general management should not be forgotten. In addition, evaluation of arterial oxygenation (via oximetry and/or arterial blood gases), acid-base status, and serum glucose, electrolytes, and osmolality should be performed.

D. Rubinstein and P.M. Buttrick: Division of Cardiology, Montefiore Medical Center, Albert Einstein College of Medicine, Bronx, New York 10467.

Another important aspect of initial management includes specific resources available to the ICU team; lists of drugs available for screening by the toxicology laboratory and available antidotes should be posted in the ICU (5). Perhaps most important, the physician should acknowledge that no amount of experience can substitute for consultation with a toxicologist; prompt phone consultation with a regional toxicology center often proves the most important first step toward accurate diagnosis and treatment (4).

Having established these basic principles, we will now review specific agents and toxicities which commonly present in an ICU (see Table 1).

## COCAINE

An alkaloid derived from the erythoxylon coca plant, cocaine can be inhaled, injected, or smoked (6). An estimated 30 million people in the United States have used cocaine, and more than 5 million currently use it on a regular basis (7). It is the illicit drug most frequently involved in emergency room visits and, despite increased awareness of its toxicities, it remains among the most frequent causes of drug-related death (8). Although cocaine is associated with a spectrum of cardiac toxicities, including myocardial infarction (MI), arrhythmias, cardiomyopathy, myocarditis, aortic dissection, and endocarditis (6, 7), we will focus on the most common clinical scenario faced by the cardiac intensivist: chest pain.

Cocaine-associated chest pain may lead to no obvious cardiac sequelae or it may herald the dramatic presentation of acute myocardial ischemia, infarction, and death. The ability to anticipate cardiac sequelae is clearly critical; however, there are few controlled studies involving large numbers of patients upon which to base clinical strategies. Despite this, the currently proposed pathophysiologic mechanisms of cocaine toxicity and the existent clinical experience do allow for the develpment of some treatment guidelines.

### Pathophysiology

Cocaine exerts multiple effects on the cardiovascular system that may result in acute myocardial ischemia and infarction (6, 7). Among the most important of these

**TABLE 1.** *Overview of treatment strategies for some common cardiotoxic agents*

| Class of agent | Indication for treatment | Initial therapy | Comments |
|---|---|---|---|
| Cyclic antidepressants | Arrhythmias, seizures; significant conduction delay; hypotension | Gastric lavage; activated charcoal; alkalinization of serum; lidocaine; volume repletion; pressors | QRS duration hallmark for assessing therapy; toxicity unlikely if QRS < 0.10; avoid type IA and IC agents |
| Methylxanthines | Nausea, vomiting; CNS[a] symptoms, seizures; tachyarrhythmias; hypotension | Activated charcoal; low-dose beta-blockers; charcoal hemoperfusion; volume repletion | Distinctions between acute and chronic ingestion |
| Cardiac glycosides | Refractory gastrointestinal symptoms, multiple arrhythmias, progressive bradycardia, hyperkalemia | Activated charcoal, digoxin-specific Fab fragments, atropine, magnesium, correct potassium imbalances | Avoid type IA agents; avoid calcium; anticipate rebound toxicity after Fab administration |
| Anthracyclines | Chronic heart failure | Supportive care, inotropic support | Anticipate toxicity |
| Calcium channel blockers | Hypotension; bradycardia and heart block; CNS: lethargy, coma | Lavage and activated charcoal, judicious fluids, calcium, glucagon | Multiple-drug interactions; follow activated calcium levels |
| Beta-blockers | Hemodynamically significant bradycardia, hypotension, atrioventricular block; seizures | Gastric lavage, activated charcoal, glucagon, adrenergic agonists | May require very high agonist dosage; variable features depending on pharmacology, lipid solubility, etc. |
| Cocaine | Tachycardia, hypertension, myocardial ischemia, myocardial infarction | Benzodiazepines, morphine, aspirin; consider thrombolysis | Avoid beta-blockers |
| Type IA antiarrhythmics, sotalol, phenothiazines, haloperidol, pentamidine (IV), organophosphates | Torsade de pointes | Magnesium sulfate, cardiac pacing, isoproterenol infusion | Certain drug-drug interactions may lead to torsade de pointes |

[a]Central nervous system.

effects are increased myocardial oxygen demand, coronary artery vasoconstriction, and coronary thrombosis.

Cocaine's most dramatic effect is its pentiation of the actions of the sympathetic nervous system. By blocking presynaptic reuptake of norepinephrine and dopamine, cocaine increases the synaptic concentration and binding of these catecholamines to adrenergic receptors, leading to increased inotropy, tachycardia, and hypertension (6). The resultant increase in myocardial oxygen, coupled with afterload mismatch from hypertension, may lead to myocardial ischemia and impaired ventricular performance as well as to supraventricular and ventricular tachyarrhythmias.

Although ergonovine challenge in the catheterization laboratory does not commonly lead to vasospasm in patients exposed to cocaine (7, 8), focal coronary artery spasm may play a role in cocaine-induced ischemia and infarction. Lange and colleagues (9) analyzed changes in coronary artery diameter after the administration of topical, intranasal cocaine to groups of non-cocaine-using volunteers. They noted small but statistically significant reductions in epicardial coronary artery diameters and in coronary blood flow despite increases in myocardial oxygen demand. These investigators hypothesized that changes in coronary artery diameter were due to alpha-adrenergic receptor stimulation, since phentolamine, an alpha-blocker, reversed the constrictive effect, while beta-blockade potentiated it (8, 9). Concomitant cigarette smoking (10) and the presence of atherosclerotic coronary artery lesions (11, 12) may also enhance the vasoconstrictive effects. These same authors have reported reversal of vasoconstriction with nitroglycerin (13), and others have suggested that phentolamine may be useful in the treatment of acute, cocaine-related, myocardial ischemia (14). Vasospasm of small-resistance coronary vessels may also contribute to myocardial ischemia and long-term ventricular dysfunction.

Thrombus formation and coronary artery occlusion have also been noted in cocaine-induced MI (15). This may be secondary to endothelial damage induced by coronary vasospasm (6, 7) or to primary hemostatic changes such as activation and aggregation of platelets, as suggested by in vitro studies (16, 17).

**Clinical Evaluation**

The difficulty in accurately diagnosing cocaine-associated chest pain is not trivial. First, it is not always cardiac in origin. Intravenous injection of cocaine or other drugs may lead to rhabdomyolysis, right-sided bacterial endocarditis with septic pulmonary emboli, or pneumothorax, all of which can present with chest discomfort. As intravenous drug use is associated with the acquisition of human immunodeficiency virus (HIV) and the subsequent development of acquired immunodeficiency syndrome (AIDS), related pulmonary infections must be included in the differential of cocaine use and chest pain. Additionally, pulmonary absorption of crack may be maximized by forceful Valsalva maneuver, possibly leading to rupture of a pulmonary bleb, pneumothorax, and associated chest pain. Crack users are also at risk for "crack lung," a syndrome notable for chest pain, dyspnea, bronchospasm, and eosinophilia (18). Cocaine use also has been associated with aortic rupture (19), and this distinctive chest pain syndrome should not be mistaken as cardiac.

When other causes of chest pain have been excluded, the diagnosis of cardiac-related chest pain may still be difficult. On the one hand is the patient with typical chest pain and electrocardiographic evidence of acute ischemia and on the other hand is the patient with an atypical history and nonspecific electrocardiographic changes or changes that are normal variants in a young patient cohort. Some generalizations and caveats which may help in the evaluation of cocaine-associated chest pain follow.

1. The route of administration, chronicity of use, and total dose of cocaine administered do not modify the potential for significant cardiac toxicity (18, 20–22). Thus, the "recreational" or "first-time" user of small amounts of cocaine is not immune to cardiac complications.

2. The average age of the presenting patient with cocaine-associated chest pain may be significantly lower than that of the more conventional patient with coronary artery disease (23), making it imperative to ask a younger patient presenting with chest pain of unclear etiology about cocaine use.

3. Although studies of cocaine-related MI show a high incidence (up to 90%) of cigarette smoking (20), there may be fewer of the usual cardiac risk factors for coronary artery disease than in the population with coronary artery disease (24).

4. Atypical chest pain does not rule out the possibility of significant cardiac toxicity (25).

5. Clinical onset is variable. While often occurring within an hour or two after use, many patients experience pain and/or siginificant ischemia up to 72 hours afterward (24, 26, 27).

6. Although an abnormal EKG may not in itself make the diagnosis of ischemia, it is unusual for patients with cocaine-associated MI to present with a normal EKG (24).

7. While rhabdomyolysis is associated with cocaine toxicity (28) and may make the finding of an elevated creatine phosphokinase (CPK) nonspecific, an elevated MB fraction in the proper clinical setting is highly suggestive of myocardial damage (18).

8. Since the differential of cocaine-associated chest pain includes pneumothorax, septic emboli, pneumonia, crack lung, or even aortic dissection as noted above, a chest radiograph should be a standard component of any initial evaluation.

**Treatment**

Cocaine's major pathophysiologic effects should be kept in mind as a guide to the treatment of myocardial ischemia/infarction. Increased sympathetic output with resultant hypertension and tachycardia may respond to therapy with morphine and benzodiazepines; these agents should be considered first-line therapy in the treatment of cocaine intoxication (18, 25). Prompt nitrate therapy is appropriate, as nitroglycerin has been shown to diminish cocaine-related coronary vasoconstriction (13). Other treatment modalities for myocardial ischemia differ somewhat from standard therapy. Due to concern that beta-blocker therapy might leave cocaine's powerful alpha-agonist vasoconstricting effects unopposed (10), therapy with beta-adrenergic antagonists should be avoided. As noted above, phentolamine, a pure alpha-blocker, has been used successfully for the initial treatment of drug-induced hypertension (14). For patients with severe and refractory hypertension, nitroprusside may also be used (21). Because of cocaine's possible effects on platelet aggregation (16), aspirin and/or other antiplatelet agents should be employed in the setting of possible ischemia and infarction (31). There are little human data to support the routine use of calcium channel blockade in the acute management of cocaine-related chest pain.

The use of thrombolytics in patients with ischemia after cocaine use is complicated by several factors. First, patients may present with elevated blood pressure. Although this can often be controlled with conventional therapy and thus does not represent a direct contraindication to thrombolysis, extreme blood pressure elevations may increase the risk of aortic dissection and intracranial hemorrhage, both of which have been reported with cocaine intoxication (19, 29). Another important issue is that many young patients with cocaine-associated chest pain have EKG variants such as early repolarization (J-point elevation) or increased voltage which make interpretation of the electrocardiogram (EKG) difficult. Attempting to acquire an old ERG or following serial EKGs is, of course, appropriate. However, in this setting, obtaining an echocardiogram to define wall motion abnormalities may be most useful. Although interpretation of segmental wall motion abnormalities can be difficult, comparison of an infarct-related territory based on electrocardiographic and echocardiographic findings may help in diagnosing myocardial infarction/ischemia and in guiding the decision as to whether thrombolytic agents should be administered.

Until recently, little data were available on the clinical safety of thrombolytic therapy in cocaine-associated MI. However, the Cocaine Associated Myocardial Infarction (CAMI) Study Group (30) recently reported a multicenter, retrospective analysis of patients who sustained cocaine-associated Q-wave MI. In this series, 25 of 66 patients received thrombolysis at the discretion of the treating physician. Although none of the patients who received thrombolysis died or sustained major bleeding complications such as intracranial hemorrhage, this analysis failed to show a significant difference in median peak creatine kinase MB (CK-MB) concentration, or time to peak CK-MB concentrations, both markers of successful reperfusion with thrombolytic therapy, between patients who did and did not receive thrombolysis. Although this suggests that the benefits of thrombolytic therapy in cocaine-associated MI are limited, the retrospective nature of the study, as well as its small population of patients, must be noted. Of interest was the fact that more than 30% of the patients in the thrombolysis group were concurrently treated with beta-blockers, leading the authors of this study to speculate that beta-blocker-associated coronary artery vasoconstriction or spasm may have limited the effect of thrombolytic agents. Therefore, while general guidelines for administration of thrombolytics may be followed, and while the CAMI study suggests that thrombolytics may be given without major bleeding complications, until larger, prospective groups of patients are analyzed, thrombolytic agents should be used cautiously.

In patients with absolute or relative contraindications to thrombolysis and clear evidence of transmural myocardial damage, acute cardiac catheterization may be considered. Findings at catheterization include areas of focal spasm as well as thrombus (8). Patients may benefit from locally administered nitrates, thrombolytic agents (i.e., urokinase or streptokinase), or even angioplasty.

Despite the dramatic presentation of acute MI in cocaine abusers, the available literature suggests that most cases of cocaine-associated chest pain and even MI will be uncomplicated, probably reflecting the absence of complex intercurrent illness in this patient population. Still, given the varied effects of cocaine and the possibility of active metabolites contributing to its toxicity, the generally recommended standard of care in the setting of chest pain and nonspecific electrocardiographic changes is to observe the patient for a 24-hour period. More precise tests for evidence of ischemia and infarction, better understanding of cocaine's toxic actions, and further epidemiologic data may allow for more specific therapeutic recommendations.

Finally, although the cardiac intensivist will likely be managing only a limited period of the cocaine abuser's course, the opportunity for impressing the patient with the potential dangers of cocaine should not be lost. While chest pain, acute MI, and myocardial damage are no guarantee that the recreational use of cocaine will stop, the drama of the ICU setting is powerful, and the intensivist should initiate the course of planned drug counseling or rehabilitation and ensure specific follow-up.

## CYCLIC ANTIDEPRESSANTS

The classic tricyclic antidepressants, such as imipramine and amitriptyline, as well as their newer cousins, the bicyclic and tetracyclic antidepressants, are important agents used by both the specialist and the generalist in the treatment of depression. Despite this, the cyclic antidepressants (CAs) are frequently misused by patients and physicians and overdoses are relatively common. Of the 2% to 3% of cases of overdoses that are fatal, the primary cause of death is cardiac related.

## Pathophysiology and Pharmacology

Cyclic antidepressants have multiple effects on the cardiovascular system. By blocking the fast sodium channel, CAs slow phase 0 of the action potential. This membrane-stabilizing, "quinidine-like" effect may potentiate arrhythmia formation in conduction tissue and also cause hypotension due to direct myocardial depression. In addition, CAs have strong muscarinic and antihistaminic effects. Anticholinergic effects can lead to tachycardia, as well as a characteristic clinical picture of hyperthermia, dry skin and mucous membranes, urinary retention, mydriasis, gastrointestinal (GI) dysmotility with intestinal ileus, and CNS alterations (including slurred speech, disorientation, hallucinations, ataxia, and seizures). The therapeutic effects of the CAs are in part due to blockade of serotonin and norepinephrine uptake and the accumulation of these substances in the CNS. However, in overdose, this may lead to systemic epinephrine depletion and hypotension. Blockade of alpha-adrenergic transmission at postsynaptic sympathetic neurons results in vasodilatation and may also contribute to hypotension (32).

Important pharmacologic properties of the CAs may alter traditional treatment approaches. The CAs are well absorbed from the intestinal mucosa, and their peak effect usually occurs 6 to 8 hours after ingestion. However, because of their potent anticholinergic effect, in the setting of overdose, ileus may lead to impaired absorption, delay in the peak onset of action, and delayed toxicity. Standard treatment with activated charcoal may need to be repeated several times in this setting. A caveat to repeated dosing regimens with activated charcoal is that patients should be followed closely on physical exam for evidence of active bowel sounds, since ileus with stercolith formation and intestinal perforation has been reported (33). Greater than 90% of CAs are protein bound in the serum and therefore not active at physiologic pH. The clinical significance of this is that acidemia and hypoalbuminemia may increase the bioavailabilty of these drugs and worsen symptoms (34). The CAs and their metabolites are lipophilic and therefore have an extensive tissue distribution. Myocardial tissue preferentially takes up CAs, leading to levels that are five times higher than in many other tissues. This large volume of distribution and long elimination half-life make dialysis or hemoperfusion ineffective treatments in overdose. Drug clearance is primarily through first-pass hepatic metabolism and demethylation or hydroxylation in the liver; thus, liver toxicity or reduced liver function with age can lead to accumulation of drug and active metabolites. As CAs and their metabolites are excreted into the gastric juice and bile, they can be reabsorbed; thus, targeting the enterohepatic circulation can be important in overdose (see below).

## Cardiac Toxicity

The most common cardiac manifestation of CA overdose, sinus tachycardia, is most likely due to the early manifestation of potent sympathetic and anticholinergic effects (32). As mentioned above, CAs cause blockade of the fast inward sodium current in Purkinje and other cardiac conduction cells, a characteristic of the type IA antiarrhythmics. Early electrophysiologic changes of slowed conduction are manifested on the surface electrocardiogram as Qtc prolongation and rightward shift in the terminal vector of the frontal plane axis of the QRS (i.e., a terminal R wave in lead aVR and a terminal S wave in leads I and aVL) (4). Prolongation of the PR and QRS intervals may occur. With worsening toxicity there is progressive widening of the QRS and ventricular ectopy. Slowed conduction in the myocardium may lead to reentrant rhythms, including ventricular tachycardia. Bundle branch block (usually of the right bundle), atrioventricular (AV) nodal block, and varied arrhythmias, including atrial and AV junctional tachycardias, atrial fibrillation and flutter, ventricular fibrillation, and asystole, have all been noted (35). Some investigators have noticed the disappearance of ectopy with advanced toxicity. This may be due to reduced membrane responsiveness; marked prolongation of the effective refractory period may abolish reentrant loops through refractory tissue (36). A wide idioventricular rhythm is seen as a terminal rhythm, often presaging death.

## Treatment

In the setting of suspected CA overdose, the presence of any major manifestation of toxicity, such as seizures, arrhythmias, or hypotension, is an indication for the initiation of general treatment measures. These include gastric lavage (which some authorities feel is indicated up to 12 hours after suspected ingestion because of the potential slow transit of drug in the gut) and the administration of multiple doses of activated charcoal with a cathartic. Although the use of syrup of ipecac to induce vomiting might seem appropriate in the setting of decreased gastric transit, the often rapid and dramatic changes in a patient's level of consciousness with significant CA overdose argue against its use.

Multiple studies have shown that neither the dose of CA ingested nor the measured plasma CA level accurately predict complications or clinical outcome (37, 38). Rather, it is the QRS duration that has become the hallmark for assessing potentially severe toxicity and the need for additional treatment (32). In an important prospective analysis of CA toxicity, Boehnert and Love-joy (37) followed 49 patients with acute CA overdose. They found that drug levels failed to predict the risk of two of the most severe forms of toxicity, ventricular arrhythmias and seizures. However, seizures were seen at a QRS duration of 0.10 or greater, and ventricular arrhythmias were seen only at a QRS interval of 0.16 or greater. Although these investigators did not study the effect of treatment on QRS duration, their analysis defines a threshold at which treatment of major toxicity seems appropriate (36), although some retrospective studies suggest that QRS duration does not correlate with toxicity (39). It should be noted that although retrospective analysis has supported the use of a right-axis deviation in the setting of toxicity, in an analysis by Wolfe (40), 17% of CA toxic patients did not have this electrocardiographic finding.

While a prolonged QRS duration predicts toxicity, an important principle of management is that patients with QRS duration below 0.10, without signs of CA toxicity, and who have received the standard activated charcoal therapy for suspected toxicity are at extremely low risk for major complications after 6 hours in a monitored setting. In a retrospective analysis of fatal cases of CA overdose, Callaham and Kassel (33) noted that, although almost half the cases presented with minor signs of toxicity, all patients developed major signs of toxicity within 2 hours of hospital arrival. This does not mean that it is impossible for major toxicity to occur after a 6-hour observational period, but without evidence of persistent tachycardia, CNS symptoms, or cardiac arrhythmias or conduction defects and with the appropriate treatment, patients in general do not progress to further toxicity.

Serum alkalinization is the mainstay of treatment of cardiac CA toxicity, whether in the setting of a widened QRS interval, arrhythmias, or hypotension (36). Treatment is usually accomplished by intravenous infusion of sodium bicarbonate; in the intubated patient, hyperventilation may be used as an adjunctive measure. There are contradictory hypotheses for the mechanism of action of bicarbonate in particular and alkalinization in general. Although hyperventilation by itself seems to decrease toxicity through alkalinization, there is a likely role for sodium bicarbonate in reversing the sodium channel blockade of CAs (although other sodium-free buffering systems also reverse CA toxicity). Alkalinization may also theoretically decrease the available CA by increasing protein binding, although this is not fully supported in the literature. Despite these controversies, it is likely that both alkalinization and reversal of sodium channel blockade play a role in reversing CA toxicity. Generally accepted guidelines for the use of sodium bicarbonate therapy include severe acidosis, hypotension, arrhythmias, prolonged cardiac conduction (increased PR or QT, or QRS

interval greater than 0.16 second), and hypotension. A general method of alkalinization would include an initial bolus administration of 1 to 2 mEq/kg followed by a continuous infusion of 150 mEq of sodium bicarbonate in 850 mL to 1 L of 5% dextrose in water (D5W), with the goal of maintaining serum pH between 7.45 and 7.50. An alternative technique is frequent bolus administrations of sodium bicarbonate to maintain the QRS below 0.16 seconds, although there is no concensus as to how rapidly bicarbonate will narrow the QRS or halt arrhythmias.

Despite alkalinization, some arrhythmias, including ventricular tachycardia and fibrillation, may persist. In this setting, lidocaine is the drug of choice. The use of type IA (quinidine, procainamide) or type IC (flecainide, encainide) agents is absolutely contraindicated, as these drugs have similar cardiotoxic profiles and anticholinergic properties to CAs. Phenytoin is also not recommended (32, 38). Beta-blockers should be used for the management of life-threatening arrhythmias only after other treatments have failed, as they may further depress cardiac function and worsen conduction (35). The role of type III (amiodarone, bretylium) and type IV agents (calcium channel blockers) is not clearly established (32).

Treatment of hypotension in CA overdose should initially consist of volume repletion with crystalloid and sodium bicarbonate. Pressors may be needed to support blood pressure. As discussed above, the causes of hypotension may be multifactorial, including catecholamine depletion, myocardial depression, and alpha-adrenergic blockade. In a dog model of amitriptyline intoxication, Vernon et al. (41) demonstrated reduced cardiac output as a primary mechanism involved in hypotension. Despite concern that CAs might block dopamine-induced release of norepinephrine, they demonstrated both dopamine and norepinephrine were effective in elevating cardiac output and blood pressure to preintoxication values. In the clinical setting, however, dopamine has proved unsuccessful in some resuscitation attempts (42). In addition, some investigators have noted a decrease in systemic vascular resistance with CA toxicity, suggesting a more prominent vasodilatory effect. Given these findings, empiric pressor therapy should probably begin with norepinephrine, with phenylephrine and high doses of dopamine as second-line alternatives (32). The use of dobutamine has not been well studied.

## METHYLXANTHINES

Despite the availability of multiple classes of drugs for the treatment of asthma and chronic obstructive pulmonary disease (COPD), the methylxanthines continue to be widely used, most commonly as the oral agent, theophylline, and the intravenous agent, aminophylline. Their exact mechanism of action is not known (43). At therapeutic levels, their most important effect is likely decreased bronchoconstriction secondary to competitive inhibition of adenosine receptors. Other effects include release of endogenous catecholamines, increased cardiac inotropy and chronotropy, inhibition of bronchoconstricting prostaglandins, calcium modulation, respiratory center stimulation, cerebrovascular vasoconstriction, increased secretion of gastric acid, and improvement of respiratory muscle performance (44, 45). At toxic levels, the drugs may increase cyclic adenosine monophosphate (cAMP) levels via inhibition of phosphodiesterase (3). For the purposes of this discussion, toxicity of theophylline will be emphasized.

## Pharmacology and Pathophysiology

Therapeutic levels of theophylline range between 10 and 20 μg/mL. Conventional oral preparations are well absorbed from the GI tract and reach peak serum concentrations in 1 to 2 hours (46). With sustained-release preparations, however, serum levels may not peak until 12 to 24 hours after ingestion (47). Theophylline displays a low volume of distribution, and approximately 60% of drug is protein bound. Metabolism is primarily hepatic, with only 10% of unmetabolized drug renally cleared. Drugs or systemic conditions that inhibit or stimulate the P-450 enzyme system may have profound effects on theophylline levels. Its metabolism can be increased by as much as 50% by cigarette smoking or by P-450 stimulating drugs such as phenobarbital and phenytoin (46). Drugs such as cimetidine (but not ranitidine), ciprofloxacin, allopurinol, and erythromycin, as well as clinical conditions such as fever, liver failure, congestive heart failure, COPD, acute viral illness, or acute ethanol intake, can decrease the metabolism of theophylline (43, 44). Elimination kinetics are first order at therapeutic levels but become zero order in overdose, leading to increased serum elimination half-life (3).

Theophylline toxicity has profound neurologic, GI, metabolic, and cardiac effects. Neurologic signs include tremor and agitation, predominantly due to increased catecholamine release, and seizures, possibly due to cerebral vasoconstriction and CNS adenosine antagonism (44). Hyperventilation is secondary to direct stimulation of the respiratory center. Direct CNS stimulation of the chemoreceptor trigger zone is responsible for nausea and vomiting, which are often severe enough to impede effective treatment (see below). Catecholamine excess leads to such metabolic complications as hypokalemia, hyperglycemia, hypophosphatemia, and hypomagnesemia (48).

Manifestations of cardiac toxicity are primarily due to excessive catecholamine release. Tachycardia is a cardinal manifestation; its absence makes theophylline toxicity unlikely, unless a concurrent ingestion with a bradycardia-inducing agent (i.e., calcium channel blockers) has occurred (47). Hypotension is likely mediated by massive peripheral beta-adrenergic stimulation (49–52), although peripheral smooth muscle dilatation may play a role (53).

As a result of catecholamine overstimulation, literally any arrhythmia may be seen, although supraventricular arrhythmias such as supraventricular tachycardia (SVT) or mulitfocal atrial tachycardia (MAT) are most common (54). Arrhythmogenic potential is enhanced by the abnormalities that may accompany catecholamine excess, including hypokalemia and acidosis (45, 55). Experimentally, theophylline decreases the fibrillation threshold (55), and it may nonuniformly affect cardiac conduction and allow for reentry arrhythmias, including ventricular tachycardia (46).

## Clinical Evaluation

It is important to recognize that toxic effects differ markedly in acute and chronic intoxication. Acute intoxication is seen primarily in younger patients with intentional, single-ingestion overdose. Compared to chronic intoxication, higher serum levels are seen before toxicity occurs, but, once toxic, patients display prominent findings, such as severe nausea and vomiting, as well as laboratory abnormalities that include leukocytosis, hypokalemia, hyperglycemia, and hypophosphatemia (3, 56). In contrast, chronic toxicity usually occurs in older patients who are receiving standing doses of theophylline. It is often due to an increase in dose, the introduction of a medication that inhibits clearance of theophylline (i.e., erythromycin, cimetidine) or a condition, such as heart failure, that impairs theophylline metabolism. Symptoms are often subtle, with nonspecific GI complaints or tremors. Metabolic changes are less frequently noted, and seizures or arrhythmias may develop suddenly (44). Toxicity is usually seen at lower serum drug levels and is more closely correlated to advancing age than to peak serum levels (57). Where acute overdose is superimposed on chronic overdose, the symptoms resemble those of acute toxicity (44).

## Treatment

If toxicity is suspected, patients should be placed on a cardiac monitor, and blood should be obtained for an emergency theophylline level. Besides the standard evaluation of serum electrolytes, glucose, and complete blood count, prothrombin time and partial thromboplastin time (PT/PTT), platelet count, and serum calcium should be obtained, as baseline and follow-up values will be important should extracorporeal drug removal via hemoperfusion or hemodialysis be required (see below) (47). Syrup of ipecac should be used only in the asymptomatic patient and within an hour of ingestion (47). Orogastric lavage should also be attempted before the onset of drug-induced emesis; this is usually 2 to 4 hours after the ingestion of standard preparations or up to 8 to 10 hours after ingestion of slow-release preparations (46).

Therapy with multiple doses of activated charcoal is crucial for reducing the serum concentration of theophylline (58–61). Not only does charcoal bind the drug in the GI tract, it also allows for back diffusion from body stores into the gut (62), since it is effective even in intravenous (aminophylline) overdose (44). Charcoal should be administered as a slurry, 1 to 2 g/kg body weight, along with a sorbitol or magnesium sulfate cathartic. In patients with advancing symptoms or increasing theophylline levels, 1 g/kg of charcoal should be readministered, without a cathartic, every hour; more stable patients should receive repeat doses every 2 hours (47). Therapy should be continued even if hemoperfusion is initiated (44). As vomiting may delay or prevent the administration of charcoal, early use of antiemetics such as metoclopramide or ondansetron should be strongly considered (63).

Although recommendations vary somewhat in the literature, the general concensus is that extracorporeal removal of theophylline should be initiated in the presence of seizures, ventricular arrhythmias, hypotension not responsive to fluids, or protracted vomiting not responsive to emetics (44, 47). Patients with acute intoxication should also undergo extracorporeal removal if serum drug levels approach 90 µg/mL at any time in their course (44, 47). Levels approaching 70 µg/L 4 hours after ingestion of a sustained-release preparation also warrant strong consideration of this treatment (47). In chronic intoxication, extracorporeal removal should be performed in the setting of major complications and a level greater than 40 µg/L (44, 47), with the understanding that a patient at high risk with other systemic conditions should undergo hemoperfusion before the onset of serious symptoms (e.g., a patient 60 or older with a history of heart failure). Charcoal hemoperfusion is the most effective method available for extracorporeal removal (44). It increases clearance rates two- to sixfold (46, 64). Despite this, the therapy is not benign. Frequent drops in platelet count and serum calcium (64, 65) may complicate hemoperfusion, and these values should be carefully followed during therapy. Patients may also sustain complications from procedure-related hypotension or heparization. If the patient cannot tolerate hemoperfusion, or if it is not available, hemodialysis may be used (3, 44, 45, 46). Since 4 hours or less of extracorporeal removal may be of significant benefit to the patient (47), every effort should be made to allow continuation of therapy, including the use of pressor agents for persistent hypotension. As emphasized above, all supportive measures, as well as multiple doses of charcoal, should be continued during treatment.

Cardiac complications of tachycardia and hypotension should initially be treated with volume repletion, as anorexia, nausea, and vomiting may lead to dehydration. As mentioned above, catecholamine excess, with beta-2-adrenergic stimulation, is felt to be responsible for the majority of findings in toxicity (49). Curry et al. (66) investigated the hemodynamics of theophylline toxicity in a dog model and found that hypotension and tachycardia were accompanied by an increased cardiac index, a decreased systemic vascular resistance index, and preserved mean pulmonary artery capillary wedge pressure. Their model suggested that toxicity involved peripheral vasodilatation and not myocardial dysfunction or dehydration. In addition to catecholamine excess, theophylline, by inhibiting adenosine, may additionally sensitize the cardiovascular system to the effects of catecholamines (66).

Studies have shown a decrease in tachycardia (50), improvement in blood pressure (52), and a reversal of hypokalemia, hypophosphatemia, hyperglycemia, and metabolic acidosis (51) with the use of beta-blockade. After fluid repletion, and while extracorporeal removal is being arranged, hypotension should be treated with low doses of a nonselective beta-blocker such as propranolol or a pressor agent with predominant alpha-adrenergic activity (i.e., norepinephrine or phenylephrine). However, as patients may have reactive airway disease, beta-blockers should be used cautiously. Again, it should be emphasized that hypotension is an indication for extracorporeal removal methods.

Supraventricular tachycardias should be treated with low doses of beta-blockade or calcium channel blockers such as diltiazem or verapamil, and electrolyte and acid-base abnormalities should be corrected (47). Propranolol or conventional doses of lidocaine should be used for ventricular arrhythmias. There is little clinical experience with the use of sotalol (47).

Additional treatment modalities should be mentioned. Although the use of whole-bowel irrigation may decrease the effectiveness of activated charcoal (67), it should be considered when serum theophylline levels continue to rise despite adequate charcoal treatment (47). In this circumstance, bowel irrigation can be alternated every 2 hours with charcoal treatment, or additional charcoal can be administered (44). Whole-bowel irrigation may also be used early in the setting of acute intoxication with a large amount of sustained-release preparation; the goal is to eliminate the drug before absorption occurs (44). The endpoint of treatment with whole-bowel irrigation is a clear rectal effluent. If serum levels continue to rise despite charcoal and irrigation, the possibility of bezoar formation or retained materials must be considered (68), and upper GI tract radiographic studies may be needed to help evaluate for possible endoscopy or laparotomy.

An agitated patient with theophylline intoxication should be evaluated for hypoglycemia and then treated with an IV benzodiazepine. Seizures, which may be refractory to therapy and are an indication for extracorporeal drug removal, should be treated with benzodiazepines followed by barbiturates and, if necessary, general anesthesia with neuromuscular blocking agents (44, 47) and CNS monitoring. Phenytoin has not proved effective in animal models and is not recommended (44).

# CARDIAC GLYCOSIDES

Cardiac glycosides are a plant-derived group of drugs that have been in clinical use for more than 200 years. Digitalis is the designated term for the entire group, which includes such drugs as digoxin, digitoxin, and oubain. Digoxin is the cardiac glycoside in most common use in the United States (69). Important pharmacologic and therapeutic differences between digoxin and digitoxin will be discussed below, but in general, the term *digitalis* will be used to refer to the cardiac glycosides as a group.

The burden of treating life-threatening cardiac glycoside toxicity has been lightened by the availability of a specific antidote, a digoxin-specific antibody fragment (Fab) that is easy to administer, rapid in its onset, and extremely effective. However, the intensivist must still have a clear understanding of the pathophysiology of digitalis toxicity, its clinical manifestations, the indications for treatment, and the potential complications that may arise once treatment is initiated.

## Pathophysiology and Pharmacology

Digitalis has direct cardiac as well as parasympathetic, sympathetic, and peripheral arterial effects. At the cellular level, digitalis binds to an inhibitory site on the alpha subunit of the enzyme NaK-adenosine triphosphatase (ATPase). The NaK-ATPase normally functions as a "sodium pump," maintaining high intracellular concentrations of potassium and low intracellular concentrations of sodium ion. With inhibition of NaK-ATPase, there is a gradual increase in intracellular sodium and extracellular potassium ion concentrations. Intracellular sodium is then exchanged for extracellular calcium, which indirectly provides the cell with more calcium for release from the sarcoplamic reticulum during each action potential, resulting in enhanced inotropy (3, 69, 70).

At therapeutic levels, most of the conduction effects of digitalis are due to its action on the autonomic nervous system (70). Digitalis enhances vagal tone by increasing the sensitivity of cardiac fibers to acetylcholine (71), especially at supraventricular sites, where the density of parasympathetic fibers is greatest (72). Digitalis also increases the sensitivity of the arterial baroreceptor reflex to parasympathetic vagal stimuli, while decreasing its sensitivity to sympathetic stimuli (71). In response to these autonomic effects, sinus node slowing is prominent, and there is an increase in the AV node refractory period and slowing of its conduction velocity (70). In the vasculature, digitalis can raise systemic and pulmonary vascular resistance. This can be clinically significant if the drug is given as an IV bolus in the setting of acute heart failure (70).

While these complex interactions tend to slow conduction and increase the refractory period of conducting tissue, digitalis has the opposite effect on heart muscle: Conduction through myocardium is more rapid, and the refractory period is shortened (70). Thus, the former effects can be noted on the EKG as prolongation of the PR interval and AV block, while the latter effects lead to a decrease in the QT interval. The effect of digitalis on repolarization can be noted by ST-segment and T-wave forces opposite in direction to QRS forces, the so-called dig effect (73).

At higher digitalis concentrations, direct cardiac, as opposed to autonomic, effects predominate. Conduction influences may lead to the suppression of normal pacemaker mechanisms and the appearance of new ones. Increased intracellular calcium ion concentrations may trigger a transient inward $Na^+$ current, leading to spontaneous afterdepolarizations (delayed afterdepolarizations) and the generation of arrhythmias. Less commonly, automatic and reentrant mechanisms may develop (72, 74).

Electrolyte imbalances, especially those involving potassium and calcium, play an important role in potentiating toxicity. With inhibition of NaK-ATPase, cells accumulate intracellular sodium and lose potassium to the extracellular environment. As intracellular potassium decreases, so does the resting membrane potential; conductance of the membrane increases. These effects lead to accelerated repolarization. Low serum potassium in and of itself tends to enhance repolarization and generate automatic rhythms; thus, the arrhythmogenic effects of digoxin are superimposed on those of hypokalemia. Potassium also competes with digoxin for membrane-binding sites. In hypokalemia, more digoxin will become bound to cells, increasing the inhibition of NaK-ATPase and thus the potential for toxicity (72). While high serum potassium values might be expected to diminish binding of digoxin to membrane receptors and thus limit toxicity, hyperkalemia, like hypokalemia, increases potassium membrane conductance and leads to accelerated repolarization. Elevated extracellular $K^+$ also acts to lower the resting membrane potential, reducing action potential amplitude and upstroke velocity and slowing conduction. These toxic effects are superimposed on digitalis (72). Additionally, both hyperkalemia and hypokalemia may enhance conduction block.

Both high and low levels of serum calcium have important modifying effects on the cardiac membrane that may exacerbate the toxic effects of digoxin. With marked increases in intracellular calcium, the trigger for the inward current that induces delayed afterdepolarizations is enhanced, as discussed above. Electrical uncoupling of cardiac fibers can also occur, leading to slowing or complete cessation of conduction (see below). Increased serum $Ca^{2+}$ can also reduce the threshold potential, decreasing the excitability of the cell and leading to conduction block. This can also augment the transient inward current that is responsible for delayed afterdepolarizations. On the other hand, reduction of extracellular $Ca^{2+}$ will increase threshold potential and increase excitability, making conduction block less likely and decreasing the magnitude of any afterdepolarizations. However, it increases the likelihood that delayed afterdepolarizations will reach threshold and induce arrhythmias (72).

## Toxicity

In addition to cardiac manifestations, digitalis toxicity has CNS and GI manifestations that are important to recognize as they may presage more life-threatening arrhythmias. The initial symptoms of toxicity may include anorexia, nausea and vomiting, and abdominal pain. In the setting of unexplained bradycardic rhythm disturbances, these findings may help distinguish acute digitalis intoxication from calcium channel blocker or beta-blocker toxicity (75). Central nervous system symptoms of headache, confusion, disorientation, lethargy, and even seizures may be seen (73). Visual disturbances include photophobia, blurred vision, and scotomata or the appearance of yellow or green halos around objects (74–76). Hyperkalemia is a common abnormality as would be predicted from the actions of the drug on the NaK-ATPase. A serum potassium greater than 5.0 mEq/L has proven to be a powerful predictor of mortality in the setting of digitalis toxicity (78). However, serum potassium concentration may be normal or decreased as a result of concomitant diuretic use.

Digitalis levels are altered by a number of clinical conditions. Hypothyroidism and renal failure both reduce the clearance of digitalis; hypothyroidism also enhances myocardial sensitivity to digitalis (79). Elderly patients may be more sensitive to digitalis due to decreased muscle mass for drug binding and decreased renal excretion (79). Myocardial ischemia may also enhance sensitivity to digitalis. Antacids and resin-binding agents reduce serum levels, and their abrupt withdrawal without adjustment of digitalis dose may lead to toxicity (80). Inactivation of digoxin by gut flora may be abolished with tetracycline or erythromycin and lead to elevated serum concentrations (72). Concomitant use of beta-blockers or calcium channel blockers may enhance AV block. In addition, quinidine, verapamil, and amiodarone all raise serum digitalis levels (79).

Clearly, there are abundant mechanisms to explain the generation of cardiac arrhythmias in digitalis toxicity, and almost any type of arrhythmia may be seen, either as a result of a disturbance in impulse formation or an impairment in impulse conduction (81). Some arrhythmias are more commonly noted, although none is truly pathognomonic. Isolated premature ventricular contractions (PVCs), although nonspecific, are the most common finding (83); bigeminal and trigeminal rhythms are more characteristic (81). Nonparoxysmal accelerated junctional tachycardia, usually at rates between 70 and 100 beats/min, is a characteristic rhythm. Paroxysmal atrial tachycardia with AV block, reflecting the combination of increased automaticity and impaired conduction,

is also highly suggestive of digitalis toxicity (83) (Fig. 1B). A regularized rhythm in the setting of atrial fibrillation suggests digitalis-induced complete AV block. A classic toxic rhythm is the uncommonly seen bidirectional ventricular tachycardia (Fig. 1A). Likely junctional in origin, it manifests as a regular alternation of two QRS complexes. Two other noteworthy electrocardiographic generalizations can be made: Since AV conduction block is supra-Hisian, digitalis toxicity is unlikely to present as a bundle branch pattern (unless there is prior His-Purkinje disease); and finally, electrocardiographic manifestations of digitalis effect, including ST-segment scooping, T-wave inversion, and QT-interval shortening, are not related to digitalis levels or digitalis intoxication and may, in fact, be absent in the setting of toxicity (81).

## Treatment

Initial management of toxicity is similar to that for other toxins. Since patients with digitalis toxicity are often taking multiple cardiac medications and may present with nonspecific symptoms, an important principle is that administration of the drug should be halted, and the development of further cardiac complications that might be treated with cardiac glycosides, such as SVT, atrial fibrillation, or congestive heart failure, should be treated with other agents. Because arrhythmias, including ventricular tachycardia or fibrillation, may be rapid in onset (81), patients should obviously be observed in a monitored setting. Serum electrolytes, including potassium, calcium, and magnesium, and blood urea nitrogen (BUN) and creatinine should be drawn and every patient with suspected digitalis toxicity should have a serum digoxin (or digitoxin) level checked. As a general rule, patients with digoxin levels less than 1.5 ng/mL in the absence of hypokalemia are unlikely to be toxic; levels less than 1.0 ng/mL with normokalemia virtually exclude the diagnosis (69).

Prevention of further GI absorption of digitalis compounds should be treated with lavage (in the setting of recent ingestion) and activated charcoal with a cathartic. Continued administration of activated charcoal (1 g/kg body weight every 2 to 4 hours) helps reduce enterohepatic recirculation (84); steroid-binding resins such as cholestyramine may be of further benefit (73). Digoxin, the most available of the cardiac glycosides in the United States, has a volume of distribution of 7 to 10 L/kg, with only 1% of drug in the serum, so methods of drug removal such as hemodialysis, forced diuresis, and hemoperfusion are not particularly effective (73).

Digoxin-specific antibody fragments (Fab) are the treatment of choice for the management of severe digitalis toxicity. Developed from the antigen-recognizing Fab moiety of sheep antibody, digoxin Fab have a high affinity for digoxin and clinically significant cross-reactivity with digitoxin. Their small size allows for a larger

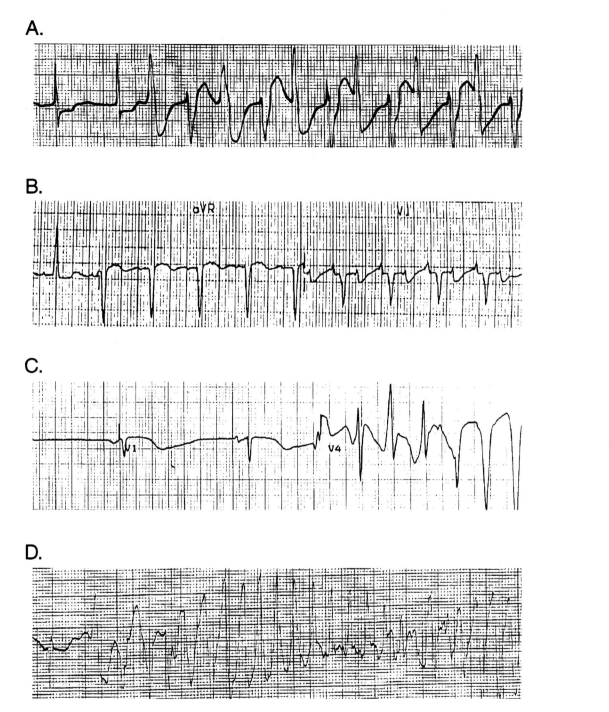

**FIG. 1.** **A:** Bidirectional tachycardia in a patient with digoxin toxicity. **B:** Paroxysmal atrial tachycardia (PAT) with block in a patient with digoxin toxicity. Note upright P waves at a rate of ~ 170 beats/min best seen in lead V1. **C:** Prolongation of the QT interval in a patient with renal failure and sotalol intoxication. Note onset of polymorphic ventricular tachycardia. **D:** Torsade de pointes in a patient with profound electrolyte disturbances.

volume of distribution, more rapid onset of action, and more rapid elimination through the kidneys than whole immunoglobulin G (IgG) antibodies (85).

The initial description of the use of digoxin Fab was by Smith and colleagues (86, 87) and the largest series was reported in 1990 by Antman et al. (88), who described the use of digoxin Fab in 148 of 150 patients with potentially life-threatening digitalis toxicity. Half the patients in this series were receiving long-term treatment with digitalis and half had taken an acute ingestion. All patients had either life-threatening cardiac arrhythmias (defined as second- or third-degree AV block, refractory ventricular tachycardia, and ventricular fibrillation) or hyperkalemia or both. At the time of study enrollment, median serum digoxin and digitoxin concentrations were eight to ten times therapeutic level. Digoxin Fab administration was calculated to be equal on a mole-for-mole basis to the amount of digoxin or digitoxin in the patient's body as estimated from the medical history or serum concentrations (see below). Following treatment, signs and symptoms of digitalis toxicity resolved in 80% of patients; an additional 10% showed improvement (resolution or improvement of some but not all of the signs of suspected toxicity), and only 10% of patients did not show a response. Time to initial response was 19 minutes, with clinically evident improvement occurring by 1 hour of termination of Fab infusion, and complete response occurring by 4 hours. In retrospective analysis, of the 10% classified as only improved, more than half were felt to have coincident medical conditions that were responsible for the signs and symptoms initially ascribed to digitalis, and the other portion consisted of patients who were moribund at the time of digoxin Fab administration, had concomitant drug toxicities, or had received an inadequate dose of Fab. Only one patient was clearly classified as a nonresponder. Noteworthy in this and other studies was a decline in serum potassium that was consistent with the rapid time course of arrhythmia response. No allergic reactions were identified. Perhaps most important, of the 56 patients in this study whose digitalis toxicity had culminated in cardiac arrest, over half survived hospitalization, as compared to a mortality approaching 100% in historical controls. Also of note was that treatment-related side effects such as increased ventricular rate in atrial fibrillation, worsening of heart failure, and clinically significant hypokalemia occurred in less than 10% of patients (88, 89).

Criteria for the administration of digoxin-specific Fab include progressive bradyarrhythmias unresponsive to atropine; ventricular tachycardia or ventricular fibrillation; a serum potassium concentration of 5 mEq/L or greater in the setting of clear drug toxicity; ingestion of more than 10 mg of digoxin; and a serum digoxin level above 15 ng/mL (75, 79, 85). In addition, rapidly progressive cardiac or GI symptoms or a rapidly rising serum potassium level warrants therapy (85). In certain patient groups, Fab therapy is more prudent than watchful waiting. Elderly patients with suspected large ingestions or patients with suspected concomitant calcium channel blocker toxicity should probably be treated promptly with Fab (85). The latter group is particularly problematic. Suspected calcium channel blocker toxicity is often empirically treated with calcium for findings such as hypotension or conduction block on EKG. Calcium, however, is contraindicated in digitalis toxicity as it aggravates preexistent intracellular hypercalcemia and may lead to intractable ventricular tachycardia or fibrillation, or asystole (73, 75, 85) In suspected mixed toxicity, or when the diagnosis is in doubt, initial therapy with digoxin Fab may allow for safer use of multiple therapies or clarify the cause of toxicity.

Digoxin-specific Fab can be dosed by (a) estimating the body load of digoxin ingested, (b) using the serum digoxin concentration (SDC), or (c) using an empiric evaluation based on the average requirement in acute or chronic overdose (85). To estimate vials of Fab needed based on ingested dose, the body load of digoxin, in milligrams, is divided by the amount of digoxin neutralized by one vial of Fab, 0.6 mg/vial. This method is most useful in acute ingestion, where a serum digoxin level would be unlikely to represent a steady-state concentration (79). A simplified formula for calculating Fab requirements (in number of vials) based on digoxin level is to multiply the patient's SDC in nanograms per milliliter by the patient's weight in kilograms and divide this number by 100 (75). This method is most useful in chronic intoxication, where the digoxin level can be assumed to be steady state (79). A conservative approach to empiric therapy would be to administer two to five vials for a chronic intoxication and 10 to 15 vials for an acute intoxication (75, 85). Emergently, digoxin Fab may be administered as a bolus (79).

After digoxin Fab administration, total serum digoxin levels rise more than tenfold due to displacement of digoxin from tissue and extracellular compartments into plasma (86, 89). Free digoxin levels approach zero immediately after Fab administration but begin to rise as early as 3 hours afterward (89). In patients with renal insufficiency, Fab-bound digoxin is more slowly eliminated, and free digoxin may rebound to therapeutic plasma levels as late as 7 to 14 days after Fab therapy (90). This raises the possibility of a secondary phase of digitalis toxicity, and it is therefore prudent in patients with renal impairment to institute prolonged monitoring and careful clinical assessment even several days after digoxin Fab administration. In the setting of rebound toxicity, free serum digoxin levels, when available, may help guide evaluation and lead to reinitiation of therapy (90). There is limited experience with the removal of Fab-bound digoxin by plasmapheresis (91).

Other treatment modalities are important in digitalis toxicity. To decrease vagal tone, atropine, in 0.5-mg IV boluses, should be given to patients with hemodynamic compromise, bradycardia, or high-degree AV block (73, 75, 79). Potassium correction should be performed cautiously: While hypokalemia sensitizes the myocardium to the effects of digitalis, hyperkalemia reduces AV conduction. Thus, serum potassium levels below 4.0 mEq/L should be corrected in the presence of PVCs, ventricular tachycardia, or SVT with AV block. With first- or second-degree AV block, greater caution should be used, and a potassium level greater than 3.5 Eq/L need not be supplemented (73). In addition to digoxin Fab as first-line therapy, marked hyperkalemia may be treated with IV insulin, dextrose, sodium bicarbonate, and ion-exchange resins. Calcium chloride as primary therapy is contraindicated in digitalis toxicity, as discussed above. Hypomagnesemia, which is often present in chronic toxicity, increases uptake of digitalis and decreases NaK-ATPase activity; it may also lead to refractory hypokalemia. Although its precise mechanism of action is unknown, magnesium may be given in the setting of digitalis-induced tachyarrhythmias (assuming normal renal function) as 2 g magnesium sulfate over 20 minutes followed by an infusion of 1 to 2 g/hr (79, 92). Patients should be followed carefully for neuromuscular dysfunction by monitoring tendon reflexes and respiratory status. Magnesium administration is contraindicated in the presence of bradycardia or AV block (73).

If digoxin Fab is not immediately available, phenytoin or lidocaine should be used to treat ventricular arrhythmias. These agents decrease ventricular irritability with minimal effect on AV nodal conduction. In addition, phenytoin may be effective in terminating digitalis-induced SVTs (73). Class IA agents (procainamide, quinidine, and disopyramide) should not be used to counteract arrhythmias as they may worsen AV block and induce arrhythmias themselves (73, 79). Cardioversion may induce intractable ventricular arrhythmias in digitalis toxicity and should only be attempted when other treatments have failed, and then at the lowest possible energy level (73, 79).

Before the availability of digoxin Fab, transvenous pacing was commonly used for digitalis-induced brady-arrhythmias (93). However, iatrogenic complications such as pacing-induced arrhythmias, infection, and delay in digoxin Fab administration have rendered this a second-line therapy that should be considered only after the administration of properly dosed digoxin Fab (91).

## MYOTOXINS (ANTHRACYCLINES)

The anthracyclines are chemotherapeutic agents used in the treatment of solid tumors and hematologic malignancies. They act by intercalating between base pairs of DNA in actively dividing cells, thus preventing DNA replication (95). Cardiac toxicity limits their clinical use. Although some degree of cardiac toxicity is common to all the anthracycline derivatives, this discussion will highlight the effects of doxorubicin (DOX), the most cardiotoxic agent of this class, and will outline a general treatment approach which is applicable to the other agents.

### Pathophysiology

Doxorubicin toxicity can be characterized as acute, subacute, or chronic, and the management of drug-associated toxicities reflects this classification. During or within hours after acute bolus administration, atrial and/or ventricular ectopic beats, SVTs, and nonspecific ST- and T-wave changes can be seen in up to 40% of patients (95, 96). Although sudden death from ventricular arrhythmia has been reported (95), it is extremely rare and the EKG changes are usually transient and do not indicate a need for discontinuation of DOX. Subacute changes include rare reports of myocarditis and pericarditis days to weeks after administration. Associated morphologic changes seen on endomyocardial biopsy in this setting include polymorphonuclear and eosinophilic infiltration of the myocardium, accumulation of hyalinelike material, contraction bands, and cytoplasmic granulation (97). This toxicity has been seen most commonly with the related chemotherapeutic agent daunorubicin (95).

Chronic effects of DOX toxicity are clinically most important and are due to cell death leading to a dilated cardiomyopathy. Characteristic histopathologic changes appear well before changes in cardiac function noted by noninvasive assessment (95) and include vacuolar degeneration with distention of the sarcoplasmic reticulum and myofibrillar loss progressing to diffuse cell damage, with loss of organelles, mitochondrial and nuclear degeneration, and loss of contractile elements (98–100). Presenting symptoms and signs are those of heart failure, with dyspnea, tachypnea, and nonproductive cough, and jugular venous distention, tachycardia, presence of S3, rales, hepatomegaly, and peripheral edema. Chronic toxicity both histologically and clinically is directly related to cumulative dose, with an incidence of greater than 20% when more than 550 mg/m$^2$ of DOX is administered (101). Other factors modify the incidence of toxicity, including peak plasma levels, prior mediastinal radiation, extremes of age, nutritional status, preexisting heart disease, and possibly the concomitant administration of other chemotherapeutic agents (95, 102). Clinical presentation usually occurs within a month of administration of the last dose but may occur weeks to months after administration (98). Although in some cases DOX toxicity is difficult to establish, long-term follow-up studies have described the development of cardiomyopathy as long as 5 to 10 years after DOX therapy, even in patients who have received less than 500 mg/m$^2$ of DOX (95).

The pathogenesis of DOX-induced cardiotoxicity is uncertain. Calcium ion influx and overload with subsequent cell membrane disturbances, carnitine depletion, inhibition of coenzyme Q10, histamine and catecholamine release, lipid peroxidation, induction of myocyte apoptosis, and free-radical formation are some of the proposed mechanisms (95, 99, 100, 103).

## Treatment

The best management of DOX cardiotoxicity is anticipation and prevention; dosages should be limited and careful noninvasive monitoring of cardiac function and/or endomyocardial biopsy performed (95, 97, 102). If large doses must be given, very slow rates of infusion decrease peak serum levels and may be beneficial. ICRF187, an iron chelator that may prevent generation of free radicals, has been approved for reducing the risks of DOX-related cardiomyopathy in women with metastatic breast cancer who have received 300 mg/m$^2$ of DOX and who would benefit from continuing DOX therapy with its attendant risks (103). Probucol, a lipid-lowering agent with antioxidant properties, has been shown to reduce cardiomyopathic changes in an animal model but has not yet been evaluated in humans (107). Once heart failure develops, treatment is supportive. Diuretics and inotropic agents such as dobutamine may be used in the acute setting, and the angiotensin-converting enzyme (ACE) inhibitors, digoxin and diuretics may be used chronically. Heart failure is often refractory to therapy, and mortality is between 30% and 60% (100, 102, 108). However, since some investigators have noted reversal of even severe dysfunction (100), a case-by-case approach is warranted.

Acute intravenous overdose of DOX with subsequent heart failure and death has been reported (109), and since many of the early histologic manifestations of toxicity are transient, an aggressive approach which includes both drug elimination and hemodynamic support is warranted (109). Enhanced elimination with hemoperfusion has been successful in a few cases, although because DOX is highly protein bound, therapy is likely to be of benefit only if initiatied within minutes of the overdose (106, 109).

## CALCIUM CHANNEL BLOCKERS

Calcium channel blockers (CCBs) have been increasingly used for a variety of cardiac and noncardiac disorders, including hypertension, angina, coronary artery spasm, Raynaud's phenomenon, stroke and migraine, and CCB toxicity has replaced both beta-blocker and cardiac glycoside toxicity as the leading cause of death secondary to cardiovascular drug overdose (110). It is therefore crucial for the intensivist to understand the important cardiac toxicities of this class of drugs and how to treat them. As is the case with other agents discussed, most of the recommendations made at present are based on animal research with only case reports or small studies available in patients.

## Pharmacology

Calcium normally enters the cells of sinoatrial and AV pacemakers during phase 0 of depolarization; it also assists in maintenance of phase 2 (the plateau phase) of the action potential in myocardial cells. This extracellular source is augmented by the intracellular release of calcium from the sarcoplasmic reticulum via calcium-dependent calcium release channels. This release is crucial for calcium-troponin binding and for excitation-contraction coupling in cardiac myocytes, as well as for the contraction of vascular smooth muscle by the binding of calcium to calmodulin. In general, CCBs block the entry of calcium into cells through attachment to the dihydropyridine receptor on the L-type calcium channel (111). Through their binding to these voltage-sensitive channels, CCBs, to varying degrees, decrease sinoatrial and AV conduction and potentiate vascular smooth muscle dilatation.

Calcium channel blockers can be divided into three classes, each with slightly different pharmacologic activities. The phenylalkylamines, such as verapamil, have potent negative chronotropic and inotropic effects, with less effect on peripheral vasodilatation. The dihydropyridines, such as nifedipine and nicardipine, have more potent vasodilatory effects and may occasionally induce a reflex tachycardia. The effects of the benzothiazepines, such as diltiazem, lie somewhere in-between, with AV node slowing, vascular smooth muscle dilatation, and intermediate effects on inotropy. As a class, CCBs are rapidly and completely absorbed from the GI tract and undergo extensive first-pass metabolism. They are highly protein bound in the serum with sizable volumes of distribution, making their removal by dialysis ineffective. Half-lives for standard preparations range from 3 to 7 hours but can be considerably longer for sustained-release preparations. This can lead to significant extention, delay, or even rebound of toxicity 24 to 36 hours after overdose (112). Several additional pharmacologic properties of CCBs are noteworthy. Their extensive hepatic metabolism makes accumulation and therefore risk of toxicity greater in patients with cirrhosis. By inhibiting hepatic drug metabolism, CCBs, particularly verapamil and diltiazem, can produce toxicity from such hepatically metabolized drugs as carbamazepine, phenytoin, and theophylline. Conversely, when other hepatic microenzyme inhibitors such as cimetidine are used with verapamil, verapamil toxicity may result (3). Finally, as discussed above, coadministration of verapamil and digoxin results in increased digoxin levels.

## Toxicity

The main effects of CCB overdose are cardiovascular and include hypotension, SA and AV node conduction abnormalities, and even pulmonary edema. In addition, CCB overdose can produce nausea, vomiting, hyperglycemia, metabolic acidosis, and CNS hypoperfusion, with lightheadedness, lethargy, change in mental status, seizures, and coma. After initiating standard treatment measures, including lavage (in the setting of early presentation or the ingestion of long-acting preparations) and activated charcoal, it is important to recognize how the pathophysiology of CCB toxicity affects the priority of treatment. The relatively few studies of CCB overdose have documented a rise in right atrial and pulmonary capillary wedge pressures associated with a decrease in peripheral vascular resistance, suggesting depressed cardiac function and peripheral vascular tone. In fact, CCB toxicity has been viewed as a form of cardiogenic shock in which normal compensatory mechanisms, such as reflex tachycardia and peripheral vasoconstriction, cannot occur. Consequently, treatment should first focus on improving myocardial inotropy and chronotropy. Excessive volume infusion that elevates preload, or pressor therapy that increases afterload alone, may only excacerbate the effects of toxicity on a depressed heart (3).

## Treatment

Although fluid overload is potentially deleterious, initial treatment in the hypotensive patient with suspected CCB toxicity should include fluid challenge (110). Calcium salts are the next treatment option for most clinicians; in animal studies and in case reports, they have reversed the negative inotropic effects associated with CCB overdose and at least partially corrected associated AV conduction abnormalities (113, 114). The usual dosage is a 1-g intravenous bolus of calcium chloride (10 mL of 10% solution, or 27% $Ca^{2+}$ by weight) administered over 5 minutes (3) or 3 g of calcium glugonate (111) which may be repeated at 10- to 20-minute intervals up to 3 to 4 times depending on the clinical response (3). As a bolus dose may only transiently elevate blood pressure and cardiac output, a continuous infusion of calcium chloride at a rate of 20 to 50 mg/kg/hr may be used, with adjustment depending upon clinical response (111).

The clinician must be aware, however, of the side effects of bolus infusion of calcium. These include nausea, vomiting, CNS alterations, and acute increases in myocardial oxygen consumption. Measurement of ionized plasma calcium concentrations should be performed 30 minutes after beginning infusion and every 2 hours thereafter (111), and the electrocardiographic manifestations of hypercalcemia, including shortening of the QT interval, high-degree AV block, ventricular tachycardia, and even asystole should be looked for. If present, these electrocardiograhic findings mandate discontinuation of therapy. Calcium should not be administered as a first-line therapy in the setting of known or suspected concomitant digitalis toxicity, as discussed above.

Although calcium is considered first-line therapy in CCB overdose, there are numerous examples in the literature of its failure to increase blood pressure or heart rate

(112, 116, 117). Glucagon, a polypeptide produced by pancreatic alpha cells, acts through nonadrenergic receptors to increase cAMP levels and enhance cardiac inotropy and chronotropy. This agent can be considered as second-line therapy (118). Animal studies have demonstrated its ability to reverse the myocardial depression induced by the three classes of CCBs (119, 120), and it has proved effective in some clinical reports, both alone and in concert with other agents (121–123). Fifty to 150 µg/kg, or an average of 3.5 to 5 mg IV, may be given as a bolus every 15 minutes, followed by a constant infusion of 1 to 5 mg/hr to maintain the effect of the bolus. Administration of greater than 2 mg of glucagon should not be performed in the provided phenol-containing diluent agent, as this may lead to phenol toxicity.

In the patient with profound hypotension and/or bradycardia unresponsive to either calcium or glucagon, it may be prudent to initiate pressor therapy despite the potential risk of increased afterload (117, 124). There is no concensus in the literature as to the most effective agent (111). Dopamine increases blood pressure and cardiac output experimentally (113) and has been the most commonly used pressor in the setting of clinical overdose (114). Epinephrine, based on its combined alpha and beta agonism, is another option (111), and there are reports of the succesful use of amrinone in combination with glucagon and isoproterenol (123, 125). Isoproterenol may increase heart rate in CCBs as well as cardiac inotropy; however, this is at the expense of increased oxygen demand and risk of arrhythmias so it should probably not be employed until other options have been exhausted. When bradycardia is prominent, atropine may be used initially (111), although it is usually ineffective, in which case external or transvenous pacing should be initiated.

## BETA-BLOCKERS

Competitive inhibitors of the beta-adrenergic receptors, beta-blockers are used in a variety of cardiac conditions, including angina, hypertension, prophylaxis following acute MI, congestive heart failure, and mitral valve prolapse syndrome, as well as in such noncardiac conditions as migraine, thyroid storm, and glaucoma (126). Although they are among the most prescribed medications in the United States, the incidence of toxicity with beta-blockers is lower than that noted with other commonly prescribed cardiotonic agents (110). However, their common use, striking chemical properties in the toxic state, and the possibility of reversing toxicity with an "antidote" (75) make it important for the intensivist to understand the principles of treatment in overdose.

## Pathophysiology and Pharmacology

When catecholamines bind to beta receptors, there is phosphorylation of a G-protein complex in the cell membrane. This second-messenger cascade results in cAMP formation within the cell, which in turn stimulates cytosolic protein kinases, leading both to an increased release of intracellular calcium and to an increase in the calcium sensitivity of the sarcomere (111). There are at least two types of beta-receptors (127), and in the cardiovascular system, these have different effects and sites of action (128). The beta-1-receptor is primarily located in the myocardium. When stimulated, it increases cardiac inotropy and conduction velocity and automaticity in the atria, ventricles, AV node, and His-Purkinje system. Beta-1 stimulation also leads to stimulation of renin and antidiuretic hormone (ADH) secretion in the kidney. Beta-2-receptor stimulation leads to dilatation of the coronary, systemic, and pulmonary vascular beds. By competitively binding to these receptor sites, beta-blockers reverse many of the above effects, with important clinical sequelae, such as reduction of cardiac inotropy, chrontropy, and automaticity, reduction of blood pressure, and (with beta-2-receptor blockade) constriction of bronchial smooth muscle.

The peak effect of standard-release beta-blocker preparations is 1 to 4 hours after ingestion, with half-lives ranging from 2 to 12 hours. As with the calcium channel blocking agents, this time frame may be significantly prolonged with sustained-release preparations. The effects of the different beta-blocking agents vary depending on the influence of four important pharmacologic variables: cardioselectivity, lipid solubility, partial agonist activity, and membrane depressant action (126). Agents such as esmolol and metoprolol are primarily beta-1 selective, and peripheral effects such as bronchospasm, glucose imbalance, and vasoconstriction are less likely to occur at therapeutic doses; however, selectivity is lost in overdose (128). Drugs with greater lipid solubility, such as propranolol and acebutolol, cross the blood-brain barrier and are more likely to manifest CNS toxicities such as decreased mentation, respiratory depression, or seizures (111, 126, 129, 130). Beta-blockers with intrinsic sympathomimetic activity, such as oxprenolol or pindolol, stimulate beta-receptors at rest while concomitantly blunting myocardial responsiveness to catecholamines (128). Toxicity with these latter agents is less commonly associated with hypotension or bradycardia, and there have even been reports of hypertensive responses to these agents in overdose (126). A prominent feature of some beta-blockers, most notably propranolol, is the ability to inhibit sodium ion transport. This "membrane stabilization" exerts a depressant effect on cardiac cells similar to that of quinidine. With the possible exception of propranolol, this effect is not seen at therapeutic concentrations (128) but in overdose patients may present with QRS widening and a terminal 40-msec axis shift that reverses with appropriate therapy (75, 130). An obvious but important characteristic of beta-blockers is that they are competitive inhibitors of the beta-receptor.

Case reports and animal studies suggest blockade can often be overcome by high doses of beta-adrenergic agonists (128). Sotalol hydrochloride is another agent with potent nonselective beta-blocking properties, although it is better recognized for its class III antiarrhythmic properties, and as such, prominent toxic manifestations include prolongation of the refractory period, lengthening of the QT interval, and torsade des pointes (see below) (111).

### Toxicity

In general, the clinical picture of beta-blocker toxicity is characterized by bradycardia, hypotension, and a low cardiac output state ultimately leading to shock (126). In a review of reported cases of beta-blocker toxicity in 1984, Weinstein et al. (129) reported that severe toxicity was seen most commonly with propranolol; bradycardia was noted in greater than 90% of patients, and severe hypotension was seen in more than 75%. Electrocardiographic manifestations included first-degree AV block, AV dissociation, right bundle branch block, and intraventricular conduction delay (111, 130). Seizures, noted in more than half of the propranolol toxicities in this series, were likely related to this agent's lipophilic and membrane-stabilizing properties, although seizures have been noted with other agents. In patients with reactive airways, bronchospasm may be a prominent toxic manifestation. Hypoglycemia is not commonly observed (111).

### Treatment

The treatment of beta-blocker toxicity begins with close observation, cardiac monitoring, and early use of lavage and activated charcoal. Syrup of ipecac to induce emesis is contraindicated because of the rapidity with which coma, seizures, and respiratory depression can occur. Volume should be replaced as clinically indicated. Atropine may be used for bradyarrhythmias, but as increased vagal stimulation is not the mechanism of bradycardia, it is unlikely to be successful (129).

Glucagon, an agent which increases myocardial cAMP concentrations independently of catecholamine stimulation, is considered an antidote by many experts (75), and its use in restoring inotropy and chronotropy is supported by case reports (129, 131–133) and animal studies (134–136). Dosage recommendations and caveats to the use of glucagon are the same as with CCB toxicity: 50 to 150 µg/kg, or an average of 3.5 to 5 mg IV, may be given by repeated bolus every 15 minutes, followed by a constant infusion of 1 to 5 mg/hr to maintain the effect of the bolus. There are no more specific therapeutic dosage recommendations, and in fact, glucagon infusions have been continued for greater than 24 hours and cumulative boluses of 30 mg have been used in rare cases (111).

If glucagon as a single agent does not effectively increase heart rate and blood pressure, use of a pressor agent to overcome the myocardial and vasodilatory effects of beta blockade is appropriate. There is no consensus on an agent of choice, and as alluded to above, the dosage that may be needed for a successful response may be much higher than that routinely used in other clinical conditions. In the presence of high serum levels of beta-blocking agents, greater than 1,000-fold increase in agonist may be necessary to overcome blockade (137). Indeed, Agura et al. (132) used 160 to 200 μg/min of isoproterenol in combination with atrial pacing before achieving a palpable blood pressure in one patient. Given these limitations, epinephrine has been successful in raising heart rate and blood pressure (129), although unopposed alpha stimulation in the periphery is a potential problem (137). Isoproterenol, a potent nonselective beta-agonist, has also been used successfully (132), and in the situation of severe toxicity, concern over beta-2-mediated systemic vasodilatation may not apply as beta selectivity is likely overwhelmed (111). Dopamine is another option, although in one series it increased heart rate and blood pressure in a minority of patients (129). There is very limited experience with the use of dobutamine and its first-line use cannot be recommended (111, 137). The cAMP-mediated effects of amrinone would seem to make it an ideal agent used singly or in combination with glucagon. Clinical experience, however, is limited (110), and in a canine model of propranolol toxicity, no increase in heart rate was seen if amrinone was used as a single agent (134), and a trend toward reduction in systemic vascular resistance (SVR) was seen when it was combined with glucagon (135). Prenalterol, a beta-1-selective agonist not available in the United States, has shown promise in experimental models and in case reports (3, 111).

Another treatment modality is insertion of a temporary transvenous pacemaker for persistent bradycardia (129). In severe toxicity, however, myocardial tissue may be refractory to pacing potentials (137). One author has even suggested cardiopulmonary bypass or the placement of an intraaortic balloon pump as temporizing measures in the setting of severe and potentially reversible toxicity (110). Hemodialysis may be considered for agents with limited protein binding, although for those, like sotalol, with a large volume of distribution it is unlikely to be successful (138).

## TORSADE DE POINTES AND TYPE IA AGENTS

Torsade de pointes ("twisting of points") is a form of ventricular tachycardia characteristic of a constellation of conditions, including drug toxicity from many different agents. Its hallmarks are the presence of a prolonged QT interval and QRS complexes of changing amplitude and morphology that appear to twist around an imaginary

baseline (Fig. 1C,D ) (140–143). Although salvos of torsade de pointes (TdP) are usually self-limited, the arrhythmia not infrequently degenerates into ventricular fibrillation. Since TdP is commonly seen in the ICU and has a different treatment approach from standard monomorphic VT, its clinical features, pathophysiology, and therapy must be familiar to the intensivist. (By definition, this discussion focuses on acquired conditions that prolong the QT interval. The reader is referred elsewhere for a discussion of the idiopathic or congenital forms of the long QT syndrome, which are also associated with premature sudden death, likely as a result of TdP (140, 141).

### Electrocardiographic Findings

The electrocardiographic findings of TdP are distinctive. The arrhythmia occurs at rates of 180 to 250 beats/min. The QT-U abnormalities, including prominent U waves, may precede the arrhythmia, and a characteristic long-short R-R sequence may initiate the episode (142). In this scenario, a brief run of tachycardia or an ectopic beat is followed by a posttachycardia pause; the following sinus beat has a proportionately prolonged QT interval. The initiating beat of TdP is then noted on the downstroke of the T wave. Although the long-short sequence is characteristic of drug-induced TdP (144), it is not an invariable finding.

### Etiology

Antiarrhythmic drugs are the most common cause of TdP in the ICU. The most commonly recognized agent is the type Ia antiarrhythmic drug, quinidine (143), although the other drugs in this class, disopyramide and procainamide, also cause TdP. Characteristically, type I toxicity manifests as prolongation of the QT interval and TdP at therapeutic or even subtherapeutic levels (144). Sotalol, a type III antiarrhythmic agent with beta-blocking properties (145), has been implicated, often in concert with predisposing factors such as bradycardia, hypokalemia, or concurrent use of other QT-prolonging drugs (145, 146). In contrast, amiodarone, also a type III agent, is associated with a low incidence of TdP (147). Likewise, type IC agents such as encainide or flecainide, although frequently associated with proarrhythmic monomorphic ventricular tachycardia in subpopulations of patients, are uncommonly a cause of TdP (141). Type IB agents have rarely been associated with TdP (146).

A number of important classes of noncardiovascular drugs cause TdP. The neuroleptic phenothiazines have electrophysiologic effects similar to class IA antiarrhythmics and induce T-wave abnormalities, QT prolongation, and TdP (140). The agent thioridazine has been implicated as a cause of sudden death in patients with schizophrenia. The butyrophenone haloperidol may also cause QT prolongation and TdP (141, 149). In addition to their many other cardiovascular effects, the cyclic antidepressants (see above), which also have class IA antiarrhythmic properties, may also cause TdP (143, 149).

Certain antibiotics have also been implicated. Pentamidine in particular, possibly due to its structural similarity to procainamide, has been associated with QT prolongation and TdP (149), although the exact incidence of this complication is undefined. Eisenhauer et al. (150) prospectively evaluated 14 patients receiving intravenous pentamidine for *Pneumocystis carinii* pneumonia, and of the 5 patients who developed QTc prolongation greater than 0.48 second on therapy, 3 developed TdP. The authors identified no baseline clinical variables or electrolyte abnormalities associated with QT prolongation or TdP. They suggested that an increase in QTc greater than 0.48 second or an absolute increase in QT of greater than 0.08 second predisposed to TdP. They recommended that all patients receiving intravenous pentamidine obtain a baseline and daily EKG for the first week of therapy, with continuous cardiac monitoring or alternate drug therapy if QT prolongation is seen. Amantadine, which has a chemical structure that is similar to the tricyclic antidepressants, has also been associated with TdP (149). Administration of erythromycin may cause TdP by modifying the metabolism of other agents (see below) or by its ability to increase action potential duration in a manner similar to that of the class IA agents (142, 149).

The nonsedating antihistamines astemizole and terfenadine can cause QT prolongation (141, 151, 152). These drugs undergo significant metabolism by P-450 oxidative pathways in the liver into inactive drug metabolites. Overdosage, hepatic disease, or concomitant drug therapy with agents that also utilize the P-450 system, such as ketoconazole or erythromycin, may lead to drug accumulation and TdP (144, 152).

Besides drugs, there are important electrolyte abnormalities, metabolic derangements, and miscellaneous conditions in which TdP can be seen. Hypokalemia and hypomagnesemia can prolong the QT interval, and these effects may act synergistically with intercurrent pharmacologic therapy to prolong the QT interval (142, 144). Hypocalcemia, although leading to QT prolongation, has rarely been associated with TdP (140). The liquid protein modified fast diet, with and without associated electrolyte abnormalities, has been associated with TdP (140, 142). Organophosphate toxicity, with enhanced parasympathetic tone, ST-T wave abnormalities, and rate-related QT prolongation, has also been implicated (140, 149). Severe bradyarrhythmias, such as complete AV block, may cause TdP (140, 141), as may medical conditions associated with enhanced autonomic tone, such as CNS insults like subarachnoid hemorrhage and stroke (141, 143).

## Pathophysiology

The mechanisms responsible for TdP are unclear, but there are several hypotheses. When conduction tissue is exposed to experimental conditions that mimic the clinical milieu of TdP (such as quinidine in combination with hypokalemia, hypomagnesemia, or bradycardia), prolongation of the action potential and repolarization abnormalities occur (153). These changes can lead to the appearance of early afterdepolarizations (EADs) originating from phases 2 or 3 of the action potential. These, in turn, can lead to triggered activity (154). El-Sherif and colleagues (155) supported the role of EADs and triggered activity by recording right ventricular monophasic action potentials in a patient with quinidine-induced long QT interval and TdP. They noted deflections during phase 3 of depolarization that were characteristic of EADs and that were synchronous with the U wave on the surface EKG.

Brachmann et al. (156) used cesium to investigate bradycardia-dependent triggered activity in a canine model. Among its other actions, cesium prolongs the action potential in Purkinje fibers by depressing outward potassium currents that normally assist in repolarization ("rectifying currents"). Cesium induced QT prolongation, ventricular ectopy and TdP-like ventricular activity in vivo, and EADs were seen in phase 3 of Purkinje fiber action potentials in vitro. These effects were more pronounced at lower heart rates and could be suppressed by pacing. In addition, EADs were abolished by tetrodotoxin, an agent known to block sodium currents. An inward-flowing, noninactivated sodium current that flows during the plateau of the action potential may have been involved in the generation of triggered activity at slow heart rates. Bailie et al. (158) studied the effect of magnesium on a similar model of cesium-induced EADs in isolated canine Purkinje fibers and noted a decrease in the amplitude of EADs and in the induction of TdP that was not rate-related. These investigators suggested that magnesium modified current flow, either by enhancing outward potassium currents or by blocking slow inward sodium or calcium currents.

Compelling evidence in support of the theory that modification of either sodium or outward rectifying potassium currents is involved in TdP comes from recent genetic linkage studies of family cohorts with congenital long QT syndrome and sudden death (158, 159). In several of these families, point mutations and/or deletions have been identified in genes expressed in the heart which encode human homologues of a delayed outward potassium channel (the so-called ether a-go-go gene) or a skeletal muscle sodium channel. These studies strongly suggest that functional abnormalities in these genes with consequent abnormalities of current flow are associated with QT prolongation and TdP.

Some additional points are noteworthy. Early afterdepolarizations have been most easily elicited from Purkinje fibers, which comprise only a small percentage of myocardial tissue. Recently, a unique subpopulation of subepicardial cells, termed M cells, have been identified that appear to share electrophysiologic properties with Purkinje fibers (143, 154). The action potential of M cells prolongs in a rate-dependent fashion and, in addition, these cells demonstrate EAD-induced triggered activity in the presence of such agents as quinidine and cesium, which suggests that similar cells might contribute to the initiation of TdP in the human heart (143, 154). Finally, it has long been noted that TdP cannot be easily generated in the electrophysiology laboratory by the administration of premature extrastimuli, arguing that reentry is not the mechanism of initiation (143). However, conditions that lead to EADs and triggered activity may also produce marked dispersion of repolarization with refractoriness between the conduction system and the myocardium, or within the myocardium itself (142, 154). This may allow for the generation of reentrant circuits that propagate the triggered rhythms of TdP.

## Treatment

Treatment of TdP differs from that of conventional monomorphic ventricular tachycardia, so the initial evaluation should include a careful review of the EKG. As many electrocardiographic leads as possible should be evaluated during tachycardia since the characteristic twisting morphology of TdP may not be apparent on a single limb or monitor lead (160). QT prolongation and T- and U-wave abnormalities should be searched for both at baseline and following extrasystoles, where they may be especially prominent (144). Keren and colleagues (161) noted that absolute QT prolongation was a more sensitive predictor of the development of TdP than the QTc: All patients in their series who eventually manifested TdP had a significant bradycardia and a QT interval longer than 0.60 second.

Initial treatment should include cardiac monitoring and immediate discontinuation of all potential etiologic agents. Serum electrolytes should be evaluated and abnormalities, especially hypomagnesemia and hypokalemia, corrected. If TdP is sustained or causes hemodynamic compromise, electrical cardioversion should be used as a temporizing measure (146), although it is unlikely to prevent recurrence of the arrhythmia (161).

Specific interventions can be divided into those that will and those that will not shorten the QT interval (144). The former includes increasing heart rate by administration of isoproterenol, or cardiac pacing. Although atropine may be used initially, it is rarely effective and may worsen His-Purkinje conduction in patients with high-degree AV block (142, 161). Isoproterenol infusion, at rates of 2 to 8 µg/min, is usually effective in suppressing TdP (146, 161). However, these

doses may precipitate other ventricular arrhythmias in patients with concurrent cardiac disorders (149). Therefore, isoproterenol should not be considered the definitive treatment of TdP (142). Temporary cardiac pacing at rates greater than 90 beats/min has also proven effective in treatment of TdP (142, 161) and avoids the potential complications associated with intravenous agents.

Intravenous magnesium suppresses recurrent drug-induced TdP without affecting the QT interval (144, 162), possibly through enhancement of potassium rectifier currents or through inhibition of calcium channels or transmembrane calcium flow (162, 163). In a series of 12 consecutive patients with acquired TdP, Tzivoni et al. (162) showed that a bolus of 2 g magnesium sulfate administered over 1 to 2 minutes abolished the arrhythmia within 5 minutes of administration in nine patients; TdP was suppressed in an additional three patients after a repeat bolus. These patients were then treated with a continuous infusion of magnesium, 3 to 20 mg/min (as well as potassium supplementation for hypokalemia), until the QT interval decreased to less than 0.50 sec and all remained in a stable rhythm. In light of this, magnesium bolus, followed by continuous infusion, may be considered either a primary therapy or an interim treatment until pacing can be initiated (162). Decreased tendon reflexes on physical exam, conduction defects on EKG, and serum magnesium levels should be followed for evidence of hypermagnesemia (163).

Finally, antiarrhythmic agents that do not prolong the QT interval, such as lidocaine, mexiletine, bretylium, and dilantin, may be used in the setting of TdP, although the treatment strategies outlined above are more likely to be successful (149, 161). Lidocaine, which blocks the sodium repolarization current and prevents EAD, has a variable effect on TdP (143), and beta-blockers, which are very effective in congenital long QT syndromes, are relatively contraindicated in the acquired variants because of the secondary bradycardia.

## CONCLUSION

From this noninclusive review, it should be clear that exposure to many drugs and environmental agents can result in profound and life-threatening cardiovascular complications. The modern-day ICU is confronted with these complications on a daily basis, and the intensivist must be familiar with a large number of specific treatment strategies, involving unique pharmacologic agents (such as digoxin-specific Fab fragments), physiologically based drug neutralization (alkalinization for cyclic antidepressants), and even mechanical interventions (pacing for TdP). A high index of suspicion, an appreciation of the physiology and pharmacology of specific toxicities, and the prompt recognition of clinical patterns of presentation are all essential first steps in the successful treatment of these toxicities.

## REFERENCES

1. Crawley IS, Schlant RC. Effect of non-cardiac drugs, electricity, poisons and radiation on the heart. In: Schlant RC, Alexander WA, O'Rourke RA, Roberts R, Sonnenblick EH, eds. *Hurst's the heart.* 8th ed. New York: McGraw-Hill; 1994:1989.
2. Wynne J, Braunwald E. The cardiomyopathies and myocarditides: toxic, chemical and physical damage to the heart. In: Braunwald E., ed. *Heart disease, a textbook of cardiovascular medicine.* 4th ed. Philadelphia: WB Saunders; 1992:1394.
3. Snook CP, Otten EJ. Effect of toxins on the heart. In: Gibler WB, Aufderheide TP, eds. *Emergency cardiac care.* St Louis, MO: Mosby; 1994:549.
4. Nelson L, Hoffman, RS. What to do when drug poisoning causes tachycardia. *J Crit Illness* 1994;9(9):831.
5. Taitelman U, Ellenhorn MJ. General management of poisoning. In: Hall JB, Schmidt GA, Wood LDH, eds. *Principles of critical care.* New York: McGraw-Hill; 1992:2051.
6. Mouhaffel AH, Madu EC, Satmary WA, Fraker TD. Cardiovascular complications of cocaine. *Chest* 1995;107:1426.
7. Kloner RA, Hale S, Alker K, et al. The effects of acute and chronic cocaine use on the heart. *Circulation* 1992;85(2):407.
8. Zimmerman FH, Gustafson GM, Kemp HG. Recurrent myocardial infarction associated with cocaine abuse in a young man with normal coronary arteries: evidence for coronary artery spasm culminating in thrombosis. *J Am Coll Cardiol* 1987;9:964.
9. Lange RA, Cigarroa RG, Yancy CW, et al. Cocaine-induced coronary-artery vasoconstriction. *N Engl J Med* 1989;321:1557.
10. Lange RA, Cigarroa RG, Flores ED, et al. Potentiation of cocaine-induced coronary vasoconstriction by beta-adrenergic blockade. *Ann Intern Med* 1990;112:897.
11. Moliterno DJ, Willard JE, Lange RA, et al. Coronary-artery vasoconstriction induced by cocaine, cigarette smoking, or both. *N Engl J Med* 1994;330:454.
12. Flores ED, Lange RA, Cigarroa RG, et al. Effect of cocaine on coronary artery dimensions in atherosclerotic coronary artery disease: enhanced vasoconstriction at significant stenoses. *J Am Coll Cardiol* 1990;16:74.
13. Brogan WC, Lange RA, Kim AS, et al. Alleviation of cocaine-induced coronary vasoconstriction by nitroglycerin. *J Am Coll Cardiol* 1991;18:581.
14. Hollander JE, Carter WA. Use of phentolamine for cocaine-induced myocardial ischemia [Letter]. *N Engl J Med* 1992;327(5):361.
15. Virmani R, Robinowitz M, Smialek JE, et al. Cardiovascular effects of cocaine: an autopsy study of 40 patients. *Am Heart J* 1988;115:1068.
16. Togna G, Tempesta E, Togna AR, et al. Platelet responsiveness and biosynthesis of thromboxane and prostacyclin in response to in vitro cocaine treatment. *Haemostasis* 1985;15:100.
17. Kugelmass AD, Oda A, Monahan K, Cabral C, Ware A. Activation of human platelets by cocaine. *Circulation* 1993;88:876.
18. Tokarski GF. Cocaine-associated chest pain. In: Gibler WB, Aufderheide TP, eds. *Emergency cardiac care.* St Louis, MO: Mosby; 1994:328.
19. Barth CW III, Bray M, Roberts WC. Rupture of the ascending aorta during cocaine intoxication. *Am J Cardiol* 1986;57:496.
20. Hollander JE, Hoffman RS. Cocaine-induced myocardial infarction: an analysis and review of the literature. *J Emerg Med* 1992;10:169.
21. Lewin NA, Goldfrank LR, Hoffman RS. Cocaine. In: Goldfrank LR, ed. *Goldfrank's toxicologic emergencies.* 5th ed. Norwalk: Appleton and Lange; 1994:847.
22. Isner JM, Estes NAM, Thompson PD, et al. Acute cardiac events temporally related to cocaine abuse. *N Engl J Med* 1986;315:1438.
23. Zimmerman J, Dellinger RP, Majid PA. Cocaine-associated chest pain. *Ann Emerg Med* 1991;20(6):611.
24. Amin M, Gabelman G, Karpel J, et al. Acute myocardial infarction and chest pain syndromes after cocaine use. *Am J Cardiol* 1990;66:1434.
25. Nelson L, Hoffman RS. How to manage acute MI when cocaine is the cause. *J Crit Illness* 1995;10(1):39.
26. Brogan WC, Lange RA, Glamann DB, et al. Recurrent coronary vasoconstriction caused by intranasal cocaine: possible role for metabolites. *Ann Intern Med* 1992;116:556.
27. Nademanee K, Gorelick DA, Josephson MA, et al. Myocardial ischemia during cocaine withdrawal. *Ann Intern Med* 1989;111:876.
28. Roth D, Alarcon FJ, Fernandez JA, et al. Acute rhabdomyolysis associated with cocaine intoxication. *N Engl J Med* 1988;319:673.
29. Bush HS. Cocaine-associated myocardial infarction: a word of caution about thrombolytic therapy. *Chest* 1988;94:878.
30. Hollander JE, Burstein JL, Hoffman RS, Shih RD, Wilson LD, Cocaine Associated Myocardial Infarction (CAMI) study group. Cocaine-associated myocardial infarction: clinical safety of thrombolytic therapy. *Chest* 1995;107:1237.
31. Hollander JE. The Management of cocaine-associated myocardial ischemia. *N Eng J Med* 1995;333:1267.
32. Pimentel L, Trommer L. Cyclic antidepressant overdoses. A review. *Emerg Med Clin North Am* 1994;12(2):533.
33. Callaham M. Epidemiology of fatal tricyclic antidepressant ingestion: implications for management. *Ann Emerg Med* 1985;14(1):29.
34. Lipper B, Bell A, Gaynor B. Recurrent hypotension immediately after seizures in nortriptyline overdose. *Am J Emerg Med* 1994;12:452.
35. Marshall JB, Forker AD. Cardiovascular effects of tricyclic antidepressant drugs. *Am Heart J* 1982;103:401.
36. Smilkstein MJ. Reviewing cyclic antidepressant toxicity: wheat and chaff. *J Emerg Med* 1990;8:645.
37. Boehnert MT, Lovejoy FH. Value of the QRS duration versus the serum drug level in predicting seizures and ventricular arrhythmias after an acute overdose of tricyclic antidepressants. *N Engl J Med* 1985;313:474.
38. Newton EH, Shih RD, Hoffman RS. Cyclic antidepressant overdose: a review of current management strategies. *Am J Emerg Med* 1994; 12:376.
39. Foulke GE, Albertson TE, Walby WF. Tricyclic antidepressant overdose: emergency department findings as predictors of clinical course. *Am J Emerg Med* 1986;4:496.
40. Wolfe TR, Caravati EM, Rollins DE. Terminal 40-ms frontal plane QRS axis as a marker for tricyclic antidepressant overdose. *Ann Emerg Med* 1989;18:348.
41. Vernon DD, Banner W, Garrett JS, et al. Efficacy of dopamine and norepinephrine for treatment of hemodynamic compromise in amitriptyline intoxication. *Crit Care* 1991;19:544.
42. Teba L, Schiebel F, Dedhia HV, et al. Beneficial effect of norepinephrine in the treatment of circulatory shock caused by antidepressant overdose. *Am J Emerg Med* 1988;6:566.
43. Rossing TH. Methyxanthines in 1989. *Ann Intern Med* 1989;110(7):502.
44. Stork CM, Howland MA, Goldfrank LR. Concepts and controversies of bronchodilator overdose. *Emerg Med Clin North Am* 1994;12(2):415.
45. Murciano D, Auclair MH, Pariente R, et al. A randomized, controlled trial of theophylline in patients with severe chronic obstructive pulmonary disease. *N Engl J Med* 1989;320:1521.
46. Gaudreault P, Guay J. Theophylline poisoning: pharmacologic considerations and clinical management. *Med Toxicol Rev* 1986;1:169.
47. Weisman RS, Goldfrank LR, Howland MA. Theophylline. In: Goldfrank LR, ed. *Goldfrank's toxicologic emergencies.* 5th ed. Norwalk: Appleton and Lange; 1994:565.
48. Hall KW, Dobson KE, Dalton JG, et al. Metabolic abnormalities associated with intentional theophylline overdose. *Ann Intern Med* 1984;101:457.
49. Vestal RE, Erickson CE, Musser B, et al. Effect of intravenous aminophylline on plasma levels of catecholamines and related cardiovascular and metabolic responses in man. *Circulation* 1983;67(1):162.
50. Gaar GG, Banner W. The effects of esmolol on the hemodynamics of acute theophylline toxicity. *Ann Emerg Med* 1987;16:1334.
51. Kearney TE, Manoguerra AS, Curtis GP, et al. Theophylline toxicity and the beta-adrenergic system. *Ann Intern Med* 1985;102:766.
52. Biberstein MP, Ziegler MG, Ward DM. Use of beta-blockade and hemoperfusion for acute theophylline poisoning. *West J Med* 1984; 141:485.
53. Rutherford JD, Vatner SF, Braunwald E. Effects and mechanism of action of aminophylline on cardiac function and regional blood flow distribution in conscious dogs. *Circulation* 1981;63(2):378.
54. Greenberg A, Piraino BH, Kroboth PD, et al. Severe theophylline toxicity: role of conservative measures, antiarrhythmic agents, and charcoal hemoperfusion. *Am J Med* 1984;76:854.

55. Horowitz LN, Spear JF, Moore EN, et al. Effects of aminophylline on the threshold for initiating ventricular fibrillation during respiratory failure. *Am J Cardiol* 1975;35:376.

56. Shannon M. Predictors of major toxicity after theophylline overdose. *Ann Intern Med* 1993;119:1161.

57. Shannon M, Lovejoy FH. The influence of age vs. peak serum concentration on life-threatening events after chronic theophylline intoxication. *Arch Intern Med* 1990;150:2045.

58. Berlinger WG, Spector R, Goldberg MJ, Johnson GF, Quee CK, Berg MJ. Enhancement of theophylline clearance by oral activated charcoal. *Clin Pharmacol Ther* 1983;33:351.

59. True RJ, Berman JM, Mahutte CK. *Crit Care Med* 1984;12(2):113.

60. Gal P, Miller A, McCue JD. Oral activated charcoal to enhance theophylline elimination in an acute overdose. *JAMA* 1984;251(23):3130.

61. Amitai Y, Yeung AC, Moye J, et al. Repetitive oral activated charcoal and control of emesis in severe theophylline toxicity. *Ann Intern Med* 1986;105(3):386.

62. Levy G. Gastrointestinal clearance of drugs with activated charcoal *N Engl J Med* 1982;307:676.

63. Henderson A, Wright DM, Pond SM. Management of theophylline overdose patients in the intensive care unit. *Anaesth Intens Care* 1992;20:56.

64. Lynn KL, Buttimore AL, Begg EJ, et al. Treatment of theophylline poisoning with haemoperfusion. *N Zealand Med J* 1988;101:4.

65. Park GD, Spector R, Roberts RJ, et al. Use of hemoperfusion for treatment of theophylline intoxication. *Am J Med* 1983;74:961.

66. Curry SC, Vance MV, Requa R, et al. Cardiovascular effects of toxic concentrations of theophylline in the dog. *Ann Emerg Med* 1985;14:547.

67. Hoffman RS, Chiang WK, Howland MA, Weisman RS, Goldfrank LR. Theophylline desorption from activated charcoal caused by whole bowel irrigation solution. *Clin Toxicol* 1991;29(2):191.

68. Bernstein G, Jehle D, Bernaski E, Braen GR. Failure of gastric emptying and charcoal administration in fatal sustained-release theophylline overdose: pharmacobezoar formation. *Ann Emerg Med* 1992;21(11):1388.

69. Marcus FI. Digitalis. In: Schlant RC, Alexander WA, O'Rourke RA, Roberts R, Sonnenblick EH, eds. *Hurst's the heart.* 8th ed. New York: McGraw-Hill; 1994:573.

70. Smith TW. Digitalis. Mechanisms of action and clinical use. *N Engl J Med* 1988;318(6):358.

71. Watanabe AM. Digitalis and the autonomic nervous system. *J Am Coll Cardiol* 1985;5:35A.

72. Rosen MR. Cellular electrophysiology of digitalis toxicity. *J Am Coll Cardiol* 1985;5:22A.

73. Lewin NA. Digitalis. In: Goldfrank LR, ed. *Goldfrank's toxicologic emergencies.* 5th ed. Norwalk: Appleton and Lange; 1994:685.

74. Smith TW, Braunwald E, Kelly RA. The management of heart failure. In: Braunwald E, ed. *Heart disease, a textbook of cardiovascular medicine.* 4th ed. Philadelphia: WB Saunders; 1992:490.

75. Nelson L, Hoffman RS. Effective strategies for drug-induced bradycardia and heart block. *J Crit Illness* 1994;9(10):916.

76. Lip GYH, Metcalfe MJ, Dunn FG. Diagnosis and treatment of digoxin toxicity. *Postgrad Med J* 1993;69:337.

77. Lee TC. Van Gogh's vision: digitalis intoxication? *JAMA* 1981;245:727.

78. Bismuth C, Gaultier M, Conso F, Efthymiou ML. Hyperkalemia in acute digitalis poisoning. Prognostic significance and therapeutic implications. *Clin Toxicol* 1973;6(2):153.

79. Karkal SS. Digitalis intoxication: dealing rapidly and effectively with a complex cardiac toxidrome. *Emerg Med Repts* 1991;12:29.

80. Smith TW. Pharmacokinetics, bioavailability and serum levels of cardiac glycosides. *J Am Coll Cardiol* 1985;5:43A.

81. Chou TC. Effect of drugs on the electrocardiogram. In: Chou TC, ed. *Electrocardiography in clinical practice.* 3rd ed. Philadelphia: WB Saunders; 1991:459.

82. Ganz LI, Friedman PL. Supraventricular tachycardia. *N Eng J Med* 1995;332:162.

83. Beller GA, Smith TW, Abelman WH, Haber E, Hood WB. Digitalis intoxication. A prospective clinical study serum level correlations. *N Engl J Med* 1971;284(18):989.

84. Lalonde RL, Deshpande R, Hamilton PP, McLean WM, Greenway DC. Acceleration of digoxin clearance by activated charcoal. *Clin Pharmacol Ther* 1985;37:367.

85. Howland MA. Digoxin-specific antibody fragments (Fab). In: Goldfrank LR, ed. *Goldfrank's toxicologic emergencies.* 5th ed. Norwalk: Appleton and Lange; 1994:685.

86. Smith TW, Haber E, Yeatman L, Butler VP. Reversal of advanced digoxin intoxication with Fab fragments of digoxin-specific antibodies. *N Engl J Med* 1976;294(15):797.

87. Smith TW, Butler VP, Haber E, et al. Treatment of life-threatening digitalis intoxication with digoxin-specific Fab antibody fragments. *N Engl J Med* 1982;307(22):1357.

88. Antman EM, Wenger TL, Butler VP, Haber E, Smith TW. Treatment of 150 cases of life-threatening digitalis intoxication with digoxin-specific fab antibody fragments. Final report of a multicenter study. *Circulation* 1990;81:1744.

89. Smith TW. Review of clinical experience with digoxin immune fab (ovine). *Am J Emerg Med* 1991;9:1.

90. Ujhelyi MR, Robert S, Cummings DM, et al. Influence of digoxin immune fab therapy and renal dysfunction on the disposition of total and free digoxin. *Ann Intern Med* 1993;119:273.

91. Rabetoy GM, Christy AP, Findlay JWA, Sailstad JM. Treatment of digoxin intoxication in a renal failure patient with digoxin-specific antibody fragments and plasmapheresis. *Am J Nephrol* 1990;10:518.

92. Reisdorff EJ, Clark MR, Walters BL. Acute digitalis poisoning: the role of intravenous magnesium sulfate. *J Emerg Med* 1986;4:463.

93. Bismuth C, Motte G, Conso F, Chauvin M, Gaultier M. Acute digitoxin intoxication treated by intracardiac pacemaker: experience in sixty-eight patients. *Clin Toxicol* 1977;10(4):443.

94. Taboulet P, Baud FJ, Bismuth C, Vicaut E. Acute digitalis intoxication-is pacing still appropriate? [Abstract]. *Clin Toxicol* 1993;31(2):261.

95. Allen A. The cardiotoxicity of chemotherapeutic drugs. *Semin Oncol* 1992;19(5):529.

96. Bristow MR, Mason JW, Billingham ME, Daniels JR. Doxorubicin cardiomyopathy: evaluation by phonocardiography, endomyocardial biopsy, and cardiac catheterization. *Ann Intern Med* 1978;88:168.

97. Kantrowitz NE, Bristow MR. Cardiotoxicity of antitumor agents. *Prog Cardiovasc Dis* 1984;27(3):195.

98. Bristow MR, Mason J, Billingham ME, Daniels JR. Dose-effect and structure-function relationships in doxorubicin cardiomyopathy. *Am Heart J* 1981;102:709.

99. Luce RK, Curran CF. Doxorubicin cardiotoxicity. In: Baskin SI, ed. *Principles of cardiac toxicology.* Boca Raton, FL: CRC; 1991.

100. Porembka DT, Lowder JN, Orlowski JP, Bastulli J, Lockrem J. Etiology and management of doxorubicin cardiotoxicity. *Crit Care Med* 1989;17(6):569.

101. Von Hoff DD, Layard MW, Basa P, et al. Risk factors for doxorubicin-induced congestive heart failure. *Ann Intern Med* 1979;91:710.

102. Rosenthal DS, Braunwald E. Hematologic-oncological disorders and heart disease. In: Braunwald E, ed. *Heart disease, a textbook of cardiovascular medicine.* 4th ed. Philadelphia: WB Saunders; 1992:1754.

103. Frishman WH, Sung HM, Yee HCM, et al. Cardiovascular toxicity with cancer chemotherapy. *Curr Probl Cardiol* 1996;21:246.

104. Speyer JL, Green MD, Kramer E, et al. Protective effect of the bispiperazinedione ICRF-187 against doxorubicin-induced cardiac toxicity in women with advanced breast cancer. *N Engl J Med* 1988;319:745.

105. Bullock FA, Gabriel HM, Jakhill A, Mott MG, Martin RP. Cardioprotection by ICRF 187 against high dose anthracycline toxicity in children with malignant disease. *Br Heart J* 1993;70:185.

106. Wang RY, Calabresi P. Antineoplastic agents. In: Goldfrank LR, ed. *Goldfrank's toxicologic emergencies.* 5th ed. Norwalk: Appleton and Lange; 1994:685.

107. Siveski-Iliskovic N, Hill M, Chow DA, Singal PK. Probocol protects against adriamycin cardiomyopathy without interfering with its anti-tumor effect. *Circulation* 1995;91:10.

108. Haq MM, Legha SS, Choksi J, et al. Doxorubicin-induced congestive heart failure in adults. *Cancer* 1985;56:1361.

109. Curran CF. Acute doxorubicin overdoses [Letter]. *Ann Intern Med* 1991;115(11):913.

110. Lewin NA. Antihypertensive agents. In: Goldfrank LR, ed. *Goldfrank's toxicologic emergencies.* 5th ed. Norwalk: Appleton and Lange; 1994:701.

111. Kerns W, Kline J, Ford MD. Beta-blocker and calcium channel blocker toxicity. *Emerg Med Clin North Am* 1994;12(2):365.

112. Horowitz BZ, Rhee KJ. Massive verapamil ingestion: a report of two cases and a review of the literature. *Am J Emerg Med* 1989;7:624.

113. Gay R, Algeo S, Lee R, et al. Treatment of verapamil toxicity in intact dogs. *J Clin Invest* 1986;77:1805.

114. Ramoska EA, Spiller HA, Winter M, et al. A one-year evaluation of calcium channel blocker overdoses: toxicity and treatment. *Ann Emerg Med* 1993;22:196.

115. Chou T. Electrolyte imbalance. In: *Electrocardiography in clinical practice*. 3rd ed. Philadelphia: WB Saunders; 1991:495.

116. Crump BJ, Holt DW, Vale JA. Lack of response to intravenous calcium in severe verapamil poisoning. *Lancet* 1982;2:939.

117. Ramoska EA, Spiller HA, Myers A. Calcium channel blocker toxicity. *Ann Emerg Med* 1990;19:649.

118. Howland MA, Glucagon. In: Goldfrank CR, ed. *Goldfrank's toxicologic emergencies*. 5th ed. Norwalk: Appleton and Lange; 1994:713.

119. Jolly SR, Kipnis JN, Lucchesi BR. Cardiovascular depression by verapamil: reversal by glucagon and interactions with propranolol. *Pharmacology* 1987;35:249.

120. Zaritsky AL, Horotwitz M, Chernow B. Glucagon antagonism of calcium channel blocker induced myocardial dysfunction. *Crit Care Med* 1988;16:246.

121. Doyon S, Roberts JR. The use of glucagon in a case of calcium channel blocker overdose. *Ann Emerg Med* 1993;22:1229.

122. Walter FG, Frye G, Mullen JT, et al. Amelioration of nifedipine poisoning associated with glucagon therapy. *Ann Emerg Med* 1993;22:1234.

123. Wolf LR, Spadafora MP, Otten ED. Use of amrinone and glucagon in a case of calcium channel blocker overdose. *Ann Emerg Med* 1993;22 (7):1225.

124. Erickson FC, Ling LJ, Grande GA, et al. Diltiazem overdose: case report and review. *J Emerg Med* 1991;9:357.

125. Goenen M, Col J, Compere A, et al. Treatment of severe verapamil poisoning with combined amrinone-isoproterenol therapy. *Am J Cardiol* 58:1142.

126. Frishman W, Jacob H, Einsenberg E, Ribner H. Clinical pharmacology of the new beta-adrenergic blocking drugs. Part 8. Self-poisoning with beta-adrenoceptor blocking agents: recognition and management. *Am Heart J* 1979;98(6):798.

127. Stiles GL. Structure and function of cardiovascular membranes, channels, and receptors. In: Schlant RC, Alexander WA, O'Rourke R, Roberts R, Sonnenblick EH, eds. *Hurst's the Heart*. 8th ed. New York: McGraw-Hill; 1994:47.

128. Clark BJ. Beta-adrenoceptor-blocking agents: are pharmacologic differences relevant? *Am Heart J* 1982;104:334.

129. Weinstein RS. Recognition and management of poisoning with beta-adrenergic blocking agents. *Ann Emerg Med* 1984;13:1123.

130. Buiumsohn A, Eisenberg ES, Jacob H, et al. Seizures and intraventricular conduction defect in propranolol poisoning. *Ann Intern Med* 1979;91:860.

131. Kosinski EJ, Stein S, Malindzak GS, et al. Glucagon and propranolol (Inderal) toxicity [Letter]. *N Engl J Med* 1971;285(23):1325.

132. Agura ED, Wexler LF, Witzburg RA. Massive propranolol overdose: successful treatment with high-dose isoproterenol and glucagon. *Am J Med* 1986;80:755.

133. O'Mahoney D, O'Leary P, Molloy MG. Severe oxprenolol poisoning: the importance of glucagon infusion. *Human Exper Toxicol* 1990;9:101.

134. Love JN, Leasure JA, Mundt DJ. A comparison of combined amrinone and glucagon therapy to glucagon alone for cardiovascular depression associated with propranolol toxicity in a canine model. *Am J Emerg Med* 1993;11:360.

135. Love JN, Leasure JA, Mundt DJ, Ganz GJ. A comparison of combined amrinone and glucagon therapy to glucagon alone for cardiovascular depression associated with propranolol toxicity in a canine model. *Clin Toxicol* 1992;30(3):399.

136. Lucchesi BR. Cardiac actions of glucagon. *Circ Res* 1968;22:777.

137. Critchley JAJH, Ungar A. The management of acute poisoning due to B-adrenoceptor antagonists. *Med Toxicol* 1989;4:32.

138. Perrot D, Bui-Xuan B, Lang J, Bouffard Y, Delafosse B, Faucon G, et al. A case of sotalol poisoning with fatal outcome. *Clin Toxicol* 1988; 26(5,6):389.

139. Adlerfliegel F, Leeman M, Demaeyer P, Kahn RJ. Sotalol poisoning associated with asystole. *Intern Care Med* 1993;19:57.

140. Jackman WM, Friday KJ, Anderson JL, et al. The long QT syndromes: a critical review, new clinical observations and a unifying hypothesis. *Prog Cardiovasc Dis* 1988;31(2):115.

141. Ben-David J, Zipes DP. Torsades de pointes and proarrhythmia. *Lancet* 1993;341:1578.

142. Napolitano C, Priori SG, Schwartz PJ. Torsade de pointes: mechanisms and management. *Drugs* 1994;47(1):51.

143. Tan TL, Hou CJY, Lauer MR, Sung RJ. Electrophysiologic mechanisms of the lung QT interval syndromes and torsade de pointes. *Ann Intern Med* 1995;122:701.

144. Roden DM. Torsade de pointes. *Clin Cardiol* 1993;16:683.

145. Hohnloser SH, Woosley RL. Sotalol. *N Engl J Med* 1994;331(1):31.

146. Kerin NZ, Somberg J. Proarrhythmia: definition, risk factors, causes, treatment and controversies. *Am Heart J* 1994;128:575.

147. Hohnloser SH, Klingenheben T, Singh BM. Amiodarone-associated proarrhythmic effects. A review with special reference to torsade de pointes tachycardia. *Ann Intern Med* 1994;121:529.

148. DiSalvo TG, O'Gara PT. Torsade de pointes caused by high-dose intravenous haloperidol in cardiac patients. *Clin Cardiol* 1995;18:285.

149. Martyn R, Somberg JC, Kerin NZ. Proarrhythmia and antiarrhytmic drugs. *Am Heart J* 1993;126:201.

150. Eisenhauer M, Eliasson AH, Taylor AJ, et al. Incidence of cardiac arrhythmias during intravenous pentamidine therapy in HIV-infected patients. *Chest* 1994;105(2):389.

151. Sakemi H, VanNatta B. Torsade de pointes induced by astemizole in a patient with prologation of the QT interval. *Am Heart J* 1993;125:1436.

152. Monaham BP, Ferguson CL, Killeavy ES, et al. Torsade de pointes occurring in association with terfenadine use. *JAMA* 1990;264:2788.

153. Davidenko JM, Cohen L, Goodrow R, et al. Quinidine-induced action potential prolongation, early afterdepolarizations, and triggered activity in canine Purkinje fibers. *Circulation* 1989;79:674.

154. Antzelevitch C, Sicouri S. Clinical relevance of cardiac arrhythmias generated by after depolarizations: role of M cells in the generation of U waves, triggered activity and torsade de pointes. *J Am Coll Cardiol* 1994;23(1):259.

155. El-Sherif N, Bekheit SS, Henkin R. Quinidine-induced long QTU interval and torsade de pointes: role of bradycardia-dependent early afterdepolarizations. *J Am Coll Cardiol* 1989;14(1):252.

156. Brachmann J, Scherlag BJ, Rosenstraukh LV, Lazzara R. Bradycardia-dependent triggered activity: relevance to drug-induced multiform ventricular tachycardia. *Circulation* 1993;68(4) 846.

157. Bailie DS, Inoue H, Kaseda S, et al. Magnesium suppression of early afterdepolarizations and ventricular tachyarrhythmias induced by cesium in dogs. *Circulation* 1988;77(6):1395.

158. Curran ME, Splawski I, Timothy KW, Vincent GM, Green ED, Keating MT. A molecular basis for cardiac arrhythmia: Herg mutations cause long AT syndrome. *Cell* 1995;80:795.

159. Wang Q, Shen J, Splawski I, et al. SCNSA mutations associated with an inherited cardiac arrhythmia, long QT syndrome. *Cell* 1995;80:805.

160. Prystowsky EN, Klein GJ. Ventricular tachycardia. In: Prystowsky EN, Klein GJ, eds. *Cardiac arrhythmias: an integrated approach for the clinician*. New York: McGraw-Hill; 1994:169.

161. Keren A, Tzivoni D, Gavish D, et al. Etiology, warning signs and therapy of torsade de pointes. A study of 10 patients. *Circulation* 1981;64(6):1167.

162. Tzivoni D, Banai S, Schuger C, et al. Treatment of torsade de pointes with magnesium sulfate. *Circulation* 1988;77(2):392.

163. Fazekas T, Scherlag BJ, Vos M, et al. Magnesium and the heart: antiarrhythmic therapy with magnesium. *Clin Cardiol* 1993;16:768.

*The Critically Ill Cardiac Patient,*
edited by V. Kvetan and D. R. Dantzker,
Lippincott - Raven Publishers, Philadelphia © 1996.

CHAPTER 18

# Cardiorespiratory Monitoring: State-of-the-Art

## Vladimir Kvetan

The following two-part discussion provides an overview of critical care monitoring of circulation using echocardiography and of lung mechanics using rapid-response pressure/flow measurements in the intensive care unit (ICU) patient population as it applies to the critically ill cardiac patient. The overview is provided by an anesthesia-based intensivist and a medicine-based pulmonary critical care specialist, even though directed at cardiologists.

Echocardiography, especially transesophageal echocardiography (TEE), is making major inroads into the critical care units. The ICU-based TEE programs are expanding, usually as collaborative projects of cardiology and anesthesiology. In general, physical examination of critically ill cardiac patients is limited in its accuracy in predicting measured physiologic data. Available studies suggest that protocol-driven pulmonary artery catheter (PAC) management will modify central venous pressure (CVP) driven management some 40% of the time, with strong suggestion of improvement in outcome. Recent data suggest that in patients with PAC-driven care, the use of TEE modifies management another 40% of the time. Diagnosis of many disease processes and pathophysiologic derangements are beyond the capabili-

ties of routine invasive monitoring techniques and can only be made by bedside echocardiography. Similar to the controversy surrounding the use of PAC in perioperative hemodynamic care as evidenced by the American Society of Anesthesiologists (ASA) Task Force statement, the utilization of TEE in perioperative intensive care remains to be clearly defined.

Lung mechanics is being rediscovered. Our ability to measure auto-positive end-expiratory pressure (PEEP) and respiratory drive parameters (i.e., $P_{0,1}$) have forced us to reconsider the issues of ventilator dependence more than 10 years ago. More recently, the awareness of positive-pressure ventilation induced pulmonary injury is forcing us to consider new methodologies of respiratory gas exchange directed at reduced exposure of parenchyma to high airway pressures, be it through permissive hypercapnia or through partial extracorporeal gas exchange. Since proper understanding of finer points of respiratory data acquisition is crucial in identifying potential for advances in therapy, this will be stressed in this section.

Proper management of the critically ill cardiac patient requires full understanding of the potential of new modes of mechanistic diagnostic approach.

V. Kvetan: Montefiore Medical Center, Division of Critical Care Medicine, Bronx, New York 10467.

# Advances in Cardiopulmonary Assessment in the Intensive Care Unit

David T. Porembka

The development and dynamics of intensive care coexisted with the physician and expansion of technology. Monitoring (continuous or continually) of these critically ill patients was part of this evolution. The use of technology is to provide information for the physician to minimize morbidity and mortality. The interaction of anesthesiologists with patient monitoring in the operating room extended to the critical care arena and perioperative medicine. Originally there was only clinical monitoring of systemic blood pressure and perfusion. The advent of continuous indwelling catheters and hardware support for cardiovascular assessment led to central intravascular (central venous and pulmonary arterial pressures) monitoring and diagnosis of varied disease states and "volume" interpretations. Even though early technology was not critically evaluated under strict investigational protocols, this technology became a standard of care. As the patient population becomes more complex because of their preexisting diseases, the need for improved technology will be demanded by the physicians (for the betterment of patient care) and the lay population (for absolute success).

This chapter will discuss the state-of-the-art monitoring (including diagnosis) of the pulmonary and cardiovascular systems. Echocardiography (particularly transesophageal echocardiography) and future developments will be discussed in the first section. The latter section will deal with the respiratory mechanics, the basic physiology, measurements, and clinical applications.

## TRANSESOPHAGEAL ECHOCARDIOGRAPHY

The most recent technology available for the critical care physician which has had an immediate impact on the management of the critically ill is transesophageal echocardiography (TEE) (1–8). This section will discuss the benefits of TEE, indications, complications,

applications of this technology, including hemodynamic assessment (ventricular function—systolic and diastolic, assessment of preload or left ventricular filling, pericardial effusion, and cardiac tamponade; aortic pathology—aortic dissection or aneurysm, aortic debris as a source of embolization; pulmonary embolism; intracardiac shunts, preexisting and acquired; valvular heart disease, native and prosthetic; and review of critical care experience).

Even though existing transthoracic echocardiography (TTE) is quite useful and has increased our appreciation of cardiovascular disease, there are many limitations with this tool (9–11). The acoustic window may be limited by both technical and physiologic constraints. Since increased depth of penetration is required with TTE, the resolution will be less when using 2.5 MHz. Body habitus is a common problem for the TTE examination (obesity, chronic obstructive lung disease, subcutaneous emphysema, and pneumothoraces). The position of the transducer cannot be maintained in a stable location for continuous evaluation or utilized intraoperatively (interferes with the surgical field). Basically, a limited examination is typical with TTE. Besides the above constraints with TTE, postsurgical patients (particularly cardiothoracic patients) will usually have dressings, tapes, and thoracostomy tubes which interfere with the acoustic window. Transesophageal echocardiography invariably obviates all of the difficulties or limitations seen with TTE (Figs. 1 to 4). Thus, TEE is an evolving powerful and diagnostic tool for the intensivist, cardiologist, surgeon, anesthesiologist, and pulmonary specialist. The only significant acoustic obstacle with TEE is the inability to have a comprehensive interrogation of the aorta (superior ascending aorta and aortic arch) (Color Plate 1). Other limitations with TEE are the size of the probe, requirement of sedation, expense of the equipment, and available innovative personnel familiar with TEE (indications and contraindications) and the principles of two-dimensional and Doppler echocardiography. In spite of the inherent conditions with TEE, the progress of ultrasound technology has yet to reach its pinnacle (8–11).

D. T. Porembka: Department of Anesthesia, University of Cincinnati Medical Center, Cincinnati, Ohio 45299.

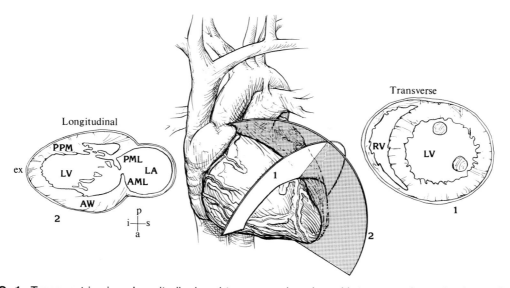

**FIG. 1.** Transgastric view. Longitudinal and transverse imaging with transesophageal echocardiography. A, anterior; AML, anterior mitral leaflet; AW, anterior wall; I, inferior; LA, left atrium; LV, left ventricle; P, posterior; PML, posterior mitral leaflet; RV, right ventricle; S, superior. Reproduced from Porembka DT, et al. In: Ayres S, et al., eds. *Textbook of critical care.* 3rd ed. Philadelphia: W.B. Saunders Company, 1995, with permission.

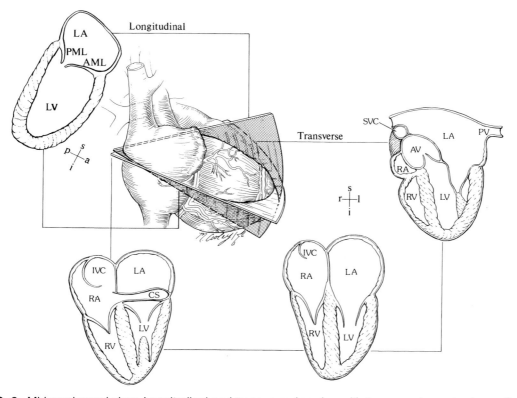

**FIG. 2.** Midesophageal view. Longitudinal and transverse imaging with transesophageal echocardiography. RA, right atrium; CS, coronary sinus; PV, pulmonary vein; IVC, inferior vena cava; SVC, superior vena cava. Reproduced from Porembka DT, et al. In: Ayres S, et al., eds. *Textbook of critical care.* 3rd ed. Philadelphia: W.B. Saunders Company, 1995, with permission.

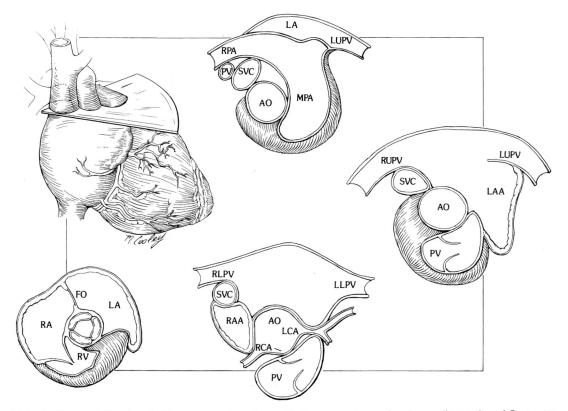

**FIG. 3.** Base of the heart. Transverse imaging with transesophageal echocardiography. AO, aorta; LAA, left atrial appendage; LLPV, left lower pulmonary vein; LUPV, left upper pulmonary vein; FO, fossa ovalis; LCA, left coronary artery; MPA, main pulmonary artery; PV, pulmonary vein; RAA, right atrial appendage; RCA, right coronary artery; RLPV, right lower pulmonary vein; RPA, right pulmonary artery; RUPV, right upper pulmonary vein. Reproduced from Porembka DT, et al. In: Ayres S, et al., eds. *Textbook of critical care.* 3rd ed. Philadelphia: W.B. Saunders Company, 1995, with permission.

## VENTRICULAR PERFORMANCE

### Global Function

Unfortunately, the most common indices used by clinicians (cardiologists) for global evaluation is the ejection fraction which is load dependent (preload, afterload, heart rate, and contractility). Ejection fraction is described as the fraction or percent of left ventricular diastolic volume that is ejected during systole. Systolic index or fraction and fractional shortening may also be assessed for global function. In stable situations or an outpatient setting these indices may be helpful. The measurements of global systolic function may be made by several means: M-mode, two-dimensional, three-dimensional, and Doppler echocardiography (10, 11).

Doppler echocardiography may be used to estimate systolic function. The determination of the aortic Doppler velocity for stroke volume is made by measuring the aortic velocity-time integral where the initial half is used to calculate the ejection force. Another method is to evaluate the mean acceleration (the slope between the onset of ejection and peak velocity). Using the modified Bernoulli equation and continuous wave Doppler, the clinician can estimate ventricular systolic function in a patient with mitral regurgitation. The measurements are made from two points along the slope of the mitral regurgitant flow where the pressure gradient is calculated between the left atrium and left ventricle. Pulsed-wave and continuous-wave Doppler may also estimate flow or cardiac output by the velocity at the pulmonary artery (10, 11). Cardiac output may be determined from the transgastric long-axis plane by the estimation of the aortic value and using Doppler for evaluation of the time-velocity flow integral (12). Stoddard et al. found a good correlation with the pulsed technique and thermodilution. In other studies various correlations have been found with the thermodilution technique. This transgastric long-axis view was recently used for estimation of cardiac output by using continuous-wave Doppler across the aortic valve (13). The investigators easily measured cardiac output via Doppler in the majority of the patients (98%) and had excellent correlation ($r = 0.94$) with thermodilution. Similar results were seen by sampling at the left ventricular

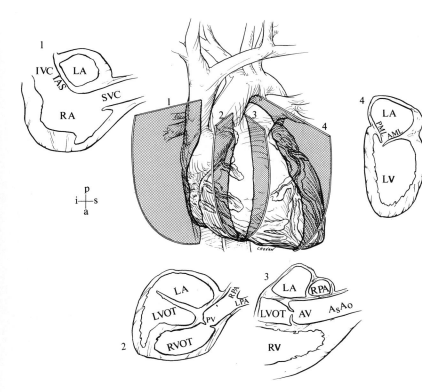

**FIG. 4.** Base of the heart. Longitudinal views with transesophageal echocardiography. AML, anterior mitral valve leaflet; AsAo, ascending aorta; AV, aortic valve; IAS , interatrial septum; IVC, inferior vena cava; LPA, left pulmonary artery; LVOT, left ventricle outflow tract; PV, pulmonary valve; RVOT, right ventricular outflow tract. Reproduced from Porembka DT, et al. In: Ayres S, et al., eds. *Textbook of critical care.* 3rd ed. Philadelphia: W.B. Saunders Company, 1995, with permission.

outflow tract with multiplane transesophageal echocardiographic Doppler imaging (stroke volume $r = 0.90$ and cardiac output $r = 0.91$) (14). It appears that continuous-wave Doppler may be more accurate than pulsed-wave echocardiography, but for clinical use it should not replace existing technology (pulmonary artery catheter) until there is more accessible and accurate echocardiographic tools (? intravascular echocardiography).

In addition to the M-mode calculations of ejection fraction, fractional shortening of the left ventricle, and circumferential shortening of the left ventricle (fraction), M-mode echocardiography can measure either the mitral E-point septal separation or the descent of the mitral annulus for systolic function estimation (10, 11).

Presently, the most common means of measuring qualitative or quantitative systolic function and volume assessment is with two-dimensional echocardiography. Areas and volume can be easily assessed with TEE by the visualization of the ventricles from the short-gastric and fore-shortened views. Generally, the end-diastolic area at the midpapillary region correlates (~87% with actual left ventricular volumes) (15). Earlier, Konstadt and others showed a good approximation between the data obtained from the TEE measurements and thermodilution (16). Beaupre and colleagues compared the stroke volume with thermodilution and the fractional short-axis changes (TEE) and described an excellent correlation (91%) (17). In their study, as expected, there was only a 23% interdependence with the pulmonary occlusion pressure and

end-diastolic short-axis change. With nuclear techniques, TEE's results were favorable (18). In a similar study, but utilizing radionuclide angiography, TEE volume estimates were excellent ($r = 0.92$) (19).

Volume interpretation can be crucial in the care of the critically ill. Can TEE be used for the estimation of volume depletion (hypovolemia)? Reich et al. (in the pediatric population) found concordant changes in 80% of the cases between ventricular dimensional changes and blood withdrawal or reinfusion (20). In a similar study (adult) by Cheung and colleagues, the left ventricular determinants of preload (TEE) correlated well with the peripheral hemodynamics in patients with either normal or abnormal left ventricular function during graded hypovolemia (21). This correlation was readily apparent at 2.5% estimated blood volume deficit. Different results were seen in a study by van Daele et al. where patients underwent acute hypervolemic hemodilution (22). Initially there was an increase in stroke volume and end-diastolic area, but as progression of hemodilution proceeded, the end-systolic area decreased. Systolic cavitary obliteration is considered as an echocardiographic sign of hypovolemia and will precede peripheral hemodynamic aberrations. However, Leung et al. found this to be the case the majority of the time but not totally inclusive (23). This is particularly the situation in patients with underlying hyperdynamic states (e.g., liver failure, systemic inflammatory distress syndrome, pancreatitis, trauma, and drugs that interfere with the cytochrome or electron transport systems) who are euvolemic and adequately resuscitated. Of particular interest in these patients, if they are severely hypovolemic, other than systolic cavitary obliteration, some patients may exhibit left ventricular outflow tract obstruction from systolic anterior motion of the anterior mitral valve leaflet (Fig. 5 ). Also, end-diastolic area has been used for the estimation of hypovolemia. If there is a decrease in this area (<5.5 cm$^2$/m$^2$), hypovolemia may be assured. However, this area is not uniform, particularly in patients where this level may coexist with actual hypovolemia which is dependent on the patient's disease state, afterload, and existing or preexisting contractility (i.e., dilated cardiomyopathy). This is one of the obvious limitations with TEE. These discrepancies are readily apparent in patients with coexisting acute lung injury and myocardial dysfunction.

The appraisal of preload is a daily controversy and a dilemma in the critically ill patient, particularly in patients with acute respiratory distress syndrome (24, 25). In patients with severe acute lung injury requiring high levels of positive end-expiratory pressure (PEEP) and ventilatory support, the appreciation of intravascular volume is enhanced with TEE. Not only can volume (dimensions) be estimated, but the ventricular interactions that occur (enlarged right atrium with abnormal atrial septal motion and bulging fossa ovalis, right ventricular dilatation with global dysfunction and septal shift, and decreased ventricular indices) may be serially evaluated during the disease and the interventions required. Schuster and Jardin's investigations revealed

the right/left interactions that occur from the addition of PEEP (24, 25). Hemodynamic assessment of cardiac patients with application of PEEP showed that at higher levels there was reduction in both systolic atrial filling of the pulmonary venous flows and early and late left ventricular inflow of the transmitral flow velocities (26). Transesophageal echocardiography was used for hemodynamic appraisal in patients with pressure-controlled inverse-ratio ventilation. We have found that the hemodynamic evaluation with TEE was no different with pressure-controlled ventilation or volume-controlled ventilation with a deceleration flow pattern (27). The authors believe that in particular circumstances the application of TEE may assist the physician in the management of these patients where apparent left- and right-sided heart interactions do occur.

To offset the inherent obstacles with the qualitative echocardiographic assessment of preload and myocardial performance, computer-enhanced images, software, and hardware development are being proposed. For example, cine-loop digitalization has greatly refined the accuracy of visual assessment of ventricular volume and function. Acoustic quantification (AQ) is another means for the assessment of left ventricular performance. In Cahalan's investigation acoustic quantification underestimated left ventricular fractional change while the real-time measurements of end-systolic and end-diastolic areas were accurate (28). Recently, acoustic quantification was contrasted with the conductance method for the development of pressure/volume loops and had a significant correlation (29). In addition to software development, probe miniaturization and multiplanar imaging is crucial for three-dimensional reconstruction. Early results have been encouraging; however, we yet have a clinical feasible tool to use (30–32).

### Regional Function

One of the most difficult dilemmas for the clinician is the accurate identification of a patient with myocardial ischemia. Existing electrocardiographic (ECG) technology, including computerized ST-segment analysis, is still limited in patients in the intensive care unit (ICU). It is not infrequent to have varied lead placements because of surgical dressings, tapes, and thoracostomy tubes. Other limiting factors for accurate ST-segment analysis are paced rhythm, intraventricular conduction delay, left ventricular hypertrophy, drug effect, and patient movement or agitation. Echocardiography is a unique tool in evaluating for myocardial ischemia at the midpapillary region of the left ventricle (8, 33, 34). This is evident from angioplastic series and animal studies (35, 36). When comparing electrocardiography with echocardiography during marginal occlusion of the coronary artery, echocardiography will invariably depict an event [regional wall motion abnormal-

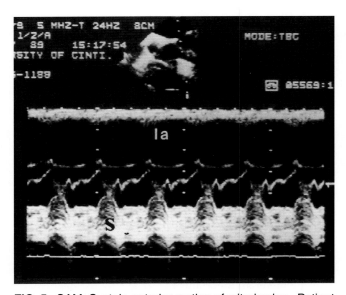

**FIG. 5.** SAM: Systole anterior motion of mitral valve. Patient in shock following Carpenter's ring placement. Systolic anterior motion of anterior lea flet of the mitral valve with M-mode echocardiography revealing systolic anterior motion of the anterior leaflet of the mitral valve and outflow tract obstruction. la, left atirum; S, septum.

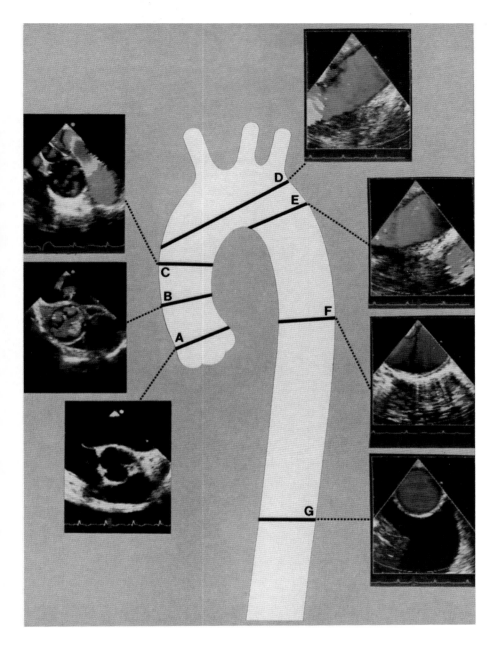

COLOR PLATE 1. Thoracic aorta. Sequential transverse imaging of the ascending, arch, and descending thoracic aorta of normal anatomy with color flow Doppler echocardiography. Reproduced with permission by Chandrasekaran K, Likoff Cardiovascular Institute, Hahnemann University Hospital, Philadelphia, PA.

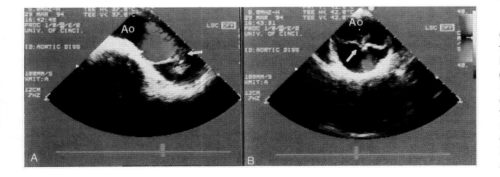

COLOR PLATE 2. Aortic dissection. A: Transverse view of the proximal descending thoracic aorta with color flow Doppler echocardiography revealing an intimal flap with an entry site and flow transversing into the lumen. B: A corresponding view (same patient) of a patient with aortic dissection with another intimal flap located in the distal thoracic aorta. Ao, aorta.

ity (RWMA)] while the ECG detection of ischemia may be delayed up to 10 minutes (37). Only when there is an acute total occlusion of the coronary artery will ECG identification approach that of echocardiography (38) (Fig. 6). Temporally, the extent of occlusion will correspond to the type of RWMA (i.e., marginal occlusion-hypokinesis, total occlusion-akinesis). In general, the most sensitive sign of myocardial ischemia is impaired systolic thickening and ventricular relaxation, followed by the appearance of RWMA, compliance changes, ST-segment changes in the ECG, and finally the presence of angina (if present at all) (38, 39). It is no wonder that echocardiography may be the ideal for serial evaluation of a patient with myocardial ischemia (RWMA) and its complications.

Numerous investigations have shown the efficacy of echocardiography over electrocardiography for the detection ischemia (33, 34, 39–43). In an earlier study by Smith and colleagues, they detected myocardial ischemia in 48% of the patients while only six patients had ST-segment changes. In contrast, patients with identifiable ECG ischemia all had concomitant RWMA (34). Comparable significance of TEE detection of ischemia was seen in Leung's study (44). In their study the detection rates for myocardial ischemia were as follows: pre-bypass 20% (TEE) vs. 7% (ECG); postbypass 36% (TEE) vs. 25% (ECG); and ICU 25% (TEE) vs. 16% (ECG). In Leung's study, 48% of the patients developed myocardial ischemia (RWMA), while only six patients had significant ECG changes. Of particular significance in this study is that the patients who developed a RWMA had an adverse outcome as compared to patients without a RWMA. Also,

73% of the patients had normal hemodynamics during the ischemic episodes (44).

Qualitative assessments of RWMA and ejection fraction are a concern (Figs. 7 and 8) In Deutch's study, 5% of the segments were graded differently by the same observer, while 39% of the patients and 9% of the segments had varied assessments by different observers (45). Obvious alterations from the norm can be easily assessed with echocardiography; however, there are major discrepancies when there are subtle changes (58%) (46, 47).

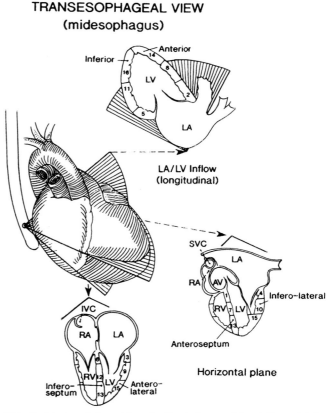

**FIG. 7.** Horizontal and longitudinal views of the left ventricle from the midesophagus (30 to 35 cm from incisors) position. Imaging planes analogous to the transthoracic apical two- and four-chamber and left ventricular outflow images are obtained. Horizontal plane: The four-chamber view visualizes the inferior septum and the anterolateral walls. Anterior angulation to the level of the outflow tract and aortic valve visualizes the anteroseptal and inferolateral walls. The true apex may be foreshortened in these views. Longitudinal plane: The left ventricular two-chamber inflow view visualizes the anterior and inferior walls. 1, Basal anteroseptum; 2, basal anterior; 3, basal anterolateral; 4, basal inferolateral; 5, basal inferior (or posterior); 6, inferobasal septum; 7, midanteroseptum; 8, midanterior; 9, midanterolateral; 10, midinferolateral; 11, midinferior; 12, midinferoseptum; 13, apical septum; 14, anteroapex; 15, lateral apex; 16, inferoapex. Reproduced from Oh JK, et al. In: Freeman WK, et al., eds. *Transesophageal echocardiography.* Boston: Little, Brown; 1994, with permission.

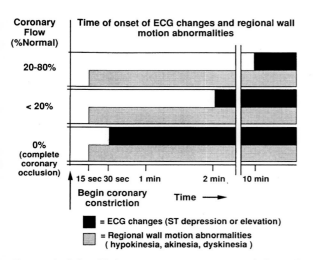

Temporal relationship between acute coronary constriction and onset of ECG changes and regional wall motion abnormalities.

**FIG. 6.** Temporary relationship of regional wall motion abnormalities and electrocardiogram (ECG) indicative of myocardial ischemia with varied coronary artery blood flow. Modified from Clements FM, de Bruijn NP. *Anesth Analg* 1987;66:249.

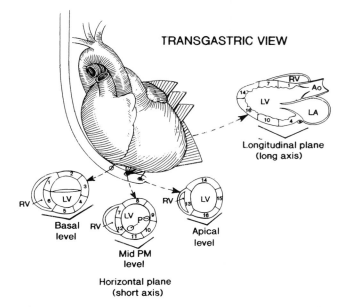

**TRANSGASTRIC VIEW**

Longitudinal plane
(long axis)

Basal level

Mid PM level

Apical level

Horizontal plane
(short axis)

**FIG. 8.** Horizontal and longitudinal transesophageal echocardiography (TEE) views of the left ventricle from the transgastric position. Horizontal plane: Depending on the position of the transducer and its angulation, short-axis views of the left ventricular basal, middle, and apical levels can be obtained. Longitudinal plane: The long-axis view of the left ventricle is visualized, similar to the transthoracic parasternal long-axis view, and shows the anteroseptal and inferolateral walls. Medial angulation would image the inferior segments and posteromedial papillary muscle. 1, Basal anteroseptum; 2, basal anterior; 3, basal anterolateral; 4, basal inferolateral; 5, basal inferior (or posterior); 6, inferobasal septum; 7, midanteroseptum; 8, midanterior; 9, midanterolateral; 10, midinferolateral; 11, midinferior; 12, midinferoseptum; 13, apical septum; 14, anteroapex; 15, lateral apex; 16, inferoapex (P, papillary muscles). (See Fig. 7 legend for key to numbered segments.) Reproduced from Oh JK, et al. In: Freeman WK, et al., eds. *Transesophageal echocardiography*. Boston: Little, Brown; 1994, with permission.

Saada showed that ejection fraction is correctly identified in 49% of the cases while preload assessment is accurately approximated 62% of the time (48). The varied sensitivities for the echocardiographic determination of RWMA and ejection fraction can easily be explained because not all RWMAs are from a ischemic nature. The situations that mimic a RWMA are aberrant ventricular contractions or conduction defects, a paced rhythm, prior tissue fibrosis, tethering of adjacent segments, and regional afterload. Many physiologic constraints occur on the ventricles in a patient in the ICU, either from the disease state itself (i.e., sepsis) or from iatrogenic involvement (i.e., application of PEEP). The clinician should always be critical about the presence of a RWMA. Is it the RWMA from myocardial ischemia? Collating all of the information from the patient, ECG, echocardiography, physiologic parameters, presentation, and laboratory results may be necessary to adequately treat the patient.

Further investigations are essential to delineate the efficacy of TEE in these difficult situations.

In spite of these limitations, stress echocardiography has come to fruition and has approximated the efficacy seen with the nuclear techniques (49–56). In Marwick's study, the sensitivity for the diagnosis of myocardial ischemia for echocardiography was 72%, while that of sestamibi scintigraphy was 76% (49). To estimate the extent of myocardial viability, the use of dobutamine stress-echocardiography has gained increasing acceptance (51). In a recent study, there was excellent agreement (90%) between fluorine-18 flurodeoxyglucose positron emission tomography and dobutamine stress echocardiography. The positive and negative predictive values for echocardiography were 81% and 97%, respectively (53). Dobutamine stress echocardiography and Doppler echocardiography have comparable results when detecting coronary artery stenosis (>70%) of the left anterior descending artery for coronary flow reserve (56). Obviously stress echocardiography will complement the nuclear techniques while having the capability of being portable and less expensive.

It is a matter of time when hardware technology (miniaturization of the probe, multiplanar or three-dimensional capabilities), software advancement, and contrast agents will increase our ability to accurately diagnose myocardial ischemia and ventricular performance (Fig. 9). Sonicated albumin has successfully been used to assess myocardial preservation (retrograde or antegrade cardioplegia) and quality of the distal anastomosis during cardiac surgery. In

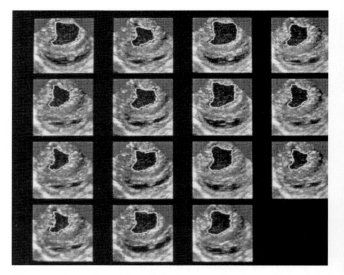

**FIG. 9.** Computer edge detection application. Automated edge detection of the left ventricle through two cardiac cycles with computer methods of artificial intelligence tracking the subendocardial edge of the ventricle. Supported by SCCM Eli Lilly Research Grant 1991-1992. Reproduced from Porembka DT, et al. In: Ayres S, et al., eds. *Textbook of critical care*. 3rd ed. *[in press]*, with permission.

addition, these agents are elucidating possible mechanisms for incomplete cardioprotection (a right-to-left shunt or aortic regurgitation) (57). An obvious question is, can these agents be used in the intensive care setting to assess myocardial perfusion, as well as perfusion in other organs? I believe that we will eventually have this capability.

### Diastolic Function

One of the major limitations of assessing cardiac performance with the pulmonary artery catheter in the critically ill is the inability to evaluate or detect diastolic dysfunction. Diastolic dysfunction may be a major component in the patient's disease process. Also, filling pressures (PAOP) will not reflect actual left ventricular volume. Because of this there are many discrepancies in the interpretation of the patient's cardiac status where the treatment may follow in error. Echocardiography is unique for this dilemma, yet not necessarily ideal for the assessment of cardiac function (including diastolic impairment) which may assist in the management. Interrogation of the pulmonary venous flow and transmitral flow patterns will allow the physician to discern if there is left ventricular diastolic compliance problems (including systolic function). Uniformly, TEE will visualize a pulmonary vein. Typically, the pattern is illustrated by four phases: systolic flow due to ventricular contractions; diastolic inflow secondary to the opening of the mitral valve; retrograde flow secondary to atrial contraction; and systolic inflow due to atrial relaxation (58–62). Classically, systolic peak flows and the diastolic component will decrease in dilated and hypertrophied hearts (63). Usually, the systolic component is influenced by systolic function while the atrial and diastolic phases are affected by diastolic dysfunction (64, 65).

Prior to the advent of TEE, TTE only evaluated the transmitral flow patterns for analysis of diastolic function. In addition to pulmonary venous flow, TEE can easily sample the velocities just proximal to the inlet of the left ventricle. This pattern is depicted as two discrete filling waves representing the instantaneous relationship between atrial and ventricular pressures. The E wave indicates the beginning of rapid atrial early in diastole while the A wave depicts the onset of atrial contraction. Typically, the E wave is larger than the A wave. Alterations in this ratio (E/A) occur from impaired ventricular function and altered loading conditions. When this ratio approximates 1.0, various etiologies may be the cause of the impaired ventricular relaxation: myocardial ischemia or injury, cardiomyopathies, left ventricular hypertrophy, systemic hypertension, and pulmonary hypertension. A second pattern (increased E/A ratio) is described as restrictive. This is illustrated in patients with systolic dysfunction and elevated ventricular end-diastolic and left atrial volumes. Normal patterns do not always represent normal physiology because this pattern is contingent on

the underlying pathophysiology, sampling, age, and more important (in the ICU) if there is any tachycardia. The latter will influence measurements and there will be a fusion of the E/A wave (66). The existence of intact pericardium (postcardiac surgical patient) will also affect the patterns over a wide range of volumes or pressures (66).

Recent attention has been given to estimation of left ventricular filling (left atrial pressure) from the evaluation of either pulmonary venous flow or transmitral patterns (67–70). As the atrial pressure increases, the systolic component of the pulmonary venous flow will decrease (70). However, in patients with altered ventricular function this inverse relationship would not always hold. Recently, we evaluated these patterns in patients with acute lung injury or systemic inflammatory response syndrome and found discouraging results (71, 72). Noninvasive assessment of left filling is attractive; however, to truly estimate this, ventricular volumes is still ideal (which can be done with echocardiography).

## PERICARDIAL EFFUSION AND TAMPONADE

The presence of a cardiac tamponade is life threatening and must be recognized early to minimize the morbidity and to avoid a possible reversible mortality. In the postsurgical cardiac patients, pericardial effusions are initially "silent" (56%) and may subsequently develop a tamponade (1.0% to 2.5%) (73–75). Pericardial effusions can arise from a variety of illnesses, including trauma. Appreciation and detection are the key.

In a patient with a suspected pericardial effusion, extensive echocardiographic examination should be performed. The majority of effusions can be visualized via the parasternal long-axis view (TTE). However, in some patients there may be an inadequate exam and TEE should be promptly initiated. The classic echocardiographic signs of tamponade are inversion of the right atrial and ventricular free walls (secondary to reversal of the transmural gradient), compression of the right ventricle or atrium at high intrapericardial pressures, and exaggerated respiratory variation of the tricuspid and mitral inflow velocities (76). These echocardiographic signs are indicative of increasing pericardial pressures or volumes. Investigations have found that there may be a critical pericardial volume of pressure or fluid when right ventricular diastolic collapse will occur. This is coexistent with a drop in the cardiac output while maintaining the systemic pressure. In profound cases, right ventricular diastolic collapse will persist throughout diastole (77).

In a dynamically unstable critical care patient, the presentation or significance of a pericardial effusion will largely depend not only on the volume of pericardial fluid but also on the presence of ventricular dysfunction and the state of preload. Consequently, the degree of right ventricular collapse is affected by the patient's hemodynamic state: preexisting right or left ventricular dysfunction, chamber compliance, and preload (78–80). In a canine model, volume replacement has been shown to decrease the extent of right ventricular collapse by increasing the transmural pressure gradient from the elevation of right intracavitary pressure (80). The presence of increased right-sided heart afterload (pulmonary artery hypertension) will detain the extent of right ventricular diastolic collapse during the hemodynamic progression of tamponade (79). However, the opposite would occur in situations where there is existing left ventricular dysfunction.

There is controversy of what is a clinically significant pericardial effusion (presence of right ventricular diastolic collapse). If cardiac tamponade is defined clinically as a decrease in the systemic pressure and pulsus paradoxus, then right ventricular diastolic pressure is not that specific. In contrast, if right ventricular diastolic inversion is the marker, then it is highly specific (76). The difficulty arises in the patient with acute lung injury requiring high levels of PEEP and elevated mean airway pressures who have a coexisting large pericardial effusion. If these patients did not need PEEP (for optimal oxygenation), the same pericardial effusion would not be clinically significant (cardiac tamponade). The effect of PEEP in this same scenario is even worse when there is concomitant left ventricular dysfunction.

Two other characteristics may assist in the determination if there is a tamponade (right atrial collapse and inspiratory variation of transmitral inflow velocities (81, 82). Right atrial inversion is another sensitive sign for cardiac tamponade (82%) (81). The sensitivity and specificity increase to 94% and 100%, respectively, when the right atrial collapse extends through the cardiac cycle from the increasing pericardial pressure (81). Normally, during inspiration, the mitral inflow velocities will decrease (10%), while velocities across the tricuspid valve will increase (17%). During the hemodynamic progression to cardiac tamponade, the flow characteristics of transtricuspid flows (80%) and transmitral velocities (40%) will be exaggerated (82). Also, it appears that prior to volume repletion in acute tamponade, the diastolic component of pulmonary venous flow is dramatically decreased. This is probably secondarily to the increased pericardial pressure constraints on diastolic filling of the left atrium (83).

In trauma and cardiac cases, one potential harbinger is the loculated effusion that may be causing regional tamponade with significant systemic effects. Transesophageal echocardiography may be the only tool to discern this diagnosis (84). There may be compression not only of cardiac chambers but also of the vena cava or the pulmonary veins. A complete TEE examination may delineate this pathology (76).

In addition, residual shunts may be depicted only with TEE in the periresuscitative phase and may result in tamponade situation if not identified early. Penetrating cardiac trauma is unfortunately increasing in today's society, and TEE will become the obvious tool for the perioperative physician. Irregular and small defects may not be visualized with standard techniques (angiography and TTE) (85). In a larger series ($n = 43$) of penetrating cardiac trauma, Skoulargis and colleagues found additional lesions in four patients that were not identified by TEE. All positive TTE ($n = 9$) results were confirmed by TEE. We have seen enlarging lesions by TEE that were totally missed by TTE (86).

## AORTIC PATHOLOGY

### Aortic Dissection and Aneurysm

Transesophageal echocardiography has revolutionized the evaluation of the aorta, particularly in the critically ill unstable patient for whom, because of TEE's quick and noninvasive nature, a diagnosis can be entertained. In aortic dissection, the goal of diagnostic strategy is an accurate and expeditious diagnosis since if it is unrecognized the mortality is quite high. The increased imaging quality (of the aorta) with TEE is because of its retrocardiac position which bypasses structures that would interfere with the acoustic windows for TTE. The only visual limitation with TEE (biplanar and omniplanar) is the superior ascending portion of the aorta because of reverberation artifacts resulting in some false-positive results.

The typical echocardiographic findings for an acute dissection are identification of a large false lumen and smaller true lumen interposed by an undulating intimal flap, identification of the entry site(s) with directional flow characterized by color flow Doppler echocardiography, accentuation of color flow into the true lumen, and thrombus in the false lumen (Color Plate 2). In addition, TEE can evaluate ventricular function, involvement of the coronary arteries with dissection, association of aortic regurgitation caused by incomplete cusp coaptation, diastolic prolapse of the cusps, or symmetrical dilatation of the aorta. Evaluation of the aortic valve and coronary arteries is crucial in the surgical plan (10, 11).

The benefit of TEE in this disease state was initially appreciated by Erbel and colleague in their multicenter European trial. This study incorporated 164 patients and compared TEE with the standard diagnostic methods (computed tomography and angiography). The results were confirmed at surgery or at autopsy. Altogether, the sensitivities and specificities were for TEE (98% and 98%), angiography (88% and 94%), and computed tomography (83% and 100%) (87). The low sensitivities seen in computed tomography were also described by Ballal et al. (88). Aortic dissections were misclassified in 33% of the patients by computed tomography while the TEE again had respectable sensitivity (97%) and specificity (100%). The advent of color flow Doppler is beneficial in the detection of the entry site(s) (100%) when compared to standard modalities (89).

Recent attention has been given to the use of magnetic resonance imaging in the diagnosis of aortic pathology. Two series from the same institution compared the imaging techniques of computed tomography, magnetic resonance imaging, TEE, and TTE. In the earlier investigation of TEE with magnetic resonance imaging, they found that both techniques had similar sensitivities (100%), but the specificities were divergent, magnetic resonance imaging (100%) and TEE (68%). These TEE false results were attributed to artifacts within an ectatic aorta with extensive plaque formation and calcification (90). The later investigation compared all of the imaging techniques and found similar results between TEE and magnetic resonance imaging. The sensitivities and specificities were for TEE (97%/77%), magnetic resonance imaging (98%/98%), computed tomography (94%/87%), and TTE (59%/83%) (91). Similar results and conclusions were depicted in Laissy's study of TEE vs. magnetic resonance imaging (92). The lower specificities for TEE are explained by the reverberation artifacts, but more importantly, these two studies only used monoplanar imaging. It is apparent that if "newer" technology was used, including Doppler echocardiography, the specificities would increase to satisfactory levels (90, 91).

Can TEE detect any prognostic indicators or affect the morbidity/mortality in patients with aortic dissection? In Roudant's study, a diameter above 35 mm of the ascending aorta was determined to be significant (93). In Erbel's recent series, the survival rates were considered to be lower as compared to historical controls: type I, 52%; type II, 69%; and type III, 70%. Other identifiable indicators of an adverse prognosis were an open false lumen with a high communication and no thrombus formation (94). The major difficulty in this study is that it was not prospective and was compared to historical controls.

Transesophageal echocardiography appears to be beneficial in atypical dissection, aortic trauma, and conditions that mimic aortic dissections. Atypical dissections occur from the spontaneous rupture of the vasa vasorum or undiagnosed intimal tears. Angiography is insufficient in this disease while TEE can invariably detect the problem (95, 96). Fusiformed aneurysms of the ascending aorta and saccular aneurysm can be easily visualized in the longitudinal planes, while sinus of Valsalva aneurysm can be detected in either planes (97). In Chan's study, TEE found multiple etiologies for situations mimicking an aneurysm while establishing the diagnosis of aortic aneurysm in 45% of the cases (98).

## Acute Aortic Trauma

In acute trauma, appropriate diagnosis is essential. The aorta can easily be interrogated for a transection, tear, or hematoma. Furthermore, other etiologies may be illustrated such as ventricular function and preload, RWMA, pericardial effusion and tamponade, and valvular insufficiency. In Kearney's investigation in suspected aortic trauma, TEE uniformly identified the injury and the existence of a mediastinal hematoma. However, angiography only detected four patients with an aortic injury and had two false-negatives and one false-positive (99, 100). Equivalent conclusions were seen in Le Bret's study (101). The subtle signs of aortic injury (mediastinal hematoma and periaortic hematoma) may only be detected by TEE, hopefully initiating a surgical exploration. To secure a more defined diagnosis, intravascular ultrasound may be the alternate or adjunct modality. One of the limitations of intravascular ultrasound is that it is invasive. However, this system detected the intimal flap in the aorta in all cases but also evaluated the distal extent of the dissection (celiac artery 100%, renal arteries 100%, and superior mesenteric arteries 80%) which other echocardiographic techniques are incapable of (102).

As echo technology improves, each diagnostic tool will have its place. The role of TEE in aortic dissection is becoming established. In acute situations where the patients may be unstable or have the propensity to rapidly decompensate, TEE should be one of the first diagnostic tools to evaluate an acute dissection. If the diagnosis is uncertain or unconfirmed, other modalities should follow (angiography, computed tomography, intravascular ultrasound, and magnetic resonance imaging).

## Aortic Debris and Thrombi: A Source for Embolism

Atherosclerotic disease is a major problem, particularly of the coronary and cerebral circulations (103, 104). Transesophageal echocardiography has unearthed and profiled the underlying pathology of the aorta (Fig. 10). Previously, angiography was limited in the evaluation of this process because of its inability to portray accurately the intimal surface, the aortic wall and adjacent structures, and the extent of atheromatous material. Plaques may be focal, smooth, and echo dense or they may be diffuse, expansive, and complex with mobile fragments within the lumen. The concerns about existing plaques is the propensity of embolization.

In a TEE study of the aorta, 7% of the patients had aortic atherosclerotic disease. The occurrence of systemic embolization was more frequent in patients who had mobile, pedunculated plaques (73%) than without (12%) (105). Proximal aortic atheroma also appears to be an independent marker for cerebral ischemia (106). In a study by Horowitz et al., 4% of the patients who had a central ischemic event were attributed to extensive and mobile plaques (107). The association between carotid disease and protruding aortic thrombi is more ominous. In Demopoulos's investigation, protruding arch athero-

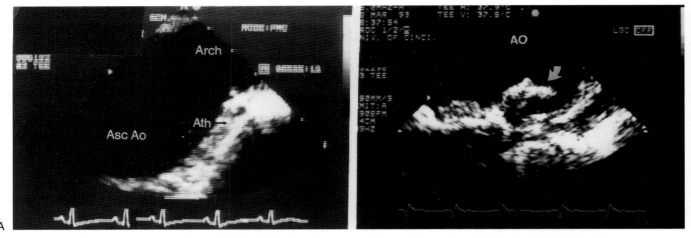

**FIG. 10.** Aortic debris. **A:** Transverse view of the ascending aorta revealing atheromatous debris. Arch, proximal aortic arch; Asc Ao, ascending aorta, Ath, atheromatous debris. **B:** Transverse view of the arch of the aorta showing large, pedunculated, free-flowing debris. Figure not marked with A and B side.

mas were present in 38% of the cases with carotid disease, while mobile atheromas were detected in 13% of the cases as compared to controls (2%) (108). Penetrating aortic ulcer is a major problem and is identified easily with TEE (109).

It is obvious that this disease process is significant and may cause considerable morbidity. Single- and multiple-organ failure may be the result of these embolic sources (110, 111). Sepsis has been caused by infective aortic masses (110). In unexplained situations, TEE may be used to interrogate the aorta for the potential problem. The question arises, who will benefit from surgery and eradication of the debris (110)? Should all patients who have unexplained strokes undergo a comprehensive TEE examination? As experience increases with TEE, the obvious answer is yes!

## VALVULAR HEART DISEASE

### Native Valvular Disease

#### *Stenosis*

Echocardiography has impacted greatly on the noninvasive evaluation of patients with valvular heart disease. In patients who are hemodynamically unstable, the cause may be a valvular abnormality. The advantages with TEE more than complements TTE in these types of patients. Transesophageal echocardiography can easily interrogate the integrity as well as the function of these cardiac valves, particularly in the mitral valve position and if it is prosthetic. The other advantages of TEE over TTE are the ability to evaluate the function and integrity of the atrial septum, identification of thrombi in the appendages, and

visualization of spontaneous echo contrast (as a prodrome to thrombus formation).

Mitral valvular stenosis is principally the consequence of rheumatic heart disease from leaflets which are immobile, thickened, deformed, and calcified. Echocardiographic hemodynamic evaluation of the mitral valve may be completed utilizing either the continuity equation, deceleration time, planimetry, or pressure half-time. From continuous-wave Doppler assessment at the inflow of the left ventricle, a pressure gradient may be generated by the application of the Bernoulli equation (maximal pressure gradient approximates four times the velocity which is equivalent to the maximal inflow velocity). An area may also be determined from the pressure half-time process (rate of decline of the diastolic pressure gradient) based on the supposition that as the severity of disease (stenosis) increases the diastolic pressure gradient is maintained longer and there is prolongation of the early diastolic signal: mitral valve area (MVA) = 220/pressure half-time (10, 11). The continuity equation presupposes that the inflow volume transversing the mitral annulus is equivalent to the left ventricular stroke volume (MVA = SV/TVIm, where TVI is the time velocity intergral of mitral inflow). In addition, the area can be estimated by the annular cross-sectional (MVA = {aortic annular cross-sectional area}TVI aorta/TVI mitral. Finally, the area may be estimated by customary planimetry (10, 11).

Transesophageal echocardiography is comparable to TTE in the estimation of the severity of mitral stenosis (112). However, the benefit of TEE may lie in the assessment of patients submitting to valvuloplasty. The perioperative complications (leaflet tear, residual mitral regurgitation, interatrial shunting, and presence of thrombus formation prior to the procedure) resulting from this procedure can readily be identified with TEE (112).

Similar techniques can also be applied to patients who have aortic stenosis (congenital bicuspid valves or acquired defects—rheumatic, degenerative, and atherosclerotic). The difference in these situations is that TEE is limited in its evaluation because of acoustic shadowing from the calcified leaflets. However, omniplanar or multiplanar probes have increased the assessment. A new approach via the transgastric (comparable to the transgastric parasternal long-axis view) appears to heighten the interrogation of both the left ventricular outflow tract and aortic valve. Planimetry may be attempted (using omniplanar imaging), but comparing to other techniques, the area could be underestimated since a true short-axis view was not achieved (113). Applying either the continuity equation or the modified Bernoulli equation via the transgastric longitudinal view, pressure gradients may be obtained (114).

### Regurgitation

The valvular disorder which has received the greatest amount of attention with TEE is mitral regurgitation. Patients' planned surgeries have been altered (27%) from the information obtained solely from TEE. The foremost impact was on mitral valve cases (40%) (115). Similarly, angiography results were also conflicting with TEE in 46% of the cases (116). The intraoperative use of TEE elucidated information on the prognosis of patients (residual ventricular impairment and residual regurgitation).

Precise decisions can only be made after complete understanding of the patient's disease process and the physiologic and technical interfaces that affect the information. It is not uncommon to have varied loading conditions on the atria or ventricles which can influence the size or extent of the regurgitant jet. Comprehensive grasp of the principles of echocardiography, including Doppler and color flow, is crucial to discern what is a significant regurgitant lesion (9–11, 117).

Mitral regurgitation is visualized as a muticolored jet within the left atrium during systole (9–11, 118). Eccentric regurgitant lesions are usually the outcome of posterior overriding, prolapsed or flailed leaflets, or the accompaniment of a vegetation or mass. Central posterior appearing jets may be the consequence of myocardial ischemia or when the leaflets are equally affected (i.e., rheumatic heart disease with annular dilatation) (9–11, 119).

Several echocardiographic principles may be applied for the assessment or the extent of severity of mitral regurgitation: area of the jet and the affected pulmonary venous flow patterns, diameter of the jet at the orifice, and proximal flow convergence. Obviously, the simplest method is measuring and averaging the maximal area of the jet (mosaic pattern) in both transverse and longitudinal planes. Transesophageal echocardiography results have been comparable with angiography, the "gold stan-

dard" (119, 120). Typically, the areas are classified as follows: trivial mitral regurgitation < 1.5 cm², mild mitral regurgitation 1.5 to 4.0 cm², moderate mitral regurgitation 4.0 to 7.0 cm², and severe mitral regurgitation > 7.0 cm² (121). To assist in the determination of the severity, evaluation of the systolic component of the pulmonary venous flow may be helpful where as the severity increases, the systolic will become blunted to systolic reversal in severe cases (122). In Lai's study, systolic reversal were excellent markers of grade 3 or 4 angiographic regurgitation (97%) (123). However, difficulty arises when the jet is of high velocity and eccentric (124, 125). To circumvent this dilemma, the pulmonary venous patterns may elucidate the severity when the affected pulmonary vein is interrogate. In other words, if the eccentric jet is posterior-lateral, the left superior pulmonary vein should be sampled (123, 125, 126).

Other methods have been used for the estimation of the severity of mitral regurgitation. The principle of flow acceleration proximal to a narrowed or regurgitant orifice is depicted by a series of proximal colored rings. These rings are produced as the signal aliases as the velocity accelerates toward a narrowed orifice. Each ring represents an isovelocity area from which all points are equidistant to the center of the orifice and is comparable in velocity. Thus, using the continuity equation, the flow (through the orifice) should approximate flow proximal to the orifice. Regurgitant flow is then calculated by the velocity at which aliasing occurs with proximal isovelocity surface area (9–11). This latter method has shown favorable results to angiography (127). Another method gaining acceptance for the estimation of regurgitation is the diameter of the jet at the orifice (128, 129). To measure regurgitant volumes, pulsed- or continuous-wave Doppler may be used (126, 130).

The extent of aortic regurgitation is not as easily determined with TEE. However, evaluating the jet width proximal to the valve with the dimensions of the left ventricular outflow tract is a reasonable method (131). Four grades have been proposed comparing the ratio of dimensions of the jet width/left ventricular outflow: grade I (mild) 0.25, grade II (moderate) 0.25 to 0.46, grade III (moderately severe) 0.47 to 0.64, and grade IV (severe) > 0.65 (131). Again using the continuity equation for the estimation of severity may be attempted (132). Also, by using the half-time method (rate of decline of the aortic regurgitant velocity) with continuous-wave Doppler may approximate the severity (133). However, as expected, when these jets are eccentric and of high velocity, the actual severity may be underestimated.

### Prosthetic Valvular Disease

One of the major benefits of TEE is the ability to interrogate the integrity and function of prosthetic valves (biological or mechanical), particularly in the mitral valve position where there is acoustic attenuation with TTE. Pathologic conditions vary from stenosis (degenerative, pannus ingrowth, thrombosis), regurgitation (transvalvular-thickening or calcification, perivalvular), leaflet perforation, tear or dihiscence, and mechanical complications of disc variance, pannus or thrombosis, endocarditis-vegetations, valve ring abscess, or fistula, hematoma, and pseudoaneurysm. Furthermore, the assessment of forward-flow hemodynamics can be completed by spectral Doppler and gradients can be determined with continuous-wave Doppler. The combination of pulsed- and continuous-wave Doppler provides the estimation of affected areas of the orifices, while color flow provides a velocity map of flow through these devices (9–11).

As one evaluates patients with prosthetic valves, the acknowledgment of what is normal is significant. For example, a St. Jude valve would have a typical pattern of three flamelike regurgitant jets, a tilting-disc prosthesis will display small holosystolic jets, and a Starr-Edwards valve will demonstrate single systolic jets (134–137).

The use of TEE has shown the inadequacies of TTE in these situations. In Khandheria's series, TEE identified abnormalities in 48% of the patients with "normal" TTE. These results were confirmed in the majority (92%) of cases at surgery (134). In van den Brink's investigation, there were varied results between the two echocardiographic techniques and TEE had similar findings with angiography (135). Color flow Doppler is an excellent tool to classify the severity of jets by estimating its direction, length and width, and appearance of mosaic pattern (138). In a prospective study, TEE easily detected perivalvular leaks (31%) and uniformly identified the normal regurgitant jets. Of interest, TEE also identified an obstruction in one patient and spontaneous echo contrast in 215 of the cases (139).

Evaluating the potential complications of prosthetic valves are crucial. However, the search for a dynamic outflow tract obstruction following placement of a Carpenter may be lifesaving. In this dynamic situation there can be turbulence in the left ventricular outflow tract (as depicted by color flow Doppler) and the presence of systolic anterior motion of the anterior mitral valve leaflet. Reversal of this dilemma is not always accomplished by volume replacement, but by removal of the ring. Systolic anterior motion as well as residual obstruction, ventricular septal defects, and sustained pressure gradients may also be discerned by TEE (140, 141).

## PULMONARY EMBOLISM

In the evaluation of patients who are critically ill and hemodynamically unstable, the clinician (in the back of his or her mind) is considering a possibility of a pulmonary embolism. The unfortunate situation in the resuscitative phase is that these patients cannot always be transported to the radiologic suite for the definite diagnosis by pulmonary angiogram. Therefore, the certain diagnosis is not made and clinical suspicion is the key. Echocardiography may be the unique tool to assist in this determination (Fig. 11).

The clinical and hemodynamic results of pulmonary embolism are dependent on the extent of the pulmonary vasculature that is obstructed in the acute event and patient's preexisting cardiac function and preload. When

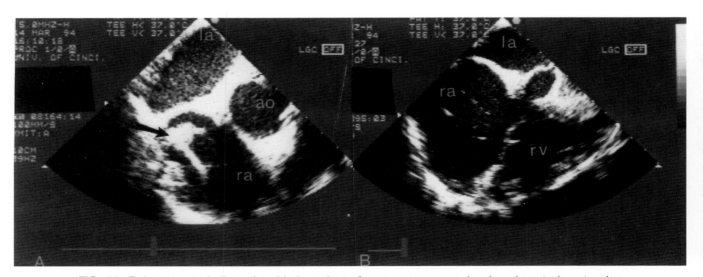

**FIG. 11.** Pulmonary embolism. An elderly patient after recent surgery developed acute hypotension and hypoxemia. **A:** Transverse view of a thrombus (in transit) identified in the right atrium. ao, ascending aorta; ra, right atrium. **B:** A corresponding transverse view of the right atrium revealing a large right atrium and bulging interatrial septum into the left atrium, indicative of a pressure overload situation. rv, right ventricle.

obstruction exceeds 25%, right ventricular afterload will increase. As pulmonary vasculature becomes impeded, right ventricular pressure will continue to rise until 40 mm Hg (in normal right ventricles) (142). Of equal value, the echocardiographic hemodynamics will occur: increased ratio of right/left ventricular dimensions, hypokinetic and enlarged right ventricle, dilated main and proximal pulmonary vasculature, paradoxical systolic septal motion and displacement toward the left ventricle, the presence of tricuspid or pulmonary regurgitation with increased velocities, and the occasional identification of either thrombotic or nonthrombotic material. The left function may be preserved. However, it can be impaired from the mechanical and pressure overload situation seen on the right side if the afterload is markedly increased (142).

Clinical and laboratory investigations have corroborated these findings. In Jardin's study, the left ventricular function was preserved (with reduced dimensions) while the right-sided indices were increased. Cardiac failure ensued in the cases with marginal preload and reduced left ventricular compliance (143). Similar findings were seen in Kasper's series: dilated pulmonary artery (77%), dilated right ventricle (75%), decreased ejection fraction (EF) slope of the mitral valve (50%), abnormal septal function (44%), and reduced left dimensions (42%). Of note, TEE identified a thrombus in 13 patients (144).

In certain situations, TEE may be extremely helpful in these critically ill patients (145, 146). However, since the emergence of TEE, a new patient population may benefit from its use, i.e., orthopedic patients. McGrath and colleagues revealed that the incidence of emboli visualized in the right cardiac chambers approached 27% (147). However, in Parmet's study, they detected echogenic material in all of their patients. A significant number of them had large echogenic masses superimposed over the millary showers. Of these patients, there were no compromised hemodynamics and three patients had a right to left paradoxical embolization (148). However, in our institution we have seen an increasing incidence of significant hemodynamics with the classic echocardiographic findings of emboli following orthopedic procedures. The question comes to fore, are some patients unable to deal with the significant right-sided afterload changes?

## INTRACARDIAC MASS AND PATENT FORAMEN OVALE: ANOTHER POTENTIAL FOR EMBOLISM

### Intracardiac Mass

A significant morbidity may result from a transit or existing mass or thrombi in the cardiac chambers. Left atrial or appendage thrombi occur more significantly than earlier appreciated. Lovett et al. concluded that there was either an indirect (23%) or direct cause (6.5%) for focal cerebral ischemia. The underlying contributing factors appear to be hypertension, preexisting cardiac disease, and particularly mitral stenosis, atrial fibrillation, and occasionally the presence of spontaneous echo contrast (149). Transesophageal echocardiography is specially suited for the evaluation of a patient with mitral stenosis, spontaneous echo contrast, and thrombi in the appendages. If the mitral valve is prosthetic, TTE would markedly be limited while TEE would not (149–153).

Several studies have shown the efficacy of TEE over TTE in these situations. In patients with ischemic stroke, TEE detected a source in 46% of the patients with a negative TTE (150, 154). In Pearson's study, TEE identified the source in 57% of the cases while TTE was beneficial in 15% (155). Divergent results were appreciated in Alber's investigation where the identification rates for TEE and TTE were 46% and 8%, respectively. In this latter study, they determined that lacunar syndromes were associated in patients with an atrial septal aneurysm and interatrial shunts were prevalent in all stroke types (156).

How significant is atrial fibrillation and mitral stenosis for the development of thrombi? In patients with an identifiable thrombus, atrial fibrillation occurred in 71% and 92% of the cases (150, 153). Forty-six percent of the patients with a thrombus had concurrent mitral stenosis. Of the patients with atrial fibrillation, thrombus was identified in 29% (150). Hwang and colleagues studied exclusively patients with mitral stenosis and found the incidence was greater (26.3%) when there was a thrombus than without (5.4%). In this study, the incidence of atrial fibrillation was quite divergent between the groups of thrombus (100%) and no thrombus formation (74.3%) (152). When the left atrial area exceeded 30 cm$^2$ and coexisted with atrial fibrillation, spontaneous echo contrast uniformly resided (a prodrome for thrombus formation?). The propensity for thrombus formation and the possibility for systemic embolization are entirely genuine. Stoddard et al. found that left atrial thrombus occurred in patients with atrial fibrillation as early as 3 days (14%). This was in contrast to patients with chronic atrial fibrillation (27%) (157). Several reports have described a significant incidence of thrombus in the atria prior to cardioversion (158–160). Cardioversion is not without risk. Grimm's evaluation of atrial function following this procedure found that its function may be worse and there was a greater propensity for spontaneous echo contrast. Do these patients require anticoagulation? The answer is not clear (161). In spite of these apparent risk factors, thrombi may still develop in patients with a sinus mechanism. This may be partly explained by an underlying abnormal atrial function (low left atrial area EF and peak emptying velocities) (162).

### Patent Foramen Ovale

If there is an existing thrombi peripherally or centrally (intracardiac), the concern for a paradoxical

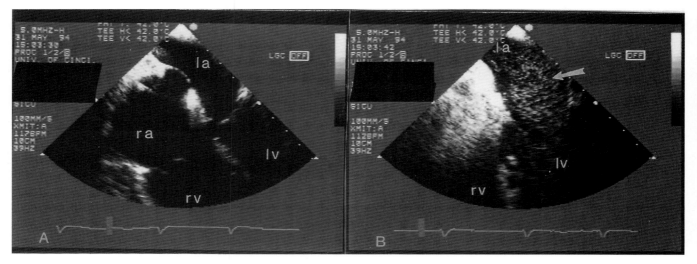

**FIG. 12.** Patent foramen ovale and paradoxical embolism. **A:** Transverse view from chamber view revealing a large right atrium and bulging fossa ovalis. lv, left ventricle. **B:** A corresponding view (transverse view) with agitated saline as a contrast agent (early injection) with multiple microbubbles in left atrium, indicative of a large right-to-left shunt.

embolism is possible. Patent foramen ovale (PFO) is a probable conduit for this event to transpire. Patent foramen ovale is a well-known entity but is achieving prominence because of its occurrence in different patient populations, particularly in the critically ill, in whom there may be coexisting hypoxia, pulmonary hypertension, acidosis, and requirement of PEEP or elevated mean airway pressure. The results of this will be increased pressure on the right side (atrial) with abnormal septal motion (bulging fossa ovalis) and propensity for interatrial pressure differential and a patent passageway (Fig. 12) (Table 1).

Comparable studies with echocardiography (TEE and TTE) have shown TEE to be a more reliable tool for the diagnosis. With TTE and TEE, the incidence of PFO at basal conditions will vary between 5% to 18% and 8% to 44%. Following augmentation maneuvers (i.e., Valsava), the incidence increases dramatically: TTE, 10% to 24%, and TEE, 22% to 63% (163–173). The importance of this may have been elaborated by Lechat and others where, in patients with strokes, the incidence of a PFO was 40%. However, in patients without a significant central event, the prevalence was only 10% (163). Hausmann's study was even more concerning. In spite of divergent detection rates for TEE and TTE, when age was highlighted, the incidence for a PFO approaching 40%. When abnormal physiology was characterized, the incidence rose to approximately 69% (164). Typically, angiography is considered the "gold" standard for the detection of a PFO. In Chen's study, the detection rate for TEE was 44% at static conditions and 63% following the Valsava maneuver. Only one PFO could not be reproduced in the catheterization laboratory (165).

Besides the propensity for paradoxical embolization, PFO may be the reason why a particular patient may have refractory hypoxia. We have experienced several cases where this was the prominent situation. In one report there was dramatic improvement in the patient's oxygenation following surgical closure (174, 175). In our institution, if there is refractory hypoxia, a TEE examination is performed to evaluate for any intracardiac pathology.

## ENDOCARDITIS

Endocarditis is a significant disease that must not be neglected, particularly in patients with prosthetic valvular devices. Occasionally, this disease state may be etiology

**TABLE 1.** *Comparative detection of vegetations with TEE and TTE echocardiography*

| Source | Number of patients | Sensitivity (%) | |
|---|---|---|---|
| | | TEE | TTE |
| Daniel et al. (137) | 33 | 82 | 36 |
| Daniel et al. (179) | 82 | 94 | 40 |
| Erbel et al. (180) | 51 | 100 | 63 |
| Mugge et al. (182) | 105 | 90 | 58 |
| Taams et al. (183) | 33 | 100 | 33 |
| Pederson et al. (184) | 24 | 100 | 50 |
| Birmingham et al. (185) | 61 | 88 | 30 |
| Shively et al. (188) | 62 | 94 | 44 |
| Shapiro et al. (190) | 30 | 87 | 60 |
| Daniel et al. (192) | 76 | 94 | 60 |

TEE, transesophageal echocardiography; TTE, transthoracic echocardiography.

for the patient's compromised hemodynamics. The use of TEE in the ICU is paramount to elucidate this dilemma (176, 177) (Fig. 13).

The usual detection rate for endocarditis and its associated complications with TTE is approximately 41% to 78%. However, inadequate imaging is not infrequent (20%). Transesophageal echocardiography circumvents all of the inadequacies that were fundamental for TTE (178–190) (Table 2). Earlier, Daniel and others revealed the divergent detection rates for infective endocarditis (TEE, 94%, and TTE, 40%). As expected, roughly 21% of these cases had inconclusive TTE images (179). Later, Erbel's results were more revealing: TTE, 63% sensitive and 98% specific; TEE, 100% sensitive and 98% specific (180). Comparable results were portrayed in Mugge's series (181). As anticipated, TEE is more suitable for the evaluation of the aortic and mitral valves but equivalent in the assessment of the tricuspid valves (188). False-negative results can be explained because of minute vegetations or acoustic shadowing of calcified valves or prosthetic devices (189).

Therefore, there would be varied detection rates for the technique utilized. The sensitivities of TTE will improve as the size of the vegetation increases (2.0 to 5.0 mm, 25%; 6.0 to 10 mm, 70%; and >10 mm, 100%). In prosthetic valvular devices, the sensitivity for TTE will only be 20% to 30%. However, consistently TEE will detect the vegetations as well as the perivalvular complications (180, 182, 191, 192). Another predictor for an embolic event is when the size of the vegetations exceed 10 mm (47%) and is mobile (38%) as compared to sessile (19%) (182). Other contributing factors are the position of the vegetation (mitral) and the association of spontaneous echo contrast. These factors can only be elucidated with TEE (183, 193, 194).

Associated complications of endocarditis (valvular and perivalvular destruction, abscess, fistula, and aneurysm) are a major concern and at times can only be detected with TEE. Invariably TEE will identify these problems, while TTE is quite limited. In this particular scenario, the detection rate for TEE was 87% as compared to TTE's detection rate of 28% (195). Subaortic structures are prin-

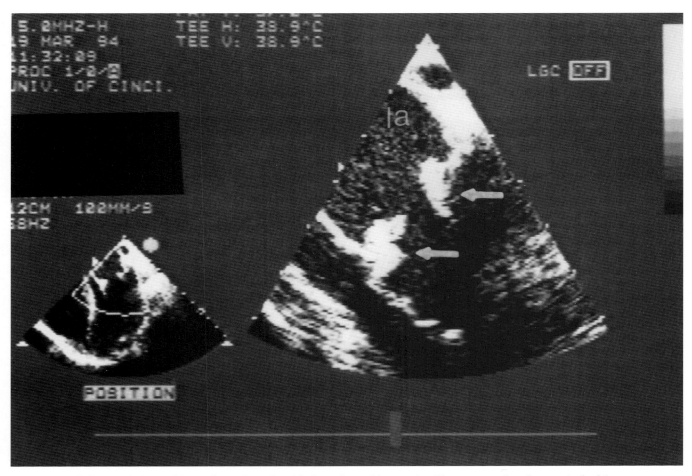

**FIG. 13.** Endocarditis: native valve. An elderly patient with a stroke. Transverse view (expanded) of the mitral valve apparatus revealing two large vegetations (with severe mitral regurgitation), as the etiology of the embolic event. la, left atrium.

**TABLE 2.** *Characterization of flow patent foramen ovale with echocardiography*

| Source | Number of patients | Modality | In vivo resting conditions (%) | Augmentation maneuvers (%) |
|---|---|---|---|---|
| Lechat et al. (163) | 100 | TTE | 5 | 10 |
|  | 60 | — | 18 | 24 |
| Hausmann et al. (164) | 198 | TTE | 8 | —[b] |
|  |  | TEE | 22 | —[b] |
| Jaffe et al. (165) | 30 | TEE | 10 | Unchanged |
| Guggiari et al. (166) | 189 | TTE | 8 | 10 |
| Chen et al. (167) | 32 | TTE | 25 | 38 |
|  |  | TEE | 44 | 63 |
| Black et al. (168) | 101 | TTE | 6 | Unchanged |
|  | 51 | TEE | 8 | —[b] |
| Konstadt et al. (169) | 50 | TEE | 10 | 22 |
| Porembka et al. (170) | 30 | TEE | 27 | —[b] |
| Siostrzonek et al. (171) | 150 | TTE | 5 | 6 |
|  | 160 | TEE | 12 | 20 |
| Stollberger et al. (172) | 264[a] | TEE | 15 | —[b] |

[a]Suspected embolic events.
[b]Not done.

cipally involved in the complicated cases that may result in significant mitral regurgitation and/or perforation. Abscess may occur in the periannular region (90%) with predominance in the aortic position (75%) (195). Transesophageal echocardiography is also quite restricted (27%) in ventricular abscesses, while TEE invariably will characterize it (195–198).

Negative identification of endocarditis does not necessarily preclude the disease process itself, even with TEE. If the result is equivocal, a high-risk patient, especially a patient with a prosthetic valvular device, should be maintained on antibiotics and may be serially evaluated with TEE. Also, a patient with an identifiable lesion who is not a candidate for surgery may undergo these serial examinations (196).

As echocardiography continues to evolve, it will become a more essential diagnostic and monitoring tool for both the cardiologist (in the ICU) and the intensivist. More research is needed to continue to show the efficacy of TEE in these critically ill patients. In the near future echocardiography as a monitoring and diagnostic tool may be as common as the pulmonary artery catheter.

# REFERENCES

1. Oh JK, Seward JB, Khandheria BK, et al. Transesophageal echocardiography in critically ill patients. *Am J Cardiol* 1990;66:1492.
2. Pavlides GS, Hause AM, Stewart JR, et al. Contribution of transesophageal echocardiography to patient diagnosis and treatment: a prospective analysis. *Am Heart J* 1990;120:910.
3. Pearson, AC, Castello R, Labovitz AJ, et al. Safety and utility of transesophageal echocardiography in the critically ill patient. *Am Heart J* 1990;119:1083.
4. Foster E, Schiller NB. The role of transesophageal echocardiography in critical care: USCF experience. *J Am Soc Echocardiogr* 1992;5:368.
5. Hwang J, Shyu K, Chen J, et al. Usefulness of transesophageal echocardiography in the treatment of critically ill patients. *Chest* 1993;104:861.
6. Wolfe LT, Rossi A, Ritter SB. Transesophageal echocardiography in infants and children: use and importance in the cardiac intensive care unit. *J Am Soc Echocardiogr* 1993;6:286.
7. Khoury AF, Afridi I, Quinones MA, et al. Transesophageal echocardiography in critically ill patients: feasibilty, safety, and impact on management. *Am Heart J* 1994;127:1363.
8. Porembka DT. Transesophageal echocardiography in the critically ill. In: *Critical care: state of the art*, vol 15. Anaheim, CA: Society of Critical Care Medicine; 1995:269.
9. Freeman WK, Seward JB, Khandheria BK, Tajik AJ, eds. *Transesophageal echocardiography*. Boston: Little, Brown; 1994.
10. Feigenbaum H. *Echocardiography*. 5th ed. Lea & Febiger; 1994.
11. Weyman AE. *Principles and practice of echocardiography*. 2nd ed. Lea & Febiger; 1994.
12. Stoddard MF, Prince CR, Ammash N, et al. Pulsed Doppler transesophageal echocardiographic determination of cardiac output in human beings: comparison with thermodilution technique. *Am Heart J* 1993;126:956.
13. Darmon P, Hillel Z, Mogtader A, et al. Cardiac output by transesophageal echocardiography using continuous-wave Doppler across the aortic valve. *Anesthesiology* 1994;80:796.
14. Feinberg MS, Hopkins WE, Davila-Roman VG. Multiplane transesophageal echocardiographic Doppler imaging accurately determines cardiac output measurements in critically ill patients. *Chest* 1995;107:769.
15. Rankin JS, McHale PA, Arentzen CE, et al. Three-dimensional dynamic geometry of the left ventricle in the conscious dog. *Circ Res* 1976;39:304.
16. Konstadt SN, Thys D, Mindich BP, et al. Validation of quantitative intraoperative transesophageal echocardiography. *Anesthesiology* 1986;65:418.
17. Beaupre PN, Cahalan MK, Kremer PF, et al. Does pulmonary artery occlusion pressure adequately reflect left ventricular filling during anesthesia and surgery? *Anesthesiology* 1983;59:A3.
18. Urbanowicz JH, Shaaban J, Cohen NH, et al. Comparison of transesophageal echocardiographic and scintigraphic estimates of left ventricular end-diastolic volume index and ejection fraction in patients following coronary artery bypass grafting. *Anesthesiology* 1990;72:607.
19. Clements FM, Harpole DH, Quill T, et al. Estimation of left ventricular volume and ejection fraction by two-dimensional transesophageal echocardiography: comparison of short axis imaging and simultaneous radionuclide angiography. *Br J Anaesth* 1990;64:331.
20. Reich DL, Konstadt SN, Nejat M, et al. Intraoperative transesophageal echocardiography for the detection of cardiac preload changes induced by transfusion and phlebotomy in pediatric patients. *Anesthesiology* 1993;79:10.
21. Cheung AT, Savino JS, Weiss SJ, et al. Echocardiographic and hemo-

dynamic indexes of left ventricular preload in patients with normal and abnormal ventricular function. *Anesthesiology* 1994;81:376.

22. Van Daele ME, Trouwborst A, Woerkens LC, et al. Transesophageal echocardiographic monitoring of preoperative hypervolumic hemodilution. *Anesthesiology* 1994;81:602.

23. Leung JM, Levine EH. left ventricular end-systolic cavity obliteration as an estimate of intraoperative hypovolemia. *Anesthesiology* 1994; 81:1102.

24. Schuster S, Erbel R, Weilemann LS, et al. Hemodynamics during PEEP ventilation in patients with severe left ventricular failure studied by transesophageal echocardiography. *Chest* 1990;97:1181.

25. Jardin F, Brun-Ney D, Hardy A, et al. Combined thermodilution and two-dimensional echocardiographic evaluation of right ventricular function during respiratory support with PEEP. *Chest* 1991;99:162.

26. Meijburg HW, Visser CA, Wesenhagen H, et al. Transesophageal pulsed-Doppler echocardiographic evaluation of transmitral and pulmonary venous flow during ventilation with positive end-expiratory pressure. *J Cardiothor Vasc Anesth* 1994;4:386.

27. Porembka D, Hoit B, McMannis D, et al. Correlation of pulmonary artery occlusion pressure with pulmonary venous flow pattern by transesophageal echocardiography. *Crit Care Med* 1993;21:S268.

28. Cahalan MK, Ionescu P, Melton HE, et al. Automated real-time analysis of intraoperative transesophageal echocardiograms. *Anesthesiology* 1993;78:477.

29. Katz WE, Mandarino WA, Gorcsan J, et al. Noninvasive pressure-volume relations to evaluate left ventricular function during dobutamine infusion. *J Am Soc Echocardiogr* 1994;7:S38.

30. Martin RW, Bashein G, Detmer PR, et al. Ventricular volume measurement from a multiplanar transesophageal ultrasonic imaging system: an in vitro study. *IEEE Trans Biomed Eng* 1990;37:442.

31. Roelandt JRT, Cate F, Vletter WB, et al. Ultrasonic dynamic three-dimensional visualization of the heart with a multiplane transesophageal imaging transducer. *J Am Soc Echocardiogr* 1994;7:217.

32. Gorcsan J, Mandarino WA, Denault AY, et al. Measurement of changes in left ventricular volume throughout the cardiac cycle: comparison of transesophageal echocardiographic automated border detection with conductance catheter techniques. *J Am Soc Echocardiogr* 1994;7:S38.

33. Beaupre DN, Kremer PF, Cahalan MK, et al. Intraoperative detection of changes in left ventricular segmental wall motion by transesophageal two-dimensional echocardiography. *Am Heart J* 1984; 107:1021.

34. Smith JS, Cahalan MK, Benefiel DJ, et al. Intraoperative detection of myocardial ischemia in high-risk patients: electrocardiography versus two-dimensional transesophageal echocardiography. *Circulation* 1985;72:1015.

35. Tennant R, Wiggers C. The effect of coronary occlusion on myocardial contraction. *Am J Physiol* 1935;112:351.

36. Alam M, Khaja F, Brymer J, et al. Echocardiographic evaluation of the left ventricle during coronary artery angioplasty. *Am J Cardiol* 1986;57:20.

37. Vatner SF. Correlation between acute reductions in myocardial blood flow and function in conscious dogs. *Circ Res* 1980;47:201.

38. Waters DD, da Luz P, Wyatt HL, et al. Early changes in regional and global left ventricular function induced by graded reductions in regional coronary perfusion. *Am J Cardiol* 1977;39:537.

39. Sunagawa K, Maughan WL, Sagawa K. Effect of regional ischemia on the left ventricular end-systolic pressure-volume relationship of isolated canine hearts. *Cir Res* 1985;86:351.

40. Rozien MF, Beaupre PN, Alper RA, et al. Monitoring with two-dimensional transesophageal echocardiography. *J Vasc Surg* 1984;1:300.

41. London MJ, Tubau MG, Wong E, et al. The "natural history" of segmental wall motion abnormalities in patients undergoing noncardiac surgery. *Anesthesiology* 1990;73:644.

42. Ellis JE, Shah MN, Briller JE, et al. A comparison of methods for the detection of myocardial ischemia during noncardiac surgery: automated ST-segment analysis systems, electrocardiography, and transesophageal echocardiography. *Anesth Analg* 1992;75:764.

43. Atkov OY, Akchurin RS, Tkachuk M, et al. Intraoperative transesophageal echocardiography for detection of myocardial ischemia. *Herz* 1993;6:372.

44. Leung JM, O'Kelly B, Browner WS, et al. Prognostic importance of post-bypass regional wall motion abnormalities in patients undergoing coronary artery bypass graft surgery. *Anesthesiology* 1989;71:16.

45. Deutsch HJ, Curtius JM, Leischik R, et al. Reproducibility of assessment of left ventricular function using intraoperative transesophageal echocardiography. *Thorac Cardiovasc Surg* 1993;41:54.

46. Doer HK, Quinones MA, Zoghbi WA, et al. Accurate determination of left ventricular ejection fraction by transesophageal echocardiography with a nonvolumetric method. *J Am Soc Echocardiogr* 1993;6: 476.

47. Berquist BD, Lemon KW, Bellows WH, et al. Real-time determination of ejection fraction by transesophageal echocardiography: how accurate are "eyeball" estimates. *Anesthesiology* 1993;79:A69.

48. Saada M, Cahalan MK, Lee E, et al. Real time evaluation of echocardiograms. *Anesthesiology* 1989;71:344.

49. Marwick T, D'hondt A, Baudhuin T, et al. Optimal use of dobutamine stress for the detection and evaluation of coronary artery disease: combination with echocardiography or scintigraphy, or both? *J Am Coll Cardiol* 1993;22:159.

50. Forster T, McNeill AJ, Salustri A, et al. Simultaneous dobutamine stress echocardiography and technetium-99m isonitrile single-photon emission computed tomography in patients with suspected coronary artery disease. *J Am Coll Cardiol* 1993;21:1591.

51. Takeuchi M, Araki M, Nakasima Y, et al. Comparison of dobutamine stress echocardiography and stress thallium-201 single-photon emission computed tomography for detecting coronary disease. *J Am Soc Echocardiogr* 1993;6:593.

52. Panza JA, Laurienzo JM, Curiel RV, et al. Transesophageal dobutamine stress echocardiography for evaluation of patients with coronary artery disease. *J Am Coll Cardiol* 1994;24:1260.

53. Baer FM, Voth E, Deutsch HJ, et al. Assessment of viable myocardium by dobutamine transesophageal echocardiography and comparison with fluorine-18 fluorodexyglucose positron emission tomography. *J Am Coll Cardiol* 1994;24:343.

54. Roger VL, Pellikka PA, Oh JK, et al. Stress echocardiography. Part I. Exercise echocardiography: techniques, implementation, clinical applications, and correlations. *Mayo Clin Proc* 1995;70:5.

55. Pellika PA, Roger VL, Oh JK, et al. Stress echocardiography. Part II. Dobutamine stress echocardiography: techniques, implementation, clinical applications, and correlations. *Mayo Clin Proc* 1995;70:16.

56. Stoddard MF, Prince CR, Morris GT. Coronary flow reserve assessment by dobutamine transesophageal Doppler echocardiography. *J Am Coll Cardiol* 1995;25:325.

57. Voci P, Bilotta F, Caretta Q, et al. Mechanisms of incomplete cardioplegia distribution during coronary artery surgery. *Anesthesiology* 1993;79:904.

58. Appleton CP, Gonzalez MS, Basnight MA, et al. Relationship of left atrial pressure and pulmonary venous flow velocities: importance of baseline mitral and pulmonary venous flow velocity patterns studied in lightly sedated dogs. *J Am Soc Echocardiogr* 1994;7:264.

59. Castello R, Pearson AC, Lenzen P, et al. Evaluation of pulmonary venous flow by transesophageal echocardiography in subjects with a normal heart: comparison with transesophageal echocardiography. *J Am Coll Cardiol* 1991;18:65.

60. Meijburg HWJ, Visser CA, Westerhof PW, et al. Normal pulmonary venous flow characteristics as assessed by transesophageal pulsed Doppler echocardiography. *J Am Soc Echocardiogr* 1992;5:558.

61. Bartzokis T, Lee R, Yeoh TK, et al. Transesophageal echo-Doppler echocardiographic assessment of pulmonary venous flow patterns. *J Am Soc Echocardiogr* 1991;4:457.

62. Akamatsu S, Terazawa E, Kagawa K, et al. Transesophageal Doppler echocardiographic assessment of pulmonary venous flow pattern in subjects without cardiovascular disease. *Intl J Cardiac Imag* 1993;9: 195.

63. Iuchi A, Oki T, Ogawa S, et al. Evaluation of pulmonary venous flow pattern in hypertrophied and dilated hearts: a new study with transesophageal pulsed Doppler echocardiography. *J Cardiol* 1991;21:75.

64. Appleton CP, Hatle LA, Popp RL. Relation of transmitral flow velocity patterns to left ventricular diastolic function: new insights from a combined hemodynamic and Doppler echocardiographic study. *J Am Coll Cardiol* 1988;12:426.

65. Pearson AC, Gudipati CV, Labovitz AJ. Effects of aging on left ventricular structure and function. *Am Heart J* 1991;121:871.

66. Lavine SJ. Left ventricular diastolic function in idiopathic cardiomyopathy: Doppler hemodynamic correlations. *Echocardiography* 1991; 8:151.

67. Hoffmann R, Lambertz H, Jutten H, et al. Mitral and pulmonary

venous flow under influence of positive end-expiratory pressure ventilation analyzed by transesophageal pulsed Doppler echocardiography. *Am J Cardiol* 1991;68:697.

68. Nishimura RA, Abel MD, Hatle LK, et al. Relation of pulmonary vein velocities by transesophageal Doppler echocardiography: effect of different loading conditions. *Circulation* 1990;81:1488.

69. Kuecherer HF, Kusumoto F, Muhiudeen IA, et al. Pulmonary venous flow patterns by transesophageal pulsed Doppler echocardiography: relation to parameters of left ventricular systolic and diastolic function. *Am Heart J* 1991;122:1683.

70. Kuecherer HF, Muhiudeen IA, Kusumoto FM, et al. Estimation of mean left atrial pressure from transesophageal pulsed Doppler echocardiography of pulmonary venous flow. *Circulation* 1990;82:1127.

71. Hoit BD, Shao Y, Gabel M, et al. Influence of myocardial contractile dysfunction on the pattern of pulmonary venous flow. *Circulation* 1991;84:369.

72. Hoit BD, Shao Y, Gabel M, et al. Influence of loading conditions and contractile state on pulmonary venous flow. *Circulation* 1992;86:651.

73. Stevenson LW, Childs J, Laks H, et al. Incidence and significance of early pericardial effusion after cardiac surgery. *Am J Cardiol* 1984; 54:848.

74. Kochar GS, Jacobs LE, Kotler MN. Right atrial compression in postoperative cardiac patients: detection by transesophageal echocardiography. *J Am Coll Cardiol* 1990;16:511.

75. Shoebrechts B, Herregods MC, Van de Werf F, et al. Usefulness of transesophageal echocardiography in patients with hemodynamic deterioration late after cardiac surgery. *Chest* 1993;104:1631.

76. Kronzon I, Cohen ML, Winer HE. Diastolic atrial compression: a sensitive echocardiographic sign of cardiac tamponade. *J Am Coll Cardiol* 1983;2:770.

77. Leimgruber PP, Klopfenstein S, Wann LS, et al. The hemodynamic derangement associated with right ventricular diastolic collapse in cardiac tamponade: an experimental echocardiographic study. *Circulation* 1983;68:612.

78. Cogswell TL, Bernath GA, Wann LS, et al. Effects of intravascular volume state on the value of pulsus paradoxus and right ventricular diastolic collapse in predicting cardiac tamponade. *Circulation* 1985; 72:1076.

79. Hoit BD, Gabel M, Fowler NO. Cardiac tamponade in left ventricular dysfunction. *Circulation* 1990;82:1370.

80. Tunick PA, Nachamie M, Kronzon I. Reversal of echocardiographic signs of pericardial tamponade by transfusion. *Am Heart J* 1990;119: 199.

81. Gillam LD, Guyer DE, Gibson TC, et al. Hydrodynamic compression of right atrium: a new echocardiographic sign of cardiac tamponade. *Circulation* 1983;68:294.

82. Appleton CP, Hatle LK, Popp RL. Cardiac tamponade and pericardial effusion: respiratory variation in transvalvular flow velocities studied by Doppler echocardiography. *J Am Coll Cardiol* 1988;11:1020.

83. Louie EK, Hariman RJ, Wang Y, et al. Effect of acute pericardial tamponade on the relative contributions of systolic and diastolic pulmonary venous return: a transesophageal pulsed Doppler study. *Am Heart J* 1995;124.

84. Berge KH, Lanier WL, Reeder GS. Occult cardiac tamponade detected by transesophageal echocardiography. *Mayo Clin Proc* 1992;67:667.

85. Porembka DT, Johnson DJ II, Hoit BD, et al. Penetrating cardiac trauma: a perioperative role for transesophageal echocardiography. *Anesth Analg* 1993;77:1275.

86. Skoularigis J, Essop MR, Sareli P. Usefulness of transesophageal echocardiography in the early diagnosis of penetrating stab wounds to the heart. *Am J Cardiol* 1994;73:407.

87. Erbel R, Engberding R, Daniel W, et al. Echocardiography in the diagnosis of aortic dissection. European Cooperative Study Group for Echocardiography. *Lancet* 1989;1:457.

88. Ballal RS, Nanda NC, Gatewood R, et al. Usefulness of transesophageal echocardiography in assessment of aortic dissection. *Circulation* 1991;84:1903.

89. Hashimoto S, Kumada T, Osakada G, et al. Assessment of transesophageal Doppler echocardiography in dissecting aortic aneurysm. *J Am Coll Cardiol* 1989;14:1253.

90. Nienaber CA, Spielmann RP, von Kodolitsch Y, et al. Diagnosis of thoracic aortic dissection. Magnetic resonance imaging versus transesophageal echocardiography. *Circulation* 1992;85:434.

91. Nienaber CA, von Kodolitsch Y, Nicholas V, et al. The diagnosis of thoracic aortic dissection by noninvasive imaging procedures. *N Engl J Med* 1993;328:1.

92. Laissy J, Blanc F, Soyer P, et al. Thoracic aortic dissection: diagnosis with transesophageal echocardiography versus MR imaging. *Radiology* 1995;194:331.

93. Roudaut RP, Marcaggi XL, Deville C, et al. Value of transesophageal echocardiography combined with computed tomography for assessing repaired type A aortic dissection. *Am J Cardiol* 1992; 70:1468.

94. Erbel R, Oelert H, Meyer J, et al. Effect of medical and surgical therapy on aortic dissection evaluated by transesophageal echocardiography. *Circulation* 1993;87:1604.

95. Wolff KA, Herold CJ, Tempany CM, et al. Aortic dissection: atypical patterns seen at MR imaging. *Radiology* 1991;181:489.

96. Mohr-Kahaly S, Erbel R, Puth M, et al. Aortic intramural hematoma visualized by transesophageal echocardiography. Follow-up and prognostic implications. *Circulation* 1991;84:II-128.

97. Blackshear JL, Safford RE, Lane GE, et al. Unruptured noncoronary sinus of Valsalva aneurysm: preoperative characterization by transesophageal echocardiography. *J Am Soc Echocardiogr* 1991;4:485.

98. Chan K-L. Impact of transesophageal echocardiography on the treatment of patients with aortic dissection. *Chest* 1992;101:406.

99. Shapiro MJ, Yanofsky SD, Trapp J, et al. Cardiovascular evaluation in blunt thoracic trauma using transesophageal echocardiography (TEE). *J Trauma* 1991;31:835.

100. Kearney PA, Smith W, Johnson SB, et al. Use of transesophageal echocardiography in the evaluation of traumatic aortic injury. *J Trauma* 1993;34:696.

101. Le Bret F, Ruel P, Rosier H, et al. Diagnosis of traumatic mediastinal hematoma with transesophageal echocardiography. *Chest* 1994;105: 373.

102. Yamada E. Matsumura M, Kyo S, et al. Usefulness of a prototype intravascular ultrasound imaging in evaluation of aortic dissection and comparison with angiographic study, transesophageal echocardiography, computed tomography, and magnetic resonance imaging. *Am J Cardiol* 1995;76:161.

103. Fazio GP, Redbers RF, Winslow T, et al. Transesophageal echocardiographically detected atherosclerotic aortic plaque is a marker for coronary artery disease. *J Am Coll Cardiol* 1993;21:144.

104. Tribouilloy C, Shen WF, Peltier M, et al. Noninvasive prediction of coronary artery disease by transesophageal echocardiographic detection of thoracic aortic plaque in valvular heart disease. *Am J Cardiol* 1994;74:258.

105. Karalis DG, Chandrasekaran K, Victor MF, et al. Recognition and emboli potential of intraaortic atherosclerotic debris. *J Am Coll Cardiol* 1991;17:73.

106. Jones EF, Kalman JM, Calafiore P, et al. Proximal aortic atheroma an independent risk factor for cerebral ischemia. *Stroke* 1995;26:218.

107. Horowitz DR, Tuhrim S, Budd J, et al. Aortic plaque in patients with brain ischemia: diagnosis by transesophageal echocardiography. *Neurology* 1992;42:1602.

108. Demopoulos LA, Tunick PA, Bernstein NE, et al. Protruding atheromas of the aortic arch in symptomatic patients with carotid artery disease. *Am Heart J* 1995;129:40.

109. Stanson AW, Kazmier FJ, Hoollier LH, et al. Penetrating atherosclerotic ulcers of the thoracic aorta: natural history and clinicopathologic correlations. *Ann Vasc Surg* 1986;1:15.

110. Porembka DT, Johnson DJ, Fowl RJ, et al. Descending thoracic aortic thrombus as a cause of multiple system organ failure: diagnosis by transesophageal echocardiography. *Crit Care Med* 1992;20:1184.

111. Coy KM, Maurer G, Goodman D, et al. Transesophageal echocardiographic detection of aortic atheromatosis may provide clues to occult renal dysfunction in the elderly. *Am Heart J* 1992;123:1684.

112. Stoddard MF, Prince CR, Ammash NM, et al. Two-dimensional transesophageal echocardiographic determination of mitral valve area in adult with mitral stenosis. *Am Heart J* 1994;127:1348.

113. Stoddard MF, Arce J, Liddell NE, et al. Two-dimensional transesophageal echocardiographic determination of aortic valve area in adults with aortic stenosis. *Am Heart J* 1991;122:1415.

114. Bengur AR, Snider AR, Meliones JN, et al. Doppler evaluation of aortic valve area in children with aortic stenosis. *J Am Coll Cardiol* 1991;18:1499.

115. Sheikh KH, deBruijn NP, Rankin JS, et al. The utility of trans-

esophageal echocardiography and Doppler color flow imaging in patients undergoing cardiac valve surgery. *J Am Coll Cardiol* 1990; 15:363.

116. Sheikh KH, Bengtson JR, Rankin JS, et al. Intraoperative transesophageal Doppler color flow imaging used to guide patient selection and operative treatment of ischemic mitral regurgitation. *Circulation* 1991;84:594.

117. Stewart WJ, Currie PJ, Salcedo EE, et al. Jet direction by color flow mapping accurately depicts the mechanism of mitral regurgitation. *Circulation* 1988;78:434.

118. Jacobs LE, Wertheimer JH, Kotler MN, et al. Quantification of mitral regurgitation: a comparison of transesophageal echocardiography and contrast ventriculography. *Echocardiography* 1992;9:145.

119. Kamp O, Dijkstra JW, Huitnink H, et al. Transesophageal color flow Doppler mapping in the assessment of native mitral valvular regurgitation: comparison with left ventricular angiography. *J Am Soc Echocardiogr* 1991;4:598.

120. Castello R, Lenzen P, Aguirre F, et al. Quantification of mitral regurgitation by transesophageal echocardiography with color flow mapping: correlation with cardiac catherization. *J Am Coll Cardiol* 1992; 19:1516.

121. Yoshida K, Yoshikawa J, Yamaura Y, et al. Assessment of mitral regurgitation by biplane transesophageal color Doppler flow mapping. *Circulation* 1990;82:1121.

122. Klein AL, Stewart WJ, Bartlett J, et al. Effects of mitral regurgitation on pulmonary venous flow and left atrial pressure: an intraoperative transesophageal echocardiographic study. *J Am Coll Cardiol* 1990; 20:1345.

123. Lai L, Shyu K, Chen J, et al. Usefulness of pulmonary venous flow pattern and maximal jet area detected by transesophageal echocardiography in assessing the severity of mitral regurgitation. *Am J Cardiol* 1993;72:1310.

124. Castello R, Fagan L, Lenzen P, et al. Comparison of transthoracic and transesophageal echocardiography for assessment of left-sided valvular regurgitation. *Am J Cardiol* 1991;68:1677.

125. Cape EG, Yoganathan AP, Weyman AE, et al. Adjacent solid boundaries alter the size of regurgitant jets on Doppler color flow maps. *J Am Coll Cardiol* 1991;17:1094.

126. Castello R, Pearson AC, Lenzen P, et al. Effect of mitral regurgitation on pulmonary venous velocities derived from transesophageal echocardiography color-guided pulsed Doppler imaging. *J Am Coll Cardiol* 1991;17:1499.

127. Chen C, Koschyk D, Brockhoff C, et al. Noninvasive estimation of regurgitant flow rate and volume in patients with mitral regurgitation by Doppler color mapping of accelerating flow field. *J Am Coll Cardiol* 1993;21:374.

128. Tribouilly C, Shen WF, Quere JP, et al. Assesment of severity of mitral regurgitation by measuring regurgitant jet width at its origin with transesophageal Doppler color flow imaging. *Circulation* 1992; 85:1248.

129. Enriquez-Sarano M, Bailey KR, Seward JB, et al. Quantitative Doppler assessment of valvular regurgittaion. *Circulation* 1993;83:841.

130. Dittrich HC, McCann HA, Walsh TP, et al. Transesophageal echocardiography in the evaluation of prosthetic and native aortic valves. *Am J Cardiol* 1990;66:758.

131. Perry GJ, Helmcke F, Nanda JC, et al. Evaluation of aortic insufficiency by Doppler color flow mapping. *J Am Coll Cardiol* 1987;9:952.

132. Nishimura RA, Vonk GD, Rumberger JA, et al. Semiquantification of aortic regurgitation by different Doppler echocardiographic techniques and comparison with ultrafast computed tomography. *Am Heart J* 1992;124:995.

133. Labovitz AJ, Ferrara RP, Kern MJ, et al. Quantitative evaluation of aortic insufficiency by continuous wave Doppler echocardiography. *J Am Coll Cardiol* 1986;8:1341.

134. Khandheria BK, Seward JB, Oh JK, et al. Value and limitations of transesophageal echocardiography in assessment of mitral valve prosthesis. *Circulation* 1991;83:1956.

135. van den Brink RBA, Visser CA, Basart DCG, et al. Comparison of transthoracic and transesophageal color flow Doppler imaging in patients with mechanical prosthesis in the mitral valve position. *Am J Cardiol* 1989;63:1471.

136. Herrea CJ, Chaudhry FA, DeFrino PF, et al. Value and limitations of transesophageal echocardiography in evaluating prosthetic or bioprosthetic valve dysfunction. *Am J Cardiol* 1992;69:697.

137. Daniel WG, Mugge A, Grote J, et al. Comparison of transthoracic and transesophageal echocardiography for detection of abnormalities of prosthetic and bioprosthetic valves in the mitral and aortic positions. *Am J Cardiol* 1993;71:210.

138. Taams MA, Gussenhoven EJ, Cahalan MK, et al. Transesophageal Doppler color flow imaging in the detection of native and Bjork-Shiley mitral valve regurgitation. *J Am Coll Cardiol* 1989;13:95.

139. Skudicky D, Skoularigis J, Essop MR, et al. Prevalence and clinical significance of mild paraprosthetic ring leaks and left atrial spontaneous echo contrast detected on transesophageal echocardiography three months after isolated mitral valve replacement with a mechanical prosthesis. *Am J Cardiol* 1993;72:848.

140. Grigg LE, Wigle D, Williams WG, et al. Transesophageal Doppler echocardiography in obstructive hypertrophic cardiomyopathy: clarification of pathophysiology and importance in intraoperative decision making. *J Am Coll Cardiol* 1992;20:42.

141. Stevenson JG, Sorensen GK, Gartman DM, et al. Left ventricular outflow tract obstruction: an indication for intraoperative transesophageal echocardiography. *J Am Soc Echocardiogr* 1993;6:525.

142. Come PC. Echocardiographic evaluation of pulmonary embolism and its response to therapeutic interventions. *Chest* 1992;101:151S.

143. Jardin F, Dubourg O, Gueret P, et al. Quantitative two-dimensional echocardiography in massive pulmonary embolism: emphasis on ventricular interdependence and leftward septal displacement. *J Am Coll Cardiol* 1987;10:1201.

144. Kasper W, Meinertz T, Henkel B, et al. Echocardiographic findings in patients with proved pulmonary embolism. *Am Heart J* 1986;112: 1284.

145. Langeron O, Goarin JP, Pansard JL, et al. Massive intraoperative pulmonary embolism: diagnosis with transesophageal two-dimension echocardiography. *Anesth Analg* 1992;74:148.

146. Heng Y, Shyu KG, Kuan, P. Expanded indication: diagnosis of pulmonary embolism by transesophageal echocardiography. *Int J Cardiol* 1993;39:91.

147. McGrath BJ, Hsia J, Boyd A, et al. Venous embolization after deflation of lower extremity tourniquets. *Anesth Analg* 1994;78:349.

148. Parmet JL, Horrow JC, Singer R, et al. Echogenic emboli upon tourniquet release during total knee arthroplasty: pulmonary hemodynamic changes and embolic composition. *Anesth Analg* 1994;79:940.

149. Lovett JL, Sandok BA, Guiliani ER, et al. Two-dimensional echocardiography in patients with focal cerebral ischemia. *Ann Intern Med* 1981;95:1.

150. Aschenberg W, Schluter M, Kremer P, et al. Transesophageal two-dimensional echocardiography for the detection of left atrial appendage thrombus. *J Am Coll Cardiol* 1986;7:163.

151. Kronzon I, Tunick PA, Colossman E, et al. Transesophageal echocardiography to detect atrial clots in candidates for percutaneous transseptal mitral balloon valvuloplasty. *J Am Coll Cardiol* 1990;16:1320.

152. Hwang J, Kuan P, Lin S, et al. Reappraisal by transesophageal echocardiography of the significance of left atrial thrombi in the prediction of systemic arterial embolization in rheumatic mitral valve disease. *Am J Cardiol* 1992;70:769.

153. Vigna C, de Rito V, Criconia GM, et al. Left atrial thrombus and spontaneous echo-contrast in non anticoagulated mitral stenosis. *Chest* 1993;103:348.

154. Lee RJ, Bartzokis T, Yeoh TK, et al. Enhanced detection of intracardiac sources of cerebral emboli by transesophageal echocardiography. *Stroke* 1991;22:734.

155. Pearson AC, Labovitz AJ, Tatineni S, et al. Superiority of transesophageal echocardiography in detecing cardiac source of embolism in patients with cerebral ischemia of uncertain etiology. *J Am Coll Cardiol* 1991;17:66.

156. Albers GW, Comess KA, DeRook FA, et al. Transesophageal echocardiographic findings in stroke subtypes. *Stroke* 1994;25:23.

157. Stoddard MF, Dawkins PR, Prince CR, et al. Left atrial appendage thrombus is not uncommon in patients with acute atrial fibrillation and a recent embolic event: a transesophageal echocardiographic study. *J Am Coll Cardiol* 1995;25:452.

158. Salka S, Saeian K, Sagar KB, et al. Cerebral thromboembolization after cardioversion of atrial fibrillation in patients without transesophageal echocardiographic findings of left atrial thrombus. *Am Heart J* 1993;126:722.

159. Manning WJ, Silverman DI, Gordon SPF, et al. Cardioversion from atrial fibrillation without prolonged anticoagulation with use of the

transesophageal echocardiography to exclude the presence of atrial thrombi. *N Engl J Med* 1993;328:750.

160. Grimm RA, Stewart WJ, Maloney JD, et al. Impact of electrical cardioversion for atrial fibrillation on left atrial appendage function and spontaneous echo contrast: characterization by simultaneous transesophageal echocardiography. *J Am Coll Cardiol* 1993;22:1359.

161. Moreyra E, Finkelhor RS, Cebul RD. Limitations of transesophageal echocardiography in the risk assessment of patients before nonanticoagulated cardioversion from atrial fibrillation and flutter: an analysis of pooled trials. *Am Heart J* 1995;129:71.

162. Hwang J, Li Y, Lin J, et al. Left atrial appendage function determined by transesophageal echocardiography in patients with rheumatic mitral valve disease. *Cardiology* 1994;85:121.

163. Lechat PH, Mas JL, Lascault G, et al. Prevalence of patent foramen ovale in patients with stroke. *N Engl J Med* 1988;318:1148.

164. Hausmann D, Mugge A, Becht I, et al. Diagnosis of patent foramen ovale by transesophageal echocardiography and association with cerebral and peripheral embolic events. *Am J Cardiol* 1992;70:668.

165. Jaffe RA, Pinto FJ, Schnittger I, et al. Aspects of mechanical ventilation affecting interatrial shunt flow during general anesthesia. *Anesth Analg* 1992;75:484.

166. Guggiari M, Lechat P, Garen-Colonne C, et al. Early detection of patent foramen ovale by two-dimensional contrast echocardiography for prevention of paradoxical air embolism during sitting position. *Anesth Analg* 1988;67:192.

167. Chen WJ, Kuan P, Lien WP, et al. Detection of patent foramen ovale by contrast transesophageal echocardiography. *Chest* 1992;101:1515.

168. Black S, Muzzi DA, Nishimura RA, et al. Preoperative and intraoperative echocardiography to detect right-to-left shunt in patients undergoing neurosurgical procedures in the sitting position. *Anesthesiology* 1990;72:436.

169. Konstadt SN, Louie EK, Black S, et al. Intraoperative detection of patent foramen ovale by transesophageal echocardiography. *Anesthesiology* 1991;74:212.

170. Porembka D, Valente J, Anderson G, et al. Postoperative detection of patent foramen ovale by transesophageal echocardiography. *Crit Care Med* 1993;21:S269.

171. Siostrzonek P, Zangeneh M, Gossinger H, et al. Comparison of transesophageal for detection of a patent foramen ovale. *Am J Cardiol* 1991;68:1247.

172. Stollberger C, Schneider B, Abzieher F, et al. Diagnosis of patent foramen ovale by transesophageal contrast echocardiography. *Am J Cardiol* 71:604;1993.

173. Louie EK, Konstadt SN, Rao TL, et al. Transesophageal echocardiographic diagnosis of right to left shunting across the foramen ovale in adults with prior stroke. *J Am Coll Cardiol* 1993;21:1231.

174. DeSio JM, Goodnough SR, Hajduczok ZD. The effect of positive end-expiratory pressure on right-to-left shunting at the atrial level as documented by transesophageal echocardiography. *Anesthesiology* 1992;77:1033.

175. Dewan NA, Gayasaddin M, Angelillo VA, et al. Persistent hypoxemia due to patent foramen ovale in a patient with adult respiratory distress syndrome. *Chest* 1986;89:611.

176. Yvorchuk KJ, Chan K-L. Application of transthoracic and transesophageal echocardiography in the diagnosis and management of infective endocarditis. *J Am Soc Echocardiogr* 1994;14;294.

177. Khanderia BK. Suspected bacterial endocarditis: to TEE or not to TEE. *J Am Coll Cardiol* 1993;21:222.

178. Gilbert BW, Haney RS, Crawford F, et al. Two-dimensional echocardiographic assessment of vegetative endocarditis. *Circulation* 1977;55:346.

179. Daniel WG, Schroder E, Nonnast-Daniel B, et al. Conventional and transesophageal echocardiography in the diagnosis of infective endocarditis. *Eur Heart J* 1987:8(Suppl J):287.

180. Erbel R, Rohmann S, Drexler M, et al. Improved diagnostic value of echocardiography in patients with infective endocarditis by transesophageal approach. A prospective study. *Eur Heart J* 1988;9:43.

181. Klodas E, Edwards WD, Khanderia BK. Use of transesophageal echocardiography for improving detection of valvular vegetations in subacute bacterial endocarditis. *J Am Soc Echocardiogr* 1989;2:386.

182. Mugge A, Daniel WG, Frank G, et al. Echocardiography in infective endocarditis: reassessment of prognostic implications of vegetation size determined by the transthoracic and transesophageal approach. *J Am Coll Cardiol* 1989;14:631.

183. Taams MA, Gussenhoven EJ, Bos E, et al. Enhanced morphological diagnosis in endocarditis by transesophageal echocardiography. *Br Heart J* 1990;63:109.

184. Pedersen WR, Walker M, Olson JD, et al. Value of transesophageal echocardiography as an adjunct to transthoracic echocardiography in evaluation of native and prosthetic valve endocarditis. *Chest* 1991;100:351.

185. Birmingham GD, Rahko PS, Ballantyne F III. Improved detection of infective endocarditis with transesophageal echocardiograpy. *Am Heart J* 1992;123:774.

186. Shapiro SM, Young E, Ginzton LE, et al. Pulmonic valve endocarditis as an underdiagnosed disease: role of transesophageal echocardiography. *J Am Soc Echocardiogr* 1992;5:48.

187. Winslow T, Foster E, Schiller NB. Pulmonary valve endocarditis: improved diagnosis with biplane transesophageal echocardiography. *J Am Soc Echocardiogr* 1992;5:206.

188. Shively BK, Gurule FT, Roldan CA, et al. Diagnostic value of transesophageal compared with transthoracic echocardiography in infective endocarditis. *J Am Coll Cardiol* 1991;18:391.

189. San Roman JA, Vilacosta I, Zamorano JL. Transesophageal echocardiography in right-sided endocarditis. *J Am Coll Cardiol* 1993;21:1226.

190. Shapiro SM, Young E, de Guzman S, et al. Transesophageal echocardiography in diagnosis of infective endocarditis. *Chest* 1994;105:377.

191. Scanlan JG, Seward JB, Tajik AJ. Valve ring abscess in infective endocarditis: visualization with wide angle two dimensional echocardiography. *Am J Cardiol* 1982;49:1794.

192. Daniel WG, Schroeder E, Mugge A, et al. Transesophageal echocardiography in infective endocarditis. *Am J Cardiol Imag* 1988;2:78.

193. Rohmann S, Erbel R, Gorge G, et al. Clinical relevance of vegetations localization by transesophageal echocardiography in infective endocarditis. *Eur Heart J* 1992;13:446.

194. Rohmann S, Erbel R, Darius H, et al. Spontaneous echo contrast imaging in infective endocarditis: a predictor of complications? *Int J Card Imag* 1992;8:197.

195. Daniel WG, Mugge A, Martin RP, et al. Improvement in the diagnosis of abscesses associated with endocarditis by transesophageal echocardiography. *N Engl J Med* 1991;324:795.

196. Karalis DG, Bansal RC, Hauck AJ, et al. Transesophageal echocardiographic recognition of subaortic complications in aortic valve endocarditis. Clinical and surgical implications. *Circulation* 1992;86:353.

197. Bansal RC, Graham BM, Jutzy KR, et al. Left ventricular outflow tract to left atrial communication secondary to rupture of mitral-aortic intervalvular fibrosa in infective endocarditis: diagnosis by transesophageal echocardiography and color flow imaging. *J Am Coll Cardiol* 1990;15:499.

198. Sochowski RA, Chan K-L. Implication of negative results on a monoplane transesophageal echocardiographic study in patients with suspected infective endocarditis. *J Am Coll Cardiol* 1993;21:216.

# Respiratory Mechanics

## N. Tony Eissa

Recently there has been renewed interest in respiratory monitoring in mechanically ventilated critically ill patients. Such monitoring would be expected to aid in clinical decision making and the management of these patients. In mechanically ventilated patients, a detailed analysis of respiratory mechanics can be performed readily with simple and commonly available equipment, namely a pneumotachograph to measure flow, an integrator to obtain volume changes from the flow signal, and a pressure transducer to measure the pressure at the airway opening or, preferably, in the trachea some distance beyond the distal end of the endotracheal tube (1). Several commercial ventilators allow direct measurements of these variables. With this equipment it is possible to determine, noninvasively, the static and dynamic elastance of the respiratory system, the flow resistance of the respiratory system, airways and thoracic tissues, and intrinsic positive end-expiratory pressure (PEEP) (2–4).

The respiratory system consists of two main parts: a gas exchanging organ, the lungs, and a pump that ventilates the lung. The pump consists of the chest wall, including the respiratory muscles, and the respiratory centers in the central nervous system which control the muscles used in moving the chest wall during breathing. Failure of any part of the system may lead to respiratory failure. Clearly, several mechanisms may account for respiratory failure in the same patient. Simplistically, however, it can be said that mechanical ventilation due to respiratory failure is required whenever the respiratory pump cannot cope with the mechanical loads that it has to overcome. In this part of the chapter, we will focus on some of the tests for assessing respiratory muscle function, and we will also discuss the various loads imposed on them (resistive, elastic, and intrinsic PEEP), together with other simple noninvasive measurements of ventilatory function.

## LUNG VOLUMES

### Functional Residual Capacity

In mechanically ventilated patients the functional residual capacity (FRC) can be measured by gas dilution techniques (5). Such measurements, however, are technically difficult, and hence few measurements have been reported (5–7). Furthermore, the above techniques do not measure the total thoracic gas volume, but rather the gas contained in airspaces with open airways. Changes in total thoracic volume (including gases, liquids, and solids) can be estimated by noninvasive methods such as radiography, computed tomography, strain gauges, magnetometers, bellows pneumographs, and inductive plethysmographs. The latter technique also allows partitioning of the respiratory movements into the motion of the rib cage and that of the abdomen-diaphragm (8).

In normal subjects at rest, the end-expiratory lung volume (FRC) corresponds to the relaxation volume ($V_r$) of the respiratory system, i.e., the lung volume at which the elastic recoil pressure of the respiratory system is zero (9, 10). In critically ill patients, however, the FRC commonly exceeds $V_r$, a condition termed dynamic pulmonary hyperinflation (11, 12).

### Dynamic Hyperinflation (ΔFRC)

Dynamic hyperinflation exists whenever the duration of expiration is insufficient to allow the lung to deflate to $V_r$ prior to the next inspiration (11, 12). This tends to occur under conditions in which expiratory flow is impeded (e.g., increased airway resistance) or when the expiratory time is shortened (e.g., increased breathing frequency or inverse I/E ratio ventilation). Expiratory flow may also be retarded by other mechanisms such as contraction of the inspiratory muscles during expiration and expiratory narrowing of the glottic aperture (10). At rest, under normal conditions, the end-expiratory elastic recoil pressure of the respiratory system ($P_{st,rs}$) is zero. When breathing takes place at lung volumes higher than $V_r$, the end-expiratory $P_{st,rs}$ is positive. This pressure has been termed auto-PEEP (13) or intrinsic PEEP (PEEPi)

N. T. Eissa: Pulmonary Branch, National Heart, Lung and Blood Institute, National Institutes of Health, Bethesda, Maryland 20892.

(14). In patients with severe airway obstruction intrinsic PEEP is an important inspiratory load (see below).

The presence of PEEPi implies that the end-expiratory lung volume during mechanical ventilation is greater than $V_r$, the difference between FRC and $V_r$ being termed $\Delta$FRC. During passive mechanical ventilation (e.g., controlled mechanical ventilation, CMV), $\Delta$FRC ($=$FRC - $V_r$) can be determined by inserting a prolonged expiratory time during a steady-state mechanical ventilation which allows the patient to exhale to $V_r$ (4, 15), as shown in Fig. 1. In patients with chronic obstructive pulmonary disease (COPD) or asthma with severe expiratory flow limitation reaching $V_r$ may require an expiratory time of up to 40 seconds (15). In patients receiving PEEP, the removal of PEEP during the prolonged expiration will allow measurement of the $\Delta$FRC due to PEEP as well (4).

### Inspiratory Capacity

The vital capacity (VC) is a simple test of thoracoabdominal mobility which is commonly measured in critically ill patients as an important index for weaning (16). In contrast, the inspiratory capacity (IC) is rarely studied in critically ill patients. This seems surprising since resting breathing usually involves only the inspiratory mus-

cles, and hence IC should be a better index than VC for predicting the patient's capacity to achieve an adequate tidal volume during spontaneous breathing.

### FLOW-VOLUME LOOPS

Measurement of flow-volume (F-V) loops during resting breathing and with maximal efforts is an integral part of routine pulmonary function testing in stable patients with respiratory disease. By comparing the F-V loops obtained during resting breathing with those obtained during forced maximal inspiratory and expiratory efforts, the ventilatory reserve can be assessed. Such measurements are particularly useful in critically ill patients in whom the ventilatory reserve is often markedly reduced due to altered respiratory mechanics and/or abnormalities in respiratory muscle function (12, 17). The respiratory status of these patients should be followed by studying their inspiratory and expiratory flow and volume reserve.

A useful way to detect for dynamic hyperinflation and hence PEEPi is the analysis of the F-V relationship during a relaxed expiration (18). When PEEPi is absent, the expiratory flow decreases smoothly to zero prior to the next mechanical inflation. By contrast, when PEEPi is present, there is flow throughout expiration which is

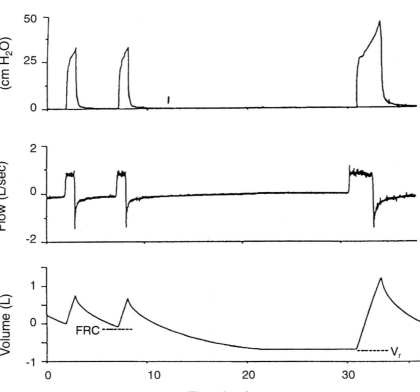

**FIG. 1.** Records of pressure at the airway opening, flow, and changes in lung volume from a sedated-paralyzed COPD patient illustrating the measurement of FRC which is the difference between end-expiratory lung volume (FRC) and relaxation volume of the respiratory system ($V_r$). A prolonged expiratory time was inserted during steady-state mechanical ventilation that allowed the patient to exhale to $V_r$. FRC in this patient amounted to 0.673 L.

abruptly terminated by the next mechanical inflation, such that the expiratory flow–time curve has a characteristic "truncated" appearance (Fig. 2).

## MAXIMAL INSPIRATORY PRESSURE

Assessment of diaphragmatic function usually requires measurement of esophageal and gastric pressures. By contrast, the inspiratory pressure developed at the mouth during a maximal inspiratory effort against an occluded airway (PI,max) is a simple noninvasive test of the contractility of the inspiratory muscles (19). A decrease in PI,max may be due to hyperinflation, change in thoracic configuration, neuromascular disease, or fatigue (19). Since PI,max represents the potential pressure which the inspiratory muscles can generate during spontaneous breathing, it has been considered a useful index to predict weaning outcome in mechanically ventilated patients (20). The test, however, proved to be unreliable in that respect (21). This can be due to several factors: (a) Although the test is simple, it requires good patient cooperation to obtain a true maximal effort. (b) The PI,max is conventionally measured with the patient making a maximal inspiratory effort at residual volume (RV) in order to maximize the mechanical advantage of the inspiratory muscles by increasing their operating length (22). Since

resting ventilation usually occurs well above RV, PI,max at FRC should be a better predictor of weaning outcome than PI,max at RV.

### Breathing Pattern

Most modern ventilators allow for direct measurement of spontaneous minute ventilation, frequency, and tidal volume (VT). The relationship between minute ventilation and arterial $P_{CO_2}$ ($Pa_{CO_2}$) provides a good index of the ventilatory demands being placed on the respiratory system (21). Since $Pa_{CO_2}$ is determined by the relationship between alveolar ventilation and $CO_2$ production ($CO_2$), a high minute ventilation in the presence of hypercapnia indicates the presence of dead-space ventilation and/or increased $CO_2$ production. Maximum voluntary ventilation (MVV) is the volume of air that can be inhaled and exhaled with maximum effort over 1 minute. The relationship between resting minute ventilation and MVV indicates the proportion of the patient's ventilatory capacity required to maintain a given $Pa_{CO_2}$ and also indicates the degree of reserve available for further respiratory demands. A resting minute ventilation of 10 L/min or less with the capability of doubling this value during a MVV maneuver is commonly considered to predict weaning success (16). Low tidal volume (less than 300

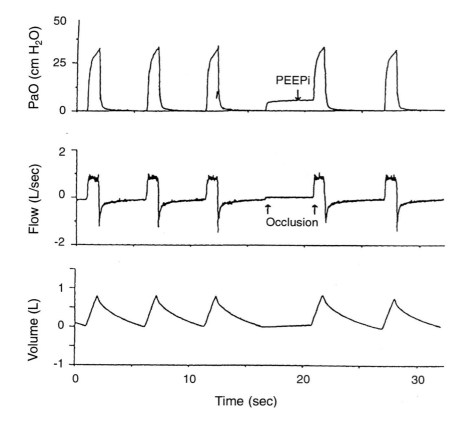

**FIG. 2.** Records of pressure at the airway opening, flow, and changes in lung volume from the same COPD patient in Fig. 1. Note that flow continues throughout expiration and is abruptly terminated by the onset of the next breath, indicating the presence of dynamic hyperinflation and intrinsic PEEP (PEEPi). PEEPi is measured by end-expiratory airway occlusion *(arrows)*. Upon occlusion, the airway pressure rises and reaches a plateau that corresponds to the static end-expiratory elastic recoil pressure of the respiratory system (= PEEPi). PEEPi in this patient amounted to 5.5 cm $H_2O$.

mL) suggests that a weaning trial is likely to be unsuccessful (21, 23). Such a low $V_T$ is often associated with tachypnea (i.e., rapid shallow breathing). Even in the absence of $V_T$ measurements, detecting a high respiratory rate (e.g., above 22 breaths/min) is a sign of respiratory failure (24). While highly sensitive, tachypnea is a nonspecific sign, and further investigation is required to determine the nature of underlying disturbance (21, 23, 24). In patients with severe airway obstruction, the fraction of inspiratory time ($T_I$) relative to the total breathing cycle duration ($T_{TOT}$) decreases (25, 26). Since the inspiratory muscles are active mainly during inspiration, a decrease in $T_I/T_{TOT}$ (also called respiratory duty cycle) will decrease the burden on the inspiratory muscles and spare them from fatigue (19, 27, 28).

## MOUTH OCCLUSION PRESSURE ($P_{0.1}$)

One of the major problems encountered in the study of the control of breathing has been to find a simple measure of the output of the respiratory center. Ventilation was originally used as a measure of this output, but it has the major disadvantage of being influenced by respiratory flow resistance, compliance, and PEEPi (if present), which may cause changes in ventilation that do not reflect variations in the respiratory center's activity. To avoid this problem, the rate of work (power) of the inspiratory muscles was proposed (29). Measurements of oxygen cost of breathing and of diaphragmatic electromyogram (EMG) have been used as well (24). These measurements, however, are technically complex, for they involve the use of esophageal electrodes, balloons, or both. Measurements of the pressure generated by the inspiratory muscles at FRC against an occluded airway have been proposed as a useful alternative (24, 30). It is a simple noninvasive measure of neuromuscular inspiratory drive (24). It consists of measurement of the pressure generated at the mouth in the first 0.1 second ($P_{0.1}$) of an inspiration made with airway occluded at FRC (24). The $P_{0.1}$ reflects the inspiratory pressure potentially available for inspiration under the conditions of neurochemical stimulation of breathing prevailing during its measurement. Its advantage is that it is independent of lung mechanics.

The primary goal of mechanical ventilation is to reduce the increased inspiratory workload which precipitates or accompanies respiratory failure. It has been shown, however, that in patient-initiated mechanical ventilation the mechanical work done by the patient frequently represented a high fraction of the total inspiratory work (31, 32). A close correlation was found by Marini et al. (31) between $P_{0.1}$ and the patient's inspiratory work per liter of ventilation, and hence $P_{0.1}$ can be used as a simple noninvasive index to evaluate the inspiratory effort performed by the patient. During patient-initiated

mechanical ventilation $P_{0.1}$ can be readily measured by virtue of the fact that delay imposed by the demand valve systems of most ventilators provides an occlusion period long enough to allow measurement of $P_{0.1}$ (6, 31). The advantage of this approach is that every breath potentially provides an estimate of $P_{0.1}$.

In healthy subjects at rest, the values of $P_{0.1}$ are generally less than 2 cm $H_2O$ (33). In patients with respiratory disease $P_{0.1}$ invariably increases (24), particularly in COPD patients with acute respiratory failure (34). In these patients, due to pulmonary hyperinflation, the inspiratory muscles operate at a mechanical disadvantage due to a decrease in their operating length (35). Furthermore, because the diaphragm is flatter, a given tension (which is related to force) will generate less pressure (19). Accordingly, the high values of $P_{0.1}$ in these patients imply very high inspiratory muscle activity. Clearly, such high levels of inspiratory muscle activity cannot be sustained for a prolonged period without development of muscle fatigue (27, 28). In fact, it has been shown that in COPD patients with acute respiratory failure, these high values of $P_{0.1}$ are associated with inspiratory muscle fatigue, as assessed by diaphragmatic EMG (36).

The use of $P_{0.1}$ as a predictor of weaning outcome has been recently examined. Murciano et al. (36) found that $P_{0.1}$ decreased from 7.4 ± 0.7 cm $H_2O$ (mean ± SE) at the time of intubation to 3.9 ± 0.4 cm $H_2O$ at the time of extubation in patients who were successfully weaned, whereas patients who failed a weaning trial showed no change in their $P_{0.1}$ values which at the time of intubation amounted to 6.6 ± 0.3 cm $H_2O$. Sasson et al. (37) found that all patients who failed a weaning trial had $P_{0.1}$ values greater than 6 cm $H_2O$, whereas all patients who were successfully weaned had $P_{0.1}$ values below 6 cm $H_2O$. In contrast, Montgomery et al. (38) failed to find a significant difference in $P_{0.1}$ values between patients who were successfully weaned and those who failed a weaning trial. Clearly, further studies are required to evaluate the use of $P_{0.1}$ in mechanically ventilated patients.

### Effective Inspiratory Impedance

It has been long been recognized that in the presence of mechanical limitations of breathing (e.g., increased elastance and flow resistance of the respiratory system), the ventilatory output reflects both how much the patient "wants" to breathe, an issue directly involving respiratory control, and how much the patient's mechanical abnormality "allows" him or her to breathe, an issue that involves control of breathing only indirectly. To distinguish between the two mechanisms, measurements of the respiratory mechanical work rate have been used in the past (24). Indeed, an increased mechanical work-rate-to-flow ratio, or increased mechanical work per liter of air ventilated, indicates the presence of mechanical abnormalities within the ventilatory pump. A simple noninvasive alternative is to measure the ratio of $P_{0.1}$ to minute ventilation or better to $V_T/T_I$. The latter $P_{0.1}/(V_T/T_I)\}$ has been termed the *effective inspiratory impedance* (24). Since this index is obtained by dividing the pressure generated during a fraction of an occluded breath by the mean inspiratory flow for an entire unoccluded inspiration, caution must be used in interpreting its significance. The effective inspiratory impedance has been found to be significantly lower in patients who are successfully weaned (37).

## RESPIRATORY LOADS

The breathing movements require work involving the following mechanisms (39): (a) elastic forces; (b) resistive forces resulting from flow of gas through the airways and viscoelastic forces attributable to stress adaptation units within the thoracic tissues (lung and chest wall) (3, 39, 40), and (c) in some patients, particularly those with airway obstruction, inspiratory work has to be exerted in order to overcome PEEPi (26, 39, 41). Since PEEPi imposes a threshold pressure which the inspiratory muscles must overcome before the onset of inspiratory flow, PEEPi can be regarded an an inspiratory threshold load (26, 41).

### Intrinsic PEEP

#### Implications of PEEPi during Spontaneous Breathing

Figure 3 illustrates the increase in pressure required to overcome the elastic recoil of the respiratory system for the same tidal volume (=20% of vital capacity, VC) inhaled from $V_r$ (=34% VC) and from end-expiratory lung volume increase to 67% VC. As shown by the hatched areas, the elastic work increases about fivefold when the breath is inhaled from 67% VC (case B) relative to the breath taken from $V_r$ (case A). Clearly, dynamic hyperinflation implies an increase of both elastic work and inspiratory muscle effort. Furthermore, as lung volume increases, there is a decreased effectiveness of the inspiratory muscles as pressure generators, because the inspiratory muscle fibres become shorter (force-length relationship) and their geometric arrangement changes (35).

Under normal conditions (case A in Fig. 3) the end-expiratory elastic recoil pressure of the respiratory system is zero. In this instance, as soon as the inspiratory muscles contract, the alveolar pressure becomes subatmospheric and gas flows into the lungs. When breathing takes place at lung volumes higher than $V_r$, the end-expiratory elastic recoil pressure (=PEEPi) is positive (15 cm $H_2O$ in case B of Fig. 3). When PEEPi is present, onset

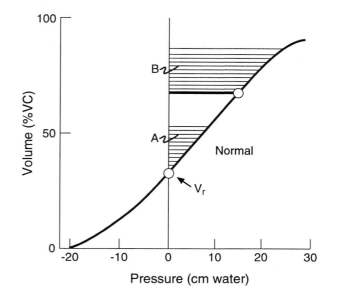

**FIG. 3.** Volume-pressure diagram of the relaxed respiratory system showing the increase in elastic work caused by dynamic hyperinflation. VC, vital capacity; $V_r$, relaxation volume of the respiratory system. *Hatched area A:* Elastic work for a breath that starts from $V_r$. *Hatched area B:* Elastic work for a similar breath that starts from a volume 29% VC higher than $V_r$. In case B, the intrinsic PEEP is 15 cm $H_2O$, as indicated by the upper circle.

of inspiratory muscle activity and onset of inspiratory flow are not synchronous: Inspiratory flow starts only when the pressure developed by the inspiratory muscles exceeds PEEPi because only then alveolar pressure becomes subatmospheric. In this respect, PEEPi acts as an inspiratory threshold load on the inspiratory muscles (12, 26, 41), which are already operating under mechanical disadvantage.

#### Implications of PEEPi during Mechanical Ventilation

As mentioned above, the putative role of mechanical ventilation is to reduce the activity of the inspiratory muscles to tolerable levels during patient-triggered mechanical ventilation (e.g., assisted mechanical ventilation, pressure support). This end is not achieved in patients who exhibit high PEEPi since the inspiratory effort required from the patient to trigger the ventilator may be excessive (41). By contrast, during controlled mechanical ventilation all of the work of breathing is done by the ventilator. Nevertheless, PEEPi must be taken into account for correct measurement of respiratory compliance (14) and more importantly in terms of adverse effects on venous return and cardiac output (13). Furthermore, patients with high PEEPi are difficult to wean from mechanical ventilation and they become ventilator dependent (12).

### Methods to Measure PEEPi

In mechanically ventilated patients, the increase in end-expiratory airway pressure will not normally register on the ventilator manometer (13). During exhalation, the ventilator manometer is exposed to ambient pressure as the exhalation valve is open. Only resistance from the valve or applied PEEP will register on the ventilator manometer. Despite the fact that distal airway pressure may be positive throughout exhalation, the manometer will not reflect the increased pressure unless the expiratory port is occluded. If the expiratory port is occluded, at end expiration distal airway pressure and circuit pressure equilibrate, and PEEPi will be reflected on the ventilator manometer. Figure 2 illustrates this method in a COPD patient. Occlusion was done at end expiration using the end-expiratory hold button on the servo 900C ventilator. The airway pressure rises and reaches a plateau which corresponds to PEEPi. An external valve will be needed to perform occlusion in patients ventilated with ventilators which are not equipped with end-expiratory hold buttons.

In spontaneously breathing patients PEEPi can be determined as the negative deflection in esophageal pressure from the start of inspiratory effort to the onset of inspiratory flow (26, 41). This pressure has been termed dynamic PEEPi (26, 41). Values of dynamic PEEPi are usually lower than those obtained by the end-expiratory occlusion technique described above (static PEEPi). Static measurement of PEEPi necessarily reflect alveolar pressure after readjustment of dynamic regional volume and pressure differences due to time constant inequalities within the lung (pendelluft). In this case, PEEPi reflects the equilibrium or static increase in end-expiratory $P_{st,rs}$ caused by dynamic hyperinflation. In the presence of pendelluft (and hence regional difference in PEEPi) static PEEPi will exceed the lowest regional alveolar pressure present at the end of an unoccluded expiration. By contrast, dynamic PEEPi should reflect the lowest regional end-expiratory alveolar pressure (or regional PEEPi) within the lung. Indeed, as soon as esophageal pressure during inspiration balances the lowest regional PEEPi, air begins to flow into the lung. In the case of a mechanically uniform lung, static and dynamic PEEPi should be identical, but in the presence of time constant inhomogeneities within the lung, static and dynamic PEEPi differ, the latter reflecting the lowest regional PEEPi. In patients with severe COPD, Petrof et al. (41) found that dynamic PEEPi represented, on average, 57% of static PEEPi.

Another approach for measuring PEEPi in spontaneously breathing patients is by monitoring changes in thoracic volume using respiratory inductive plethysmography while adding continous positive airway pressure (CPAP) (41). The level of CPAP where thoracic volume starts to increase should correspond to PEEPi .

## COMPLIANCE

### Static Compliance of the Respiratory System ($C_{st,rs}$)

Reduced $C_{st,rs}$ implies an increase in the elastic load on the respiratory muscles. The $C_{st,rs}$ in mechanically ventilated patients is conventionally measured by dividing $V_T$ by end-inspiratory $P_{st,rs}$ obtained by end-inspiratory airway occlusion until a plateau is reached (usually several seconds). In this case the adequacy of respiratory muscle relaxation is indirectly assessed by the presence of a plateau in airway pressure during the occlusion. This approach assumes that the end-expiratory lung volume during mechanical ventilation corresponds to the relaxation volume of the respiratory system. This assumption, however, is often not valid (see above). This problem can be easily overcome by performing airway occlusion at end expiration (Fig. 1) in addition to end inspiration (Fig. 4). The $C_{st,rs}$ is then computed as $V_T$ divided by the difference in airway pressure between end-inspiratory and end-expiratory occlusions (14). Failure to recognize and measure PEEPi will lead to underestimation of $C_{st,rs}$ measurements. The above measurements require patients to be relaxed; otherwise the use of an esophageal balloon to measure pleural pressure is needed. The esophageal balloon technique has been validated in critically ill patients (36, 42, 43). The $C_{st,rs}$ varies considerably with changes in tidal volume (3, 44). Therefore its measurement becomes mainly useful to follow the progress of a given patient at a given ventilation settings. Increase in $C_{st,rs}$ in this case can be taken as a sign of improvement and vice versa.

### Static Volume-Pressure (V-P) Relationship of the Respiratory System

The elastic properties of the respiratory system are best assessed by constructing the static V-P relationship of the respiratory system obtained under conditions in which airflow is absent and respiratory muscle relaxation is complete. This measurement can be readily performed in relaxed mechanically ventilated patients using the rapid airway occlusion technique (4, 42, 43, 45). In this procedure $V_T$ is changed for one breath (test breath), and end-inspiratory airway occlusion for 2 to 5 seconds will give rise to a plateau pressure which corresponds to the end-inspiratory $P_{st,rs}$ (Fig. 4). If a series of end-inspiratory airway occlusions is performed at different $V_T$'s, the static V-P relationship can be constructed by plotting $P_{st,rs}$ against the corresponding inflation volume. Relaxation of the respiratory muscles can be achieved by administration of muscle relaxants and/or sedatives. The use of mechanical hyperventilation to relax patients by reducing their $Pa_{CO_2}$ and hence their respiratory drive should be avoided since hypocap-

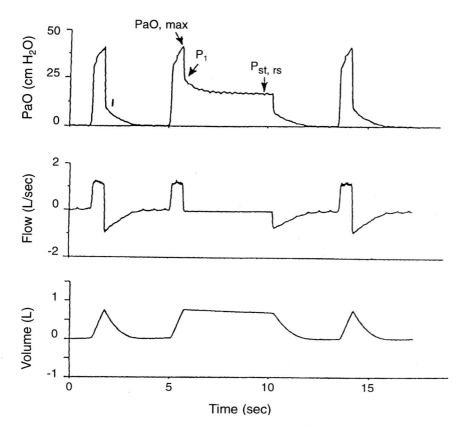

**FIG. 4.** Records of pressure at the airway opening, flow, and changes in lung volume from a sedated-paralyzed ARDS patient which illustrate the technique of rapid airway occlusion. After end-inspiratory airway occlusion there is an immediate drop in pressure from Pao,max to $P_1$, followed by a slow decay to a plateau value that represents static elastic recoil pressure of the respiratory system ($P_{st,rs}$). The decrease in pressure from Pmax to $P_1$ includes resistive pressure attributable to the endotracheal tube.

nia will lead to increased airway resistance (46). The airway occlusion technique is an appealing approach compared to the earlier method ("supersyringe technique") used to construct static V-P curves in mechanically ventilated patients (47) for it is simple, does not require disconnecting the patient from the ventilator, and minimizes the artifact due to continued gas exchange during the procedure (4, 45).

## Dynamic Compliance of the Respiratory System ($C_{dyn,rs}$)

"Effective" $C_{dyn,rs}$ is commonly determined in by dividing VT by the difference between peak airway pressure (Pao,max) and end-expiratory airway pressure (48). This variable clearly does not represent the true $C_{dyn,rs}$, as Pao,max includes a resistive pressure component (3, 48). Furthermore, this measurement does not take into account PEEPi. It is a useful index, however, of the effective inspiratory *impedance* of the respiratory system (49). The true $C_{dyn,rs}$ is obtained by dividing VT by the difference in pressure between the end-inspiratory and end-expiratory points of zero flow. The end-inspiratory point of zero flow corresponds to the airway pressure immediately following end-inspiratory occlusion ($P_1$) (Fig. 4) (3), while the end-expiratory point of zero flow corre-

sponds to dynamic PEEPi (41, 43). The $P_1$ can be readily measured breath by breath by applying a brief end-inspiratory pause (e.g., 0.1 second) available on most ventilators. In both normal subjects (2) and critically ill patients (3) $C_{dyn,rs}$ is markedly flow, volume, and TI dependent. It should be noted that compliance is simply the reciprocal of elastance.

## FLOW RESISTANCE

There are four approaches available for measuring flow resistance: (a) the elastic subtraction method (50), (b) the interrupter method (50), (c) the forced oscillation method (51), and (d) the plethysmographic method (1). For obvious reasons, the last of these cannot be applied in mechanically ventilated patients. In the past, the forced oscillation technique could not be applied in these patients because of technical problems caused by the tracheal tube; however, a possible solution has been proposed recently (52). The technique of rapid airway occlusion during constant-flow inflation, previously described in detail (2, 3), is essentially a combination of two of the basic approaches for measuring flow resistance described in 1927 by von Neergaard and Wirz: the interrupter and the elastic subtraction methods (50). This technique was originally proposed by Rattenborg in 1956 (53). A virtue of the technique is that flow resistance can be measured at a fixed inspiratory flow but different tidal volumes, or at fixed tidal volumes but different inflation flows. Furthermore, with this approach the measurements can be carried out with any preselected previous lung volume history. This technique is appealing both for its simplicity and because it provides a comprehensive on-line assessment of respiratory mechanics. It can not only be applied in patients with relaxed respiratory muscles but also in patients who trigger the ventilator provided that most of the inspiration is passive (relaxed). Furthermore, if pleural pressure is measured by the use of an esophageal balloon, measurements could be partitioned into lung component and chest wall component (36, 42, 43).

This technique allows for measurements of the interrupter resistance, which in humans is thought to reflect airway resistance (40), and the effective additional resistance due to viscoelastic properties of the respiratory system and time constant inequalities. The latter is also called tissue resistance (54) and is flow, volume, and $T_I$ dependent (2, 13).

### Endotracheal Tube Resistance

It should be stressed that in mechanically ventilated patients the endotracheal tube contributes markedly to total flow resistance (18, 55). The flow resistance offered by the endotracheal tubes increases markedly with increasing flow and varies with the size of the tube (18).

### CLINICAL IMPLICATIONS

Monitoring and management of patients should be tailored to individual patients. Therefore we will discuss separately two common disorders, namely COPD and adult respiratory distress syndrome (ARDS).

### Chronic Obstructive Pulmonary Disease

The PEEPi and dynamic hyperinflation is almost invariably present in patients with severe COPD and appears to play a paramount role in causing hypercapnic respiratory failure. In COPD patients there is a vicious circle: The inspiratory flow resistive work is invariably increased due to airway obstruction, which in turn promotes dynamic hyperinflation with a concomitant increase in elastic work and impaired mechanical performance of the inspiratory muscles (35). With increased severity of COPD a critical point is eventually reached at which the inspiratory muscles become fatigued (25).

### PEEPi in Stable COPD Patients

Haluszka et al. (26) have recently studied the prevalence and magnitude of PEEPi, and its correlation to pulmonary mechanics and $Pa_{CO_2}$, in 96 COPD patients with varying degrees of airway obstruction. The PEEPi was determined as the negative deflection in esophageal pressure from the start of inspiratory effort to the onset of inspiratory flow. A significant correlation was found between PEEPi and forced expired volume in 1 second and between PEEPi and pulmonary flow resistance ($R_L$). These results confirm that increased $R_L$ promotes the development of dynamic hyperinflation. Although $R_L$ is paramount in determining dynamic hyperinflation, other factors, such as respiratory frequency, $V_T$, and the braking action of the glottis and of the inspiratory muscles during expiration should also play a role (26). In the presence of a high $R_L$, an increase in respiratory frequency and $V_T$ makes COPD patients especially prone to develop dynamic hyperinflation with a concomitant increase in the work of breathing. When the magnitude of the inspiratory efforts approaches the critical level, causing fatigue (25), the patients reduce their $V_T$ and hence hypoventilate. This results in chronic hypercapnia (33). If such patients are asked to voluntarily restore $V_T$ to normal values, they invariably develop diaphragmatic fatigue (25), indicating that the shallow breathing pattern is an adaptive strategy which is used to avoid inspiratory muscle fatigue.

### PEEPi in COPD Patients with Acute Respiratory Failure

The highest values of PEEPi observed in stable COPD patients range between 7 and 9 cm $H_2O$ (26). In COPD patients with acute respiratory failure higher values have been reported: up to 13 cm $H_2O$ during spontaneous breathing (41) and 22 cm $H_2O$ during mechanical ventilation (56). Such high values of PEEPi have profound consequences on the energetics of breathing, as shown schematically in Fig.5. Acute ventilatory failure in COPD patients is usually triggered by a predisposing event (e.g., airway infection). As a result, there is an acute increase in airway resistance and expiratory flow limitation becomes more severe. The increased resistance causes increased work of breathing and promotes dynamic hyperinflation. The latter is further exacerbated by the tachypnea, which is invariably present in acutely ill COPD patients. Dynamic hyperinflation promotes an increase of elastic work of breathing which is due to PEEPi and decreased lung compliance. The latter is reduced because at high lung volume the slope of the static V-P curve of the lungs decreases (Fig. 3) (17). The increased resistive and elastic work of breathing and increased work due to PEEPi, in association with the

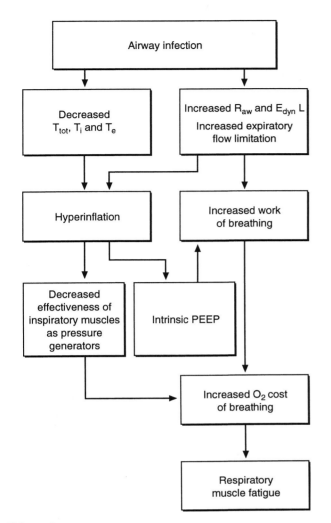

**FIG. 5.** Scheme of the pathophysiology causing acute ventilatory failure in COPD patients. $T_{TOT}$, total breathing cycle duration; $T_I$ and $T_E$, inspiratory and expiratory times; $R_{aw}$, airway resistance; $E_{dyn}$, L lung elastance (reciprocal of lung compliance).

impaired inspiratory muscle performance, lead eventually to inspiratory muscle fatigue. As a result, the patient needs to be mechanically ventilated.

### Strategies to Reduce the Inspiratory Load Caused by PEEPi

As implied in Fig. 5, treatment of COPD patients with respiratory failure should be aimed at reducing the respiratory frequency (and hence increasing expiratory time) and decreasing the flow resistance. To the extent that tachypnea is due to fever and/or airway infection, a resolution of these by conventional treatment should be beneficial. Similarly, administration of bronchodilator drugs may be useful in reducing both flow resistance and

PEEPi. A less conventional but promising approach to deal with PEEPi is the external application of positive pressure. Indeed, CPAP has been found to reduce the magnitude of the inspiratory muscle efforts and the work of breathing in stable patients with severe COPD (41). In addition, CPAP administered through a face or nasal mask (57) may also be of therapeutic benefit during an acute exacerbation of COPD in nonintubated patients. The early use of CPAP in this setting may preclude the need for intubation and mechanical ventilation in some COPD patients. It should also be noted that application of external PEEP during patient-initiated mechanical ventilation can counterbalance and reduce the inspiratory load imposed by PEEPi (41, 58). To avoid pulmonary hyperinflation with increasing PEEP, lung volume can be monitored using a magnetometer or respiratory inductance plethysmography (41, 58).

### Adult Respiratory Distress Syndrome

Reduced $C_{st,rs}$ (increased stiffness) is generally considered a hallmark of the syndrome (47, 59). Reduced lung compliance in ARDS has been attributed to pulmonary edema, loss of ventilated lung units, and increased lung surface tension (60).

Slutsky et al. (61) noted that after inducing pulmonary edema with oleic acid in dogs, the V-P curves of the lungs were shifted downward and to the right (i.e., reduced compliance). However, when volume was determined in terms of rib cage expansion (anteroposterior diameter) using a magnetometer, the pre- and post-oleic acid curves were virtually superimposed. Since the changes in rib cage magnetometer signal reflect the changes in total volume of the thorax (gas, liquid, and solid), these findings are consistent with the notion that the presence of pulmonary edema does not alter the intrinsic compliance of the lung tissue, but rather that the excess edematous fluid simply competes with gas for space. In fact, recent work by Gattinoni et al. (62) using computed tomography has demonstrated that the lungs in ARDS patients are not homogeneously affected and that V-P curves performed on theses patients investigate only healthy or recruitable zones which have essentially normal intrinsic properties. Thus in ARDS, the clinician might be effectively dealing with a functionally small lung ("baby lung"), rather than with a stiff lung of normal dimensions.

The above findings have important clinical implications. Large tidal volumes (10 to 15 mL/kg) and high levels of PEEP (10 to 15 cm $H_2O$) are often used in the management of ARDS patients to improve arterial oxygenation (59). Several mechanisms have been postulated to account for this effect: recruitment of previously collapsed alveolar units, reduction of cardiac output, improvement in ventilation-perfusion mismatch, and redistribution of lung water (60). In the absence of significant alveolar recruitment, application of PEEP will result in hyperinflation of the functional lung units and increased risk of pulmonary barotrauma (4, 44, 59). Application of high levels of PEEP and/or large tidal volumes in patients whose lungs are severely affected (i.e., with baby lungs) will be expected to result in dangerous alveolar overdistension (4, 44). In eight ARDS patients studied on zero end-expiratory airway pressure (ZEEP) and with variable $V_T$'s, six patients showed evidence of alveolar overdistension (i.e., reduced compliance) when they were ventilated with $V_T$'s within the conventionally recommended range (10 to 15 mL/kg). The stiffer the patient's respiratory system was, the less $V_T$ needed to reach alveolar overdistension (44y).

Figure 6 illustrates the static V-P curves in two ARDS patients obtained both on ZEEP and on PEEP of 10 cm $H_2O$. Lung volume is expressed relative to the FRC on ZEEP. Changes in FRC due to PEEP were determined using the procedure shown in Fig. 1. In the patient of panel A the static V-P curve on ZEEP exhibited a convexity toward the x-axis indicating progressive alveolar recruitment with increasing inflation pressure. Application of 10 cm $H_2O$ of PEEP in this patient resulted in an upward shift of the static V-P curve which reflects mostly recruitment of new lung units (4, 48). By contrast, in the patient of panel B the static V-P curve on ZEEP reflected a curvilinear relationship, with concavity toward the x-axis indicating that this patient was already operating on the flat portion of her V-P curve. With application of PEEP the data points moved along a fixed V-P relationship, indicating no alveolar recruitment but rather overdistension of lung units with increased risk of pulmonary barotrauma. The above results imply that measurement of the static V-P curve can provide useful information about the potential response to added PEEP in terms of alveolar recruitment and risk of pulmonary barotrauma (4).

Apart from pulmonary barotrauma, severe alveolar overdistension has been shown to cause acute lung injury characterized by pulmonary edema through epithelial and endothelial damage (63). Surfactant deficiency was also produced in dog lungs by ventilation with large $V_T$'s (64). Since the same end-inspiratory lung volume can be reached by various combinations of PEEP and $V_T$'s, further studies are needed to elucidate the optimal combination of PEEP and $V_T$.

### PEEPi in ARDS Patients

Moderate values of PEEPi (up to 6.5 cm $H_2O$) have also been reported in patients with no history of chronic airway obstruction during mechanical ventilation, including patients with ARDS (4, 65). While in COPD

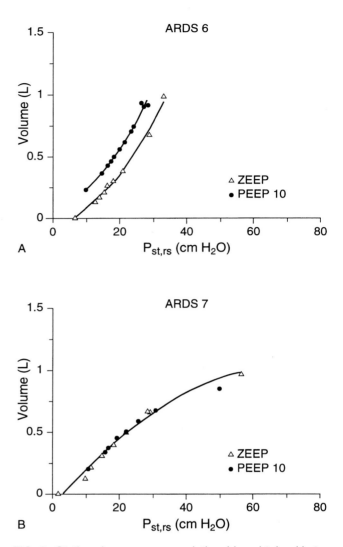

**FIG. 6.** Static volume-pressure relationships obtained in two ARDS patients on ZEEP and on PEEP of 10 cm $H_2O$. Volume is expressed relative to end-expiratory lung volume on ZEEP. $P_{st,rs}$, static elastic recoil pressure of the respiratory system.

patients PEEPi is caused primarily by expiratory flow limitations (26, 41), the nature of PEEPi in ARDS patients is not clearly understood. In the absence of respiratory muscle activity, the rate of lung deflation is determined by the elastic recoil pressure stored during the preceding lung inflation and the opposing total flow resistance offered by the respiratory system (including endotracheal tube, ventilator tubing, and additional equipment, if any) (55). Accordingly, the stiffer the respiratory system (i.e., decreased compliance), the faster will be the rate of lung emptying. Conversely, increased flow resistance will impede the rate of lung deflation. From the above, it seems likely that PEEPi in ARDS should be due to increased expiratory flow resistance.

### Flow Resistance in ARDS Patients

Adult respiratory distress syndrome is not only a disease characterized by reduced compliance but it also entails increased flow resistance. Indeed, recent work has shown that patients with ARDS have an increase of both airway and tissue flow resistance (3, 40, 56, 65, 66). Factors leading to increased airway resistance in ARDS include airway flooding, reduced lung volume, vagal reflexes, and bronchial hyperreactivity (40). Tissue resistance is markedly flow, volume, and $T_I$ dependent (2, 3). It is particularly prominent at low respiratory frequencies (<15 breaths/min) where it accounts for most of the total resistance of the respiratory system (3). At high frequencies (>30 breaths/min), it becomes negligible (3).

## PEAK AIRWAY PRESSURE (PAO,MAX)

The $P_{AO,max}$ is the sum of (a) the end-inspiratory $P_{st,rs}$, (b) the pressure losses due to viscoelastic mechanisms and/or time constant inequalities within the respiratory system, and (c) the resistive pressure dissipations due to the resistance of the airways, endotracheal tube, and tubing connecting the patients to the ventilator. Figure 7 illustrates the relationship between $P_{AO,max}$ and several of its components with flow in an ARDS patient during constant-flow inflations with a fixed $V_T$ of 0.683 L delivered at the same end-expiratory lung volume but at different inspiratory flows. The $P_{tr,max}$ is the tracheal pressure measured 3 cm past the carinal end of the endotracheal tube. The end-inspiratory lung volume was

fixed, as evidenced by the constancy of the end-inspiratory $P_{st,rs}$. By contrast, $P_{AO,max}$ increased markedly with increasing flow, reflecting in part the increase in the resistive pressure due to the endotracheal tube (represented by the difference between $P_{AO,max}$ and $P_{tr,max}$). The $P_1$ is the airway pressure immediately following end-inspiratory airway occlusion. The difference between $P_{tr,max}$ and $P_1$ is the resistive pressure offered by the airways. The difference between $P_1$ and $P_{st,rs}$ reflects the pressure losses due to viscoelastic mechanisms and/or time constant inequalities within the respiratory system (2, 3). From the above, it appears that under changing conditions of inspiratory flow $P_{AO,max}$ will be a poor parameter for monitoring. For instance, an increase in $P_{AO,max}$ in a patient could be due to change in one or more of its components described above: (a) reduced compliance with a concomitant increase in $P_{st,rs}$; (b) increased viscoelastic pressure dissipations and/or time constant inequalities within the respiratory system with an increase in the difference between $P_1$ and $P_{st,rs}$; (c) increased airway resistance with an increase in the difference between $P_{tr,max}$ and $P_1$ ; and (d) increased endotracheal tube resistance due to accumulations of bronchial secretions or tube kinking with an increase in the difference between $P_{AO,max}$ and $P_{tr,max}$. Therefore, making a correct diagnosis requires examining each component which can readily be obtained using the technique of rapid airway occlusion (Fig. 4). Nevertheless, in a given patient the $P_{AO,max}$ is useful to follow if ventilator settings remained unchanged. Mean ariway pressure, measured at the oral end of the endotracheal tube, has been advocated as a useful parameter for monitoring during mechanical ventilation. This is based on the assumption that the mean airway pressure is a good approximation of the mean alveolar pressure. The validity of this assumption, however, has been challenged (67).

## CARDIAC FAILURE

Many abnormalities in pulmonary functions can occur as a consequence of heart failure. With the onset of left-sided heart failure and accumulation of fluid in the peribronchial interstitium, several changes occur in lung ventilation (68). The caliber of the airway is reduced, leading to early airway closure during expiration with air trapping and an increase in residual volume. Edema fluid accumulation can cause reflex constriction of bronchial smooth muscle cells, leading to the syndrome of "cardiac asthma." This reflex bronchoconstriction is thought to be mediated through nonmyelinated nerves in the alveolar interstitium called J fibers. Airway collapse and bronchoconstrition lead to decrease in flow rates, total lung capacity, and FEV1 while ventilatory dead space increases. With chronic congestive heart failure total lung capacity is decreased along with vital capacity and peak

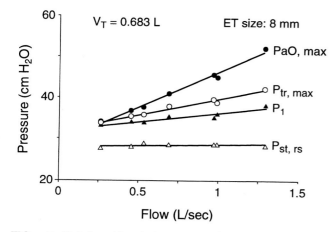

**FIG. 7.** Relationship between peak airway pressure ($P_{AO,max}$) and its components with flow in a sedated-paralyzed ARDS patient during constant-flow inflations with a fixed $V_T$ of 0.683 L delivered at the same end-expiratory lung volume but at different inspiratory flows. $P_{tr,max}$, peak tracheal pressure; $P_1$, airway pressure immediately following end-inspiratory airway occlusion; $P_{st,rs}$, static elastic recoil pressure of the respiratory system.

flow rates (restrictive defect) while residual volume is increased (obstructive defect).

Progression of pulmonary function abnormalities usually parallels worsening of congestive heart failure. With mild heart failure, lung function is only slightly compromised. There is a slight decrease in vital capacity and widening of the alveolar-arterial oxygen gradient. With severe heart failure there is significant fall in vital capacity while residual volume remains normal. Forced expiratory flows and FEV1 decrease. Fluid in the interstitium causes a fall in measurements of both static and dynamic lung compliance, producing "stiff" lungs. It has been shown that dynamic compliance varies inversely with pulmonary capillary wedge pressure (69). The above abnormalities lead to both obstructive and restrictive ventilatory disease. In symptomatic patients in New York Heart Association functional class 4, vital capacity averages 60% of normal value while diffusion capacity and dynamic compliance average 33% of normal (70). The ventilatory defects in heart failure increase the work of breathing, as more negative pleural pressures are needed for air movement. Breathing efficiency is greatly reduced and compensatory mechanisms to reduce caloric expenditure on respiration are instituted. Under these circumstances breathing work is best accomplished by lowering tidal volume and increasing respiratory rate.

Ventilatory defects can improve, however, with treatment of congestive heart failure. In fact, vital capacity has been proposed as a monitor of therapy for congestive heart failure (71). Further, following mitral valve replacement for mitral stenosis, FEV1, vital capacity, and diffusion capacity improve. Persistent postoperative decrease in vital capacity, total lung capacity, FEV1, and diffusion capacity are most likely to occur in those patients with preoperative pulmonary hypertension and tricuspid insufficiency (72). In the Framingham Study a reduced vital capacity was a significant risk factor for the development of congestive heart failure during follow-up (73).

## POSTCARDIAC SURGERY

Clinically, maximum pulmonary impairment is seen 24 hours postoperatively, gradually improving over the following 7 to 10 days. There is about 50% reduction in vital capacity by day 3 which does not return to preoperative values for 2 weeks. There is 25% to 40% reduction in diffusion capacity for the first 2 weeks following surgery. Total lung capacity, inspiratory capacity, and FRC are also reduced in the postoperative period. The reduction in FRC is further exacerbated by poor lung reexpansion after cardiopulmonary bypass, small tidal volumes, and fixed tidal volumes not interrupted by sighs or not adding PEEP. Static compliance is reduced in patients following open-heart surgery. The reduction in static compliance can be explained by reduced lung volume, altered surfac-

tant function due to residual effects of anesthesia, reduced chest wall compliance, and atelectasis.

Postoperative pulmonary atelectasis was first described in 1908 by Pasteur (74). Atelectasis, mainly left lower lobe, occurs in 60% to 85% of patients undergoing open-heart surgery due to the effects of cariopulmonary bypass, anesthesia, secretions, and persisting lung disease. Further insight concerning atelectasis stems from recent work of Brismar et al. (75). Utilizing computed tomography, they showed that in supine subjects atelectasis occurred within 5 minutes of induction of anesthesia in the dependent parts of both lungs. The atelectasis was most pronounced in the caudal segments of the lung. Application of 10 cm $H_2O$ of PEEP reduced substantially the degree of atelectasis, which, however, was rapidly reinstated after removal of PEEP. This results in a reduction in FRC, increase in intrapulmonary shunt and ventilation perfusion mismatching, widening of the alveolar-arterial oxygen gradient, and hypoxemia. Since most evidence suggests that arterial hypoxemia following cardiopulmonary bypass results from airway collapse, the application of PEEP following open-heart surgery has been widely advocated and its efficacy in reducing atelectasis documented.

Recently, Valta et al. (76) studied the effects of different levels of PEEP on respiratory mechanics in mechanically ventilated open-heart surgery patients in the immediate postoperative period. Positive end-expiratory pressure was studied in increasing increments and in decreasing increments. Static compliance was determined using the rapid airway occlusion technique. Changes in end-expiratory lung volume were measured with respiratory inductive plethysmography. Recruitment of lung units was estimated as the difference in lung volume between PEEP and ZEEP for the same static inflation pressure (15 cm $H_2O$). Static compliance was found to be significantly reduced. While PEEP of 5 cm $H_2O$, commonly used in routine postoperative management after open-heart surgery, did not cause significant recruitment, higher levels of PEEP (10 to 15 cm $H_2O$) were effective. Static compliance and lung volume were higher during stepwise PEEP decrease. Importantly, at the end of the procedure, there was a small but persistent increase in lung volume and static compliance at base line (ZEEP). The above study suggests that in the postoperative period PEEP less than 10 cm $H_2O$ may not be effective to reopen atelectatic lung units. Furthermore, the fact that there was a persistent increase in lung volume following the procedure suggests that the practice of introducing sighs during mechanical ventilation may be particularly useful in these patients.

It has been shown that a minimum critical opening transpulmonary pressure (PL) is needed before any gas could enter gas-free lungs. In humans this minimum critical opening pressure is about 20 cm $H_2O$ (77). Since atelectasis occurs preferentially in the dependent lung zones where the end-expiratory values of PL at ZEEP are around zero in the supine position, the end-expiratory static pressure required to reopen the atelectatic alveoli should exceed 20 cm $H_2O$. In most patients following open-heart surgery static end-inspiratory pressure is lower than the critical reopening pressure (76) even on PEEP of 5 cm $H_2O$. With PEEP of 10 cm $H_2O$ or more end-inspiratory pressure exceeds the critical reopening pressure and alveolar recruitment occurs. The adverse effects of high PEEP, however, on ventricular performance and cardiac output and hence oxygen transport must be taken into consideration in managing these patients. An alternative approach is to periodically perform large sustained lung inflations. In this connection, it should be noted that in spontaneously breathing postoperative patients, performing periodic deep breaths, in the form of incentive spirometry, is an effective and common modality for treating atelectasis. Recently, however, with the advent of large tidal volumes (10 to 15 mL/kg) ventilation and PEEP, the use of sighs has been generally abandoned. The study of Valta et al. (76) indicates that, in postoperative open-heart surgery patients, even when relatively large tidal volumes are used in association with low levels of PEEP, large periodic inflations (sighs) might still be beneficial in reopening atelectatic units.

# REFERENCES

1. Dubois AB, Botelho SY, Comroe JH Jr. A new method for measuring airway resistance in man using a body plethysmograph: values in normal subjects an in patients with respiratory disease. *J Clin Invest* 1956;35:322.
2. D'Angelo E, Calderini E, Torri G, et al. Respiratory mechanics in anesthetized paralyzed humans: effects of flow, volume, and time. *J Appl Physiol* 1989;67:2556.
3. Eissa NT, Ranieri VM, Corbeil C, et al. Analysis of behavior of respiratory system in ARDS patients: effects of flow, volume, and time. *J Appl Physiol* 1991;70:2719.
4. Ranieri MV, Eissa NT, Corbeil C, et al. The effect of PEEP on alveolar recruitment and gas exchange in ARDS patients. *Am Rev Respir Dis* 1991;144:544.
5. Ramachandran PR, Fairly HB. Changes in functional residual capacity during respiratory failure. *Can Anaesth Soc J* 1970;17:359.
6. Fernández R, Benito S, Sanchis J. Inspiratory effort and occlusion pressure in triggered mechanical ventilation. *Intensive Care Med* 1988;14:650.
7. Suter PM, Schlobohm RM. Determination of functional residual capacity during mechanical ventilation. *Anesthesiology* 1974;41:605.
8. Sackner MA, Krieger BP. Noninvasive respiratory monitoring. In: Scharf SM, Cassidy SS, eds: *Heart-lung interactions in health and disease.* New York: Marcel Dekker; 1989:663.
9. Agostoni E, Mead J. Statics of the respiratory system. In: Fenn W, Rahn H, eds. *Handbook of physiology. Respiration.* Sect 3, vol 1, chapt 13. Washington, DC: American Physiological Society; 1965:387.
10. Shee CD, Ploy-song-sang Y, Milic-Emili J. Decay of inspiratory muscle pressure during expiration in conscious humans. *J Appl Physiol* 1985;58:1859.
11. Gottfried SB, Rossi A, Milic-Emili J. Dynamic hyperinflation, intrinsic PEEP, and the mechanically ventilated patient. *Intensive Crit Care Dig* 1986;5:30.
12. Kimball WR, Leith DE, Robins AG. Dynamic hyperinflation and ventilator dependence in chronic obstructive pulmonary disease. *Am Rev Respir Dis* 1982;126:991.
13. Pepe PE, Marini JJ. Occult positive end-expiratory pressure in mechanically ventilated patients with airflow obstruction. *Am Rev Respir Dis* 1982;126:166.
14. Rossi A, Gottfried SB, Zocchi L, et al. Measurement of static compliance of the total respiratory system in patients with acute respiratory failure during mechanical ventilation. *Am Rev Respir Dis* 1985;131:672.
15. Tuxen DV, Lane S. The effects of ventilatory pattern on hyperinflation, airway pressure, and circulation in mechanical ventilation of patients with severe air-flow obstruction. *Am Rev Respir Dis* 1987;136:872.
16. Sahn SA, Lakshminarayan S. Bedside criteria for discontinuation of mechanical ventilation. *Chest* 1973;63:1002.
17. Pride NB, Macklem PT. Lung mechanics in disease. In: Macklem PT, Mead J, eds. *Handbook of physiology, mechanics of breathing.* Sect. 3, vol 3, chapt 37. Bethesda, MD: American Physiological Society; 1986:659
18. Gottfried SB, Rossi A, Higgs BD, et al. Noninvasive determination of respiratory system mechanics during mechanical ventilation for acute respiratory failure. *Am Rev Respir Dis* 1985;131:414.
19. Derenne J-PH, Macklem PT, Roussos C. State of the art. The respiratory muscles: mechanics, control, and physiopathology. *Am Rev Respir Dis* 1978;118:113(Pt 1);373(Pt 2);581(Pt 3).
20. Black LF, Hyatt RE. Maximal respiratory pressures: normal values and relationship to age and sex. *Am Rev Respir Dis* 1968;99:696.
21. Tobin MJ. State of the art. Respiratory monitoring in the intensive care unit. *Am Rev Respir Dis* 1988;138:1625.
22. Marini JJ. Monitoring during mechanical ventilation. *Clin Chest Med* 1988;9:73.
23. Tobin MJ, Perez W, Guenther SM, et al. The pattern of breathing during successful and unsuccessful trials of weaning from mechanical ventilation. *Am Rev Respir Dis* 1986;134:1111.
24. Milic-Emili J. Recent advances in clinical assessment of control of breathing. *Lung* 1982;160:1.
25. Bellemare F, Grassino A. Force reserve of the diaphragm in patients with chronic obstructive pulmonary disease. *J Appl Physiol* 1983;55:8.
26. Haluszka J, Chartrand DA, Grassino AE, et al. Intrinsic PEEP and arterial $P_{CO_2}$ in stable patients with chronic obstructive pulmonary disease. *Am Rev Respir Dis* 1990;141:1194.
27. Fitting J-W, Grassino A. Diagnosis of diaphragmatic dysfunction. *Clin Chest Med* 1987;6:91.
28. Grassino A, Macklem PT. Respiratory muscle fatigue and ventilatory failure. *Ann Rev Med* 1984;35:625.
29. Cherniac RM. The oxygen consumption and efficiency of the respiratory muscles in health and emphysema. *J Clin Invest* 1959;38:494.
30. Grunstein MM, Younes M, Milic-Emili J. Control of tidal volume and respiratory frequency in anesthetized cats. *J Appl Physiol* 1973;35:463.
31. Marini JJ, Rodriquez RM, Lamb V. The inspiratory workload of patient-initiated mechanical ventilation. *Am Rev Respir Dis* 1986;134:902.
32. Ward M, Corbeil C, Gibbons W. Optimization of respiratory muscle relaxation during mechanical ventilation. *Anesthesiology* 1988;69:29.
33. Sorli J, Grassino A, Lorange G. Control of breathing in patients with chronic obstructive lung disease. *Clin Sci Mol Med* 1978;54:295.
34. Aubier M, Murciano D, Fournier M, et al. Central respiratory drive in acute respiratory failure of patients with chronic obstructive pulmonary disease. *Am Rev Respir Dis* 1980;122:191.
35. Sharp JT, Lith PV, Nuchprayoon CV, et al. The thorax in chronic obstructive lung disease. *Am J Med* 1968;44:39.
36. Murciano D, Aubier M, Bussi S, et al. Comparison of esophageal, tracheal, and mouth occlusion pressure in patients with chronic obstructive pulmonary disease during acute respiratory failure. *Am Rev Respir Dis* 1982;128:837.
37. Sasson CSH, Te TT, Mahutte CK, et al. Airway occlusion pressure: an important indicator for successful weaning in patients with chronic obstructive pulmonary disease. *Am Rev Respir Dis* 1987;135:107.
38. Mongomery AB, Holle RHO, Neagley SR, et al. Prediction of successful weaning using airway occlusion pressure and hypercapnic challenge. *Chest* 1987;91:496.
39. Eissa NT, Ranieri VM, Corbeil C, Chassé M, Braidy J, Milic-Emili J. Effects of positive end-expiratory pressure on the work of breathing in adult respiratory distress syndrome patients. *J Crit Care* 1992;7:142.
40. Eissa NT, Ranieri VM, Corbeil C, Chassé M, Braidy J, Milic-Emili J. Effects of positive end-expiratory pressure, lung volume, and inspira-

tory flow on interrupter resistance in patients with adult respiratory distress syndrome. *Am Rev Respir Dis* 1991;144:538.

41. Petrof BJ, Legaré M, Goldberg P, et al. Continuous positive airway pressure reduces work of breathing and dyspnea during weaning from mechanical ventilation in severe obstructive pulmonary disease. *Am Rev Respir Dis* 1990;141:281.

42. Coussa ML, Guérin G, Eissa NT, et al. Partitioning of work of breathing in mechanically ventilated COPD patients. *J Appl Physiol* 1993;75:1711.

43. Guérin G, Coussa ML, Eissa NT, et al. Lung and chest wall mechanics in mechanically ventilated COPD patients. *J Appl Physiol* 1993;74:1570.

44. Eissa N, Ranieri M, Corbeil C, et al. The effects of inflation volume on the elastic properties of the total respiratory system and the risk of pulmonary barotrauma in ARDS patients. *Intensive Care Med* 1990;16(S1):S39.

45. Levy P, Similowski T, Corbeil C, et al. A method for studying the static volume-pressure curves of the respiratory system during mechanical ventilation. *J Crit Care* 1989;4:83.

46. Don HF, Robson JC. The mechanics of the respiratory system during anesthesia. The effect of atropine and carbon dioxide. *Anesthesiology* 1965;26:168.

47. Metamis D, Lemaire F, Harf A, et al. Total respiratory pressure volume curves in the adult respiratory distress syndrome. *Chest* 1984;86:54.

48. Fairly HB. Respiratory monitoring. In: Blitt CD, ed. *Monitoring in anesthesia and critical care medicine.* New York: Churchill Livingstone; 1985:229

49. Milic-Emili J, Ploysongsang Y. Respiratory mechanics in the adult respiratory distress syndrome. *Crit Care Clin* 1986;2(3):573.

50. Neergaard K von, Wirz K. Die Messung der Strömungswiederstande in der Atemwege des Menschen, insbesondere bei Asthma und Emphysem. *Zeitschrift für Klimische Medizin* 1927;105:51.

51. Dubois AB, Brody AW, Lewis DH, et al. Oscillation mechanics of lungs and chest in man. *J Appl Physiol* 1956;8:587.

52. Navajas D, Farré R, Rotger M, et al. Recording pressure at the distal end of the endotracheal tube to measure respiratory impedance. *Eur Respir J* 1989;2:178.

53. Rattenborg C. In: Lassen HCA, ed. *Basic mechanics of artificial ventilation in management of life-threatening poliomyelitis.* London: Livingstone; 1956:23.

54. Milic-Emili J, Robatto FM, Bates JHT. Respiratory mechanics in anesthesia. *Br J Anaesth* 1990;65:4.

55. Behrakis PK, Higgs BD, Baydur A, et al. Respiratory mechanics during halothane anesthesia and anesthesia-paralysis in humans. *J Appl Physiol* 1983;55:1085.

56. Broseghini C, Brandolese R, Poggi R, et al. Respiratory mechanics during the first day of mechanical ventilation in patients with pulmonary edema and chronic airway obstruction. *Am Rev Respir Dis* 1988;138:355.

57. Petrof BJ, Kimoff RJ, Levy RD, Cosio MG, Gottfried SB. Nasal continuous positive airway pressure facilitates respiratory muscle function during sleep in severe chronic obstructive pulmonary disease. *Am Rev Respir Dis* 1991;143:928.

58. Smith TC, Marini JJ. Impact of PEEP on lung mechanics and work

of breathing in severe airflow obstruction. *J Appl Physiol* 1988;65:1488.

59. Falke KJ, Pontoppidan H, Kumar A, et al. Ventilation with end-expiratory pressure in acute lung disease. *J Clin Invest* 1972;51:2315.

60. Eissa NT, Milic-Emili J. Effects of positive end-expiratory pressure on adult respiratory distres syndrome. In: Potchen EJ, Grainger RG, Greene R, eds. *Pulmonary radiology.* Philadelphia: WB Saunders; 1993:169.

61. Slutsky AS, Scharf SM, Brown R, et al. The effect of oleic acid-induced pulmonary edema on pulmonary and chest wall mechanics in dogs. *Am Rev Respir Dis* 1980;121:91.

62. Gattinoni L, Pesenti A, Avalli L, et al. Pressure-volume curve of total respiratory system in acute respiratory failure. *Am Rev Respir Dis* 1987;136:730.

63. Dreyfuss D, Soler P, Basset G, et al. High inflation pressure pulmonary edema: respective effects of high airway pressure, high tidal volume, and positive end-expiratory pressure. *Am Rev Respir Dis* 1988;137:1159.

64. Greenfield LJ, Ebert PA, Benson DW. Effects of positive pressure ventilation on surface tension properties of lung extracts. *Anesthesiology* 1964;25:312.

65. Valta P, Takala J, Eissa NT, Milic-Emili J. Does alveolar recruitment occur with positive end-expiratory pressure in adult respiratory distress syndrome patients? *J Crit Care* 1993;8:34.

66. Eissa NT, Ranieri VM, Corbeil C, et al. Effects of PEEP on the mechanics of the respiratory system in ARDS patients. *J Appl Physiol* 1992;73:1728.

67. Eissa NT, Kenyon C, Milic-Emili J. Relationship of mean alveolar pressure to mean airway pressure: model analysis and clinical implications. *J Crit Care* 1992;7:158.

68. Remetz MS, Cleman MW, Cabin HS. Pulmonary and pleural complications of cardiac disease. *Clin Chest Med* 1989;10:545.

69. Saxton GA Jr, et al. The relationship of pulmonary compliance to pulmonary vascular pressures in patients with heart disease. *J Clin Invest* 1965;35:611.

70. Nery LE, Wasserman K, French W, et al. Contrasting cardiovascular and respiratory responses to exercise in mitral valve and chronic obstructive pulmonary disease. *Chest* 1983;83:446.

71. Light RW, George RB. Serial pulmonary function in patients with acute heart failure. *Arch Intern Med* 1983;143:429.

72. Ohno K, Nakahara K, Hirose H, et al. Effects of valvular surgery on overall and regional lung function in patients with mitral stenosis. *Chest* 1987;92:224.

73. Kannel WB, Seidman JM, Fercho W, Castelli WP. Vital capcity and congestive heart failure. The Framingham study. *Circulation* 1974;49:1160.

74. Pasteur W. Massive collapse of the lung. *Lancet* 1908;7:1352.

75. Brismar B, Hendenstierna G, Lundquist H, Strandberg A, Svensson L, Tokies L. Pulmonary densities during anesthesia with muscular relaxation: a proposal of atelectasis. *Anesthesiology* 1985;62:422.

76. Valta P, Takala J, Eissa NT, Milic-Emili J. Effects of PEEP on respiratory mechanics after open heart surgery. *Chest* 1992;102:227.

77. Radford EP Jr. Static mechanical properties of mammalian lungs. In: Fenn WO, Rahn H, eds. *Handbook of physiology. Respiration*, vol 1. Washington, DC: American Physiological Society; 1964:429.

*The Critically Ill Cardiac Patient,*
edited by V. Kvetan and D.R. Dantzker,
Lippincott-Raven Publishers, Philadelphia © 1996.

## CHAPTER 19

# Cardiac Complications of Invasive Procedures

Yehuda Ginosar, Leonid A. Eidelman, and Charles L. Sprung

The assessment of complications in this chapter is considered in isolation from the indications and contraindications and general techniques of each procedure.

While most attention will be focused upon the cardiac complications of the pulmonary artery catheter (PAC), the multidisciplinary approach of intensive care unit (ICU) management dictates a broader view and the cardiac complications of other invasive ICU procedures are also included.

## CARDIAC COMPLICATIONS OF INVASIVE CARDIAC PROCEDURES

### Diagnostic Procedures: The Pulmonary Artery Catheter

As might be expected from an invasive procedure, the PAC is associated with complications. The nature of the adverse effects may be (1) the direct result of central venous access (such as pneumothorax), (2) the direct result of PAC insertion or maintenance [such as ventricular dysrhythmias or pulmonary artery (PA) rupture], or (3) the indirect consequence of the measurement of data using the PAC (such as the initiation of inappropriate therapy as a result of errors in cardiac output determination).

The incidence of overall complications is difficult to assess, as it depends largely upon the experience of the physicians involved and upon the types of patients selected. The assessment of likely harm is best considered in the context of acceptable risk, assessed by the balance between risk and benefit, an equation that varies from patient to patient (1). This is a matter of considerable controversy.

Y. Ginosar, L.A. Eidelman, and C.L. Sprung: Department of Anesthesiology and Critical Care, Hadassah University Hospital, Hebrew University Medical School, Ein Karem, Jerusalem, Israel 91120.

### Complications of Central Venous Cannulation

The potential complications of central venous cannulation include pneumothorax, bleeding or hematoma, arterial or tracheal puncture, air embolism, chylothorax, arrhythmias, and nerve injury. Thrombosis, colonization, infection, and generalized sepsis are complications of catheter maintenance (2).

The traumatic complications associated with central venous cannulation (principally pneumothorax and hemorrhage) are functions of the anatomic site of catheterization. Although not the most comfortable or convenient route for hemodynamic monitoring, brachial cannulation enables the insertion of central venous and PACs without risks of pneumothorax and is the site at which hemorrhage may be most easily controlled. The femoral vein route is also free of the danger of pneumothorax but may rarely be associated with retroperitoneal hematoma or intra-abdominal trauma (2). The external jugular vein provides relatively safe access to the central veins, although the passage of a wire or catheter may be difficult.

In general, the central veins (internal jugular and subclavian) are the most commonly used sites for PAC access. Of the central veins used for direct access, the internal jugular vein is generally associated with the fewest complications, although carotid artery puncture and, rarely, tracheal puncture and pneumothorax may occur. The subclavian vein is more frequently associated with pneumothorax and also with subclavian artery puncture and is a difficult site at which to control bleeding (making it an unwise choice for patients with coagulopathies).

### Complications of PA Catheterization

#### Arrhythmias

The occurrence of cardiac arrhythmias is the most common complication of PA catheterization. Arrhythmias may be atrial or ventricular, isolated, transitory, or sustained and may be life threatening (3–5). Swan et al. (6) noted a 13% incidence of transient premature ventricular contractions in their original report. Although the original series did not report any ventricular tachycardia (VT), subsequent investigations have shown an incidence of VT ranging between 12% and 53%, particularly in critically ill patients (4–7). Studies of elective catheterizations in stable patients (8) disclosed a much lower incidence of arrhythmias than similar studies in critically ill patients (5, 9). Prophylactic lidocaine has been advocated in certain high-risk critically ill patients (5, 10), and the availability of lidocaine and a defibrillator should be assured before commencing PA catheterization. Catheter-induced arrhythmias are typically resistant to drug treatment but often respond to catheter withdrawal (4, 5).

Arrhythmias are usually due to direct mechanical stimulation of the atrium or ventricle. The development of arrhythmias is lessened by the design of the catheter (when inflated correctly, its protective balloon reduces the contact between the stiffer, more arrhythmogenic catheter and the myocardium). Factors that increase the susceptibility of the myocardium to arryhthmogenic stimuli include myocardial ischemia or infarction, shock, hypoxemia, and acid-base or electrolyte disorders (11). Any of these underlying factors should be corrected, where possible, prior to PA catheterization.

In addition, prolonged insertion times may increase the occurrence of arrhythmias due to an increased arrhythmogenic stimulus (4). Conditions that predispose to prolonged insertion times include reduced cardiac output states (particularly poor myocardial contraction), dilated right ventricle, tricuspid regurgitation, and pulmonary hypertension.

### Conduction Defects

The mechanical effect of the catheter impinging upon the conduction system is believed to be the cause for conduction defects occasionally observed during and after catheterization. Right bundle branch block (RBBB) is the most typical conduction defect seen, with a reported incidence between 3% and 6% (5, 9, 12). The obvious danger of this complication is in a patient with preexisting left bundle branch block (LBBB), who is at risk of developing complete heart block (CHB) (13). Akhtar et al. suggested that patients with baseline LBBB were more likely to develop subsequent conduction defects than were other patients (23%, as compared with 5% for control patients) (14). Morris et al. differentiated between old and new cases of LBBB and concluded that only those with new-onset LBBB were at greater risk of developing further conduction defects (15).

The issue of prophylactic transvenous pacing in patients with preexisting LBBB is controversial. The advantage for the occasional patient who might develop CHB must be offset by the disadvantage of delayed catheterization and possible interference between the pacing wire and the catheter. External transcutaneous pacing equipment "on standby" as an alternative to prophylactic pacing has been recommended (5), although transvenous pacing should also be available under these circumstances.

### Pulmonary Infarction

Pulmonary infarction in the critically ill might be expected to occur as the result of pulmonary emboli arising from a deep vein thrombosis, precipitated by the combination of immobilization, a low output state, hypercoagulability, and, possibly, trauma, sepsis, and abdominal or pelvic surgery. In patients with a PAC in situ, pulmonary infarction may occur by a local disturbance to the pulmonary circulation. Continuous inflation of the balloon in the PA will eventually lead to widespread distal ischemia and, subsequently, infarction (11, 16–18). In addition, distal migration of the catheter tip may occlude one of the smaller branches of the PA, even with the balloon deflated.

Thromboembolic phenomena may occur despite the catheter being situated in the correct position. Thrombi within or surrounding the catheter may form and embolize to the distal pulmonary circulation. The pulmonary endothelium may be damaged by the catheter and may thus trigger the formation of thrombi, which could either block the PA directly or cause emboli (resulting in distal pulmonary infarction).

Even if none of these events occur, parenchymal infarction distal to the catheter may occur because of local reduction in pulmonary blood flow around the catheter in a critically ill patient with the risk factors for thrombosis mentioned above. This may be further aggravated by pulmonary venous congestion in a patient with left ventricular failure. The incidence of pulmonary infarction was as high as 7% (16) in early reports, but a later study showed no cases occurring in 320 catheterizations (19).

The most important factor in preventing pulmonary infarction is to avoid persistent occlusion of the PA ("permanent wedge"), which may be detected by the presence of a PA occlusion pressure (PAOP) trace despite an apparently deflated balloon. This may occur due to distal migration of an initially correctly positioned catheter or due to failure to deflate the balloon after PAOP measurements. To avoid this preventable complication, it is essential to display the PA tracing continuously. If a low-amplitude trace is seen, the balloon should be deflated and the catheter withdrawn to a more central position. The balloon should only be inflated intermittently and not for more than 15 seconds. When measuring PAOP, it is important to make certain that no less than 1.25 mL of air is required to obtain PA occlusion. Performing daily chest X-rays to check the balloon position and to confirm the absence of air within it is part of the routine maintenance of the catheter (20).

The use of a continuous heparin flush device appears to reduce the incidence of intracatheter thrombi (16). The introduction of heparin-coated catheters may further reduce the incidence of thrombus formation; however, both heparin flushes and heparin-coated catheters have been reported to be occasionally associated with the development of thrombocytopenia (21).

### Pulmonary Artery Rupture

This is the most serious and most immediately life threatening of the complications associated with the PAC (16, 22). Fortunately it is uncommon, with a reported incidence between 0.06% and 0.2% of catheterizations (23, 24). The reported mortality, however, is between 45% and 65% (23) with many of the deaths occurring within 30 minutes of diagnosis. The patients may present with a range of symptoms from cough and dyspnea to overt shock. Hemoptysis, however, is the classical symptom and is present in 90% of cases (although it should be remembered that hemoptysyis may also be the presenting feature of pulmonary infarction).

Treatment is generally guided by the severity of the patient's condition. The patient should be placed with the affected side down to prevent aspiration of blood to the unaffected lung. Intubation of the unaffected bronchus or double-lumen intubation should be undertaken if hemoptysis is severe. Venous blood injected through the distal PAC port, PA balloon occlusion, or the use of a Fogarty catheter to both create tamponade and isolate the bleeding focus are examples of non-surgical remedies that have been described to reduce bleeding (25). Pulmonary angiography with embolization has also been recommended (23). Nevertheless, definitive surgical treatment with emergency thoracotomy and resection of the affected lobe is usually required (11, 26).

Pulmonary artery rupture occurs as a result of local trauma by the PAC, its tip, or the balloon. Factors that make perforation more likely include rapid balloon inflation, catheter advancement without balloon inflation, distal catheter position, poorly compliant pulmonary vessel walls, and rigid catheters. Clinical conditions in which these factors predominate include (a) pulmonary hypertension (distended pulmonary vasculature, hence, distal PA occlusion position, in conjunction with poorly compliant walls); (b) heparinization; (c) advanced patient age; and (d) poor catheterization technique (17). Cardiac surgery is a particular hazard where all of the above factors may be compounded by cardiac manipulation (pushing the catheter into a more distal position without the balloon inflated) together with hypothermia (where the catheter becomes more rigid). It is generally recommended to withdraw the PAC to the right atrium during cardiopulmonary bypass.

### Knotting and Catheter Entrapment

Catheters may become knotted upon themselves or become entangled with other intracardiac structures, such as papillary muscles, valves, or intracardiac pacing wires. They may also be inadvertently sutured to the heart during cardiac surgery.

Knotting is usually a consequence of looping of the catheter within the right atrium or right ventricle and may be due to excessive length of catheter inserted into the heart, a dilated right ventricle, or failure to fully inflate the balloon. This latter factor deprives the catheter of its flow-directed property and increases the chance of entrapment in the chordae tendinae (11, 18).

To remove an entrapped catheter, gentle traction alone may suffice. Use of invasive procedures may, however, be required. These may include the passage of a wire within the catheter, a large-bore sleeve over the wire, snaring the distal portion and removing it through the inferior vena cava, and thoracotomy.

Care should be taken not to use excessive force when removing the catheter, whether entrapped or not, as this may cause damage to or avulsion of the tricuspid valve, chordae tendinae, or papillary muscles.

### Balloon Rupture

The reported incidence of balloon rupture is between 1% and 23% (6, 9–11, 19) and seems to have decreased significantly since the PAC was first introduced. The potential sequelae of balloon rupture are embolization of air or of fragments of the balloon. Although some have recommended that carbon dioxide or helium, which are more soluble than air, be used for inflation, most physicians use air.

Adherence to the routine precautions for catheter management should reduce the likelihood of this complication. The balloon should be tested for patency prior to insertion, no more than 1.5 mL air should ever be injected for PA occlusion, the balloon should be passively and not actively deflated, and the catheter should always be withdrawn with the balloon deflated. Furthermore, the latex balloon becomes progressively less elastic (and hence more liable to rupture) with prolonged exposure to blood lipoproteins; this is another reason why a catheter should be removed from a patient as soon as the clinical situation permits. Signs of balloon rupture include loss of resistance to balloon inflation, absence of PAOP tracing despite attempted inflation, and the ability to withdraw blood from the balloon port (although this may not be present if the remnants of the balloon collapse on attempted aspiration and create a one-way valve). Once the diagnosis has been made, the catheter may be left in situ to monitor PA pressure, to measure cardiac output, and to sample mixed venous blood, but air should not be injected to measure PAOP.

*Infection*

Infection is a hazard with any indwelling catheter, particularly if its use involves repeated breaks in an otherwise sterile and closed system (e.g., mixed venous aspiration and cardiac output determinations) (27). The danger of infection in a catheter traversing the right side of the heart and in intimate contact with the tricuspid and pulmonary valves is that endocarditis might ensue, possibly with vegetations and septic embolization (28). Myocardial abscess has also been described after PA catheterization (29). The infected catheter may also be a source for generalized sepsis (9, 28–30).

Several studies have demonstrated an increased infection rate when transparent as opposed to gauze dressings are used (31–33). The use of triple-antibiotic ointment at the catheter site has been noted to reduce the infection rate, whereas the use of povidine-iodine did not confer a statistically significant improvement over control (no agent) (34). Daily dressing changes have been demonstrated not to reduce infection rates (35). There is no consensus concerning the recommended duration of a central venous or PAC in situ. Concerning PACs, infection rates in critically ill patients have been noted as 0.3% to 0.5% per day (36). Based on the same report (36), some physicians support the practice of retaining the PAC in situ for as long as 1 week (when indicated), although more typically the PACs are changed after 3 or 4 days, but this does not preclude the possibility of exchanging the catheter over a wire (37).

A functional approach to the degree of colonization or infection of indwelling PACs was described by Elliott et al. (9). Contamination was defined as the isolation of a typical nonpathogen from one of a series of blood cultures but where no growth was observed from the catheter tip itself. Colonization was defined as a positive culture from the catheter tip. Colonization may be with or without signs of local infection; if there is infection, the PAC can be implicated as a cause if (in the absence of any other sources of sepsis) there is bacteriologic or other evidence that the organism is the same as that cultured from the catheter tip.

The reported incidence of colonization depends on the microbiologic status of the patient prior to catheterization. Applefeld et al. (30) reported a difference of colonization rates between 46% and 9%, respectively, in patients with and without sepsis prior to catheterization. In addition, those with colonization had catheters in situ for longer periods of time (particularly beyond 72 hours), had more frequent catheter manipulations, and were more likely to have had repeated catheterization over their clinical course.

Advancing the catheter is a risk factor for catheter infection. The use of sterile outer sleeves has reduced the need for time-consuming preparations prior to catheter manipulation and may improve the short-term sterility of the catheter (38). The effects of these sleeves on the long-term sterility of the catheter is as yet unsubstantiated.

The use of an existing central venous line for PAC insertion over a wire is not ideal because of the possibility that the lumen of the central line may already be colonized by organisms, although one recent study did not show an increased infection rate (36). Nevertheless, the perceived need for invasive monitoring in a patient with difficult venous access or with a coagulopathy, for example, may override this relative contraindication. However, under all circumstances, the insertion and subsequent use of the PAC must be undertaken with the greatest possible commitment to sterility.

### Indirect Complications Associated with the Measurement of Data Using the PAC

The indirect complications associated with the use of the PAC include (1) errors in data collection and (2) the inappropriate application of the physiologic assumptions upon which rational use of the PAC is based to patients in whom these assumptions do not apply. The most important sequel to inaccurate data is the incorrect assessment of the patient's condition and the potential use of inappropriate treatment regimens (39).

The technical errors that occur in pressure measurement include (1) the presence of air in the transducer dome or tubing, (2) a faulty transducer, (3) poor calibration, (4) changing the patient's position without recalibration, (5) pressures not being measured in end-expiration, and (6) the catheter tubing being either too long (resonance) or too soft (damping).

The technical errors that occur in cardiac output measurement include (1) the inaccurate assessment of injectate volume, (2) too slow an injection of fluid, (3) the temperature of the injectate not being equal to the measured "injectate" temperature, (4) a faulty thermistor, (5) the cardiac output not being measured in end-expiration, and (6) the cardiac output computer being programmed with an incorrect constant.

The technical artifacts in the PAC waveform which may lead to errors in interpretation and diagnosis include the following:

1. *Waveform absent.* This is invariably a technical problem that may be due to one of the following: catheter clotted, catheter closed by stopcock or external sliding clamp, faulty transducer, incorrectly calibrated amplifier, inappropriate gain of amplifier, or monitor failure.

2. *Damped waveform.* This phenomenon may be related to the presence of air or blood in the transducer dome or tubing, partial obstruction of the catheter by a blood clot, kinking of the catheter or tubing, the loss of pressure from the flush system or the use of an amplifier that is either not correctly calibrated or that has an inappropriate gain. This should be distinguished from the

"damped" permanent PAOP tracing that is seen when the catheter is in too distal a PA or when the balloon is not deflated after PAOP determination. A damped trace may also be seen in patients in whom the catheter is located in too distal a PA or in a non–zone III position (best seen on lateral chest X-ray as the catheter tip being placed incorrectly above the left atrium) or when the balloon is not deflated after PAOP determination.

3. *Inability to obtain PAOP tracing on balloon inflation.* This problem may be due to the catheter being in too proximal a position or due to balloon rupture. Catheter position may be verified by chest X-ray. The catheter should be advanced with the balloon inflated with 1.5 cc air until a PAOP tracing is observed. If the catheter is correctly positioned, the diagnosis of balloon rupture should be considered, particularly if no resistance to balloon inflation is encountered and if there is a high resistance to attempted aspiration or if blood is aspirated from the balloon port. No further air should be injected.

4. *Excessive variations in pressures with respiration.* This phenomenon is common to all intrathoracic pressure measurements, where the pressure rises during a mechanical breath and falls during a spontaneous breath. Excessive variations may be seen in the hypovolemic patient ventilated with peak end-expiratory pressure (PEEP) but most clearly in the patient ventilated with high inspiratory pressures [e.g., asthma, adult repsiratory distress syndrome (ARDS)]. One should remember to measure all intrathoracic pressures as well as the cardiac output at end expiration.

5. *Excessive noise.* The presence of the PAC within the heart may lead to catheter whip artifact where the mechanical shock of cardiac contraction causes catheter oscillation. This is worse the nearer the catheter tip is to the pulmonary valve and may be improved after catheter advancement. This may also be modified by adjusting the high-frequency filter on the amplifier (37).

6. *Abnormal PAOP trace.* Papillary muscle dysfunction or mitral regurgitation may lead to the presence of abnormal "V" waves in the PAOP tracing. Prominent "A" waves are usually the result of the left atrium contracting against a closed mitral valve (CHB). In addition, the overdistension of the balloon may create a rising low-amplitude trace.

The physiologic conditions which invalidate the assumptions upon which PA catheterization data are interpreted include (1) the presence of the catheter tip in non–zone III conditions in the lung, where the pulmonary vasculature distal to the catheter tip is not patent (catheter tip above the right atrium on a lateral chest X-ray, high levels of PEEP, absolute hypovolemia); (2) abnormal left ventricular pressure-volume relationships (low compliance: myocardial ischemia, aortic stenosis; high compliance: vasodilator therapy, severely failing heart); and (3) failure to equalize pressures between the left ventricle and left atrium at end diastole (mitral stenosis: pressure gradient; aortic regurgitation: premature closure of the mitral valve)

### Therapeutic Procedures

#### Synchronous Direct Current Cardioversion and Defibrillation

Synchronous direct current (DC) cardioversion is the synchronization of the electric shock with the R wave of the QRS complex when it exists [for rhythms other than ventricular fibrillation (VF)], so as to avoid R on T stimulation with the induction of VF as a complication of the procedure.

Principal complications of synchronous DC cardioversion include the induction of dysrhythmias and systemic embolization. Other complications include chest wall burns, myocardial trauma, and electrical injury to the staff.

Transient brady- or tachydysrhythmias may occur after synchronized DC cardioversion and generally do not warrant therapy. Occasionally, patients with sick sinus syndrome (bradycadia-tachycardia syndrome) may develop severe bradycardia or asystole following DC cardioversion (40). Severe dysrhythmias may occur in patients in whom synchronized DC cardioversion was performed in the presence of clinical or ECG evidence of digoxin toxicity. Ventricular fibrillation has been observed in up to 5% of all patients following synchronized DC cardioversion and is generally due to failure of adequate synchronization with consequent R on T stimulation (40).

Clinically evident systemic embolization of thrombus has been described in 1% to 2% of all patients following DC cardioversion and is a particular risk in patients with ventricular or atrial mural thrombus, dilated chambers, or mitral valvular disease (41). In such patients, anticoagulation should be initiated prior to the procedure where possible.

Chest wall burns may occur as a result of the delivery of excessive, focused or repeated electrical shock, particularly if chest wall impedance is low or if there is a track of electrical jelly short circuiting the intrathoracic contents.

Myocardial electrical burns may occur following DC shock, although clinical sequelae are rare; transient ST-segment elevation (42) and rises in serum creatinine phosphokinase (43) have been described. The reasons for this low incidence of electrical injury are due to the fact that (1) the electrical energy is transmitted through all the tissues in proportion to their conductivity and the plane through which the current travels and (2) the density of the energy reaching the heart is considerably lower than that applied to the body surface. However, patients with a direct, narrow, low-impedance pathway to the heart (such as a patient with a transvenous pacemaker device or with central venous saline infusions) may be at risk for microshock, where the transmitted electrical signal may emerge at the surface of the heart over a very small cross-sectional area, thereby producing a relatively large current density at the heart which may produce VF (44). Care should be taken to provide the electrical stimulation along an axis perpendicular to the passage of the pacing wires and as far removed from them as possible. Other complications of DC cardioversion for patients with indwelling permanent pacemakers include interference with the sensing and pacing programs which should be checked prior to and following the procedure. Temporary pacemakers should be disconnected from the wires, where possible, immediately prior to the procedure.

All personnel in the vicinity of the procedure, including the operator, should be isolated from electrical contact with the patient and the bed. Accidental electrical stimulation of staff is obviously not synchronized to their own QRS complex and has been associated with the development of VF (40).

Failure to successfully reverse VF with defibrillation is also regarded as a life-threatening complication of defibrillation. Failure may reflect underlying medical problems such as continuing severe myocardial ischemia, hypoxia or hypercarbia, or disturbances in electrolyte, acid-base, or temperature balance. However, technical problems may often be the cause of a seemingly refractory VF, particularly basic errors in the provision of cardiopulmonary resuscitation, and poor familiarity with the defibrillator (not charged, inappropriately in synchronous mode, poor paddle application etc.).

### Cardiac Pacing

Cardiac pacing delivers an electric stimulus to the heart in order to depolarize the myocardium and impose an exogenous rhythm to replace a preexisting abnormal rhythm. Cardiac pacing may be performed via one of several routes; transcutaneous, transthoracic, transesophageal, and transvenous. Cardiac pacing is associated with complications, some of which are common to all routes of pacing, some peculiar to specific routes of pacing only.

#### General Complications of Cardiac Pacing

Complications of pacing include (a) the hemodynamic consequences of paced conduction and (b) failure of the pacemaker.

*Hemodynamic Consequences of Paced Conduction:* Cardiac pacing imposes an exogenous but otherwise almost normal rhythm in a situation where an abnormal rhythm existed prior to intervention. As a consequence of improved rate or rhythm, cardiac output generally improves. In the presence of an intact AV conduction system, atrial pacing may take place with almost normal myocardial mechanics. The atrial contraction contributes approximately 20% to the total stroke volume, and the generation of the electrical impulse throughout the ventricles is via the AV node and along the bundle of His which provides an optimally fast and coordinated ventricular component of contraction. During ventricular pacing neither of these factors are preserved, and the improvement in cardiac output due to pacing is proportionately less. As a consequence, atrial pacing is almost invariably preferred in the presence of an intact AV conduction system.

*Pacemaker Failure.* Pacemaker failure may occur for several reasons: (1) undersensing, (2) oversensing, and (3) failure to capture.

1. *Undersensing.* The failure to sense the endogenous QRS complex may lead to inappropriate pacing stimuli with the genesis of dysrhythmias. Poor lead position, lead fracture, inappropriate sensitivity adjustment, or weak endogenous electrocardiographic signals may all cause undersensing; the latter may be due to myocardial ischemia or failure or disturbances in acid-base or electrolyte balance. The intracardiac signal may be enhanced when using transvenous cardiac pacing by transferring the pacing lead from bipolar to unipolar (by the use of a surface electrode to the positive terminal of the pacemaker and the intracardiac electrode to the negative terminal, with the second intracardiac lead being isolated within a rubber sheath) (40).

2. *Oversensing.* The sensing of extraneous signals may be hazardous for pacemakers where the mode of action is inhibition, typically permanent VVI pacemakers or temporary pacemakers in the demand mode. If the pacemaker senses a signal that mimics an intrinsic R wave and when the apparent R-R interval is shorter than that programmed into the pacemaker as the automatic interval, then the pacing function will be suppressed. Myopotentials (exercise, fasciculation due to succinylcholine administration during anesthesia, shivering) and electrocautery (intraoperative diathermy) may lead to the suppression of inhibition-based cardiac pacemakers. In addition the sensing of endogenous T waves as R waves may lead to inappropriate inhibition. The response to such an occurrence when using a temporary transvenous pacemaker should be to turn the sensitivity function to asynchronous; in permanent pacemakers a magnet may be used to reprogram the pacemaker to VOO function with similar results.

3. *Failure to capture.* Failure to capture may be due to purely technical problems such as lead malposition, disconnection, or fracture or pulse generator or battery failure. In transvenous pacing it may be due to myocardial perforation. It may be possible to change the pacing current and so resume, at least temporarily, adequate cardiac pacing. However, it should be remembered that failure to capture may reflect changing myocardial pacing thresholds which may in turn be due to myocardial ischemia or infarction or due to electrolyte or acid-base imbalance.

*Complications of Specific Pacemakers:*

These may be divided into the routes of pacing that is (1) transcutaneous, (2) transthoracic, (3) transesophageal, and (4) transvenous.

1. *Transcutaneous cardiac pacing.* In early models of transcutaneous pacing, the pain associated with stimulation of underlying muscles and nerves made its use unacceptable in the conscious patient. Design modifications allow its use to be better tolerated, although patients frequently require sedation (45). Transcutaneous cardiac pacing has been found to be successful in the majority of patients studied (46) with a similar hemodynamic response. The majority of failures reported were after prolonged cardiac arrest, at which stage the poor myocardial substrate may have hampered successful cardiac pacing by any route (40).

2. *Transthoracic cardiac pacing.* This technique, where external pacing suture wires are placed through the chest wall and into the ventricular or atrial muscle directly, is a common procedure that is used during cardiac surgery, prior to chest closure. The wires may be left in place for a few days after surgery and atrial, ventricular, or AV sequential modes of pacing used. The principal complications of transthoracic pacing include the dislodgment of pacing wires and bleeding from the suture site.

3. *Transesophageal cardiac pacing.* This is a relatively noninvasive mode of pacing with consequently few specific adverse effects. Gastrointestinal discomfort, brachial plexus, and phrenic nerve stimulation are occasional problems. Close apposition of the esophagus with the left atrium provides reasonable atrial but poor ventricular pacing. The esophageal electrode is prone to be dislodged and so leads to pacing failure (40).

4. *Transvenous cardiac pacing.* The specific complications due to transvenous cardiac pacing may be due to (a) the central venous access or (b) the insertion and maintenance of the pacing wires.

(a) *Venous cannulation.* The complications discussed above for central venous access for the PAC in the section Complications of Central Venous Cannulation are equally applicable here; thus, bleeding, hematoma, arterial puncture, air embolism, pneumothorax, nerve injury, or deep vein thrombosis are the principal complications due to venous access.

(b) *Pacing wire insertion and maintenance: dysrhythmias.* As for any intracardiac stimulus, ventricular dysrhythmias may occur (see Complications of PA Catheterization above). Hypoxia, acidosis, electrolyte disturbance, or continued myocardial ischemia may all promote the genesis of dysrhythmias and should be avoided or corrected where possible prior to the procedure. Prolonged mechanical irritation of the right ventricle inflow or outflow tracts should be avoided; however, low cardiac output,

dilated cardiomyopathies, poor operator experience, and emergency conditions may all hamper successful passage of the pacing wires and so lead to repeated dysrhythmic stimuli.

*Myocardial perforation* with or without pericardial tamponade is a rare but serious complication of transvenous cardiac pacing. The clinical presentation is of chest pain or a pericardial friction rub following wire insertion, associated with a failure to capture or sense, or a change in the paced QRS configuration. The diagnosis may be made by proximal and distal unipolar electrograms and by electrocardiography. The catheter should be pulled back to the right atrium and repositioned with the aid of fluoroscopy.

*Complications of the pacing wires* include lead fracture, which causes pacing failure and requires the replacement of pacing wires, and microshock, where seemingly insidious electrical currents may be inadvertently passed down the low-impedance pathway to the heart and, due to the high current density at the pacing wire—cardiac interface, may generate dysrhythmia or result in myocardial electrical burns (see Synchronous Direct Current Cardioversion and Defibrillation).

### Intra-aortic Balloon Counterpulsation Pump

The complications due to this procedure include (1) malfunction of the apparatus and (2) direct complications due to the balloon pump.

*Intra-aortic Balloon Counterpulsation Pump (IABCP) Malfunction*

(a) *Patient signal.* Problems due to poor patient triggering signal include faulty electrocardiographic connections, low-amplitude QRS complexes, arrhythmias, tachycardia, and cardiac arrest.

(b) *Pump malfunction*

(i) *Maladjustment of the inflation-deflation cycle.* Inflation of the IABCP prior to closure of the aortic valve may cause aortic regurgitation or premature valve closure, paradoxical increases in afterload, and its correlates (increased left ventricular wall stress, left ventricular end diastolic volume, and pressure). The reduction in all of these determinants of myocardial oxygen consumption is one of the goals of a normally functioning IABCP. Thus premature inflation is a serious malfunction.

Delayed inflation of the IABCP well after the closure of the aortic valve reduces the period of enhanced diastolic pressure that is associated with a normally functioning IABCP. Coronary blood flow, which is principally diastolic, will be less enhanced than might be expected.

Premature deflation of the IABCP not only limits the enhancement of diastolic pressure and coronary flow as discussed above, but may even lead to retrograde coronary artery flow. This, combined with the reduced impact on afterload reduction (thus raising myocardial oxygen consumption), may lead to myocardial ischemia .

Delayed deflation of the IABCP until almost the onset of systole leads to a reduction in the time available for afterload reduction. Indeed, very delayed deflation of the balloon may lead to paradoxical rises in afterload as the left ventricle attempts to eject blood against the resistance of the balloon.

(ii) *Technical problems with the apparatus.* The balloon may be partially entrapped within the sheath. There may be kinks or disconnections in the gas line, leak or rupture of the balloon, or electrical or pneumatic malfunction of the IABCP itself.

### Direct Complications to the Patient of the IABCP

Ipsilateral leg ischemia is the most common serious complication of the use of the IABCP; pulses usually return following removal of the device (47). Occasionally thrombectomy or even cross-over femoral grafting may be required to restore flow and avoid tissue necrosis and amputation.

Heparin is a standard antithromboembolic prophylaxis in the presence of the IABCP, despite concerns regarding excessive bleeding from the femoral artery puncture site. This bleeding, while occasionally excessive, may usually be controlled by external pressure, although occasionally surgical repair is required.

Rare complications include the perforation or dissection of the aorta (usually lethal) or femoral artery and embolization of the gas within the balloon (usually carbon dioxide or occasionally helium so as to maximize gas diffusion and hence minimize the adverse effects of gas embolism) . Thrombocytopenia due to the effect of the balloon on platelet consumption has been reported but is rarely severe enough to warrant any specific therapy.

## CARDIAC COMPLICATIONS OF INVASIVE, NONCARDIAC PROCEDURES

### Respiratory Procedures

The cardiac complications of laryngoscopy and endotracheal intubation include (1) the cardiac implications of failed airway management and (2) the cardiac manifestations of reflex sympathetic and parasympathetic stimulation in the richly innervated upper airway (particularly the larynx).

### Cardiac Implications of Failed Airway Management

Endotracheal intubation, if not successful within a short period of time and particularly if associated with general failure of airway management, may lead to hypoxemia and hypercarbia. Both hypoxemia and hypercarbia have implications for cardiac physiology, particularly in the cardiac compromised patient.

The cardiovascular effects of hypoxemia are both direct and indirect, the latter mediated by both humoral and neural reflex mechanisms. Cardiac output initially increases as heart rate, stroke volume, and myocardial contractility all rise in response to sympathetic activation and the release of circulating catecholamines. As hypoxemia worsens, systemic vascular resistance falls (direct vasodilatation) and myocardial contractility diminishes (direct myocardial depression), with an associated marked reduction in arterial pressure. The cumulative effect is of impaired myocardial oxygen supply (reduced oxygen delivery, tachycardia leading to reduced diastolic filling time, and eventually, lowered diastolic pressure) and increased myocardial oxygen consumption (tachycardia, initially raised systemic arterial pressure with raised afterload). This impaired myocardial oxygen balance is further aggravated in the presence of coronary artery disease and hypoxemia-induced arrhythmias. Eventually, shock, bradycardia, and cardiac arrest (either asystole or VF) intervene. Hypoxemia also increases pulmonary vascular resistance which may exacerbate an intracardiac right-to-left shunt which in turn intensifies the hypoxemia, thus perpetuating positive feedback.

The cardiovascular response to hypercapnia follows a pattern similar to that described above for hypoxemia, with direct systemic vasodilatation and myocardial depression and both neural and humoral sympathetic cardiovascular stimulation. The overall impairment of myocardial oxygen balance is as described above. In addition, the metabolic effects of hypercarbia and the associated acidosis include redistributional hyperkalemia and a shift in the oxyhemoglobin dissociation curve to the right (so facilitating tissue uptake of oxygen).

### The Cardiac Manifestations of Reflex Sympathetic and Parasympathetic Stimulation During Endotracheal Intubation

The base of the tongue, oropharynx, epiglottis, larynx, and trachea are structures with a rich sensory and autonomic innervation. Accordingly, there is a profound response to the instrumentation of the airway in awake subjects, and most conscious patients require systemic or local anesthesia prior to tracheal intubation. Potential cardiac sequelae of tracheal intubation include sympathetic and vagal responses to the stimulation, in addition to the general depressant effects of anesthetic drugs given to ablate these responses.

Reflex sympathetic-mediated responses to tracheal intubation include hypertension and tachycardia, particularly excessive in chronically hypertensive patients. The cardiac implications of these responses are a reduction in myocardial oxygen supply (reduced diastolic filling time) and a raised myocardial oxygen demand (raised afterload, tachycardia). This impaired myocardial oxygen balance may lead to myocardial ischemia in susceptible individuals.

Reflex vagal-mediated responses to tracheal intubation include hypotension and bradycardia (even cardiac arrest), which are dominant early responses in children but are generally masked by the sympathetic response in adults. Further local responses to tracheal intubation which have a parasympathetic input include laryngeal spasm and bronchospasm, which may lead to hypoxia whose cardiac sequelae have been discussed above.

In order to minimize these reflex responses, particularly the hypertension and tachycardia, various drugs have been advocated, many of which may cause systemic vasodilation and negative inotropism and thus a reduction in arterial pressure and, hence, in coronary perfusion. Examples include sodium thiopentone, benzodiazepines, propofol, and volatile anesthetics. Ketamine has an opposite effect; narcotics confer the greatest hemodynamic stability but often lead to the need for mechanical ventilation due to profound respiratory depression. The use of local anesthetic drugs, either topically or intravenously, has been widely advocated to suppress both the reflex sympathetic and the vagal responses to intubation. The use of beta-adrenergic blocking drugs, particularly the ultra-short acting esmolol to block the sympathetic response, and of anticholinergic agents to block the vagal response (particularly in children) enables more control of these autonomic responses. However, all of these pharmacologic interventions carry with them their own benefits and risks.

## Mechanical Ventilatory Support

The heart and great vessels lie within the thoracic cavity and are thus affected by the changing intrathoracic pressures induced by positive-pressure ventilation. The single most important cardiac effect is the decrease in cardiac output due to the reduction in venous return. The consequence of this effect may be to limit, or even reverse, the projected rise in oxygen delivery, which is often the main indication for the various ventilatory techniques (48). The scope of this reduction in cardiac output is itself determined by underlying cardiac function. A severely hypovolemic patient with a critically preload-dependent left ventricle is much more sensitive to the reduced venous return induced by positive-pressure ventilation than is a normovolemic patient. Stroke volume, cardiac output, and systemic blood pressure all fall much more markedly in the presence of absolute hypovolemia. Indeed, the exaggerated phasic variations in the arterial pressure wave in ventilated patients have been used as a most sensitive indicator of volume status (48). The presence of continuous positive airway pressure (CPAP) or PEEP or a too rapid ventilatory rate may all exacerbate this adverse hemodynamic effect.

Positive-pressure ventilation also increases pulmonary vascular resistance which may exacerbate an intracardiac right-to-left shunt. This phenomenon is exacerbated in the presence of hypoxemia and may be sustained by the positive feedback described above.

The provision of appropriate mechanical ventilation may reduce the work of breathing, particularly in patients with impaired lung mechanics. This is generally accompanied by an improvement in the myocardial oxygen balance. However, high levels of CPAP may significantly increase the expiratory work of breathing due to a markedly increased lung volume. A similar rise in the work of breathing may occur if a conscious patient "fights" controlled mandatory ventilation, if tidal volume or the ventilatory rate is too low, or if the sensitivity of the demand valve is low (or its response is too slow), thus forcing the patient to generate excessive and spontaneous inspirtory effort. In all of these cases, the potential benefits on myocardial oxygen balance may be diminished or even reversed.

Hypercarbia and hypoxemia as consequences of technical failures of mechanical ventilatory support have been discussed above in relation to their implications for cardiovascular pathophysiology. The principal complications of hyperoxia in adults are generally restricted to the respiratory system (pulmonary oxygen toxicity and the removal of the hypoxic drive in chronically hypercarbic patients). However, hypocarbia, due to excessive mechanical ventilation has several significant cardiac sequelae (apart from an exaggerated ventilation-related reduction in venous return, as discussed above). Hypocarbia may cause negative inotropism, mediated both by a reduction in sympathetic tone and also by a reduction in ionized calcium due to raised plasma pH. In addition, hypocapnia and the associated alkalosis, tend to shift the oxygen dissociation curve to the left, increasing the affinity of hemoglobin for oxygen and thus impairing oxygen unloading at the tissue level, including the myocardium. Hypocapnia may inhibit the hypoxic pulmonary vasoconstriction response, which may in turn exacerbate the ventilation-perfusion (VA/Q) abnormalities associated with an extracardiac right-to-left shunt and thus cause hypoxemia, so reducing further myocardial oxygen delivery. Furthermore, both hyperoxia and hypocarbia may cause coronary vasoconstriction and thus impair myocardial oxygen delivery.

Noncardiac complications of mechanical ventilatory support may have cardiac implications. Foremost among these is barotrauma and, particularly, tension pneumothorax, which causes life-threatening circulatory collapse due to critical reduction in venous return to the right atrium. Ventilation with low tidal volumes may cause atelectasis, which leads to VA/Q abnormalities and an extracardiac right-to-left shunt with consequent hypoxemia and reduced myocardial oxygen delivery.

## Bronchoscopy

Many of the cardiac complications associated with bronchoscopy are related to hypoxemia, reflex vagal and/or sympathetic stimulation, and the use of sedative or anesthetic drugs to ablate these responses. These have all been discussed in relation to the complications following endotracheal intubation.

The reported incidence of major complications following diagnostic fiberoptic bronchoscopy is between 0.08% (49) and 1.7% (50) with a mortality between 0.01% (49) and 0.1% (50). In a different study (51) hypoxemia was implicated in nearly half of the deaths. Indeed, even in patients without recognized complications of bronchscopy, a degree of hypoxemia has been demonstrated with a mean reduction in $PaO_2$ of between 20 mm Hg (52) to 34 mm Hg (53). In a separate study of cardiac rhythm disturbances following bronchoscopy, severe hypoxia ($PaO_2 < 60$ mm Hg) was found to be the only variable that correlated with the development of major cardiac arryhthmias (54). In this study, the incidence of major and minor arrhythmias during bronchoscopy were 70% and 11%, respectively, which compared with 49% and 7% in the "baseline" hour prior to the procedure.

It should be noted that these complication rates refer to overall statistics from bronchoscopies performed in relatively low risk patients. In the ICU environment, the complication rates may be expected to exceed the quoted data. Indeed, in one study (51), mortalities were only observed in patients with underlying cardiovascular disease, severe chronic obstructive pulmonary disease, pneumonia, or cancer, diseases which figure prominently in the ICU population.

When bronchoscopy is performed as part of bronchoalveolar lavage (BAL), the complication rates rise somewhat, partly due to the higher risk population involved. Complication rates up to 2.3% have been reported (55). These general complications include transient alveolar infiltrates, crepitations, and fever, the incidence of which are all correlated with the volume of lavage fluid instilled and the number of lung segments lavaged (55).

For transbronchial lung biopsy complication and mortality rates of 7% and 0.2%, respectively, have been reported which compare with 13% and 1.8% for open-lung biopsy (55).

## Hemodialysis

Hemodialysis is associated with changes in systemic blood pressure, extracellular fluid volume, pH, and serum concentrations of potassium, sodium, calcium, and magnesium. The consequence of these changes on cardiac output include effects on preload, afterload, heart rate, and contractility. However, the clinical correlates of these cardiac effects vary between patients and depend to a large degree on the underlying cardiac condition.

Changes in preload in patients with normal cardiac function may be well tolerated, but the effects on patients with diastolic dysfunction (ischemic or hypertrophied myocardium) are particularly marked, as these patients are critically preload dependent.

The decrease in systemic vascular resistance that may accompany hemodialysis may dramatically lower coronary perfusion pressure and cardiac output. Tissue ischemia is one important cause of reduced afterload during hemodialysis (56). In addition, the use of acetate as the dialysate may reduce systemic vascular resistance, and its replacement with bicarbonate is recommended for high-risk patients (57). The use of a dialysate with a high calcium concentration is thought to reduce dialysis-associated hypotension, but its influence on the frequency of chest pain has not been evaluated. Other specific measures advocated to prevent or treat intradialytic hypotension include the maintenance of an acceptable hematocrit, crystalloid or colloid fluid loading, Trendelenburg position, and the use of pressurized leg boots. Inotropic or vasoactive pharmacologic support may also be required.

Chest pain occurs not infrequently during hemodialysis. In one study between 80% and 97% of patients experienced hypotension, and more than one-third of patients complained of chest pain during hemodialysis over a 5-month period of observation (58). Myocardial ischemia may be caused or aggravated by hypoxemia and hypotension, which not infrequently accompany hemodialysis. Cardiac patients experiencing angina during hemodialysis should be given oxygen routinely, blood pressure should be corrected, and nitroglycerin administration should be considered.

Inadequate dialysate electrolyte composition can cause either acidosis or alkalosis as well as either hyponatremia or hypernatremia. Significant hypokalemia may also occur due to both potassium washout and the influx of potassium into the intracellular compartment following the rapid correction of metabolic acidosis during hemodialysis. In addition, hypophosphatemia may occur during hemodialysis. All of these metabolic derangements may cause severe cardiac arrhythmias. Patients treated with digoxin are particularly susceptible.

## CONCLUSION

A thorough knowledge of the cardiac complications of invasive procedures in the ICU setting is important for several reasons. It enables the early recognition of complications once they have arisen and facilitates prompt and appropriate therapy. It focuses attention on the importance of the adoption (and occasionally the adaptation) of accepted procedural technique so as to avoid the complications arising in the first place. Furthermore, it enables a cost-benefit approach to be prepared for each procedure in each patient where the potential complications may be weighed against well-founded indications.

# REFERENCES

1. Matthay MA, Chatterjee K. Bedside catheterization of the pulmonary artery: risks compared with benefits. *Ann Intern Med* 1988;109:826.
2. Venus B, Mallory DL. Vascular cannulation. In: Civetta JM, et al., eds. *Critical care,* 2nd ed. Philadelphia: Lippincott; 1992:149.
3. Patel C, Laboy V, Venus B, et al. Acute complications of pulmonary artery catheter insertion in critically ill patients. *Crit Care Med* 1986; 14:195.
4. Sprung CL, Jacobs LJ, Caralis PV, et al. Ventricular arrhythmias during Swan-Ganz catheterization of the critically ill. *Chest* 1981;79: 411.
5. Sprung CL, Marical EH, Garcia AA, et al. Prophylactic use of lidocaine to prevent advanced ventricular arrhythmias during pulmonary artery catheterization: prospective, double-blind study. *Am J Med* 1983;75:906.
6. Swan HJC, Ganz W, Forrester J, et al. Catheterization of the heart in man with the use of a flow-directed balloon tipped catheter. *N Engl J Med* 1970;283:447.
7. Moore CH, Lombardo TR, Allums JA, et al. Left main coronary artery stenosis: hemodynamic monitoring to reduce mortality. *Ann Thorac Surg* 1978;26:445.
8. Steele P, Davies H. The Swan Ganz catheter in the cardiac laboratory. *Br Heart J* 1973;35:647.
9. Elliot CG, Zimmerman GA, Clemmer TP. Complications of pulmonary artery catheters in the care of critically ill patients. *Chest* 1979;76:647.
10. Shaw TJI. The Swan Ganz pulmonary artery catheter. *Anaesthesia* 1979;34:651.
11. Sprung CL. Complications of pulmonary artery catheterization. In: Sprung CL, ed. *The pulmonary artery catheter: methodology and clinical applications.* Rockville: Aspen; 1983:73.
12. Thomson IR, Dalton BC, Lappas DG, et al. Right bundle branch block and complete heart block caused by the Swan Ganz catheter. *Anesthesiology* 1979;51:359.
13. Abernathy WS. Complete heart block caused by the Swan Ganz catheter. *Chest* 1974;65:349.
14. Akhtar M, Damato RN, Gilbert-Leeds CJ, et al. Induction of iatrogenic electrocardiographic patterns during electrophysiologic studies. *Circulation* 1977;56:60.
15. Morris D, Mulvihill D, Lew WY. Risk of developing complete heart block during bedside pulmonary artery catheterization in patients with left bundle branch block. *Arch Intern Med* 1987;147:2005.
16. Foote GA, Schabel SI, Hodges M. Pulmonary complications of the flow directed balloon tipped catheter. *N Engl J Med* 1974;290:927.
17. Hines,R, Barash PG. Pulmonary artery catheterization. In: Blitt CD, ed. *Monitoring in anesthesia and critical care medicine,* 2nd ed. New York: Churchill Livingstone; 1990:221.
18. Kaplan JA. Hemodynamic monitoring. In: Kaplan JA, ed. *Cardiac anesthesia.* Philadelphia: WB Saunders; 1987:179.
19. Sise MJ, Hollingsworth P, Brimm JE, et al. Complications of the flow directed pulmonary artery catheter: a prospective analysis in 219 patients. *Crit Care Med* 1981;9:315.
20. Civetta JM. Pulmonary artery catheter insertion. In: Sprung CL, ed. *The pulmonary artery catheter: methodology and clinical applications.* Rockville: Aspen; 1983:21.
21. Laster J, Silver D. Heparin-coated catheters and heparin induced thrombocytopenia. *J Vasc Surg* 1988;7:667.
22. Barash PG, Nardi D, Hammond G, et al. Catheter induced pulmonary artery perforation: mechanisms, management, and modifications. *J Thorac Cardiovasc Surg* 1981;82:5.
23. Carlson TA, Goldenberg IF, Murray PD, et al. Catheter induced delayed recurrent pulmonary artery hemorrhage: intervention with therapeutic embolism of the pulmonary artery. *JAMA* 1989;261: 1943.
24. McDaniel DD, Stone JG, Faltas AN, et al. Catheter-induced pulmonary artery hemorrhage. *J Thorac Cardiovasc Surg* 1981;82:5.
25. Fleisher AG, Tyers GFO, Manning GT, et al. Management of massive hemoptysis secondary to catheter-induced perforation of the pulmonary artery during cardiopulmonary bypass. *Chest* 1989;95:1340.
26. Pellegrini RV, Macelli G, Di Marco RF, et al. Swan Ganz catheter induced pulmonary hemorrhage. *J Cardiovasc Surg* 1987;28:646.
27. Yonkman CA, Hamory BH. Sterility and efficiency of two methods of cardiac output determination: closed loop and capped syringe methods. *Heart and Lung* 1988;17:121.
28. Greene JF, Fitzwater JE, Clemmer TP. Septic endocarditits and indwelling pulmonary artery catheters. *JAMA* 1975;233:891.
29. Ehrie M, Morgan AP, Moore FD, et al. Endocarditis with the indwelling balloon tipped pulmonary artery catheter in burn patients. *J Trauma* 1978;18:664.
30. Applefeld JJ, Caruthers TE, Reno DJ, et al. Assessment of the sterility of long term cardiac catheterization using thermodilution Swan Ganz catheters. *Chest* 1978;74:377.
31. Anderson PT, Herlevesen P, Schaumburg H. A comparative study of "Op-site" and "Nobecutan" gauze dressings for central venous line care. *J Hosp Infect* 1986;7:161.
32. Craven DE, Lichtenberg DA, Kunches LM, et al. A randomised study comparing a transparent polyurethane dressing to a dry gauze dressing for peripheral intravenous catheter sites. *Infect Control* 1985;6: 361.
33. Katich M, Band J. Local infection of the intravenous cannula wound associated with transparant dressings. *J Infect Dis* 1985;151:971.
34. Maki DG, Band JD. A comparative study of polyantibiotic and iodophore ointments in prevention of vascular catheter-related infection. *Am J Med* 1981;70:739.
35. Maki DG, Ringer M. Evaluation of dressing regimens for prevention of infections with peripheral intravenous catheters: gauze, a transparent polyurethane dressing and an iodophore-transparent dressing. *JAMA* 1987;258:2396.
36. Eyer S, Brummitt C, Crossley K, et al. Catheter related sepsis: prospective, randomized study of three methods of long term catheter maintenance. *Crit Care Med* 1990;18:1073.
37. Kett DH, Schein RMH. Techniques for pulmonary artery catheter insertion. In: Sprung CL, ed. *The pulmonary artery catheter: methodology and clinical applications,* 2nd ed. Closter, NJ: Critical Care Research Associates; 1993:43.
38. Johnston WE, Prough DS, Royster RL, et al. Short term sterility of the pulmonary artery catheter inserted through a sterile plastic shield. *Anesthesiology* 1984;61:461.
39. Iberti TJ, Fischer EP, Leibowitz AB, et al. A multicenter study of physicians' knowledge of the pulmonary artery catheter. *JAMA* 1990; 264:2928.
40. Hahn SM, Goldschlager N. Treatment of cardiac dysrhythmias. In: Benumof JL, ed. *Clinical procedures in anesthesia and intensive care.* Philadelphia: Lippincott; 1992:507.
41. Mancini J, Goldberger AL. Cardioversion of atrial fibrillation: consideration of embolisation, anti-coagulation, prophylactic pacemaker and long term success. *Am Heart J* 1982;104:617.
42. Chun PKC, Davia JE, Donohue DJ. ST segment elevation with elective DC cardioversion. *Circulation* 1981;63:220.
43. Ehsanin A, Ewy GA, Sobel BE. Effects of electric countershock on serum creatinine phosphokinase isoenzyme activity. *Am J Cardiol* 1976;37:12.
44. Starmer CF, Whalen RE. Current density and electrically induced ventricular fibrillation. *Med Instrum* 1973;7:158.
45. Hedges JR, Syverud SA, Dalsey WC, et al. Prehospital trial of emergency transcutaneous cardiac pacing. *Circulation* 1987;76:1337.
46. Falk RH, Zoll PM, Zoll RH. Safety and efficacy of non-invasive cardiac pacing: a preliminary report. *N Eng J Med* 1983;309:1166.
47. Bolooki H. Current status of circulatory support with an intra-aortic balloon pump. *Cardiol Clin* 1985;3:123.
48. Perel A, Pizov R. Cardiovascular effects of mechanical ventilation. In: Perel A, Stock MC, eds. *Handbook of mechanical ventilatory support.* Baltimore: Williams & Wilkins; 1992:51.
49. Credle WF, Smiddy JF, Elliott RC. Complications of fibreoptic bronchoscopy. *Am Rev Resp Dis* 1974;109:67.

50. Pereira W, Kovnat DM, Snider GL. A prospective co-operative study of complications following flexible fibreoptic bronchoscopy. *Chest* 1978;73:813.

51. Surratt PM, Smiddy JF, Gruber B. Deaths and complications associated with fiberoptic bronchoscopy. *Chest* 1976;69:747.

52. Albertini RE, Harrell JH, Kurihara N, Moser KM. Arterial hypoxemia induced by fiberoptic bronchoscopy. *JAMA* 1974;230:1666.

53. Lindholm CE, Ollman B, Snyder JV, et al. Cardiorespiratory effects of flexible fiberoptic bronchoscopy in critically ill patients. *Chest* 1978;74:362.

54. Shrader DL, Lakshminarayan S. The effect of fiberoptic bronchoscopy on cardiac rhythm. *Chest* 1978;73:821.

55. Klech HH, Pohl WW. Use of bronchoalveolar lavage in interstitial lung disease. In: Bone RC, ed. *Pulmonary and critical care medicine.* St Louis: Mosby Year-Book; 1993:1.

56. Bregman H, Daugirdas JT, Ing TS. Complications during dialysis. In: Daugirdas JT, Ing TS, eds. *Handbook of dialysis*, 2nd ed. Boston: Little, Brown; 1994:146.

57. Maher JF. Cardiac complications of uremia and dialysis. In: Maher JF, ed. *Replacement of renal function by dialysis.* Dordrecht, Holland: Kluwer Academic; 1989:788.

58. Levin NW, et al. Complications during hemodialysis . In: Nissenson AR, Fine RN, Gentile DE, eds. *Clinical dialysis*, 2nd ed. Norwalk, CT: Appleton & Lange; 1990:172.

*The Critically Ill Cardiac Patient,*
edited by V. Kvetan and D. R. Dantzker,
Lippincott-Raven Publishers, Philadelphia © 1996.

CHAPTER **20**

# Critical Care Radiology

Arfa Khan and Daniel F. Settle

A portable chest radiograph (PCR) is integral in the management of intensive care unit (ICU) patients. Routine daily radiographs, which are customary at most ICUs, frequently demonstrate unexpected or changing abnormalities, many of which prompt changes in diagnostic management. The efficacy of this practice has been studied in the recent literature, and its continuation is justified by the data collected (1, 2). The incidence of abnormal radiographic findings in ICUs is reported to be between 43% and 70% (3–6). Beckmeyer et al. (1) reported a study of 1,300 PCRs in 167 ICUs, in which 35% of PCRs showed new or progressive cardiopulmonary disease or tubes and catheters in an unexpected position leading to a change in management in 30% and a change in tube and catheter in 20%. Over the last several decades, the imaging of the critically ill has expanded beyond the bedside radiograph to include several other bedside examinations, including ultrasound and nuclear medicine techniques (6). Other procedures require the patient to be transported to the radiology department, such as computed tomography (CT), magnetic resonance imaging (MRI), and nuclear medicine scintigraphy. The role of CT in the care of the critically ill is well established (7, 8).

Storage phosphor computed radiography (CR) and film digitization with automated density correction have replaced conventional radiography in a small number of ICUs in the United States (9), and the number is expected to increase to 50% by the turn of century (10). Computed radiography involves a plate coated with photostimulable phosphor housed in a cassette which is exposed to x-rays. The latent image is scanned by a laser to generate digital images. The digitized image is processed and can be viewed on a video display terminal (VDT) or recorded on film. In contrast to conventional film, CR has greater sensitivity and latitude, consistent film density, opportunity

for image processing to enhance diagnostic information (Figs. 1, 2), rapid electronic image transmission, and compact digital storage. The advantage of CR, particularly in portable applications, is the complete elimination of repeat examinations caused by exposure error, thus leading to a reduction in film cost and decrease in radiation exposure both to the patient and to the technologist. The VDT can be placed in strategic locations in the ICU and radiology departments for prompt viewing of the computed radiograph. The overall diagnostic quality of CR is equal to conventional radiography (10). At our institution, CR has been used instead of conventional radiography in the ICU for the last 2 years with favorable results (11).

Communication between the radiologist and ICU staff leads to better imaging and diagnosis. Daily review conferences between radiologist and clinician aid in planning future studies and decrease hospital stay (12). This chapter will discuss the radiology of thoracic catheters, wires, and tubes, acute cardiopulmonary diseases in the ICU, abnormal air and fluid collections, and acute aortic dissection. The role of radiologic procedures like CT, ultrasonography (US), and MRI will be emphasized.

## RADIOLOGY OF THORACIC CATHETERS, WIRES, AND TUBES

In the ICU, various types of catheters and tubes are used routinely. Proper placement of these is essential if their monitoring or support goals are to be achieved. Each piece of equipment may cause complications, many of which can be recognized on the chest radiograph and prevented before they cause clinical problems. Knowledge of the purpose of each device, its ideal position, and potential complications facilitate better interpretation of the radiograph obtained in the ICU and early detection of any problems.

A. Khan and D.F. Settle: Department of Radiology, Long Island Jewish Medical Center, New Hyde Park, New York 11040.

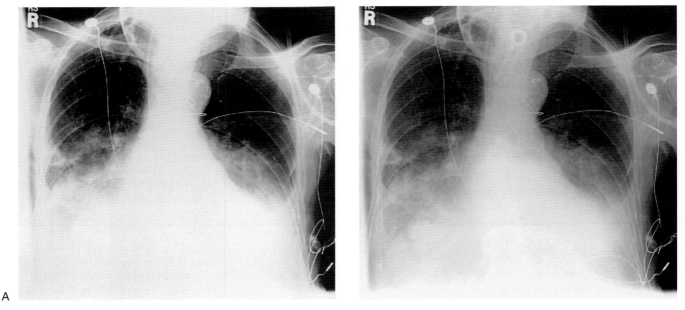

**FIG. 1.** Computed radiograph (CR) image processing. **A, B:** Film density can be altered to enhance diagnostic information.

## Endotracheal Tube

The normal adult trachea is 10 to 13 cm in length from cricoid cartilage to the carina. The ideal endotracheal tube (ETT) position is in the midtrachea, 5 to 7 cm from the carina with head in neutral position, which allows a safe margin for tube tip movements. With flexion of the neck, the tip of the tube will move down the trachea a maximum of 3 cm, and when the neck is extended, it will move up a maximum of 2 cm (13, 14) (Fig. 3). If the carina is not visible, its position may be estimated relative to the thoracic spine. On 95% of portable radiographs, the carina projects over T5 to T7 (13). If the vertebral bodies cannot be counted, one may count the posterior ribs and follow them medially. The tip of the ETT should project over the T2 or T3 level. The position of the chin relative to the vertebral bodies is a clue to the neck position. The chin is usually projected over T1 or T2 with flexion, at C5 to C6 in the neutral position, and above C4 with neck extension (14). A number of potential complications exist with ETTs (15).

### Aberrant Positioning

Right mainstem bronchus intubation resulting from overinsertion occurs in 10% to 15% intubations and is associated with an increased patient mortality. The chest radiographs will demonstrate the tube in the right mainstem bronchus with atelectasis of the left lung (Fig. 4). If the ETT is in the intermediate bronchus, right upper lobe collapse will be evident as well. Hyperinflation of the intubated lung ensues, increasing the risk of barotrauma. Fifteen percent of patients with right mainstem bronchus intubation develop pneumothorax. Left mainstem bronchus intubation is much less common due to its more oblique course. A tube placed close to the larynx may cause ventilatory difficulties and extubation (Fig. 5). An ETT inserted into the esophagus at the time of intubation is usually diagnosed clinically.

### Laceration or Rupture

Laceration or rupture of the airway is a less common but very serious complication of intubation. It is more common in infants and elderly patients and characteristically involves the membranous portion of the trachea. When the tear extends beyond the pleural reflection of the main bronchus, pneumothorax, pneumomediastinum, and subcutaneous emphysema make the diagnosis obvious at an early stage (6). If the tear is confined to the mediastinum, perforation may be clinically silent for hours, with emphysema of the deep cervical fascia and pneumomediastinum occurring later. If tracheal laceration is suspected, cross-table lateral views and chest CT are helpful in confirming the diagnosis. An early radiographic sign of tracheal rupture is the presence of an overinflated balloon of the ETT while still registering normal intracuff pressures. The large balloon extends through the tracheal laceration and is now free in the mediastinum, offering no resistance to overinflation. A second sign is an oblique direction of the distal portion of the ETT to the right relative to the tracheal lumen. The

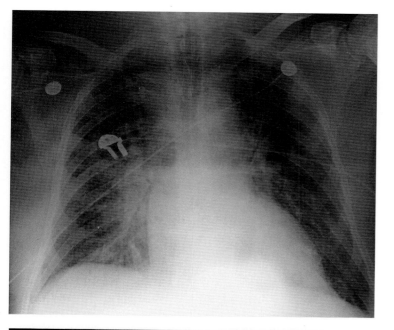

A

**FIG. 2.** A CR image manipulation. **A–C:** Image manipulation of a single exposure to optimally visualize the lung, mediastinum, and monitoring devices.

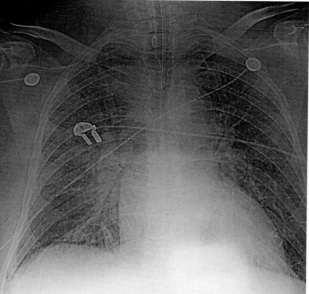

B

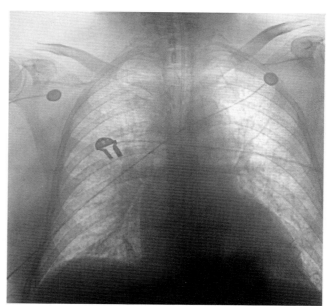

C

tube is anchored in that peculiar direction by the balloon herniated through the laceration. The ETT and nasogastric tubes as seen on the PCR may form an acute angle instead of being parallel (16).

## Tracheal Stenosis and Tracheomalacia

Cuffed tracheostomy tubes developed for use with positive-pressure respirators in a closed system can cause tracheal damage resulting in tracheomalacia and tracheal stenosis. The high pressure of the balloon cuff is respon-

sible for the focal necrosis. Overinflation of the cuff usually is not manifest clinically but is visible radiographically. The size of the balloon should be evaluated in daily radiographs when checking the position of the ETT. The cuff-trachea ratio as measured on the radiograph is a valuable predictor of tracheal damage. Marked tracheal damage is seen in patients who have a cuff-trachea ratio over 1.5 (17) (Fig. 6). In such patients, tracheal damage may be prevented by decreasing cuff pressure and volume, changing the tube or early extubation. However, with the routine use of high-volume, low-pressure cuffs, these complications are rare.

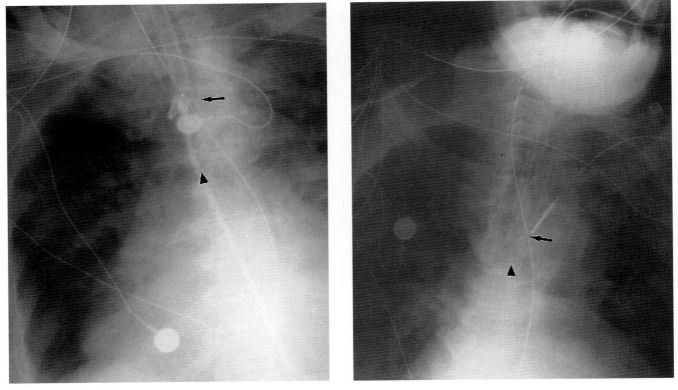

**FIG. 3.** Alteration of endoctracheal tube (ETT) position. **A:** Extension. **B:** Flexion of neck. (*Arrow*, tip of ETT; *arrowhead*, carina.)

### Pleural Drainage Tube

In the bedridden patient, intrapleural air collects beneath the sternum and intrapleural fluid collects posteriorly. The ideal position for the thoracotomy tube is, therefore, anterosuperior for a pneumothorax and posteroinferior for a hydrothorax. When in doubt, a cross-table lateral radiograph will demonstrate the position of the tube relative to air or fluid. After removal of the tube, residual pleural lines often delineate the former tube position. They are not significant but may be confusing.

Following placement of a chest tube, improvement in effusion or pneumothorax should be evident within several hours. Lack of improvement suggests tube malposition. The tube may become malpositioned within the major or minor fissures, intraparenchymally, or within the extrapleural soft tissues. At times, the frontal and cross-table lateral radiographs are inadequate and oblique views or CT are necessary to confirm the tube position. Pleural adhesions, empyema, and bleeding from intercostal vessels may complicate tube insertion and impede drainage of the pleural space. Spleen, liver, and stomach lacerations have been reported by inadvertent passage of the tube through the diaphragm.

Pulmonary complications due to tube thoracotomy include lung laceration (with or without the development of a bronchopleural fistula), unilateral pulmonary edema following rapid removal of fluid or air from pleural space, and rarely infarction of a peripheral segment of lung aspirated into the drainage opening of the tube (18). Iatrogenic Horner's syndrome has been reported as a result of the chest tube lying near the first and second thoracic ganglion (19). An extrathoracic location of the tube should be suspected if both walls of the tube are not visualized in the portions thought to be in the pleural space.

### Nasogastric Tubes

Nasogastric tubes are commonly used for suctioning gastric contents as well as for tube feeding. These tubes should generally terminate within the stomach beyond the cardia. Clinical assessment of nasogastric tube position is usually inadequate, and a radiograph is often necessary for this purpose. The most frequent misplacements are incomplete insertion and tube coiling within the esophagus. Inadvertent nasogastric tube insertion into the tracheobronchial tree may occur in the obtunded

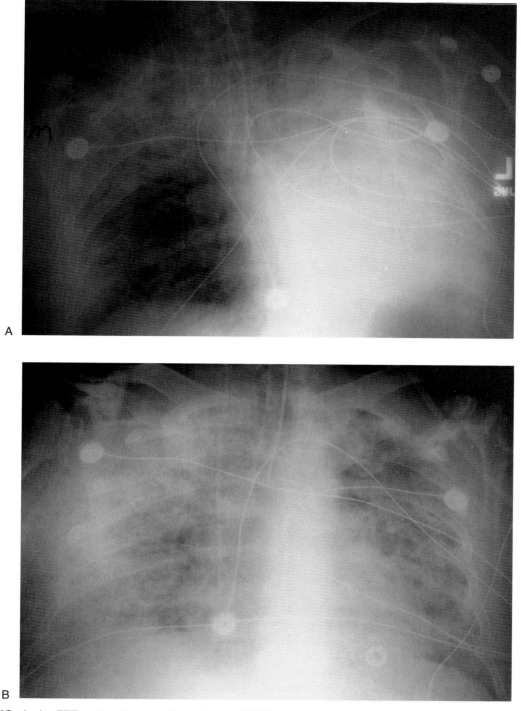

**FIG. 4.** An ETT malposition **A:** Malposition of ETT in right mainstem bronchus with atelectasis of left lung. **B:** Reexpansion of left lung after ETT repositioning.

patient (Fig. 7). The presence of a cuffed ETT does not prevent this misplacement, especially with the currently used high-volume, low-pressure cuff. Transpleural tube passage, resulting in pneumothorax, may also occur (20, 21) (Fig. 8).

Esophageal perforation is a rare, potentially fatal complication of nasogastric tube insertion. Radiographic clues of this complication include the rapid appearance of pleural effusion with the initiation of tube feeding, pneumomediastinum, extraesophageal location of the naso-

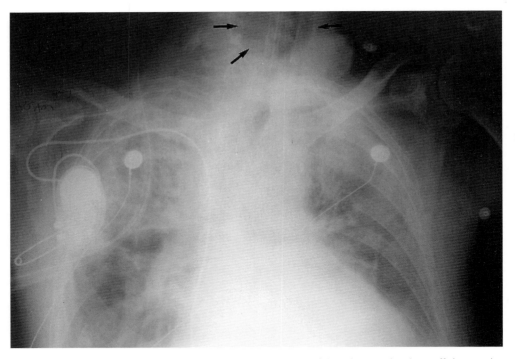

**FIG. 5.** Malposition of ETT in the larynx with distention of the pharynx by the cuff *(arrows).*

gastric tube, mediastinal widening, and mediastinal air-fluid levels. An esophagram with water-soluble contrast medium and thoracic CT are indicated in cases of suspected esophageal rupture.

### Central Venous Pressure Catheters

Central venous pressure (CVP) catheters are most often employed in the setting of hypotension or complicated intravascular volume and pressure states. Central venous catheters provide a means for administration of medications and for hyperalimentation. These catheters are usually inserted into the subclavian or internal jugular vein. In order for the catheter to monitor CVP accurately, it must lie medial to the last valve in the subclavian vein, which is approximately at the level of the first anterior rib. On a chest radiograph, if the catheter extends medial to the anterior first rib, it is safely proximal to the valves (22). The optimal location of the CVP catheter is at the junction of the brachiocephalic veins or within the superior vena cava itself. About one-third of CVP catheters are incorrectly positioned at the time of insertion (22). The most common locations of malposition include placement in the internal jugular vein (Fig. 9), the right atrium or ventricle, or various extrathoracic locations including the upper extremities or the hepatic veins. Less common locations of malpositioned catheters are the azygos, superior intercostal, pericardiophrenic, or internal mammary veins. Complications in these veins include

inaccurate CVP measurement and thrombosis. Although most catheters can be localized on the frontal radiograph, there are occasions when the lateral film is necessary even if it must be obtained with a portable technique. Malposition in the right atrium leads to an increased incidence of cardiac perforations by the catheter. Infusion of fluid through the catheter into the pericardial space can rapidly produce a fatal cardiac tamponade (23). Positioning in the right ventricle often causes cardiac arrhythmias because of irritation of the endocardium. Cannulation of a persistent left superior vena cava has a characteristic appearance on radiographs on the frontal film, and a catheter in this vein resembles one in the internal mammary vein. However, on the lateral film, it is located along the posterior aspect of the heart (Fig. 10). The catheter may extend through the coronary sinus into the right atrium. The persistent left superior vena cava results from failure of the left cardinal vein to obliterate, and the reported incidence varies from 0.3% to 4.4% (18).

### Pneumothorax

The complication most frequently detected by radiologists after CVP insertion is pneumothorax. The incidence of pneumothorax ranges from 1% to 12% depending on the experience and expertise of the individual placing the catheter (24). A chest film (upright, with patient in expiration, if possible) should always be obtained whenever placement of a catheter has been attempted. Since the portable chest radiographs are made in the supine position

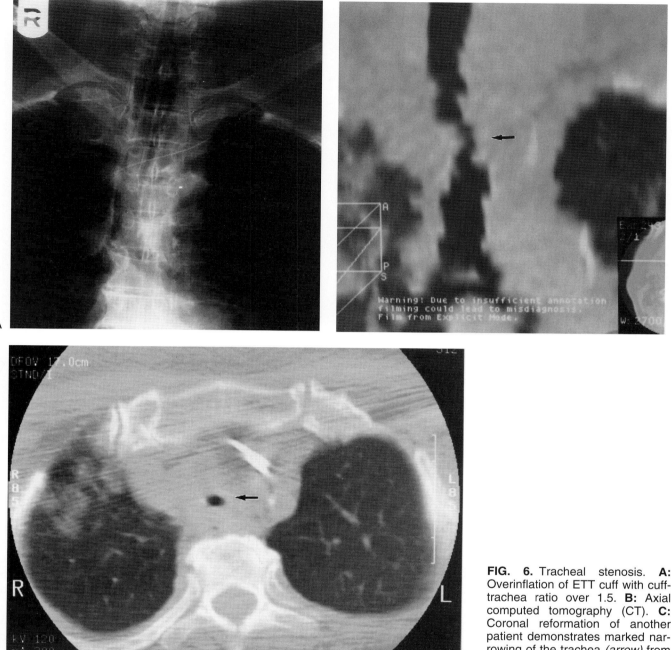

**FIG. 6.** Tracheal stenosis. **A:** Overinflation of ETT cuff with cuff-trachea ratio over 1.5. **B:** Axial computed tomography (CT). **C:** Coronal reformation of another patient demonstrates marked narrowing of the trachea *(arrow)* from previous intubation.

in the majority of cases, the pneumothorax may be difficult to detect. Pneumothorax should be sought in the anteromedial and subpulmonic recesses because these are the nondependent regions in the supine patient (25) (Fig. 28).

### Vascular Injury and Perforation

Another serious complication of intravenous catheter placement is perforation of the superior vena cava with hemorrhage into the mediastinum, and if infusion therapy is started, hydromediastinum can result. A catheter inserted into a vessel must run parallel to the wall of that vessel. A gentle curve at the tip of the catheter suggests that it may lie against the vessel wall, predisposing the vessel to perforation. Sometimes it is also possible for these catheters to perforate into the pleural space, and consequent infusion of solutions can cause severe pain and discomfort (18).

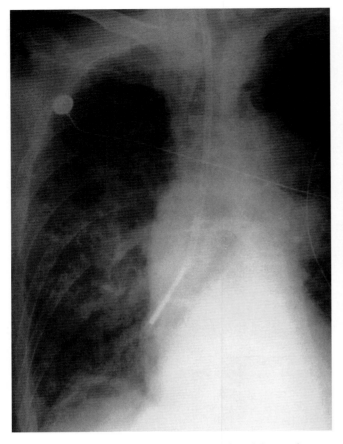

FIG. 7. Malposition of feeding tube in right mainstem bronchus.

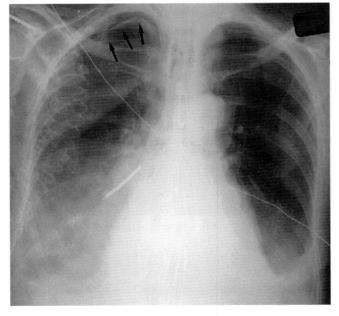

FIG. 8. Transpleural passage of feeding tube resulting in pneumothorax *(arrows)*.

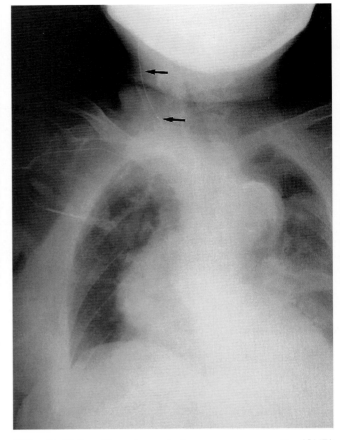

FIG. 9. Malpositioned central venous pressure (CVP) catheter in right internal jugular vein *(arrows)*.

### Thrombosis

The incidence of detectable thrombosis occurring from CVP catheters is 7% to 28% and up to 71% in patients having a catheter in place for more than seven days (26). Roentgen findings of superior vena cava obstruction include enlargement of the cava, pleural effusions, and the presence of dilated collateral vessels, such as the azygos and superior intercostal veins. Dilatation of the left superior intercostal vein is seen as an "aortic nipple" on frontal radiographs (27).

### Infectious Complications

The CVP catheters, particularly those used for long periods of time, may cause infectious complications. The incidence of catheter-related infections such as septicemia, osteomyelitis, septic arthritis, and endocarditis ranges from 8% to 32% (28, 29).

### Catheter Knotting and Fragmentation

A potential serious complication is catheter breakage and embolization. This can result from laceration of the

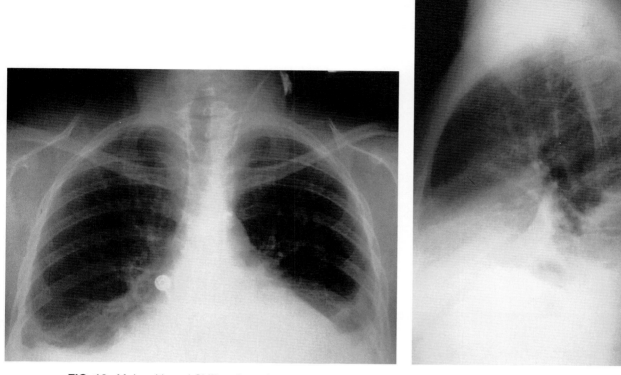

**FIG. 10.** Malpositioned CVP catheter in persistent left superior vena cava. **A:** Frontal film demonstrates catheter adjacent to left side of mediastinum. **B:** Lateral film. The catheter is directed posteriorly.

catheter by the needle used to insert it, fracture at a point of stress, or detachment of the catheter from its hub. Following such an event, the catheter fragments may lodge in the vena cava, in the right side of the heart, or in the pulmonary artery. They may provoke fatal arrhythmias or result in thrombosis, infection, or perforation. Frequently it is possible to retrieve catheter fragments under fluoroscopic control, with the use of specially designed snares (Fig. 11), although on occasion thoracotomy is required. A 71% incidence of fatal complications has been reported with cases of embolized catheters that have not removed (30). Other rare complications of CVP catheters include air embolism, brachial plexus or phrenic, vagus, or recurrent laryngeal nerve injury, injury to thoracic duct, internal mammary, carotid, or ascending cervical artery lacerations, and venobronchial fistula (31–33). All these complications result from improper puncture technique.

### Swan-Ganz Catheters

The Swan-Ganz (SWG) catheter, introduced in 1970, is a balloon-tipped flow-directed catheter used for the accurate management of intravascular volume. The catheter is introduced via the antecubital, jugular, or subclavian vein. Its ideal position is within the left or right

pulmonary artery with the balloon deflated. In order for pulmonary arterial wedge pressure to reflect the left atrial pressure and left ventricular end-diastolic pressure, there must be a continuous column of blood between the catheter tip and the left atrium (34). This only occurs in zone 3 (of West) where both the pulmonary artery and venous pressure exceed alveolar pressure. A catheter placed in zone 1 or 2 will record alveolar pressure, not left atrial pressure (34, 35). In supine patients, zone 3 is in the lower zone. A SWG catheter in the upper or middle lobe must be repositioned in order to give an accurate reading. The tip of the SWG catheter should lie distal to the pulmonary valve, yet proximal enough not to occlude the vessel lumen. A catheter tip distal to either interlobar artery should be repositioned to a more proximal vessel to reduce the probability of thrombosis. A number of complications may occur, of which infarction is the most significant (Fig. 12).

Infarction occurs as a result of occlusion of the pulmonary artery by the catheter itself or as a result of clot formation in or about the catheter. The radiographic patterns of pulmonary infarction are similar to those seen with infarctions from other causes. Most consist of patchy air space infiltrates involving the area of the lung supplied by the pulmonary artery in which the catheter lies. Occasionally, the classical Hampton's hump configuration

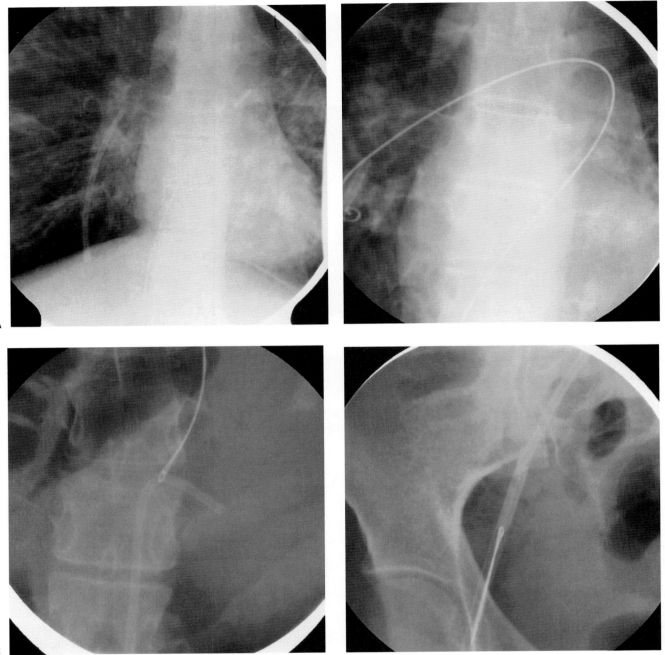

**FIG. 11.** Catheter fragmentation and retrieval. **A:** Catheter fragment in right descending pulmonary artery. **B–D:** Catheter retrieval with the use of specially designed snare catheter.

with a wedge-shaped pleural-based density is identified. Often, however, no radiographic manifestation of infarction is noted (36, 37). If recognized or suspected, the pulmonary infarction is treated by removal of the SWG catheter; systemic heparinization is not required. A rare, potentially fatal complication of catheter malposition is pulmonary artery rupture. Although pulmonary artery rupture may result in minor pulmonary hemorrhage, a 53% mortality rate from this complication has been

reported (38). Other complications of SWG catheters include endocarditis, septic emboli, catheter knotting, and cardiac arrythymias (18).

### Intra-Aortic Counterpulsation Balloon

The intra-aortic counterpulsation ballon (IACB) was first introduced in the 1960s for treatment of cardio-genic shock, and this continues to be a major indication

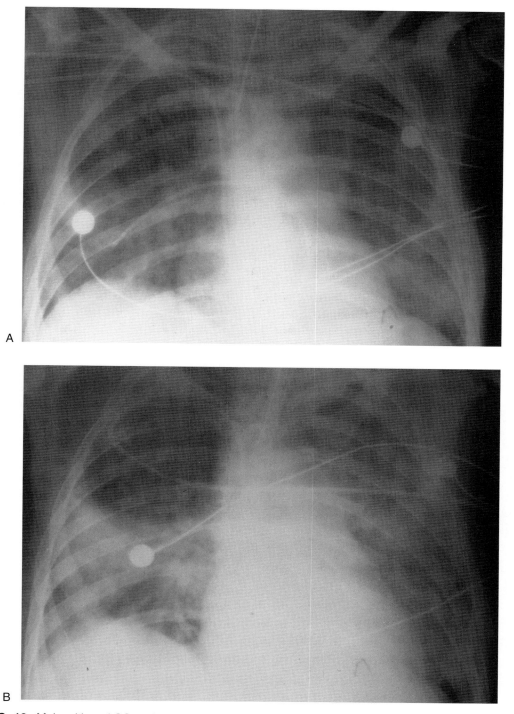

A

B

**FIG. 12.** Malpositioned SG catheter with resultant infarction. **A:** Tip of SG catheter too far in the right lower lobe segmental pulmonary artery. **B:** Infarction in the area supplied by the segmental artery.

for its use. The IACB is a large catheter introduced via the common femoral artery. It is advanced retrograde to the upper descending thoracic aorta. The device consists of a 25-cm-long, fusiform balloon that is inflatable and surrounds the distal end of the catheter. The balloon is inflated by gas to a volume of approximately 40 mL

during diastole and forcibly deflated during systole. The timing of inflation-deflation is gated to the electrocardiogram. The end result is improved oxygen delivery to the myocardium and diminished left ventricular workload, which in turn results in improved cardiac function (39, 40). The ideal position of the IACB is in the proximal aorta, just distal to the left subclavian artery origin (Fig. 13). On the chest radiograph, the tip of the device, therefore, should be at the level of the aortic arch. This position allows maximum augmentation of diastolic pressure in the proximal aorta and decreases the risk of embolization of the cerebral vessels. A number of complications have been noted.

If the catheter is advanced too far, it may enter the left subclavian artery or may lie in the aortic arch and increase the risk of cerebral embolism (Fig. 14). If positioned too distal, it may obstruct the major abdominal vessels.

Aortic dissection may occur at the time of insertion. A history of difficulty in inserting the device or complaints of pain by the patient during the procedure should alert the clinician to this potential complication.

## Transvenous Pacemaker

Pacemakers were introduced in the late 1950s as the method of choice to control and maintain cardiac rhythm in patients with heart block and certain other bradyarrhythmias. The pacemaker electrode is inserted into the internal jugular or subclavian vein and directed

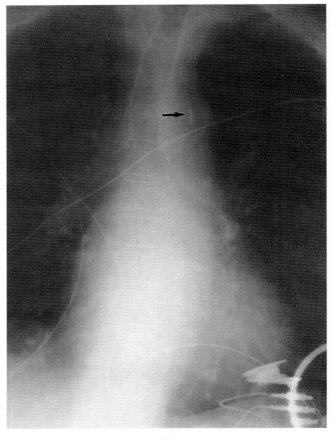

**FIG. 14.** Malposition of IACB in the aortic arch *(arrow).*

to the apex of the right ventricle under fluoroscopic guidance. Ideally, the catheter is positioned in the apex of the right ventricle. Radiographs in both frontal and lateral projections are required to assess positioning completely. On the frontal view, the catheter should project at the apex of the right ventricle, and on the lateral view the tip of the catheter should lie anteriorly 3 to 4 mm posterior to the epicardial fat stripe (41). Potential complications are numerous.

### Aberrant Positioning

The most common abnormality recognized radiographically is malpositioning. Common aberrant locations include the coronary sinus, the right atrium, the pulmonary outflow tract, and the pulmonary artery. Of these, the most difficult to assess radiographically is placement in the coronary sinus. In this location, the catheter appears to be ideally positioned on the frontal projection but is directed posteriorly on the lateral projection. If only a frontal view is available, a clue to ectopic placement in the coronary sinus is an upward deflection of the catheter tip as it follows the sinus around the posterior atrioventricular groove (42).

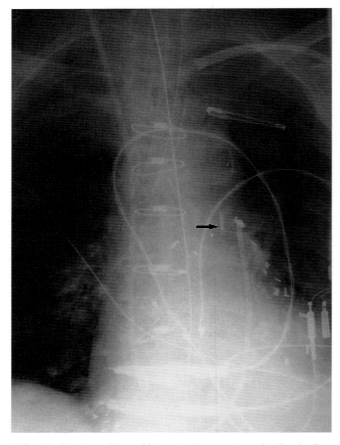

**FIG. 13.** Ideal position of intra-aortic counterpulsation ballon (IACB) in the proximal aorta *(arrow).*

## *Myocardial Perforation*

Another potential complication is perforation of the myocardium by the catheter itself. Perforation usually occurs at the time or within a few days after insertion. Perforation may be difficult to recognize unless the catheter clearly projects outside the myocardium or anterior to the epicardial fat stripe (42). Computed tomography may be helpful in identifying the position of the catheter tip (Fig. 15).

## *Mechanical Problems*

Inadequate pacing may result from fracture of the electrode, detachment of the pacemaker wires from the pulse unit, or battery failure. Whereas detachments can be readily recognized on the chest radiograph, electrode fracture may be more difficult to define because the insulating sheaths can hold the broken ends close enough together to escape detection. Although initial reports outlined radiographic criteria by which battery failure could be determined, in actual practice such techniques are difficult to apply. It is easier to measure the electronic output of the pacer directly in order to determine battery failure (42, 43).

## RADIOLOGY OF ACUTE CARDIOPULMONARY DISEASES

Determining the cause of lung disease in the critically ill is often a frustrating task. Many of the radiographic changes are nonspecific and require careful attention to the time of onset, speed of progression, and distribution of lesions. An ongoing and timely dialogue between the radiologist and the referring physician is vital for optimal interpretations. Among critically ill patients a new pulmonary opacity may reflect aspiration pneumonia, atelectasis, pneumonia, pulmonary edema, the adult respiratory distress syndrome (ARDS), embolism, or any combination of these entities. The most common ones are considered below.

## Aspiration Pneumonia

Aspiration pneumonia is a frequent cause of acute pulmonary disease in the ICU. The clinical and radiographic course depends on the nature and volume of the aspirated material. There are three separate aspiration syndromes (44): (a) aspiration of toxic fluids, (b) aspiration of bland fluids or particles, and (c) aspiration of infected material. Although this division is helpful in understanding the various patterns caused by aspiration, overlap may occur (44, 45).

## *Aspiration of Toxic Fluids*

The most frequently aspirated toxic fluid is gastric juice with a pH of less than 2.5 (Mendelson's syndrome). Within seconds, the aspirated acid crosses both the alveolar epithelium and the capillary endothelium, causing a capillary permeability edema. The typical patient history includes an observed episode of aspiration. Symptoms are present within minutes and radiographic evidence of consolidation is usually present within hours. Consolidation usually progresses for the first 24 hours followed by a brief period of stability. By 48 to 72 hours, there is usually evidence of clearing (46). Depending on the severity of the chemical pneumonitis, total clearing may take a week or two (47). The lung pattern may vary from diffuse interstitial infiltrates to focal dense air space consolidation. Following massive aspiration, the pneumonitis may progress to a full-blown ARDS. In approximately 25% of patients, the chemical pneumonitis is complicated by bacterial infection, and abscess or empyema formation is frequent. Infection usually causes a reversal of the patient's recovery. This is usually evidenced by an area of worsening consolidation 3 to 7 days after injury, at a time when the radiograph should be improving.

Other liquids, such as hydrocarbons, animal fats, alcohol, and water-soluble contrast agents, can also induce chemical pneumonitis.

## *Aspiration of Bland Fluids or Solids*

The aspiration of neutral pH gastric contents, food, blood, water, etc., does not cause a chemical pneumonitis. Transient respiratory distress is either due to volume of aspirated fluid or due to bronchospasm caused by the foreign substance (44). The lungs may be normal or show evidence of some consolidation due to flooding. If consolidation is present, it rapidly disappears following coughing, suctioning, or positive-pressure therapy. Particles or clots may cause areas of atelectasis or focal hyperinflation. In general, with prompt removal of the obstructing material, the lung returns to normal rapidly.

## *Aspiration of Infected Material*

Infected secretions may be aspirated from the sinuses, the pharynx, or the tracheobronchial tree. Aspiration of pathogenic bacteria is usually unobserved, but it may be suspected when a patient at risk for aspiration shows signs of fever, purulent sputum, and opacities in dependent areas of the lungs. In a supine patient, the opacities typically appear in the posterior segments of the upper lobe or the superior segments of lower lobe. The radiographic appearance of pneumonia due to aspirated infected secretions may vary from a focal indolent basilar

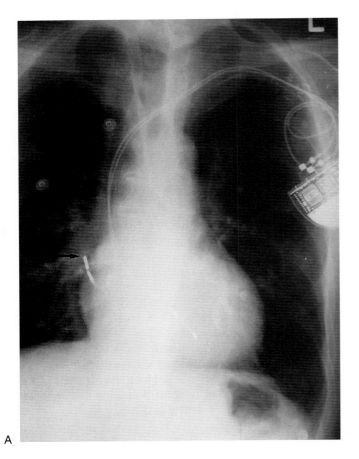

A

**FIG. 15.** Myocardial perforation. **A:** PA chest shows catheter tip *(arrow)* projecting beyond the right-sided heart border. **B:** CT scan shows catheter tip in pleural space adjacent to right atrium *(arrow)* and presence of pneumothorax. The catheter was withdrawn into right atrium without complication.

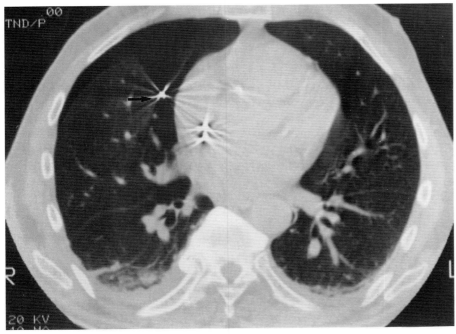

B

consolidation, abscess, or empyema to rapidly progressive bilateral symmetrical consolidations, often mimicking pulmonary edema in both its distribution and its rapidity of appearance (Fig. 16). This diffuse pattern is most frequently associated with *Pseudomonas* and other anaerobic organisms (6).

### Atelectasis

The most frequent chest radiographic abnormality in the ICU is atelectasis. It may vary from linear, subsegmental atelectasis to lobar collapse. Atelectasis of an entire lung may also occur (Fig. 17). Atelectasis usually appears rapidly and may change from film to film, especially following physical therapy. Various factors, sometimes multiple in a given case and the most common being hypoventilation or secretions, lead to atelectasis in a critically ill patient. The radiographic appearance of atelectasis varies markedly from that of clear lungs to one of total opacification and volume loss. The most direct evidence of volume loss is displacement of an interlobar fissure. Other signs of atelectasis are crowding of vessels and bronchi in the involved area, elevation of the ipsilateral diaphragm, ipsilateral shift of the mediastinum, and hyperinflation of the remainder of the lung. The presence or absence of air bronchograms may indicate the cause of atelectasis, the approximate site of obstruction, and appropriate therapy. Presence of air bronchograms within a segmental or lobar atelectasis strongly suggests that the etiology is not an endobronchial obstruction, e.g., mucus

plug, clot, tumor. Conversely, absence of the air bronchogram in an area of atelectasis suggests endobronchial obstruction and is an indication for tracheobronchial suctioning or bronchoscopy (6, 48). Atelectasis is most frequent and most severe at the lung bases, especially the left-lung base (49). In the supine bedridden patient, the heart may press on the left lower lobe bronchus, impeding drainage. In addition, blind suctioning of the left lower lobe bronchus is more difficult than that of the right lower lobe bronchus (50). The radiographic diagnosis of left lower lobe atelectasis may be difficult through the cardiac silhouette. Suggestive signs of left lower lobe atelectasis are presence of a triangular density in the retrocardiac area with its apex at the hilum and base along the medial aspect of the left hemidiaphragm which is obscured, downward displacement of the left hilum, and elevation of the left hemidiaphragm (Fig. 18).

### Pneumonia

Hospital-acquired or nosocomial pneumonia is an infection that appears beyond the third day of hospitalization. Infection occurs in about 10% of all ICU patients and in about 30% to 60% of patients with ARDS (6). *Staphylococcus* and aerobic gram-negative bacilli are most frequent. Polymicrobial infection is very common. Pneumonia is not easy to diagnose in ICU patients. The hallmarks of pneumonia such as fever, pathogens in the sputum, altered white blood cell count, and x-ray evidence of consolidation may be present for multiple other reasons and

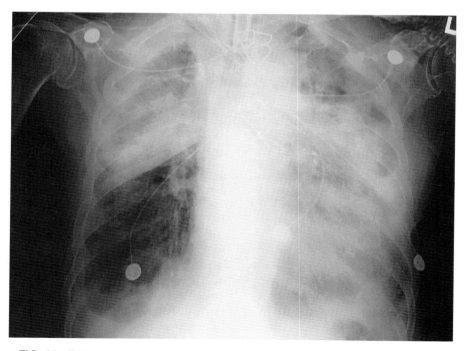

**FIG. 16.** Bilateral *Pseudomonas* pneumonia due to aspirated infected secretions.

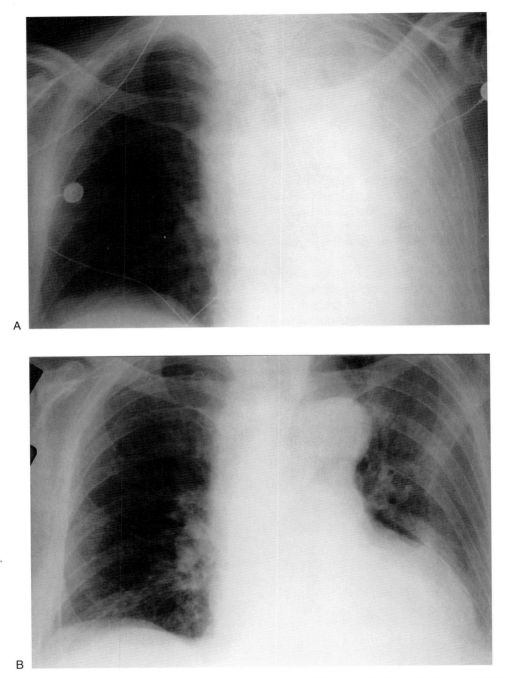

**FIG. 17.** Atelectasis secondary to mucus plug. **A:** Acute left-lung atelectasis. **B:** Reexpansion of left lung after removal of a large mucus plug by bronchoscopy.

lead to the inappropriate diagnosis of pneumonia. Parenchymal consolidation in ICU patients is commonly due to noninfectious causes such a atelectasis, aspiration pneumonitis, pulmonary edema, or infarction. Roentgenographic clues to the presence of pneumonia include the following: air space opacities that contain air bronchograms with segmental or lobar involvement, asymmetric localized areas of consolidation, ipsilateral pleural effusions, and absence of volume loss. New areas of pulmonary opacity or existing ones that become worse may also raise the question of pneumonia. Specifically, areas that are focal, multifocal, and asymmetric are suspect. Although signs on chest films may be suggestive of pneumonia, they are not necessarily conclusive in ICU patients receiving mechanical ventilation. The diagnostic accuracy of the chest film is only 52% (51) because of the high rate of

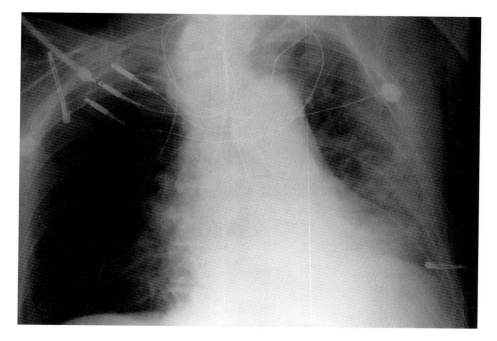

FIG. 18. Left lower lobe atelectasis, typical signs on portable chest radiograph (PCR).

false-negative and false-positive interpretations. False-negative interpretations occur in cases of ARDS with superimposed pneumonia while false-positive ones are secondary to noninfectious disorders like atelectasis, pulmonary hemorrhage, infarction, and asymmetric edema which can mimic focal patterns of pneumonia (51, 52). The abnormal chest film must be considered in context with other clinical criteria, including fever, leukocytosis, and change in respiratory symptoms. Fiberoptic bronchoscopy may be indicated to help select appropriate antibiotic therapy. Pleural effusions associated with nosocomial infections may lead to empyema or bronchopleural fistula. On portable radiography, it may be difficult to differentiate pulmonary consolidation or abscess from loculated pleural effusion or empyema. Computed tomography is helpful in both diagnosing the underlying condition and planning therapy (8) (Figs. 19, 20).

## PULMONARY EDEMA

Pulmonary edema is a common cause of acute respiratory failure in critically ill patients. Pulmonary edema, or the accumulation of extravascular lung water, may be due to either increased hydrostatic pressure, known as cardiac pulmonary edema (CPE), or increased permeability of capillary wall, known as noncardiac pulmonary edema (NCPE). In some instances, both etiologies may coexist. Cardiogenic pulmonary edema is characterized by an increase in extravascular lung water due solely to an abnormally elevated hydrostatic pressure, the latter mea-

sured clinically as the pulmonary capillary wedge pressure (PCWP) or left atrial pressure. An elevated hydrostatic pressure results from left ventricular failure or intravascular volume overload. Cardiac pulmonary edema usually has two distinct stages. The first, which is characterized by interstitial edema, leads to dilated lymphatic vessels, widened alveolar septa, engorged perivascular and peribronchial spaces, and thickening of interlobular septa (septal or Kerley lines). A chest radiograph at this time may show perihilar and perivascular haziness, peribronchial cuffing, increased arterial-bronchial ratio, and presence of septal lines (Fig. 21A). The second stage, alveolar edema, causes alveolar flooding. Chest radiography at this time may show a central alveolar pattern of edema with air bronchograms (53) (Fig. 21B).

Noncardiac pulmonary edema is a catastrophic and frequently unanticipated complication of acute illness. The extravascular lung water in NCPE originates from an acute injury to the capillary membrane which separates the vascular compartment from the pulmonary interstitium and alveoli. A variety of clinical conditions, including diffuse lung infection and traumatic or septic shock, are associated with damage to the capillary membrane. In addition, endothelial damage can result from circulating inhaled toxins or aspiration of gastric contents. In contrast to CPE, NCPE fills the alveoli rapidly. Therefore, roentgenographic signs of interstitial edema are usually absent (54).

To optimally treat acutely ill patients with pulmonary edema, it is important to differentiate CPE from NCPE. Chest radiography is the most commonly used noninvasive technique for assessing pulmonary edema in critically ill

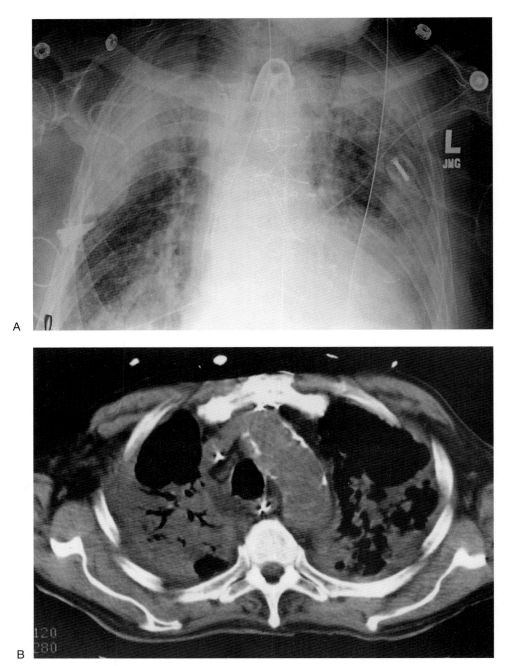

**FIG. 19.** Consolidation vs. empyema. **A:** Chest radiograph demonstrates right upper lung opacity believed to be loculated fluid. **B:** CT scan shows presence of consolidation with air bronchograms without loculated fluid.

patients. An accurate diagnosis of CPE is possible in 87% of patients using radiographic criteria (55–57). Cardiac pulmonary edema is characterized by a central distribution of pulmonary edema (Fig. 21), peribronchial cuffing, septal lines, air bronchograms, pleural effusions, and cardiomegaly. An accurate diagnosis of NCPE is possible in only 60% of patients. The single most discriminating criterion is a patchy peripheral distribution of pulmonary edema

(Fig. 22). Peribronchial cuffing, septal lines, air bronchogram, and pleural effusions are notably absent in NCPE.

The presence of existing pulmonary disease and concomitant therapy will influence the radiographic estimation of edema severity. For example, the presence of pulmonary emphysema or pulmonary embolism will underestimate the severity of edema. Positive end-expiratory pressure (PEEP) increases lung volume and gives a

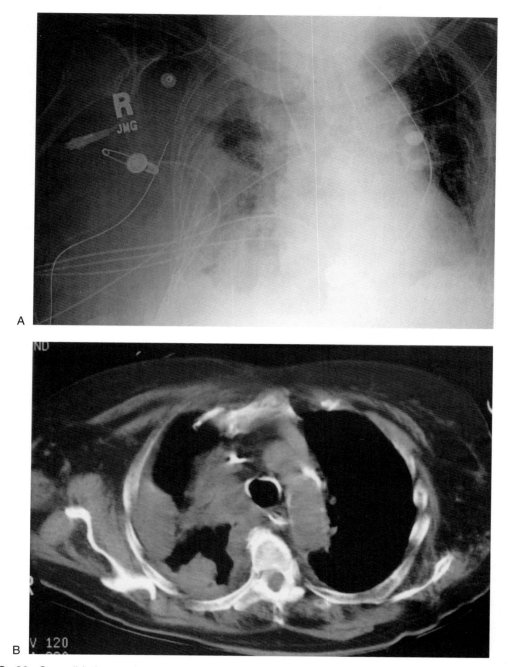

**FIG. 20.** Consolidation and empyema vs. neoplasm. **A:** Chest radiograph shows right pleural and parenchymal opacity believed to be consolidation and loculated pleural effusion. **B:** CT scan shows right upper lobe neoplasm and pleural metastases.

false impression of improvement on the radiograph (58) (Fig. 23). The chest radiograph needs to be interpreted with respect to the clinical data.

## Adult Respiratory Distress Syndrome

Adult respiratory distress syndrome is a clinical situation characterized by a profound increase in pulmonary capillary permeability accompanied by progressive arterial hypoxia and reduced lung compliance. Adult respiratory distress syndrome is a common response of the lung to a variety of insults; e.g., sepsis, aspiration of gastric contents, ingestion of poisons, inhalation of noxious gases, near drowning, and massive trauma. As it progresses, ARDS manifests a variety of clinical and radiographic changes which are nonspecific (6, 54, 59–61).

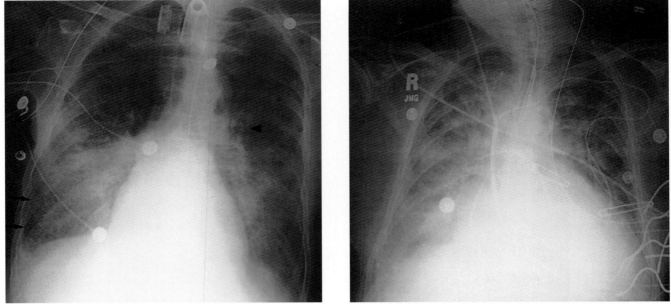

A                                                                                          B

**FIG. 21.** Cardiogenic pulmonary edema. **A:** Interstitial pulmonary edema with peribronchial cuffing *(arrowhead)*, thickening of interlobular septa *(arrows)*, and perihilar and perivascular haziness. **B:** Alveolar pulmonary edema, with bilateral pleural effusions and cardiomegaly.

**STAGE I.** The chest film remains normal for the first 12 to 24 hours after the onset of respiratory distress. Thus, in this stage, radiologic diagnosis lags behind clinical diagnosis. Any pulmonary opacities that do occur usually reflect an inciting event or condition, such as aspiration into the dependent areas of the lungs, pulmonary contusion, or pneumonia. Lung volumes are often slightly diminished.

**STAGE II.** This stage usually begins at day 2 and ends at day 5. Fluid leakage produces pulmonary consolidation, which is the radiographic hallmark of this stage of ARDS (Fig. 22). Patchy zones of alveolar opacity yield to uniform consolidation at a rate dependent on type and severity of lung injury. Although the alveolar opacities appear uniformly distributed on chest films, CT of the chest may show gravitationally dependent densities, which result, in

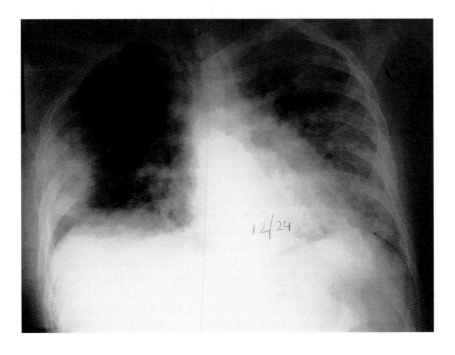

**FIG. 22.** Noncardiogenic pulmonary edema. Adult respiratory distress syndrome (ARDS) with bilateral patchy and peripheral infiltrates.

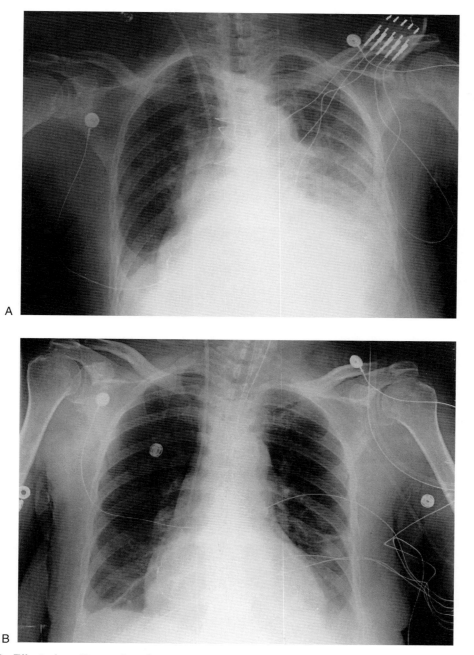

**FIG. 23.** Effect of positive end-expiratory pressure (PEEP) on PCR. **A:** Chest x-ray (CXR) shows bilateral interstitial pulmonary edema and effusions. **B:** Same day, after intubation and PEEP, there is an increase in lung volume giving a false impression of improvement.

part, from compression atelectasis caused by increased pulmonary weight (62, 63). Air bronchograms may be prominent as airway pressures increase. The heart size remains normal. The presence of pleural effusion should raise the question of superimposed cardiac edema, pulmonary infarction, or complicating pulmonary infection.

**STAGE III.** After 5 days, consolidation becomes less dense and more ground glass in appearance. The high

pressures required for ventilation may cause barotrauma, which is a major complication of late ARDS.

Barotrauma is most likely to occur in areas of lung necrosis, that is, in sites damaged by pulmonary infarction and infection.

Evidence of barotrauma, including interstitial emphysema, subpleural air cysts, pneumomediastinum, subcutaneous emphysema, pneumothorax, and even pneumoperitoneum, may be visible on the chest film (Fig. 24).

The radiographic findings of the post-ARDS chest have been described and include findings which vary from the completely normal to evidence of pneumatoceles, interstitial "infiltrates," reduced lung volumes, and increased lung volumes (64). The diagnostic accuracy of portable chest radiography for ARDS is 89%, compared to 52% for pneumonia, probably reflecting the well-defined radiographic appearance of this disorder (51).

## ABNORMAL AIR AND FLUID COLLECTIONS

Iatrogenic trauma to the thorax may be caused by several procedures: barotrauma from positive-pressure ventilation or trauma after placement of catheters, tubes, pacemaker electrodes, or counterpulsation balloons (65).

### Barotrauma

Barotrauma is defined as damage that results from increased intra-alveolar pressure causing air leaks in

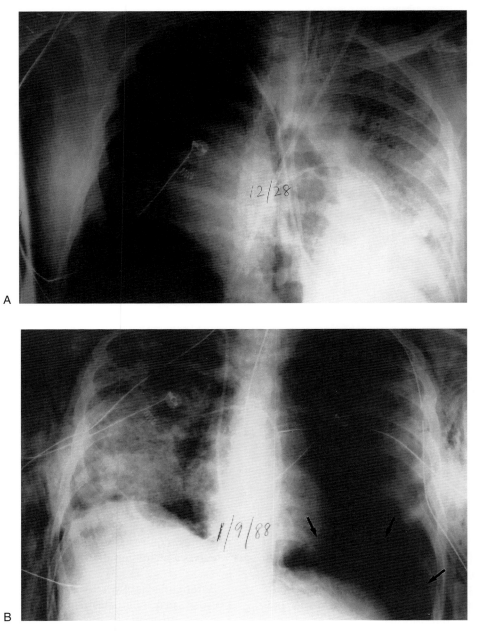

**FIG. 24.** ARDS with barotrauma. **A:** Tension pneumothorax with mediastinal shift. **B:** Subcutaneous emphysema and pneumoperitoneum *(arrows)*.

the connective tissue of the lung, mediastinum, and subcutaneous tissues (66). The incidence of barotrauma has increased greatly with more aggressive management of the critically ill patient. Barotrauma is a frequent and potentially lethal problem in the ICU. Positive-pressure therapy, closed-chest massage, and subclavian vein catheterization are the most frequently implicated procedures. While the reason for sudden deterioration of the patients' condition may not be apparent at the bedside, the portable supine radiograph offers necessary information concerning the location and severity of abnormal air collections. Knowledge of the subtle and early radiographic findings of extra-alveolar air and prompt communication with the attending medical staff minimize the deleterious effect that extra-alveolar air has on the critically ill. The incidence of barotrauma in patients receiving mechanical ventilation is 5% to 15% (6).

### Interstitial Emphysema

Following rupture of the alveoli, air dissects along the interstitial tissues and appears radiographically as irregular radiolucent mottling and linear shadows likened to a "disorganized" air bronchogram. These do not decrease in caliber or branch in the peripheral lung zones, differentiating them from air bronchograms. A pathognomonic but rare sign is the visualization of a radiolucent "halo" of air around a pulmonary vessel seen on end (67) (Fig. 25). The interstitial air may accumulate in the loose connective tissue beneath the pleura and present as round or oval subpleural air cysts on radiographs. Rupture of these cysts may lead to pneumomediastinum and pneumothorax (67). Interstitial pulmonary emphysema characteristically changes rapidly; frequently it appears and disappears within several hours. When it persists for several days, it often proves to be irreversible (67). At times, interstitial pulmonary emphysema may be difficult to distinguish from consolidation in a lung with previously existing emphysema. However, most cases of interstitial pulmonary emphysema are seen in younger age groups, and it is characteristically more extensive in the central and lower portions of the lungs—unlike emphysema, which is most severe in the upper lobes (68).

### Pneumomediastinum

Pneumomediastinum is often the first radiographic sign of existing pulmonary interstitial emphysema, which has dissected medially to the hilar regions. Thirty-eight percent of patients with pulmonary interstitial emphysema in Woodring's study (69) developed pneumomediastinum, while pneumothorax occurred in

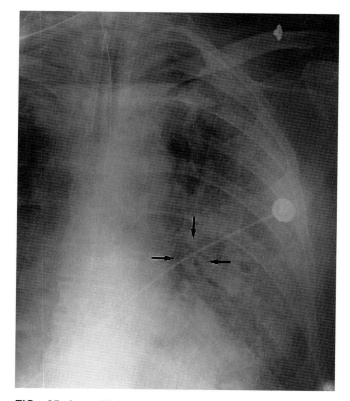

FIG. 25. Interstitial pulmonary emphysema. Chest radiograph shows "disorganized" air bronchograms and pathognomonic radiolucent halo sign (arrows).

77% of patients. Other than barotrauma, etiologies include perforation of the esophagus, trachea or bronchus, blunt chest trauma, labor, and diabetic ketoacidosis (70). Radiographic signs of pneumomediastinum include a thin, sharp, radiolucent line around the heart and mediastinum with a pleural reflection delineating it laterally (Fig. 26). A similar appearance may be produced by a "kinetic halo," a radiolucency seen around the heart border, caused either by the milking action of structures in motion against the lung or by the "Mach" effect (71). This halo can be differentiated from pneumomediastinum by the absence of sharp lateral borders produced by displaced visceral and parietal pleura. A crescent of air outlining the aortic arch may be present. Air may dissect between parietal pleura and diaphragm, outlining the undersurface of the heart and crossing the midline. The latter sign can also be present in pneumopericardium but not pneumothorax (72). Decubitus radiographs are often of benefit to delineate the location of the air. On lateral radiographs, a sharp radiolucent line outlining the ascending aorta, the great vessels, thymus, and prevertebral soft tissues may be seen. Because the mediastinum is continuous with the retroperitoneum, a posterior pneumomediastinum can outline the crura of the diaphragm and extend to cause a

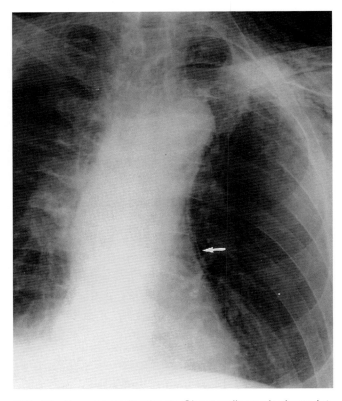

**FIG. 26.** Pneumomediastinum. Chest radiograph shows lateral displacement of the pleura along the left side of mediastinum *(arrow)*.

pneumoretroperitoneum. This is one route of extra-alveolar air into the peritoneum in patients with barotrauma. Pneumothoraces often follow a pneumomediastinum, but the reverse is not seen.

### Pneumothorax

Pneumothorax is common in patients who require high pressures to maintain satisfactory oxygenation and is a major cause of morbidity and mortality. Incidence rates as high as 25% have been reported (73). Pneumothorax can also be a complication of invasive procedures, such as central venous catheterization, endotracheal intubation, and feeding tube placement. Air may reach the pleural space following pneumomediastinum or may enter directly into the pleural space from rupture of the alveoli or pneumatocele (6). Pneumothorax may be especially difficult to detect in patients who are supine. The radiographic diagnosis of pneumothorax in the supine patient requires a detailed knowledge of the anatomy of the pleural recesses and mediastinal structures (74) and an understanding of the forces governing the movement of pleural air, that is, gravity and lung compliance (75). The radiographic hallmark of pneu-

mothorax is displacement of the visceral pleura from the parietal pleura by air within the pleural space. The visceral pleura appears as a thin, white line outlined by air in the pleural surface on one side and air in the lung on the other side (Fig. 8). This radiodense visceral pleural line helps in differentiating pneumothorax from other conditions which may mimic it, e.g., emphysematous bullae or skin folds (Fig. 27). If the patient is radiographed in the supine position, the typical appearance of pneumothorax is altered. Pleural air in the supine position collects anteriorly and may not be seen on the radiograph or may mimic pneumomediastinum or pneumopericardium. In a study of 88 ICU patients, the distribution of the pneumothorax in the supine radiograph was mainly in the anteromedial and subpulmonic location, and apicolateral pneumothorax was relatively uncommon (74). Pleural air in the anterior costophrenic sulcus produces hyperlucency over the upper abdominal quadrants and the deep costophrenic sulcus sign (75–78) (Fig. 28). When in doubt, a lateral decubitus film with the side in question elevated will show air between the lung and ribs. If the patient cannot be moved, horizontal cross-table lateral radiographs will show increased retrosternal radiolucency and may show air in the sternodiaphragmatic angle. All pneumothoraces detected on supine radiograph should be promptly evaluated because the size of pneumothorax in the ICU patient correlates poorly with its clinical significance.

Tension pneumothorax should be diagnosed clinically and treated immediately. If not discovered until the chest has been radiographed, diagnosis is late and the condition is even more urgent. The radiograph usu-

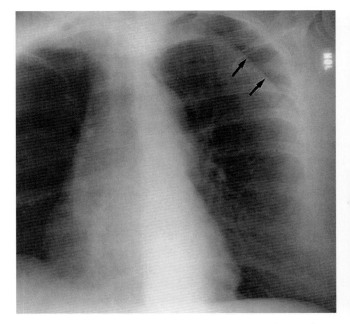

**FIG. 27.** Skin fold mimicking pneumothorax *(arrows)*.

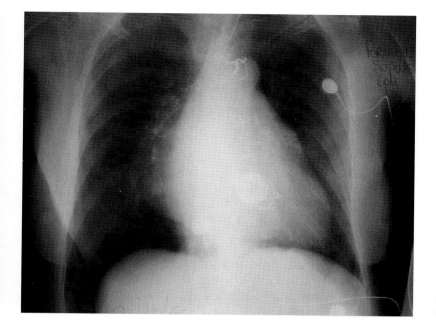

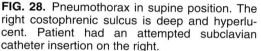

**FIG. 28.** Pneumothorax in supine position. The right costophrenic sulcus is deep and hyperlucent. Patient had an attempted subclavian catheter insertion on the right.

ally shows total collapse of lung with shift of the mediastinum to the contralateral side (Fig. 24A). Additional findings of a flat or inverted hemidiaphragm confirm the diagnosis (68). Patients with stiff lungs frequently have tension pneumothorax without complete collapse of the lung. This is because of the rigidity of the lung itself and also because frequent adhesions may fix the lung to the chest wall.

### Pneumopericardium

Pneumopericardium is a rare complication of positive-pressure ventilation and usually occurs in infants. Diagnosis rests on demonstrating air around the entire circumference of the heart outlined by the parietal pericardium (Fig. 29); air along the left, right, or inferior border of the heart is usually due to pneumomediastinum or anteromedial pneumothorax (79). Lateral views may be helpful in patients in whom sagittal views are not diagnostic. On the upright radiograph the air extends to surround the pulmonary artery and proximal ascending aorta but does not extend above this level in the absence of tamponade. Pneumopericardium does not always cause ill effects, but if the pericardial air is under tension, rapid and fatal cardiac tamponade may occur.

### Subcutaneous Emphysema

From the mediastinum, air can travel along fascial planes into subcutaneous tissues of the neck and chest wall as well as the abdominal wall (6). The presence of subcutaneous emphysema in patients receiving mechanical ventilation is often the first radiographic sign of extra-alveolar air. Air in the soft tissues of the neck in the absence of pneumomediastinum signifies possible injury to the upper airway during intubation or during blind attempts at placement of the feeding tube (80). Although it presents a dramatic clinical picture, subcutaneous emphysema is a benign event that resolves as pneumomediastinum and pneumothorax improve. The progressive increase in subcutaneous air indicates the presence of bronchopleural fistula or a malfunctioning chest tube. Radiographically, subcutaneous emphysema appears as sharply etched linear radiolucencies that parallel the tissue planes or as multiple lucent bubbles in the soft tissues. Individual muscle masses or muscle slips are often visible (Fig. 24B). Extensive air in the soft tissues of the chest may mimic or obscure pulmonary parenchymal disease. Computed tomography of the chest can add important information regarding the presence of pneumothorax and parenchymal disease in patients with severe subcutaneous emphysema, particularly in cases of blunt chest trauma (81).

### Pleural Effusion

Pleural effusions, common in critically ill patients, arise from a variety of causes. These include congestive heart failure, renal disease, pneumonia, and therapeutic interventions. However, pleural fluid on the supine radiograph may not be readily detected. In the supine position the most dependent pleural spaces are the apex of the hemithorax and the posterior basilar space (82). Fluid in

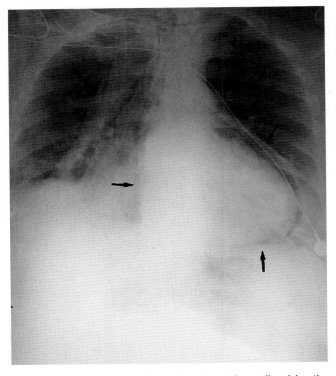

**FIG. 29.** Pneumopericardium. The heart is outlined by the air separated from the lung by parietal pericardium *(arrows)*.

these locations may be difficult to detect. In an analysis of 34 radiographs, 12 of 36 effusions present in decubitus films could not be identified on corresponding supine radiograph (83). The presence of fluid in the posterior basilar pleural space is first reflected by a homogeneous increase in density of lower hemithorax, without obliteration of the normal bronchovascular markings, in the absence of radiographic signs of parenchymal disease or collapse (84). Blunting of the costophrenic angle, decreased visibility of the lower lobe vessels behind the density of the diaphragm, loss of diaphragmatic contour, and apparent elevation of the diaphragm are helpful radiographic signs of pleural effusion in the upright radiograph. In the supine radiograph, however, the difficulty in detecting pleural effusion is not only due to the position of the patient but also due to multiple technical factors including poor centering, rotation, underpenetration, respiratory motion, and poor inspiration. A careful analysis of the radiographic findings and detection of fluid in other locations such as the paraspinal location, fissures, and apex of hemithorax increase the predictive value of initial observation (6).

Several bedside techniques to confirm or rule out the presence of pleural effusion are available. Decubitus radiographs can be obtained. Whenever possible, bilateral decubitus radiographs are obtained to rule out an unsuspected effusion on the opposite side. If decubitus

radiographs cannot be obtained, supine and erect radiographs may be obtained demonstrating a generalized increased density on the supine film that disappears when the patient sits erect (Fig. 30). A supine oblique radiograph may also demonstrate fluid between the lung and the lateral chest wall (6).

Ultrasonography can readily detect free effusions and can locate loculated collections. Ultrasonographically guided thoracentesis greatly increases the chance of a successful tap and has one-sixth of the pneumothorax rate of nonguided aspirations (85). Computed tomography is very accurate in evaluation of the presence, extent, and loculations of pleural fluid and can be helpful in differentiating empyema from pneumonia (Fig. 19).

## AORTIC DISSECTION

Aortic dissection is a life-threatening emergency in which prompt diagnosis and treatment directly influence patient survival (86). Approximately 2,000 cases of acute aortic dissection are estimated to occur in the United States each year (87). Untreated aortic dissection leads to death in 20% of patients within 1 day, 62% within 1 week, 74% within 2 weeks, and more than 90% of patients within 3 months of diagnosis (88). More than 95% of patients have chest pain, which can be anterior or posterior (89). Hypertension, the most common predisposing condition, is present in 90% of patients. Other factors include cystic medial necrosis, coarctation, congenital aortic stenosis, bicuspid aortic valve, and pregnancy (89). Iatrogenic injury, secondary to thoracic surgery or cannulation for aortic bypass, can also lead to aortic dissection (90).

Aortic dissection usually begins as a tear in the intima. The tear allows blood to enter the aortic wall, separating the layers of the media. This separation results in a true lumen that is distinguishable from the false lumen on the basis of an intimal flap.

DeBakey (91) classified aortic dissection into three types, based on the site of the intimal tear and the extent of the false channel. DeBakey type I dissection involves the ascending aorta, arch, and descending aorta. Type II dissections involve only the ascending aorta, and type III dissections involve only the descending aorta distal to the origin of the left subclavian artery. Daily (92) proposed a simpler classification (also known as the Stanford Classification) whereby type A dissection involves the ascending aorta and type B dissection is limited to the descending aorta. DeBakey type I and II dissections or type A dissections are considered surgical emergencies because they may dissect proximally to cause pericardial effusion and tamponade, acute aortic insufficiency, or acute myocardial infarction. The optimal care of patients with aortic dissection requires that the diagnosis be made promptly and that its site of ori-

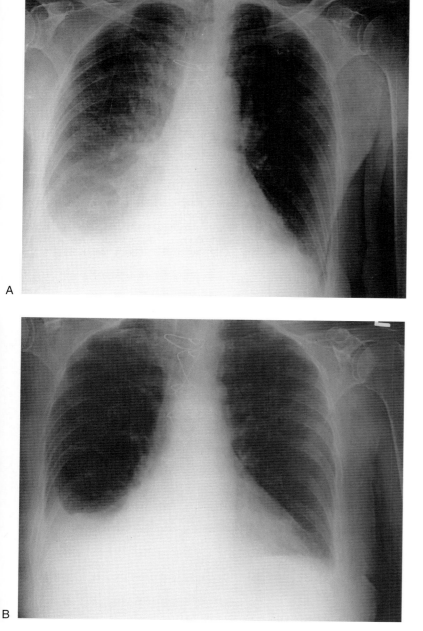

A

B

**FIG. 30.** Pleural effusion movement in supine and upright position. **A:** Supine radiograph shows increased density of the right lower hemithorax and normal bronchovascular markings. **B:** Upright radiograph. The fluid has gravitated inferiorly with disappearance of hazy density.

gin and extent be identified as rapidly as possible. The diagnostic information sought in patients with aortic dissection includes confirming the presence of dissection, involvement of the ascending aorta, extent of dissection, sites of entry and reentry, thrombus in the false lumen, branch-vessel involvement, aortic insufficiency, pericardial effusion, and coronary artery involvement (93). Plain chest radiographs are often nonspecific in the diagnosis of aortic dissection. Mediastinal widening is the most common abnormality encountered. Displacement of intimal calcification of more than 6 mm may be helpful in suggesting the diagnosis (94) (Fig.

31). Other findings include disparity in size between ascending and descending aorta, indistinct aortic contour, double aortic knob, or localized aneurysm formation. Displacement of mediastinal structures or pleural effusion may also occur (95). Occasionally the chest radiograph may be entirely normal (89).

There are four imaging techniques available at the present time for evaluation of patients with suspected aortic dissection, namely, aortography, CT, MRI, and echocardiography (particularly by a transesophageal approach). None of these diagnostic procedures are ideal for all patients, and deciding which to choose for a given patient

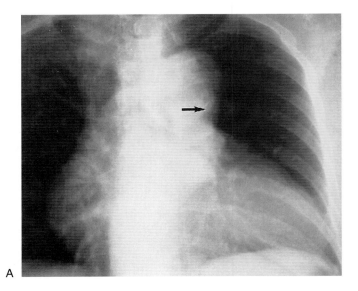

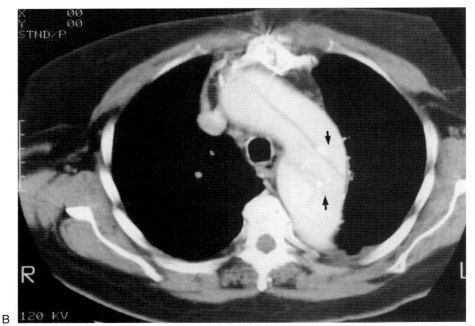

**FIG. 31.** Displacement of intimal calcification. **A:** Chest radiograph shows medial displacement of intimal calcification *(arrow)*. **B:** Contrast-enhanced CT scan at level of aortic arch confirms displacement of intimal calcification *(arrows)* and shows the intimal flap as a radiolucent linear density.

requires an understanding of the accuracy and limitation of each technique.

Aortography is an accurate technique for evaluating patients with aortic dissection (96). Angiographic findings can be divided into direct and indirect signs of aortic dissection. The direct signs, which are considered diagnostic, include visualization of a double lumen separated by an intimal flap (Fig. 32). The indirect signs, which are considered suggestive of dissection, include a thickening of the aortic wall greater than 5 mm, ulcerlike projections, compression of the true lumen by the false lumen, aortic insufficiency, occlusion of branch vessels, and the abnormal position of the catheter (97).

Aortography has a sensitivity of 88% and a specificity of 94% for the identification of aortic dissection (98). False-negative angiograms may occur in cases of thrombosis of the false channel, equal and simultaneous opacification of both the true and false lumens when the intimal flap is not tangential to the x-ray beam and is therefore not visualized (99). False-positive results may be caused by layering of contrast material within the aorta, thickening of the aortic wall, or branch occlusions from other preexisting conditions (97). Angiography is invasive and not without complications. At present, angiography is reserved for patients who have indeterminate findings on other imaging modalities.

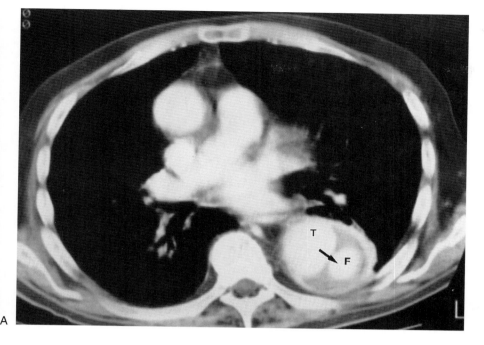

A

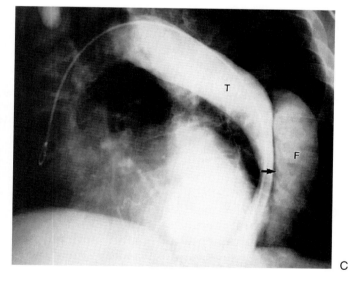

**FIG. 32.** Type B aortic dissection (T, true lumen; F, false lumen). **A:** Contrast-enhanced CT scan at level of midascending aorta shows an intimal flap *(arrow)* separating the true and false lumen in the descending aorta. The ascending aorta is normal. **B:** Aortogram early phase. The descending aorta is narrowed *(arrow)*. The ascending aorta is normal. **C:** Aortogram late phase. There is opacification of false lumen which is separated from true lumen by the intima *(arrow)*.

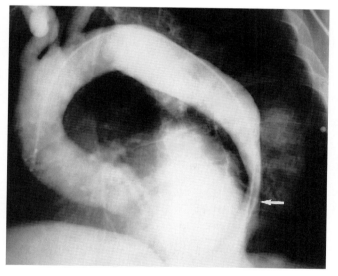

B

C

Currently, in many institutions, CT is the diagnostic method of choice in evaluation of patients with suspected aortic dissection (6). A number of investigators evaluating the effectiveness of contrast-enhanced CT scanning in the diagnosis of aortic dissection have demonstrated a sensitivity of 83% to 100% and a specificity of 90% to 100% (98, 100). In evaluating patients with suspected aortic dissection, the CT technique is extremely important. A single-level dynamic scan series is obtained at the level of aortic arch, midascending aorta, and aortic root. The diagnosis of aortic dissection is made if two contrast-filled channels separated by intimal flap are identified within the aorta. The true lumen opacifies with the contrast earlier than the false lumen

when observed on the single-level dynamic scan series (Fig. 33). Other nonspecific findings in aortic dissection include aortic widening, medial displacement of peripheral intimal calcifications (Fig. 31), spiraling of the false lumen around true lumen as it proceeds distally down the aorta, and extra-aortic fluid collections in the mediastinum, pericardium, and pleural spaces. Pericardial effusions are found in approximately 50% of patients with type A dissection (101).

There are, however, some limitations of CT in the evaluation of the aortic dissection. Computed tomography does not depict the site of the intimal tear, the presence of aortic insufficiency, involvement of the coronary arteries, or branch vessel occlusion.

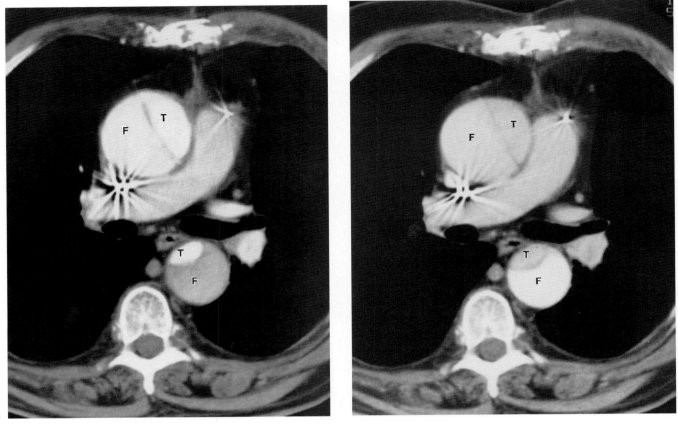

**FIG. 33.** Type A aortic dissection. Single-level dynamic CT scan at level of midascending aorta (T, true lumen; F, false lumen). **A:** Early phase. **B:** Late phase. Opacification of true and false lumen separated by intimal flap involving both the ascending and descending aorta. The true lumen opacifies earlier than the false lumen.

Magnetic resonance imaging has been shown to be an effective imaging method of evaluating patients with aortic dissection. It is noninvasive and does not require contrast media. Furthermore, MRI can provide high-quality images in the transverse, coronal, sagittal, and oblique planes of the aorta, which facilitates the diagnosis of dissection, provides better definition of its location and extent, and may reveal involvement of arch vessels (102). With the use of spin-echo imaging, a standard MRI technique for evaluating anatomic abnormalities, rapidly flowing blood produces no intraluminal signal and appears as a signal void, whereas slowly moving blood produces an increased intraluminal signal (99, 103). The criterion used to diagnose an aortic dissection by MRI is, as with contrast CT, the presence of the intimal flap seen as a linear structure of medium signal intensity between a signal void of flowing blood in the true and false channels (Fig. 34). Other nonspecific findings in aortic dissection include widening of the aorta, thickening of the aortic wall, thrombosis of the false lumen, or spiraling of a thrombosed false lumen (104, 105). The sensitivity and specificity of MRI in evaluat-

ing patients with aortic dissection are 96% and 90%, respectively (102, 104).

A thrombosed false lumen and slow flow are the main problems in differentiating dissection from a thrombosed aneurysm. Cine-MRI is one of the more recent advances and is designed to study dynamic cardiac function. This technique rapidly supplies images that are referenced to a simultaneously recorded electrocardiogram and then used to simulate real-time cardiac imaging. Cine-MRI can identify aortic regurgitation with a sensitivity of 85% (105).

Although MRI seems to be a reliable screening procedure, a major limitation is its inability to study the hemodynamically unstable patient requiring life support equipment. The MRI may provide some information about the presence of arch vessel involvement, but the imaging of these vessels is poorer in quality than that obtained with aortography (99). The MRI does not reliably provide information about the involvement of the coronary arteries (106).

Transesophageal echocardiography (TEE) and transthoracic ultrasonography (TTUS) are noninvasive modal-

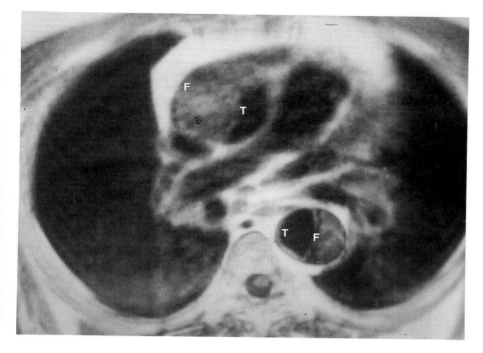

**FIG. 34.** Type A aortic dissection. Axial T1-weighted magnetic resonance image at the level of midascending aorta shows intimal flap separating true and false lumen. The difference in luminal signal intensity is caused by differences in blood flow between true and false lumen (T, true lumen; F, false lumen).

ities that provide both physiologic color flow information and anatomic detail (93). Tranesophageal echocardiography is superior to TTUS, although it is not as readily available, is more costly, and requires patient sedation and intubation. Approximately 90% to 95% of the thoracic aorta is seen regularly by TEE (107). It accurately detects aortic regurgitation and may evaluate the coronary ostia and possible hemopericardium (107). Tranesophageal echocardiography can be readily performed in the emergency room, in the coronary care unit, during resuscitation efforts, and even intraoperatively to assess the repair while the patient is still on bypass. It is generally superior to TTUS with sensitivity/specificity for detection of aortic dissection of 85% to 95%/68% to 90% versus 59% to 85%/63% to 96% for TTUS, respectively (105, 107–109).

The echocardiographic criteria of aortic dissection are aortic dilatation in excess of 42 mm and detection of an intimal flap, combined with high-frequency oscillation of this structure (6). Two-dimensional echocardiography combined with Doppler can detect differential flow in the true and false channels, determine the site of intimal tear, and detect the presence or absence of aortic insufficiency (110). Transesophageal echocardiography is contraindicated in patients with known esophageal disease, including varices, strictures, and tumors and may not be tolerated in up to 3% of patients (98).

Selecting a method of imaging in suspected acute aortic dissection depends on the clinical condition of the patient, the diagnostic information needed, the accuracy of the diagnostic information obtained, and the availability, length of time, safety, and cost of the study. In some institutions, TEE is the preferred method of choice because of its accuracy, safety, speed, and convenience. Although MRI may be less practical than TEE for evaluation of patients with suspected aortic dissection, it is nonetheless very well suited for patients with stable or chronic dissections. In many community hospitals, CT is the diagnostic method of choice in the evaluation of patients with suspected dissection, with a sensitivity and specificity comparable to TEE and MRI. Aortography, an accurate technique for evaluating patients with aortic dissection, should be reserved for patients who have indeterminate noninvasive imaging techniques. In the final analysis, each institution determines its own best method of approaching the diagnosis of aortic dissection on the basis of available human and material resources.

## REFERENCES

1. Bekemeyer WB, Crapo RO, Calhoon S, et al. Efficacy of chest radiography in a respiratory intensive care unit—a prospective study. *Chest* 1985;88:691.
2. Greenbaum DM, Marschall KE. The value of routine daily chest x-rays in intubated patients in the medical intensive care unit. *Crit Care Med* 1982;10:29.
3. Henshke CL, Pasternack GS, Schroeder S, et al. Bedside chest radiography: diagnostic efficacy. *Radiology* 1983;149:23.
4. Janower ML, Jennas-Nocera Z, Makai J. Utility of portable chest radiographs. *AJR* 1984;142:265.
5. Strain DS, Kinasewitz GT, Vereen LE, George RB. Value of routine daily chest x-rays in the medical intensive care unit. *Crit Care Med* 1985;13:534.
6. Goodman LR, Putnam CE. *Critical care radiology,* 3rd ed. Philadelphia: Saunders; 1992.
7. Mirvis SE, Tobin KD, Kostrubiak I, Belzberg H. Thoracic CT in

detecting occult disease in critically ill patients. *AJR* 1987;148:685.

8. O'Moore PV, Mueller PR, Simeone FJ, et al. Sonographic guidance in diagnostic and therapeutic interventions in the pleural space. *AJR* 1987;149:1.

9. Aberle DR, Hansell D, Huang HK. Current status of digital projectional radiography of the chest. *J Thorac Imag* 1990;5(1):10.

10. Fraser RG, Sanders C, Barnes GT, et al. Digital imaging of the chest. *Radiology* 1989;171:297.

11. Maguire WM, Herman PG, Khan A, Simon-Gabor M, Cruz V, Eacobacci T. Interobserver agreement using computed radiography in the adult intensive care unit. *Acad Radiol* 1994;1:10.

12. Baker SR, Stein HD. Radiologic consultation: its application to an acute care surgical ward. *AJR* 1986;147:637.

13. Conrady PA, Goodman LR, Lainge F, Singer M. Alteration of endotracheal tube position: flexion and extension of neck. *Crit Care Med* 1976;4:8.

14. Goodman LR, Conrady PA, Lainge F, et al. Radiologic evaluation of endotracheal tube position. *AJR* 1976;127:433.

15. Zwillick CV, Pierson DJ, Creagh CE, et al. Complications of assisted ventilation: a prospective study of 354 consecutive episodes. *Am J Med* 1974;57:161.

16. Rollins RJ, Tocino I. Early radiographic signs of tracheal rupture. *AJR* 1987;148:695.

17. Khan F, Reddy N, Khan A. Cuff-trachea ratio as an indicator of tracheal damage. *Chest* 1976;70:431(abst).

18. Wechsler RJ, Steiner RM, Kinori I. Monitoring the monitors: the radiology of thoracic catheters, wires and tubes. *Semin Roentgenol* 1988;23:61.

19. Fleishman JA, Bullock JD, Rosset JS, Beck RN. Iatrogenic Horner's syndromes secondary to chest tube thoracostomy. *J Clin Neurol Ophthalmol* 1983;3:205.

20. Woodall BH, Winfield DF, Bisset III GS. Inadvertent tracheobronchial placement of feeding tubes. Radiology 1987;165:727.

21. Stark P. Inadvertent nasogastric tube insertion into tracheobronchial tree. *Radiology* 1982;142:239.

22. Langston CS. The aberrant central venous catheter and its complications. *Radiology* 1971;100:55.

23. Kline IK, Hoffman WI. Cardiac tamponade from CVP catheter perforation. *JAMA* 1968;206:1794.

24. Giuffrida DJ, Bryan-Brown CW, Lumb PD, et al. Central vs peripheral venous catheters in critically ill patients. *Chest* 1986;90:806.

25. Touno IM, Miller MH, Fairfax WR. Distribution of pneumothorax in the supine and semirecumbent critically ill adult. *AJR* 1985;144:901.

26. Lazarush M, Lowder JN, Herzig RH. Occlusion and infection in broviac catheters during intensive cancer therapy. *Cancer* 1983;52:2342.

27. Carter MM, Tarr RW, Carter MM, et al. The "aortic nipple" as a sign of impending superior vena caval syndrome. *Chest* 1985:775.

28. Mitchell SE, Clark RA. Complications of central venous catheterization. *AJR* 1979;133:467.

29. Jacobs MB, Yeager M. Thrombotic and infectious complications of Hickman-Brovial catheters. *Arch Intern Med* 1984;144:1597.

30. Fisher RG, Ferreyro R. Evaluation of current techniques for non surgical removal of intravascular iatrogenic foreign bodies. *AJR* 1978;130:541.

31. Ryan JA, Abel RM, Abbott WM, et al. Catheter complications in total parenteral nutrition. *N Engl J Med* 1974;290:757.

32. Flanagan JP, Gradisar IA, Gross RJ, et al. Air embolus-a lethal complication of subclavian venipuncture. *N Engl J Med* 1969;281:488.

33. Epstein EJ, Quereshi MSA, Wright JS. Diaphragmatic paralysis after supraclavicular puncture of subclavian vein. *Br Med J* 1976;1:693.

34. Henry DA, LeBolt S. Invasive hemodynamic monitoring: radiologist's perspective. *Radiographics* 1986;6:535.

35. Kubicka RA, Smith C. A primer on the pulmonary vasculature. *Med Radiogr Photogr* 1985;61:14.

36. McCloud TC, Putman CE. Radiology of the Swan-Ganz catheter and associated pulmonary complications. *Radiology* 1975;116:19.

37. Ravin CE, Putman CE, McCloud TC. Hazards of the ICU. *AJR* 1976;128:915.

38. Kelly TF, Morris GC, Crawford ES, et al. Perforation of the pulmonary artery with Swan-Ganz catheters: diagnosis and surgical management. *Ann Surg* 1981;193:686.

39. Hyson EA, Ravin CE, Kelly MJ, Curtis AM. Intraaortic counter pulsation balloon: radiographic considerations. *AJR* 1977;128:915.

40. Pasternack G, O'Cain CF. Thoracic complications of respiratory intensive care. In: Herman PG, ed. *Iatrogenic thoracic complications.* New York: Springer-Verlag; 1983.

41. Ormond RS, Rubenfire M, Anbe DT, et al. Radiographic demonstration of myocardial perforation by permanent endocardial pacemakers. *Radiology* 1971;98:35.

42. Hall WM, Rosenbaum HB. The radiology of cardiac pacemakers. *Radiol Clin North Am* 1971;9:343.

43. McHenry MM, Grayson CE. Roentgen diagnosis of pacemaker failure. *AJR* 1970;109:94.

44. Bartlett JG, Gorbach SL. The triple threat of aspiration pneumonia. *Chest* 1975;68:560.

45. Wynne JW. Aspiration pneumonitis: correlation of experimental models with clinical disease. *Clin Chest Med* 1982;3:25.

46. Landay MJ, Christensen EE, Bynum LJ. Pulmonary manifestations of acute aspiration of gastric contents. *AJR* 1978;131:587.

47. Bynum LJ, Pierce AK. Pulmonary aspiration of gastric contents. *Am Rev Respir Dis* 1976;114:1129.

48. Marini JJ, Pierson DJ, Hudson LD. Acute lobar atelectasis: a prospective comparison of fiberoptic bronchoscopy and respiratory therapy. *Am Rev Respir Dis* 1979;149:971.

49. Shevland J, Hirleman MT, Huang KA, Kealey GP. Lobar collapse in the surgical intensive care unit. *Br J Radiol* 1983;56:531.

50. Friedman AP, Goodman LR. Suctioning of left bronchial tree in the intubated adult. *Crit Care Med* 1982;10:43.

51. Winer-Muram HT, Rubin SA, Ellis JV, Jennings SG, et al. Pneumonia and ARDS in patients receiving mechanical ventilation: dianostic accuracy of chest radiography. *Radiology* 1993;188:479.

52. Ruiz-Santana S, Jimenez AG, Esteban A, et al. ICU pneumonia: a multi-institutional study. *Crit Care Med* 1987;15:930.

53. Milne ENC, Pistolesi M, Miniati M, et al. The radiologic distinction of cardiogenic and non-cardiogenic edema. *AJR* 1985;144:879.

54. Chiles C, Putman CE. Techniques for interpreting pulmonary opacities in ICU. *J Crit Illness* 1994;9:198.

55. Aberle DR, Wiener-kronish JP, Webb WR, et al. Hydrostatic versus increased permeability edema: diagnosis based on radiographic criteria in critically ill patients. *Radiology* 1988;168:73.

56. Smith RC, Mann H, Greenspan RH, et al. Radiographic differentiation between different etiologies of pulmonary edema. *Invest Radiol* 1987;22:859.

57. Sibbald WJ, Cunningham DR, Chin DN. Non-cardiac or cardiac pulmonary edema? A practical approach to clinical differentiation in critically ill patients. *Chest* 1983;84:452.

58. Zimmerman JE, Goodman LR, Shahvari MBG. Effect of mechanical ventilation and positive end-expiratory pressure (PEEP) on chest radiograph. *AJR* 1979;133:811.

59. Iannuzi M, Petty TL. The diagnosis, pathogenesis and treatment of adult respiratory distress syndrome. *J Thorac Imaging* 1986;1:1.

60. Green R. Adult respiratory distress syndrome: acute alveolar damage. *Radiology* 1987;163:57.

61. Aberle DR, Brown K. Radiologic considerations in the adult respiratory distress syndrome. *Clin Chest Med* 1990;11:737.

62. Gattinoni L, Presenti A, Torrisin S, et al. Adult respiratory distress syndrome profiles by computed tomography. *J Thorac Imaging* 1986; 1:25.

63. Zapol WM. Understanding images: correlation between computerized tomographic scans of lung structure with impaired function in ARDS. *Anesthesiology* 1988;69:812.

64. Elliott CG. Pulmonary sequelae in survivors of the adult respiratory distress syndrome. *Clin Chest Med* 1990;11:789.

65. Khan A, Noma S, Herman PG. Iatrogenic diseases of the lung. *Postgrad Radiol* 1990;10:219.

66. Ovenfors CO. Iatrogenic trauma to thorax. *J Thorac Imaging* 1987;2:18.

67. Westcott JL, Cole SR. Interstitial pulmonary emphysema in children and adults. Roentgenographic features. *Radiology* 1974;111:367.

68. Westcott JL, Cole SR. Barotrauma in iatrogenic thoracic complications. In: Herman PG, ed. *Iatrogenic Thoracic Complications.* New York; Springer-Verlag; 1974:79.

69. Woodring JH. Pulmonary interstitial emphysema in the adult respiratory distress syndrome. *Crit Care Med* 1985;13:199.

70. Cylark D, Milne ENC, Imray TJ. Pneumomediastinum: a diagnostic problem. *Crit Rev Diag Imaging* 1984;23:75.

71. Lane EF, Proto AV, Philips TW. Mach bands and density perception. *Radiology* 1976;121:9.
72. Levin B. The continuous diaphragm sign. *Clin Radiol* 1973;24:337.
73. Greene R, McLoud TC, Stark P. Pneumothorax. *Semin Roentgenol* 1977;12:313.
74. Tocina IM, Miller MH, Fairfax WR. Distribution of pneumothorax in supine and semirecumbent critically ill adult. *AJR* 1985;144:901.
75. Lams PM, Jolles H. The effect of lobar collapse on the distribution of free intrapleural air. *Radiology* 1982;142:309.
76. Rhea JT, Van Sonnenberg E, McCloud TC. Basilar pneumothorax in the supine adult. *Radiology* 1979;133:593.
77. Gordon R. The deep sulcus sign. *Radiology* 1980;136:25.
78. Ziter FM, Westcott JL. Supine subpulmonary pneumothorax. *AJR* 1981;137:699.
79. Varano LA, Maisels MJ. Pneumopericardium in the newborn: diagnosis and pathogenesis. *Pediatrics* 1974;53:941.
80. Woodall BH, Winfield DF, Bisset GS. Inadvertent tracheobronchial placement of feeding tubes. *Radiology* 1987;165:727.
81. Tocino I, Miller MH. Computed tomography in blunt chest trauma. *J Thorac Imaging* 1987;2:45.
82. Raasch BN, Carsky EW, Lane EJ, et al. Pleural effusion; explanation of some typical appearances. *AJR* 1982;139:899.
83. Ruskin JA, Gurney JW, Thorsen MK, et al. Detection of pleural effusion on supine chest radiographs. *AJR* 1987;148:681.
84. Woodring JH. Recognition of pleural effusion on supine radiographs: How much fluid is required? *AJR* 1984;142:59.
85. Raptopoulos V, Davis LM, Lee G, et al. Factors affecting the development of pneumothorax associated with thoracentesis. *AJR* 1991;156:917.
86. Sorenson HR, Olsen H. Ruptured and dissecting aneurysms of the aorta: incidence and prospects of surgery. *Acta Chir Scand* 1964;128:644.
87. Anagnostopoulos CE, Prabhakar MJ, Kittle CF. Aortic dissection and dissecting aneurysms. *Am J Cardiol* 1972;30:263.
88. Hirst AE Jr, Johns VJ Jr, Kime SW Jr. Dissecting aneurysm of the aorta: a review of 505 cases. *Medicine* 1958;37:217.
89. Slater EE, DeSanctis RW. The clinical recognition of dissecting aortic aneurysm. *Am J Med* 1976;60:623.
90. Thorsen MK, Goodman LR, Sagel SS, Olinger GN. Ascending aorta complications of cardiac surgery: CT evaluation. *J Comput Assist Tomogr* 1986;10:219.
91. DeBakey ME, Henly WS, Cooley DA, et al. Surgical management of dissecting aneurysms of the aorta. *J Thorac Cardiovasc Surg* 1965;49:130.
92. Daily PO, Trueblood HW, Stinson EB, Wuerflein RD. Management of acute aortic dissections. *Am Thorac Surg* 1970;10:234.
93. Cigarroa JE, Isselbacher EM, De Santis RW, Eagle KA. Diagnostic imaging in the evaluation of suspected aortic dissection. *New Engl J Med* 1993;328:35.
94. Eyler WR, Clark MD. Dissecting aneurysms of the aorta: roentgen manifestations including a comparison with other types of aneurysms. *Radiology* 1965;85:1046.
95. Smith DC, Jang GC. *Radiologic diagnosis of aortic dissection.* New York: McGraw-Hill; 1983.
96. Stein HL, Steinberg I. Selective aortography, definitive technique for diagnosis of dissecting aneurysm of the aorta. *AJR* 1968;102:333.
97. Hayashi K, Meaney TF, Zelch JV, Tarar R. Aortographic analysis of aortic dissection. *AJR* 1974;122:769.
98. Erbel R, Engberding R, Daniel W, et al. Echocardiography in diagnosis of aortic dissection. *Lancet* 1989;1:457.
99. Petasnick JP. Radiologic evaluation of aortic dissection. *Radiology* 1991;180:297.
100. Vasile N, Mathieu D, Keita K, Lellouche D, Bloch G, Cachera JP. Computed tomography of thoracic aortic dissection: accuracy and pitfalls. *J Comput Assist Tomogr* 1986;10:211.
101. Thorsen MK, Dan Dretto MA, Lawson TL, Foley WD. Dissecting aortic aneurysms: accuracy of computed tomographic diagnosis. *Radiology* 1983;148:773.
102. Geisinger MA, Risius B, O'Donnell JA, et al. Thoracic aortic dissections: magnetic resonance imaging. *Radiology* 1985;155:407.
103. Goldman AP, Kotler MN, Scanlon MH, Ostrum BJ, Parameswaran R, Parry WR. Magnetic resonance imaging and two-dimensional echocardiography: alternative approach to aortograph in diagnosis of aortic dissecting aneurysm. *Am J Med* 1980;80:1225.
104. Kerstig-Sommerhoff BA, Higgins CB, White RD, et al. Aortic dissection: sensitivity and specificity of MR imaging. *Radiology* 1988;164:687.
105. Nienaber CA, Spielmann RP, von Kodolitsch Y, et al. Diagnosis of thoracic aortic dissection: magnetic resonance imaging versus transesophageal echocardiography. *Circulation* 1992;85:434.
106. Paulin S, von Schulthess GK, Fossel E, Krayenbuehl HP. MR imaging of the aortic root and proximal coronary arteries. *AJR* 1987;148:665.
107. Ballal RS, Nanda NC, Gatewood R, et al. Usefulness of transesophageal echocardiography in assessment of aortic dissection. *Circulation* 1991;84:1903.
108. Nienaber CA, von Kodolitsch Y, Nicolas V, et al. The diagnosis of thoracic aortic dissection by non-invasive procedures. *N Engl J Med* 1993;328:1.
109. Adachi H, Omoto R, Kyo S, et al. Emergency surgical intervention of acute aortic dissection with rapid diagnosis by transesophageal echocardiography. *Circulation* 1991;84(Suppl III):14.
110. Illiceto S, Nanda NC. Rizzon petal. Color doppler evaluation of aortic dissection. *Circulation* 1987;75:748.

*The Critically Ill Cardiac Patient,*
edited by V. Kvetan and D. R. Dantzker,
Lippincott-Raven Publishers, Philadelphia © 1996.

# CHAPTER 21

# Severity Scoring for the Cardiovascular Patient

Daniel Teres and Jay S. Steingrub

Severity scoring and outcomes assessment will play an increasingly important role in the evaluation of hospitalized patients. General intensive care unit (ICU) severity scores have paved the way for the development of stable, robust, statistically sophisticated models for a heterogeneous patient mix and are widely discussed for aggregate patient application such as comparison of one ICU to another as well as for individual patient bedside clinical decision making. Although still in its infancy, similar approaches are being applied to cardiovascular patients who have highly visible, technical, and costly procedures and are under intense public scrutiny in our new era of cost containment and health care reform.

In this chapter, we will review the general issues related to the development and potential application of severity scoring and probability estimates and we will describe the reasons that these models should be applied with caution for individual patients or for political or economic reasons.

## GENERAL ISSUES ABOUT SEVERITY MEASURES

There has been a long understanding that the overall crude mortality rate for any disease process or therapeutic intervention is insufficient by itself when applied for global quality-of-care comparisons. While approaches to risk assessment and associated comorbid conditions are well understood medical concepts, case-mix adjustment, use of large administrative databases, and sophisticated mathematically derived multiple logistic regression models are less well understood. Since we are now in a new medical arena which can be described under the general heading of managed competition, physicians and hospitals are under close scrutiny by the public, the business community, government, and third-party payors. We will need to become familiar with issues related to case-mix adjustment, statistical models, and outcomes assessment as they bear directly on highly political issues such as third party-contract negotiations, economic credentialing, and cost reduction. There is no doubt that severity systems will be used. Is there sufficient understanding of the technical factors related to the quality of the data being collected, who inputs the data, who checks the data collector, and what safeguards are there so that the scoring system is not "gamed" by the players? What about confidentiality of the patient? Is there concern about due process for the physician or hospital ranked as a negative outlier?

There are also statistical concepts that must be understood when probability theory is applied as a quality-of-care measure or as a prognostic adjunct to bedside clinical decision making (1). For quality-of-care and cost-effectiveness comparisons, the appropriate term to be applied to such a probability is that it provides an *estimation* of the outcome for that *group* of patients. The term *prediction* is what is imposed by use of an arbitrary cutpoint from a probability model as it may apply for an individual patient (2).

General severity measures relate to hospital mortality. There may be other important endpoints. The direction in prediction models for coronary patients has been to predict the likelihood that a patient with chest pain has a myocardial infarction. For cardiac surgery patients, the outcome is postoperative hospital mortality. There should be skepticism when the same unmodified general models are utilized to predict length of ICU stay, nurse or resource utilization, or post–cardiac surgery infection complication.

A cardiologist or cardiac surgeon is quite comfortable discussing options with a patient who has chest pain and a possible myocardial infarction or a patient being considered for coronary artery bypass graft (CABG) surgery. Prognosis and risk factors are spelled out both in general terms and based on specific factors for that individual patient. However, if two validated models are applied to the same patient to generate a probability of hospital mor-

D. Teres and J. S. Steingrub: Baystate Medical Center and Tufts University School of Medicine, Springfield, Massachusetts 01199.

tality, it is quite likely that the prediction for that individual patient may be different from each other (3, 4).

There also should be a clear understanding that for an outcome measure to be clinically useful for quality comparisons, the relevant variables should be collected early in the course of the illness (prior to the procedure), rather than throughout the patient's hospital course and before complications that occur during the procedure (4). There may be subtle differences in retrospective data collection by quality assurance nurses or record room personnel versus prospective or concurrent data entered directly by the cardiologist or cardiac surgeon team, including bedside cardic surgery nurses. For cardiac surgery the outcome measure is considered vital status at hospital discharge rather than the traditional 30-day postoperative mortality since many patients go home and may have other medically related critical illnesses not directly attributable to the cardiac surgery. Medicare is interested in 90-day mortality because they are interested in related medical illnesses. There may be some valid distinction between *preoperative risk assessment* and immediate *postoperative severity adjustment*.

It should also be recognized that cardiac surgery models apply to patients who undergo the procedure. There should not be any inference as to whether the procedure was appropriate or not. Appropriate guidelines are quite different and include a clinical as well as a policy dimension. For example, as a society do we want to promote having complicated coronary artery bypass and cardiac valve procedures universally available for the elderly. There is no doubt that clinical series have demonstrated that elderly patients may do well following coronary artery bypass surgery (5). These studies include the clinical caveat that the patients have been carefully selected and presumably represent the "healthy elderly." However, there obviously is an incremental "cost" for wider application of a high-technology procedure to "all" elderly patients. Appropriate guidelines may require complex cost-benefit analyses or the input of broad-based consensus panels. Risk assessment studies based on current patient outcomes may be a part of the evaluation process. Probability modeling, with the endpoint of hospital mortality, however, is limited in such analyses. The next generation of severity models will be looking at estimating morbidity, and ultimately the equation will incorporate the more comprehensive term *quality-adjusted life years*.

## GENERAL SEVERITY SCORES

General ICU severity scores include the APACHE system (Acute Physiology and Chronic Health Evaluation) (6), the Mortality Probability Model (MPM II) (7), the Simplified Acute Physiology Score (SAPS II) (8), and the Pediatric model (PRISM) (9). All four systems are now considered stable or robust models for estimating hospital mortality for heterogeneous groups of general medical/surgical ICU patients after collecting relevant variables at admission or within the first 24 hours. The Therapeutic Intervention Scoring System (TISS) is a technique for estimating resource consumption of general medical/surgical ICU patients and is based on scoring of nursing and medical procedures done during the first 24 hours after ICU admission (10). The general trauma scores are used for registry purposes and have not been applied as prediction instruments (11). There are no widely accepted statistical models for measuring nursing assignments.

The general medical/surgical ICU severity models have been developed on patients of age greater than 18, with *exclusion* of burn, *cardiac surgery*, and *coronary care* unit patients. The general methodology for the physiology-based systems is to collect a score with an increasing numerical value for deviation from normal. The score is summed and the higher the score, the higher the general reflection of physiologic instability and, therefore, mortality. There are no direct assumptions related to resource consumption, nurse assignment, or length of ICU or hospital stay. The worst variable or most extreme deviation from normal is recorded during the first 24 hours. In the early models the worst variable could have included values several hours prior to ICU admission (12). At the end of 24 hours, the severity score is totaled (13).

It has been pointed out that selection of the worst variable could depend on the details of nurse charting during periods of extreme instability or for a transient drop in vital signs which may occur during suctioning or turning, or the score could be influenced by the frequency of laboratory tests and monitoring (14). If an ICU philosophy was to measure blood gas and electrolytes primarily at times when patients become "stabilized," a patient would have a lower score than the same patient where the ICU philosophy is to measure frequent blood gases and electrolytes, especially if patients were briefly unstable. There are also differences related to whether a patient is stabilized in the emergency department or in the ICU prior to going to the operating room. Also during the operation, the anesthesiologist and surgeon try to normalize or stabilize physiology. In the 24-hour-based models, it is also problematic about what to do with patients who die or are transferred out before 24 hours. It is unclear what to do with the small number of patients who have multiple ICU admissions. Which one counts?

Some of these same issues would apply to physiology scoring in postoperative cardiac surgery patients. If in one program patients were moved directly from the operating room to the ICU and there was a long distance for the transport, it is possible that the patient might show more *physiologic instability* upon arrival than a similar patient who was stabilized in a postanesthesia care unit and then moved a shorter distance to a closer ICU later that day.

In the development of the MPM, the goal was to have a probability of mortality as the output rather than a physiology score (15). The methodology included using multiple logistic regression techniques for variable selection and weighting. In the MPM system, there are a small number of physiologic variables, but these are listed as extreme variables such as heart rate above 150 rather than intervals with a different score for each level of heart rate abnormality. All of the general ICU systems are now based on large databases (approximately 20,000 patients) from multiple hospital settings and have followed strict methods which include developmental dataset, validation, and interrater reliability of data collection. The models also meet high standards for discrimination using the area under the receiver/operator characteristic (ROC) curve and for calibration using the goodness-of-fit test (16). The physiology scores now also use multiple logistic techniques for converting a score to a probability. In the APACHE system, there is a different equation for each of 79 primary precipitating diagnoses causing ICU admission plus the physiology score, age, and chronic health evaluation (1, 6). In the SAPS system, logistic regression was used to determine the point score for the physiologic variables plus a limited number of diagnoses as well as conversion of the score to produce a probability estimate of hospital mortality (1, 8).

The main use of these ICU severity scores is the aggregate evaluation of quality-of-care comparisons. By measuring the individual prediction of death for each patient and then following that patient to hospital discharge to determine vital status (whether the patient lived or died) and summed over a large number of consecutive ICU admissions, it is possible to determine the severity-adjusted expected mortality. This severity-adjusted expected mortality can be compared to what is published in the literature or what is available in an on-going databases for the observed mortality (17). There could also be separate comparisons among hospitals with similar case-mix and demographic characteristics. The ICUs with low observed-to-expected mortality rates would be considered high-performance units (17).

The models are now being extended out to different time periods. There is an expanding database utilizing daily APACHE scores to look at daily risk of death (18). The MPM system has developed a simple approach at 48 and 72 hours, and these researchers are continuing work on looking at the change in probability over time or dynamic modeling (19). The MPM is the only system that has developed a unique probability estimate *at the time of ICU admission* (7). However, the authors have cautioned that this presentation probability should not be used to deny patients admission to the ICU because the probability estimate is based on patients *having been treated* in the ICU. There is on-going debate and discussion regarding individual patient application, triage deci-

sions, and admission criteria regarding all of these severity models (20–24).

## GENERAL SEVERITY MODELS AND CORONARY CARE UNIT/ CARDIAC SURGERY PATIENTS

As stated before, coronary care patients and post-CABG patients were excluded from APACHE II, III, MPM II, and SAPS II model development. APACHE III does include a primary precipitating diagnosis of postoperative procedure for cardiac valve surgery. However, this APACHE III logistic equation is not in the public domain (6).

There are published studies looking at application of APACHE II to cardiac surgery patients. In one study, the authors felt that APACHE was applicable to risk assessment of cardiac surgery patients; however, the sample size was small and appropriate calibration tests were not included (25). The histogram showing observed-to-expected mortality comparisons at different levels of APACHE score did not demonstrate appropriate correspondence, suggesting that, in this sample, APACHE II did not appropriately describe the mortality experience of these cardiac surgery patients.

In another attempt at using APACHE scores for cardiac surgery patients, the authors measured daily APACHE scores. If the APACHE score remained elevated beyond 48 hours, this physiologic instability was felt to be consistent with high risk for postoperative sepsis in cardiac surgery patients (26). The rationale is that the physiologic variables should normalize quickly, generally within 24 or 48 hours. Noninfectious post–cardiac surgery complications such as stroke or prolonged respiratory failure would not yield high physiology points. Rebleeding would be identified and corrected without having a sustained physiologic instability. Therefore, persistently high physiology scores could point to postoperative infection. However, physiologic instability or the systemic inflammatory reaction system can have multiple etiologies, not just sepsis. For complicated patients it is unlikely that an elevated APACHE score would be clinically useful. It is unclear why immunoglobulins would be considered as a therapy (27).

Since cardiac surgery and coronary care unit (CCU) patients share many characteristics with general medical/surgical ICU patients, it is not inconceivable that APACHE, MPM, or SAPS might "fit" for these two groups of patients, even though models were not developed on these subsets (Table 1). There is no APACHE III equation for coronary artery bypass surgery patients. If Knaus and co-workers follow their established pattern, they presumably will develop a CABG model using the same APACHE III physiology variables and weights with a unique logistic regression equation for postoperative

**TABLE 1.** *Cardiovascular modeling approaches*

1. General severity models (APACHE, MPM, SAPS)
   Standard, unmodified
   Modified
   "Customized"
2. Administrative database
3. Unique models
   Parsonnet Model
   New York State Cardiac Surgery Model
   Northern New England State Model
   Society for Thoracic Surgeons National Cardiac Surgery
     Database

APACHE, Acute Physiology and Chronic Health Evaluation; MPM, Mortality Probability Model; SAPS, Simplified Acute Physiology Score.

coronary bypass graft patients. In the European/North American study (ENAS) of severity of illness, there were 13,000 patients collected in 137 different ICUs in North America and Europe. Several ICUs routinely collected data on CCU and cardiac surgery patients, but these patients were not included in ENAS study from which MPM II and SAPS II were refined and enhanced. In a separate analysis of these patients (Table 2) MPM II, SAPS II, and APACHE II did provide good discrimination for these two groups of patients as demonstrated by a large area under the ROC curve (28). Discrimination as measured by the area under the ROC curve is defined as the model's tendency to assign higher probabilities of mortality to those patients who actually die than to those who actually live. The physiology-based scores have sur-

**TABLE 2.** *General ICU severity models and the cardiovascular patient*

| Model | n | $C^a$ | p-Value | Area under ROC curve |
|---|---|---|---|---|
| Coronary patients | | | | |
| MPM0 | 532 | 17.33 | 0.08 | 0.83 |
| MPM 24 | 523 | 17.12 | 0.07 | 0.89 |
| SAPS II | 528 | 6.07 | 0.81 | 0.87 |
| APACHE II | 529 | 12.23 | 0.30 | 0.84 |
| Cardiac surgery patients | | | | |
| MPM0 | 131 | 7.46 | 0.70 | 0.82 |
| MPM24 | 131 | 6.97 | 0.54 | 0.88 |
| SAPS II | 131 | 6.60 | 0.76 | 0.89 |
| APACHE II | 131 | 7.07 | 0.72 | 0.85 |
| Customized models for all coronary and cardiac surgery patients | | | | |
| MPM0 | 662 | 11.82 | 0.29 | 0.85 |
| MPM24 | 653 | 5.48 | 0.86 | 0.90 |
| SAPS II | 658 | 5.64 | 0.84 | 0.88 |

Courtesy of J. Klar and S. Lemeshow, School of Public Health, University of Massachusetts, Amherst.
$^a C$ statistics from Hosmer-Lemeshow goodness-of-fit tests.
ICU, intensive care unit; ROC, receiver/operator characteristic.

prisingly good calibration for coronary patients. (In the goodness-of-fit test, a poor calibration is defined by a low *p* value.) Calibration is the degree of correspondence between the estimated probabilities and the actual mortality experience of the patients. All three models accurately described the cardiac surgery patients, although the sample size was small.

## POTENTIAL APPLICATION OF GENERAL SEVERITY MODELS

It is unclear how to interpret the above findings or how to apply them. In many settings, the CCU is part of the medical ICU and, therefore, perhaps the general severity model could apply to all of these medical ICU/CCU patients. Similarly, many cardiac surgery patients are treated in general surgical ICUs, and perhaps general severity models could be applied to all surgical ICU patients. Since many elective cardiac surgery patients are "fast tracked" out of the ICU to a telemetry area in under 24 hours, the residual patients remaining 24 or 48 hours postoperatively would have a comparable range of ICU-related problems (29).

Since cardiac surgery procedures are done in such large numbers, it might be useful to abstract administrative databases to come up with case-mix adjusted severity (30). For general applications, this approach might have some value, especially when looking at postoperative length of stay, 6-month or 1-year mortality, and readmission to hospital. For the application of quality-of-care comparisons of individual surgeons or hospitals providing high-volume cardiac surgery procedures, it would ***not*** seem reasonable to utilize standard or unmodified general ICU severity models. It would make much more sense to use modified severity models or to develop unique models based on variables related to the risk of the procedure (Table 1) and to look at relevant outcomes such as hospital mortality, reoperation rates, and relevant morbidity such as stroke.

## CARDIAC SURGERY MODELS

### General Comment

Since the Health Care Financing Administration first published mortality rates of Medicare patients having cardiac surgery (1986), there has been active development of severity models that identify factors that could risk stratify patients undergoing open-heart procedures. Such a strategy would provide a more realistic approach to assessing the operative mortality of these patients than simply providing crude mortality rates or rates modified with some adjustment for age and other general risk factors. In Table 3, there is a brief description of seven models which use mathematical modeling to risk stratify by

**TABLE 3.** *Preoperative severity models for cardiac surgery*

| Model | Location | Method | Type | n | Years of cases |
|---|---|---|---|---|---|
| Parsonnet | Newark, NJ | LR | All | 3,500 | 1982–1987 |
| Williams | Five Philadelphia hospitals | Disease staging | DRG 106 | 4,613 | 1985–1987 |
| Lyer | Adelaire, Australia | LR | Uncomplicated CABG | 12,003 | 1978–1990 |
| O'Connor | Northern New England | LR | CABG | 3,055 | 1987–1989 |
| Higgins | Cleveland Clinic | LR | All CABG[a] | 501 | 1986–1988 |
| | | | | 4,169 | 1988–1990 |
| Hannan | New York State: 30 hospitals | LRA | All open heart | 7,596 | 1989 |
| | | | Isolated CABG | 57,187 | 1989–1992 |
| Edwards | Walter Reed "National" | Bayesian | Urgent CABG | 700 | 1984–1989 |
| | | | Isolated CABG | 80,881 | 1984–1990 |

[a]Includes concomitant value or carotid endarterectomy.
LR, logistic regression; CABG, coronary artery bypass graft.

severity of disease. These models are based on a large number of patients and are primarily geared to a statistical assessment of postoperative mortality by evaluating preoperative risk factors. Even the earlier collaborative study in Coronary Artery Surgery (CASS) developed a risk equation which incorporated left main coronary artery stenosis (≥90%), female sex, and left ventricular dysfunction using ejection fraction, wall motion, and end-diastolic pressure (30). A great deal has been learned by these studies about risk assessment, and the sample sizes are now large enough so that it may be possible to compare one hospital or surgeon's experience to a "national average." It is recognized that the Parsonnet model overpredicts the mortality of current patients. In addition, by strictly defining the clinical variables, by providing an *external audit* to assure accurate data entry, it is possible to provide a "score card" for individual hospitals as well as individual surgeons regarding a consumer report that could be made available to third-party payors or to the public (31).

There are several general comments regarding these models. First of all it is not clear what is meant by postoperative mortality. Is this the traditional 30-day mortality? Is it cardiac surgery ICU mortality? In most cases, it appears to be hospital mortality. Medicare analysts are also interested in 90-day postdischarge mortality. There are also models based on distinct clinical subsets of patients undergoing open-heart procedures. Several models include all open-heart patients, including patients having gunshot wounds to the heart (32). Most studies have focused on patients with CABG, ranging from isolated uncomplicated procedures to all coronary bypass operations, including concomitant procedures.

The most common statistical methods are *multiple logistic regression* techniques, which afford the ability to incorporate continuous as well as categorical variables and do not require that the response variable be normally distributed. A normally distributed response variable is required for linear regression techniques. Logistic regression has become the predominant methodology in general severity scores, for scaling physiologic variables, for assessing whether a variable should be included, as well as for assigning statistical weights for these variables (1). Interaction of variables can also be assessed using logistic regression. Adequate field testing and external validation of the current cardiac surgery models have now been satisfactorily performed. There is also the addition problem of constantly changing anesthetic and surgical techniques and cardioplegia.

## Risk Stratification

For general risk stratification approaches and for placing patients in broad risk categories, strict statistical validation techniques are probably not necessary. However, for quality assessment comparisons, the models should be externally validated, meet high criteria for discrimination by the area under the ROC curve, as well as calibration by using formal goodness-of-fit testing (16). In general, the models that have utilized sophisticated model evaluation demonstrate that models work better for isolated, uncomplicated coronary artery bypass procedures and are less accurate for higher risk procedures (33).

Much has been learned about various risk factors. In Tables 4, 5, and 6 the risk factors from the Cleveland Clinic (33), the Society of Thoracic Surgery (34), and the New York State models (32, 35) are listed by their relative weights. Obviously, preexisting left ventricular dysfunction and acute cardiac instability by myocardial infarction, unstable angina, or cardiac catheterization complication are major risk factors. In addition, it has been learned that low body weight (36) and female gender are associated with higher risk factors (35). It may well be that there is an interaction between small body surface and female gender since individuals with small-caliber vessels may have added technical problems when coronary artery bypass procedures are performed.

The outcome of the risk stratification technique is to provide broad categories for patients *preoperatively*.

**TABLE 4.** *Cleveland Clinic model (high score variables)*

| | |
|---|---|
| Emergency | 6 |
| Creatinine > 1.8 mg/dL | 4 |
| Severe LV dysfunction | 3 |
| Reoperation | 3 |
| Operative mitral value insufficiency | 3 |
| Age ≥ 75 | 2 |
| Prior vascular surgery | 2 |
| COPD on bronchodilating drugs | 2 |
| Hct < 34 | 2 |

LV, left ventricular; COPD, chronic obstructive pulmonary disease; Hct, hematocrit.2

**TABLE 6.** *New York State cardiac surgery prediction model*

Cardiac risk factors:
  Preoperative myocardial infarction
  Unstable angina
  Congestive heart failure/low ejection fraction
  ≥90 Left main coronary stenosis
  Valve operation
  Reoperation
  Catheter laboratory crash
Noncardiac risk factors
  Age/female
  Diabetes
  Dialysis
  "Disaster"[a]
  Noncardiac operation

[a]ATN (Acute tubular necrosis), cardiogenic shock, gunshot, cardiac structural change.

These broad categories are generally in the range of *very, low risk* (<2% predicted mortality), *low risk* (2% to 4% predicted mortality), *intermediate risk*, which may range from 4% to 7%, and *high risk*, which may be even broader in its probability range. These categories are not precise and vary from one study group to another but are generally satisfactory for assigning a preoperative mortality assessment for a given clinical patient. The Cleveland Clinic approach converts the logistic weights to a numerical score for simplicity purposes. For a score up to 5, the model is well calibrated and the predicted mortality is less than 3%. There is much wider discrepancy for scores of 6 or more between the observed and expected mortality (33).

The study by Williams comparing the outcome of five Philadelphia hospitals used *disease staging* as their severity adjustment (37). This incorporates a subjective assessment, with stage I being an asymptomatic patient, stage II one with *stable angina*, and stage III one with *unstable angina or recent MI*. The logistic regression models would be expected to provide a much better approach to variable selection than subjective disease staging. It is interesting that the Philadelphia group studied patients with *DRG 106* as their clinical subset. These are patients who have a cardiac catheterization at the same hospitalization as the CABG. Such a patient would generally be considered sicker than a patient who has a coronary angiogram, is discharged home, and is electively scheduled for CABG at a later hospitalization or

different hospital. In this study as well as in several others, there was wide variability in the observed-to-expected outcome by hospital and individual surgeon (37, 38). In the Philadelphia study, there was no relationship between surgical volume and the severity-adjusted outcome. However, the observed-to-expected outcome did shift in an expected direction when individual surgeons moved from one hospital to another, suggesting a quality-of-care relationship.

The Society of Thoracic Surgeons has by far the largest database, with over 80,000 patients enrolled (34). They utilize a different statistical modeling approach, the *Bayesian method* (39). This technique allows the research group to predict future events based on associated past events. They developed a conditional probability matrix for assessing important clinical findings. Each variable must be independent for the Bayesian technique to work. In the Society of Thoracic Surgeons database, participation is voluntary and there is no external technique for evaluating the quality of the data input. The original modeling by Edwards was performed at the Walter Reed Hospital on urgent coronary artery graft patients and included both a development and validation dataset (39). The larger database is focused on patients who have isolated CABGs (34). The risk stratification variables in descending order of importance are shown in Table 5. Other methods of model development such as neural networks or artificial intelligence will be utilized in future evaluations. Performance comparisons among models on the same patients should be evaluated next.

**TABLE 5.** *Society for Thoracic Surgery risk factors (decreasing importance)*

Cardiogenic shock
Reoperation
Renal failure
Cardiomegaly
Angioplasty emergency
Female
Stroke
Left main disease
Age

## Postoperative Mortality/Morbidity

None of the above models incorporate intraoperative factors such as bypass time. For preoperative risk and for comparing the performance of one hospital or an individual surgeon, it would be inappropriate to "adjust" for intraoperative technical aspects of care. However, for *postoperative mortality* and selected complications it might be appropriate to incorporate *bypass time, cross-clamping time*, and *method of cardioplegia*. There has been one attempt by the Cleveland Clinic Group to develop a risk stratification model for postoperative morbidity as opposed to mortality. However, the calibration of this model was not satisfactory (33). Since uncomplicated and isolated CABGs now have such a low postoperative mortality, it would be important to incorporate the morbidity risks of such an operation. Incorporating a discussion of morbidities would be important for patients and families in preoperative assessment since their clinical decision making may hinge as much on quality of outcome as simply on survival. Such complications would include both minor and major neurologic complications, pneumonia, and prolonged respiratory failure, mediastinitis, and other complications that occur during any major invasive procedures. With such large sample sizes available for these high-risk cardiac procedures, the future direction would be to improve preoperative mortality probability models for higher risk open-heart procedures and to develop and enhance preoperative morbidity assessment and postoperative morbidity and mortality severity models.

Two current approaches are worthy of mentioning. The first is the Computerized Severity Index, which is being extended to CABG patients (40). This approach is directed by Susan Horn, who is now at the Intermountain Health Care Institute. The focus is on postoperative severity adjustment but entails extensive data collection. An even more audacious program is envisioned by the Academic Medical Center Consortium, which is located in Rochester, NY. They have put together prominent clinical teams to develop the Quality Measurement and Management Initiative and data instruments or tools for angioplasty and coronary artery bypass procedures (41).

## QUALITY-OF-CARE COMPARISONS: SCORE CARD APPROACH

A sophisticated approach has been published by Hannan et al. representing the efforts of the New York State Department of Public Health in using mathematical models for a comprehensive quality-of-care program (35). The initial models were based on all patients having an open-heart procedure, including patients with gunshot wounds (32). There was also concern in the medical community when the media published *individual* hospital and surgeon severity-adjusted outcomes. Although the public does presumably have a right to know this information, there must be an appropriate context for evaluating such complex information. First, a simple rank ordering is not appropriate since there may be no statistical difference between hospitals that differ by one or two rankings. It would be more appropriate to use confidence or probability intervals to separate hospitals or individual surgeons into three broad groupings that are statistically distinct: those above the average, those within the range of average (the confidence interval includes one), and those below average (20). Furthermore, Richard Orr at the Fallon St. Vincent Health Care System has compared the probability of mortality based on four probability models calculated on over 1,000 procedures done at St. Vincent's Hospital, Worcester, Massachusetts (42). The Parsonnet model provided the highest predicted mortality, but this model was developed many years ago, before generally accepted surgical improvements had occurred (43). The other models provided similar probabilities with wide overlap. It is not surprising that, by incorporating different models with different risk stratification variables, predicted outcomes would not be identical.

Hannan also compared a model based on an administrative database using the SPACS (the State-Wide Planning and Research Corporation System) and showed that the model using bedside tabulated clinical risk factors in the Cardiac Surgery Reporting System provided a better system (44).

In the subsequent organization of 4-year mortality outcome of this mandated New York State Department of Health quality assessment program, there was substantial input by the Cardiac Advisory Committee of New York State (35). This committee included cardiologists and cardiac surgeons. The updated models focused on coronary artery bypass procedures and demonstrated an impressive reduction, year by year, in risk-adjusted mortality. In 1992, the risk-adjusted mortality rate was 2.45%. Since lower risk patients today often have angioplasty techniques rather than open bypass procedures, it is not surprising that the expected mortality over time increased. The main explanation for the small number of outlier institutions and surgeons with higher than expected mortalities was related to the number of procedures done per year. Hospitals and surgeons with low surgical volumes had worse than expected outcomes (45).

We are now in a new era of external review of all aspects of medical care (Joint Commission on Accreditation of Healthcare Organizations, Peer Review Organizations, state, federal agencies, third-party payors) with particular focus on high-volume expensive technology. Although there are many critics of such programs, it may be suggested that such a score card method has indirect benefits (31). The public should have confidence that 27 of the 30 participating hospitals in New York State had an impressive and steady reduction of risk-adjusted mortality rates (35). There does not appear to be "gaming" of the *expected* mortality, since there was *external review* of records from one-third of the participating hospitals. Hospitals and surgeons did seem to respond in a generally positive way regarding the external oversight. Referral patterns did change. Many programs had internal reviews. Some programs were reorganized. It has been suggested that some higher risk patients were transferred from some institutions to others. Some hospitals improved their stabilization of emergency patients prior to operative procedure. There may also have been a faster learning curve for adopting newer techniques for intraoperative anesthesia management, assessment, and correction of postoperative bleeding, testing of different cardioplegic approaches, and fast-track extubations.

To have such a program work, it is important to have involvement by participating physicians. There must be good-quality input of clinical data and there should be open discussion of statistical models and results. In the future, it is also likely that regular feedback of information to the participating institution would also be useful. An additional approach might be to provide some "artificial" adjustment for higher risk patients so that patients are not turned away by surgeons who are unduly concerned by "excessive" oversight. Additional modeling may be necessary for the more complicated procedures. Models can also be customized or recalibrated for the higher risk patient. However, it is not unreasonable to encourage quaternary referrals for the sickest patients.

The cost of additional data collection should be incorporated into the assessment of any program. There should be a clear focus on the high-performance units including hospital process and surgeon components as well as ICU and other postoperative care aspects to determine what they are doing correctly, rather than focusing on the other type of outlier. A positive approach would encourage physician participation. Since surgical volume seems to play such an important role, one concern would be how to support a recently trained surgeon so the learning curve will be kept within clinically acceptable limits. It would be unfortunate to penalize highly trained recent graduate cardiac surgeons who might have difficulty starting up their own practice.

## SUMMARY

It is recognized that there is a variation in medical practice that remains unexplained regarding length of hospital stay, resource use, and mortality for many of our clinical practices, including open-heart procedures. Preoperative risk assessment and postoperative severity-adjusted mathematical models provide approaches to reducing or explaining these variations. It has been suggested that a cardiac surgery unit with "excess" risk-adjusted mortality may represent an outlier in a true quality-of-care measure. Before reaching such a conclusion, it must be recognized that there may be random variation, poorly recorded or measured risk factors, or unknown case-mix or patient mix factors that are difficult to exclude. Some important components of excess mortality could also be contributed to by anesthesia, cardiology, or postoperative ICU care.

## ACKNOWLEDGMENT

The authors thank Janelle Klar and Stanley Lemeshow for reviewing the manuscript, Richard Engelman and Richard Orr for helpful suggestions, and Mark Kennedy for literature search. We also thank Suzanne Allen and Maureen Harbilas for manuscript preparation.

## REFERENCES

1. Lemeshow S, Le Gall JR. Update on ICU severity measures. *JAMA* 1994;272(13):1049.
2. Lemeshow S. Individual outcome prediction: the case for and against. *Rean Urg* 1994;3(2):223.
3. Lemeshow S, Klar J, Teres D. Outcome prediction for individual intensive care patients: useful, misused or abused? *Int Care Med* 1995;21:770.
4. Teres D, Lemeshow S. Severity of illness modeling. In: Rippe JM, ed. *Intensive care medicine*, 3rd ed. Boston: Little, Brown; 1994.
5. Krumholz H, Forman DE, Kuntz RE, et al. Coronary revascularization after myocardial infarction in the very elderly: outcomes and long-term follow-up. *Ann Intern Med* 1993;119(11):1084.
6. Knaus WA, Wagner DP, Draper EA, et al. The APACHE III prognostic system. Risk prediction of hospital mortality for critically ill hospitalized adults. *Chest* 1991;100(6):1619.
7. Lemeshow S, Teres D, Klar J, et al. Mortality probability models (MPM II) based on an international cohort of intensive care unit patients. *JAMA* 1993;270(20):2478.
8. Le Gall JR, Lemeshow S, Saulnier F. A new simplified acute physiology score (SAPS II) based on a European/North American multicenter study. *JAMA* 1993;270:2957.
9. Pollack MM, Urrimann UE, Getson PR. The pediatric risk of mortality (PRISM) score. *Crit Care Med* 1988;16:1110.
10. Cullen DJ, Nemeskal AR, Zaslavsky AM. Intermediate TISS: a new therapeutic intervention scoring system for non-ICU patients. *Crit Care Med* 1994;22:1406.
11. Teres D, Lemeshow S. Why severity models should be used with caution. *Crit Care Clin* 1994;10(1):93.
12. Knaus WA, Zimmerman JE, Wagner DP, et al. APACHE—acute physiology and chronic health evaluation: a physiologically based classification system. *Crit Care Med* 1981;9:591.
13. Knaus WA, Draper EA, Wagner DP, et al. APACHE II: a severity of disease classification system. *Crit Care Med* 1985;13:818.
14. Teres D. Calculating the odds. In: *Pathways in critical care*. Greenwich: Clinical Communications 1995;203:629.
15. Lemeshow S, Teres D, Pastides, et al. A method for predicting survival and mortality of ICU patients using objectively derived weights. *Crit Care Med* 1985;13:519.
16. Hadorn DC, Keeler EB, Rogers WH, et al. Assessing the performance of mortality prediction models. Santa Monica, CA: RAND; 1993.
17. Teres D, Lemeshow S. Using severity measures to describe high performance intensive care unit. *Crit Care Clin* 1993;9(3):543.
18. Wagner DP, Knaus WA, Harrell Fe, et al. Daily prognostic estimates for critically ill adults in intensive care units: results from a prospective, multicenter, inception cohort analysis. *Crit Care Med* 1994;22(9):1359.
19. Lemeshow S, Klar J, Teres D, et al. Mortality probability models for patients in the intensive care unit for 48–72 hours: a prospective, multicenter study. *Crit Care Med* 1994;22(9):1351.
20. Rapoport J, Teres D, Lemeshow S, et al. A method for assessing the clinical performance and cost effectiveness of intensive care units: a multicenter inception cohort study. *Crit Care Med* 1994;22(9):1385.
21. Vassar MJ, Holcroft JW. The case against using the APACHE system to predict intensive care unit outcome in trauma patients. *Crit Care Clin* 1994;10(1):117.
22. Cerra FB, Negro F, Abrams J. APACHE II score does not predict multiple organ failure or mortality in post-operative surgical patients. *Arch Surg* 1990;125(4):519.
23. Civetta JM. The clinical limitations of ICU scoring systems. *Problems Crit Care* 1989;3(4):681.
24. Watts CM, Knaus WA. The case for using objective scoring systems to predict ICU outcome. *Crit Care Clin* 1994;1:73.

25. Turner J, Mudalier YM, Chang RW, et al. Acute physiology and chronic health evaluation (APACHE II) scoring in a cardiothoracic intensive care unit. *Crit Care Med* 1991;19(10):1266.
26. Kreuzer E, Kääb S, Pilz G, Werdan K. Early prediction of septic complications after cardiac surgery by APACHE II score. *Eur J Cardiothorac Surg* 1992;6:524.
27. Pilz G, Kreuzer E, Kääb S, Appel R, Werdan K. Early sepsis treatment with immunoglobulins after cardiac surgery in score-identified high-risk patients. *Chest* 1994;105:76.
28. Courtesy of J. Klar and S. Lemeshow, School of Public Health, University of Massachusetts.
29. Engelman RM, Rousou JA, Flack JE. Fast track recovery of the coronary bypass patient. *Ann Thor Surg* 1994;58:1742.
30. Kennedy JW, Kaiser GC, Fisher LD, et al. Multivariate discriminant analysis of the clinical and angiographic predictors of operative mortality from the Collaborative Study in Coronary Artery Surgery (CASS). *J Thorac Cardiovasc Surg* 1980;80:876.
31. Topol EJ, Califf RM. Scorecard cardiovascular medicine. *Ann Intern Med* 1994;120;65.
32. Hannan EL, Kilburn H, O'Donnell JF, Lukacik G, Shields EP. Adult open heart surgery in New York State: an analysis of risk factors and hospital mortality rates. *JAMA* 1990;264(21):2768.
33. Higgins TL, Estafanous FG, Loop FD, Beck GJ, Blum JM, Paranandi L. Stratification of morbidity and mortality outcome by preoperative risk factors in coronary artery bypass patients: a clinical severity score. *JAMA* 1992;267:2344.
34. Edwards FH, Clark RE, Schwartz M. Coronary artery bypass grafting: the Society of Thoracic Surgeons national database experience. *Ann Thorac Surg* 1994;57:12.
35. Hannon EL, Kilburn H, Racz M, Shields E, Chassin MR. Improving the outcomes of coronary artery bypass surgery in New York State. *JAMA* 1994;271:761.
36. Iyer VS, Russell WJ, Leppard P, Craddock D. Mortality and myocardial infarction after coronary artery surgery: a review of 12,003 patients. *Med J Austral* 1993;159:166.
37. Williams SV, Nash DB, Goldfarb N. Differences in mortality from coronary artery bypass graft surgery at five teaching hospitals. *JAMA* 1991;266(6):810.
38. O'Connor GT, Plume SK, Olmstead EM, et al. Multivariate prediction of in-hospital mortality associated with coronary artery bypass graft surgery. *Circulation* 1992;85:2110.
39. Edwards FH, Albus RA, Zajtchuk R, et al. Use of a Bayesian statistical model for risk assessment in coronary artery surgery. *Ann Thorac Surg* 1988;45:437.
40. Hopkins DSP, Carroll RJ. Severity adjustment models for CPI. In: *Clinical practice improvement: a new technology for developing cost-effective quality health care.* New York: Faulkner & Gray; 1994:91.
41. Academic Medical Center Consortium. Quality measurement and management initiative: Coronary revascularization project protocol. In: Curtis LH, ed. Rochester, NY: 1994.
42. Orr RK, Maini BS, Sottile FD, Dumas EM, O'Mara P. A comparison of four severity adjusted models to predict mortality after coronary artery bypass graft surgery. *Arch Surg* 1995;130:301.
43. Parsonnet V, Dean D, Bernstein AD. A method of uniform stratfication of risk for evaluating the results of surgery in acquired adult heart disease. *Circulation* 1989;79(Suppl I):1-3.
44. Hannan EL, Kilburn H, Lindsey ML, Lewis R. Clinical versus administrative data bases for CABG surgery: does it matter? *Med Care* 1992;30:892.
45. Hannan EL, Kilburn H, Bernard H, O'Donnell JF, Lukacik G, Shields EP. Coronary artery bypass surgery: the relationship between inhospital mortality rate and surgical volume after controlling for clinical risk factors. *Med Care* 1991;29(11):1094.

*The Critically Ill Cardiac Patient,*
edited by V. Kvetan and D. R. Dantzker,
Lippincott - Raven Publishers, Philadelphia © 1996.

CHAPTER 22

# Post-Myocardial Infarction Risk Stratification: Current State-of-the-Art

Jay S. Steingrub and Daniel Teres

Economic considerations are prompting physicians to examine the usage of expensive and potentially harmful resources. Current medical ethics behooves clinicians to reflect on both the potential benefits and risks of therapy in the context of the individual versus the community when the cost is high and resources are considered to be limited. The ability to answer these questions is predicated on our ability to estimate outcome of therapy in individual patients, preferably before therapy is initiated or at least soon after admission to an ICU. Lacking sufficient precision and reliability in describing patient outcome, physicians have relied on their clinical experiences. Although the decision to institute or discontinue intensive care treatment will for the foreseeable future be a matter for clinical judgment, the use of objectively derived prognostic information will give that judgment a sound basis. Recognized variations of both practice patterns of quality and utilization of service have encouraged the development of severity scoring systems to study case mix and to develop risk stratification methodology for different clinical entities.

Treatment regimens and prognosis of patients who have survived an initial acute myocardial infarction (AMI) have been widely studied, and methods of assessing the risk of future events in survivors of infarctions have been well documented (1). Newer therapies available to improve the prognosis are due to an overgrowth of clinical trials investigating predictors of outcome of AMI. Since the survival of patients with AMI has been associated with hemodynamic, electrophysiologic (EP), structural, biochemical, and functional measurements, risk is determined through the pathophysiologic assessment of the patient. Risk stratification allows the physi-

cian to identify low-risk patients requiring no invasive therapy and high-risk patients who may require intervention. The primary value of risk stratification, or for that matter any approach to decision making, is to identify a group of patients who are at such low risk that even if they have a serious coronary event the survival will probably not be prolonged by interventional procedures. Assigning a postinfarction population into severity groups is appealing because classification has implications for management and is easily remembered. However, classifying infarction survivors into high risk, low risk, and moderate risk may be hindered by oversimplification implicit in dividing a large prognostically diverse cohort of patients into two or three theoretically homogeneous subgroups. A prognostic score or a probability can provide a more objective measure of baseline risk than a formal clinical assessment and might provide a more rational basis for selecting patients who would benefit from referral for further invasive intervention.

## RISK STRATIFICATION

Survivors of AMI can be categorized into high-, low-, and moderate-risk groups. The Multicenter Postinfarction Research Group found four factors that were independent predictors of mortality, including an ejection fraction below 40%, ventricular ectopy with greater than ten ventricular premature beats per hour, cardiovascular disability prior to infarction conforming to classes II through IV of the New York Heart Association classification, and evidence of heart failure in the coronary care unit (CCU) (2). Those at *high* risk for subsequent cardiac events, including recurrent myocardial infarction (MI), death, postinfarction angina requiring revascularization, and ventricular arrhythmias, have a postinfarction first-year mortality rate of approximately 25%. The *low*-risk

J. S. Steingrub and D. Teres: Adult Critical Care Division, Baystate Medical Center and Tufts University School of Medicine, Springfield, Massachusetts 01199.

group with an annual mortality of between 2% and 5% will have no evidence of myocardial ischemia or complex ventricular arrhythmias at hospital discharge. The remaining population with a first-year mortality rate of approximately 10% constitutes a group at *moderate* risk, usually having one or more of the above risk factors. Identification of these clinical groups is an important first step toward reducing post-MI morbidity and mortality (Fig. 1).

Ideally, risk stratification should satisfy several criteria, including the identification of patients at high risk and the specific mechanism by which death or reinfarction occurs so that treatment can be targeted. Results should be readily available prior to hospital discharge, allowing decisions regarding treatment or further investigation to be undertaken in an opportune fashion. Since survival curves demonstrate that the majority of arrhythmic events occur in the days or weeks immediately after discharge, many events can be overlooked by risk stratification schemes that are deferred (requiring patients to return for outpatient investigation) or whose results are not immediately available before discharge.

Historically, the momentum for developing post-MI risk stratification resulted from the observations that most studies of in-hospital morbidity/mortality of acute infarct patients also noted increased mortality in the postinfarction period following hospital discharge regardless of the patient's status. This recognition of the postinfarction state for the coronary patient has served to focus attention on this particular time period. Although risk assessment from early hospital admission to discharge can add substantial independent prognostic information to the clinical assessment, this chapter will foremost review aspects of the pre–hospital discharge risk stratification literature, including concepts regarding application of risk stratification to clinical practice and the role of a variety of tests employed in risk assessment. Clinically significant pathophysiologic considerations form the conceptual framework for postinfarction risk stratification including size of infarction, ventricular

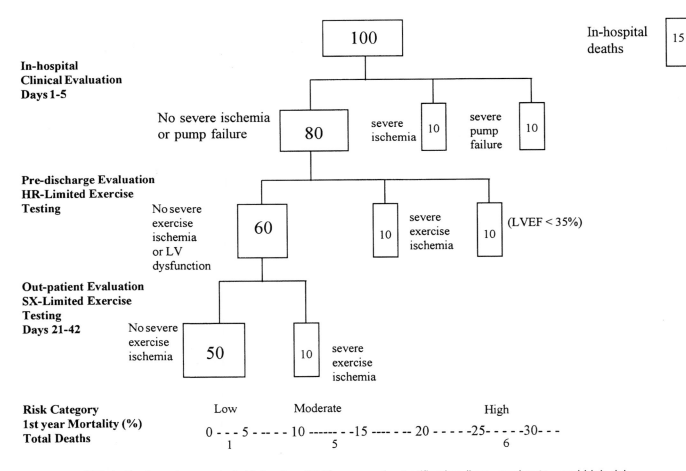

**FIG 1.** Post–acute myocardial infarction (AMI) prognostic stratification (low-, moderate-, and high-risk categories based on degree of myocardial ischemia and left ventricular (LV) dysfunction. Number in boxes indicates size of patient subsets. LVEF, left ventricular ejection fraction. Adapted from the American College of Physicians. *Ann Intern Med* 1989;110:485.

function, ventricular arrhythmias, anginal status, stress testing response, and coronary angiography. Although recognized as major prognostic factors for outcome, only recently have these factors been incorporated into pragmatic treatment strategies. Provided with this information, clinicians are now able to alter the natural history of MI with appropriate intervention in high-risk patients.

## ELECTROCARDIOGRAM

The electrocardiogram (ECG) may be beneficial in predicting both acute complications and the long-term prognosis of an AMI. The height of ST-segment elevation correlates with a large infarction and poor survival. Willems and co-workers showed that in patients not receiving thrombolytic therapy, high admission ST-segment elevation (>20 mm) had a greater in-hospital mortality (10%) than did patients with ST sums measured from 12 to 20 mm (3.8%) and those with sums of 12 mm or less (2.3%) (3). Patients with anterior wall infarcts and ST depression of greater than 2 mm in leads II, III, or AVF had an in-hospital mortality of 14.3% compared with 6.7% of patients with anterior infarcts in the absence of marked inferior ST depression. Several reports have found that thrombolytic therapy was most beneficial in those patients with associated large electrocardiographically determined infarctions (3, 4). Reperfusion therapy, although most effective in patients with the greatest amount of ST-segment elevation, does not appear to benefit the population of patients presenting with primarily ST depression. Patients presenting with ST-segment depression alone have a poor prognosis and are characterized by triple-vessel disease without total occlusion of any single vessel.

## SIZE OF INFARCTION

The relevance of infarct size in determining the prognosis after a MI was established from autopsy studies in patients who were diagnosed with left ventricular (LV) failure. Interestingly, the timing of such cardiac necrosis was found not to be as important as the amount of nonviable myocardium existing (a single episode causing infarction of 40% of the left ventricle was equivalent to an old 20% infarct and a recent 20% infarct). The keystone of risk stratification today is the definitive relationship between infarct size and mortality. Echocardiography or radionuclide ventriculography can assist in confirming the extent of LV damage. Factors reflecting the degree of LV damage include new Q-wave location (anterior versus inferior), congestive heart failure severity, and creatinine phosphokinase (CPK) elevation in the absence of thrombolysis.

## VENTRICULAR FUNCTION

One of the most reliable and strongest predictors of cardiac mortality postinfarction is the degree of LV dys-

function, an alternative reflection of infarct size. The mortality rate in the first year increases dramatically when resting LV ejection fraction (EF) is less than 30%. A combination of significant ventricular dysrhythmias and a diminished EF leads to a more unfavorable outcome (1, 5, 6). LV function as measured by multiple gated image acquisition (MUGA) measurement of EF correlates with the size of the infarct. A landmark multicenter study in 1983 demonstrated a curvilinear relationship between the first-year postinfarction cardiac mortality and predischarge MUGA ejection fraction (2). A decreasing level of EF down to the 40% range had minimal impact on mortality. A dramatic increase in mortality was noted at an EF level below 35%. This higher risk is independent of other clinical factors such as overt congestive heart failure.

Patients with LV dysfunction are prone to develop arrhythmia events during the first year after their infarction. However, in the absence of other risk factors, the rate of arrhythmic events in these patients with a depressed EF, in contrast to patients with normal EF postinfarction, is similar. In comparison to small infarcts, hearts with large infarcts may be more likely to incorporate interventricular reentrant circuits. However, impaired ventricular function per se does not necessarily identify an arrhythmogenic substrate. Major goals of therapy in patients who have encountered an AMI are to minimize the extent of damage by obviating the development of hemodynamic decompensation and extend prognosis by managing arrhythmias. Importantly, impaired ventricular function does not identify a specific mechanism by which patients will die; rather a variety of reasons might be responsible including ventricular tachyarrhythmias, intractable congestive heart failure, reinfarction, and asystole or bradycardiac arrest.

## ARRHYTHMIA

The major cause of death in the first year after an AMI is attributed to malignant ventricular tachyarrhythmias. Therefore, investigators have attempted to identify high-risk groups in which further investigation or intervention is necessary. The risk for sudden death is highest within the first 6 to 7 months post-AMI. Although this risk decreases, it continues to be sustained for up to 3 years.

Several studies analyzing the correlation between ventricular dysfunction and ventricular premature beats (VPBs) suggest that VPBs are illustrative of myocardial scar and, accordingly, ventricular dysfunction. Moss et al. found that repetitive VPBs (more than 10 per hour) significantly correlated with mortality even after adjusting for ventricular dysfunction (1). In other postinfarction trials, the presence of VPBs themselves, regardless of frequency and multiformity, did not increase risk of death. Evidence exists that special types of VPBs, specifically, runs of nonsustained ventricular tachycardia (VT) (more than three sequential VPBs) increase the risk for sudden death post-AMI. A majority of acute infarction patients experience infrequent ventricular arrhythmias. For patients considered to be at low risk for sudden death, infrequent VPBs (less than 30 per hour) without runs of nonsustained VT are observed in 60% of cases. The moderate-risk group encompassing approximately one-third of postinfarction patients, have fairly frequent VPBs (more than 30 per hour) or infrequent runs of nonsustained VT. Their risk for sudden death is about twofold that for the low-risk group. The high-risk population, with a probability of sudden death of about two to five times that of patients without arrhythmias, are characterized by frequent VPBs (more than 60 per hour) in combination with runs of nonsustained VT. Although seen in 1% of patients, at highest risk for sudden death are those with frequent runs of VT in the prehospital and CCU phases of AMI (7, 8). The occurrence of VT in the period of 10 to 20 days postinfarction is associated with an increased risk of sudden death. Other associated clinical findings included previous infarction, heart failure, atrial fibrillation, VT, or ventricular fibrillation in the CCU (7). Both VPBs and ventricular dysfunction have been shown to be independent contributors to postinfarction mortality with the predicted patient mortality with both VPBs and ventricular dysfunction being greater than the arithmetic sum of each individual risk factor (9). The generation of complex ventricular ectopy, sustained VT, or fibrillation during the acute phase of MI does not imply a poor long-term prognosis. In the late postinfarction period a strong correlation exists between spontaneous ventricular ectopy (defined as greater than 10 VPBs per hour) or nonsustained VT whether symptomatic or not and long-term risk of sudden cardiac death (10).

## SIGNAL-AVERAGED ELECTROCARDIOGRAPHY

In the Multicenter Post Infarction Study of AMI, Bigger and colleagues analyzed the relationship among ventricular arrhythmias, ventricular dysfunction, and mortality within 2 years of infarction (11). Although 1-year mortality was highest in those with ventricular dysfunction and nonsustained VT (35%), over 60% of those classified as high risk were alive at a follow-up of 3 years. Identifying postinfarction patients at highest risk for sudden death from among those with ventricular dysfunction and nonsustained VT has encouraged an expansion of new technology.

A technique has recently been employed to potentially predict the generation of ventricular arrhythmias in postinfarction patients. This signal-averaged electrocardiogram is not based upon the presence, absence, or inducibility of ventricular ectopic activity (VEA). Rather, the signal-averaged ECG enables the noninvasive detection of ventricular late potentials. These regions of delayed potentials may represent the area of slow conduction which is a prerequisite for a reentrant mechanism of arrhythmia. This capability of detecting the presence of late potentials can provide important prognostic information in identifying patients who may have the EP substrate for ventricular reentry and subsequent arrhythmic events.

Several studies have found that the presence of ventricular late potentials in patients with an AMI is an independent predictor of sudden cardiac death (9, 12). A recent analysis has determined that an abnormal signal-averaged ECG compared to controls independently predicted an eightfold increase in the risk of arrhythmic events (9). An abnormal signal-averaged ECG combined with the presence of clinical factors such as ventricular arrhythmias on ambulatory monitoring and depressed ventricular function can identify a population at very high risk for arrhythmic events in the first year after infarction (30%). Conversely, patients with a normal signal-averaged ECG are at low risk for arrhythmic events (≤5%) (13). While the absence of late potentials is associated with low risk, the presence of late potentials is of less predictive value.

## INDUCIBLE VENTRICULAR TACHYARRHYTHMIA

Since the occurrence of malignant ventricular tachyarrhythmias after hospital discharge is the major cause of death in postinfarction patients after the first year, greater efforts to identify high-risk groups are necessary. Recent experience with EP testing has demonstrated predictive value to stratify survivors of infarction patients into a large group at low risk and a smaller group at high risk of late arrhythmias during follow-up. Most studies have demonstrated that the absence of inducible ventricular tachyarrhythmia portends a good prognosis independent of the extent of LV dysfunction, but the predictive value of a positive test remains controversial. Nevertheless, many centers have been unwilling to apply risk stratification with EP testing after infarction. Programmed ventricular stimulation probably identifies a specific mechanism for malignant ventricular tachyarrhythmias, but it is an invasive procedure and not ideally suited as a screening test in a large number of patients. Pedretti and co-workers have identified a small subgroup of patients characterized by a low EF, ventricular late potentials, and repetitive VEA on ambulatory monitoring (14). In these preselected patients with a high prevalence of events, programmed ventricular stimulation was useful in improving prognostic accuracy. Consequently, combined use of noninvasive tests and EP studies selected with a good sensitivity (81%) a group of postinfarction patients at high arrhythmic risk (65% event rate) to be considered candidates for therapy guided by EP testing or use of an implantable cardioverter defibrillator.

Noninvasive factors like depressed EF, high-grade ventricular ectopic activity on ambulatory monitoring, and ventricular late potentials appear to be useful in identifying a group of surviving infarction patients with a significantly higher incidence of late malignant ventricular tachyarrhythmias. Although stratification on the basis of noninvasive risk factors could be applied to diminish the proportion of surviving acute infarction patients receiving EP, few data are available regarding the usefulness of all these prognostic variables in combination to evaluate arrhythmic propensity (Fig. 2). Inducible VT by EP study, an EF below 40% by MUGA, and an abnormal signal-averaged ECG accounted for nearly all the increased risk of cardiac death in postinfarction patients in a study reported by Richards and co-workers (15). Stress testing to induce arrhythmias in the exercise state did not predict outcome in this population. Current research does not support the stratification of patients into different risk categories depending on whether VT can be induced in asymptomatic patients with recent infarction (16).

## HEART RATE VARIABILITY

The use of ambulatory electrocardiographic monitoring to assess heart rate over 24 hours has been suggested

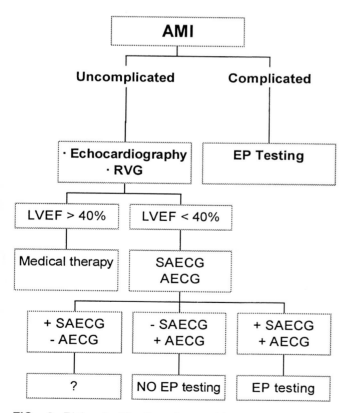

**FIG. 2.** Risk stratification for sudden cardiac death. SAECG, signal-averaged electrocardiogram; AECG, 24-hour ambulatory ECG; EP, electrophysiology; RVG, radio-nuclide ventriculography.

as a means of identifying high-risk patients. The normal variation in heart rate routinely measured by an RR interval on ambulatory monitor may be caused by sympathovagal influences on the heart. Several adult models of MI with sudden death have stressed the protective function of vagally mediated reflex heart rate responses to acute ischemia. Animals with well-preserved vagal reflexes are much less likely to develop ventricular fibrillation. The loss of normal heart rate variability in patients surviving an infarction has been closely associated with subsequent sudden death and all cause mortality (17). Therefore, analysis of heart rate variability provides additional predictive power. The combination of analysis of signal-averaged ECG and heart rate variability may hold significant promise as a risk stratification strategy in that it identifies patients with a potential anatomic substrate for ventricular tachyarrhythmias in whom the presence of abnormal autonomic tone may initiate ventricular arrhythmias. However, until the two techniques are studied adequately, their use remains uncertain of proven clinical utility. Further investigations are necessary to determine whether decreased heart rate variability is an independent predictor of arrhythmic death.

The value of prognostic tests must be judged against the cost and benefits of therapy. Noninvasive assessment offers a relatively inexpensive and simple method of risk stratification. If more expensive strategies such as an implantable defibrillator or EP testing are to be used, a highly specific test that minimizes false-positive results is required, and the choice of selection criteria will reflect this. The combination techniques of assessing heart rate variability and late potentials may be an appropriate method of selecting patients at high risk in whom such strategies could be applied.

## POSTINFARCTION ANGINA

In the prethrombolytic era, early postinfarction angina generally implied an unfavorable short- and long-term prognosis. Herlitz and co-workers showed that the quantity of analgesics used to relieve angina pain correlated with mortality and cardiac complications (18). Those patients requiring more analgesics had a 2-year mortality of 29% and a probability of developing heart failure of 63.6%, compared to 2.7% and 29.6%, respectively, for those requiring less. Being free of pain, nevertheless, did not indicate reperfusion of the infarct-related artery. More recently, the timely administration of thrombolytic therapy has been shown to improve both survival and ventricular function in patients with an AMI. Silva and colleagues showed that recurrent ischemia (24 hours postinfarction) after thrombolytic therapy identified a subgroup of patients who were at greater risk of early reinfarction, other hospital cardiac events, and emergency revascularization (19). Clinical or angiographic characteristics appear not to predict recurrent ischemic events in postthrombolytic therapy patients. In all probability, the long-term prognostic implications of angina symptoms in the immediate postinfarction period is not likely to be thoroughly investigated due to the introduction of thrombolytics, the widespread availability of percutaneous transluminal coronary angioplasty (PTCA), and the universally held perception that postinfarction angina implies a need for revascularization. The consensus that infarction patients with angina are at greater risk than those without such angina is based upon limited data.

## EXERCISE STRESS TESTING

The benchmark of any stress test is defined by its ability to noninvasively select a patient population at high risk for subsequent cardiac events so that interventions to prevent them may be considered. The safety of exercise testing prior to hospital discharge is now established. Within 1 month of infarction, exercise testing reveals an overall complication rate of 0.02%, with nonfatal, nonsustained VT being the most commonly encountered problem. The utility of stress testing is largely attributed to the use of standardized protocols for test performance and interpretation. Pre–hospital discharge submaximal exercise testing after an uncomplicated AMI has greater predictive power (higher risk ratios) than does postdischarge maximal testing. That is, predischarge testing at low work loads is better able to determine which patients are at increased risk after infarction. In contrast, postdischarge abnormal exercise responses obtained at higher work loads have less predictive value. Although most clinicians recommend a submaximal exercise test prior to discharge, a maximal test probability is usually done when the patient is able to return to full activity. Patients excluded from either predischarge or postdischarge exercise testing for clinical reasons have the highest short-term mortality, the 1-year death rate ranging from 18% to 32% (20). Correspondingly, the 1-year mortality is approximately 5% in patients undergoing exercise testing (21). Current practice is to attempt to resolve residual ischemia as detected by stress testing through cardiac catheterization and institution of appropriate medical interventional and/or surgical therapy.

Confirmation of postinfarction ischemia via exercise testing indicates that additional cardiac muscle is in jeopardy of being infarcted. Correlation of this finding is not available from other risk stratification techniques of postinfarction patients. Numerous studies document as much as a tenfold increase in mortality in patients with a positive exercise test soon after an AMI. Prior to reperfusion therapy, a first-year 27% total mortality rate in patients with ST depression had been observed, in contrast to a 2% total mortality in patients without ST depression (22). Sudden death mortality in patients with

and without ST depression was 16% and 17%, respectively. Patients with symptoms or signs of myocardial ischemia during exercise testing have usually been found on coronary angiography to have severe multivessel disease. In those patients established to be at high risk for increased mortality and morbidity, additional testing can be undertaken to determine whether or not revascularization procedures would be beneficial. Those at low risk can avoid unnecessary further testing. In postinfarction patients, interpretation of exercise test results can be confounding. Uncertainty exists concerning which variables (ST shifts, systolic blood pressure response, angina, exercise capacity, and VEA) have the most predictive value. In Froelicher's study, exercise-induced ST depression, angina, and VEA were not consistent predictors of cardiovascular death (20). Despite the limitation of the study, they concluded that poor exercise capacity, an abnormal systolic blood pressure response, and ventricular dysfunction are the variables that best predict outcome in patients with Q-wave infarctions. Exercise-induced ST depression was most predictive in patients with a first non-Q-wave infarction and could be used to determine which patients with non-Q-wave infarction have a significant risk of cardiovascular death. Generally, angina and ST depression during exercise testing are markers for the presence of ischemia, whereas abnormalities in the maximal systolic blood pressure response, heart rate response, and exercise capacity are markers for both ventricular dysfunction and ischemia (Fig. 3).

To determine the mortality of postinfarction patients, other prognostic factors including age, clinical status, history of previous infarctions, presence of resting ST-segment abnormalities, type and location of the index infarction, and amount of LV damage need to be considered when interpreting a patient's response to exercise testing.

## AGE

An important risk predictor for mortality is age. Mortality in the first year postinfarction is estimated to be approximately 25% in patients older than 75 years and less than 5% in those under 50. Roubin and colleagues demonstrated overall survival rates of 96% and 95% in the first and second years, respectively, in survivors aged 60 or younger (23). The high survival rates in younger patients can be attributed to the prevalence (58%) of single-vessel disease. The effect of age on prognosis can be explained by the greater chance of multivessel disease, underlying LV dysfunction, or cardiac arrhythmias present. All these factors may complicate the postinfarction course. Furthermore, in the elderly, reduced cardiovascular reserve, noncompliant ventricles with greater predisposition to high LV end-diastolic pressure and pulmonary edema, as well as a greater chance of not recognizing infarction can increase mortality. Finally,

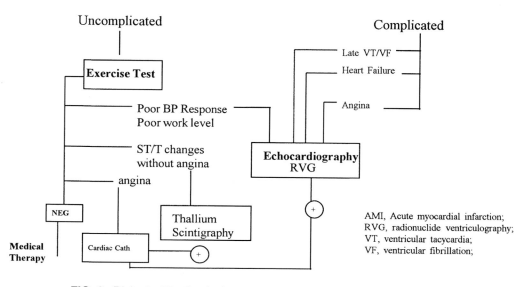

AMI
(Post thrombolysis)

**FIG. 3.** Risk stratification before hospital discharge in patients with AMI.

certain treatment modalities such as contrast studies carry a higher risk in the elderly in whom multiple comorbidities can compound the clinical problems that might arise. Selecting the optimal therapy for the elderly patient is difficult, weighing the risks of thrombolysis or PTCA against the risk of a conservative medical approach. The use of thrombolytic agents must be weighed against the potential risk of intracranial bleeding, the risk for bleeding being approximately three times greater than for younger patients. Many of the large studies have excluded the elderly in the selection criteria, and thus we have little information of various approaches in the elderly. Less than 5% of elderly are actually given thrombolytics for AMI. Recent data pooled from several large trials suggesting an overall mortality reduction of approximately 20% in the elderly are similar to the results in patients less than 65 (14% to 34%) (24). Potentially, the elderly may receive the greatest survival benefit from thrombolysis, due to the large numbers of infarctions observed in the elderly and the overall higher mortality rate.

## CLINICAL STATUS

Patients at highest risk for early death are those with evidence of extensive myocardial damage. Those with findings that suggest extensive areas of ischemia have an increased risk of angina and reinfarction but a lower risk of early death. The myocardial damage is more serious in the high-risk group, but the extent of distribution is fixed.

In the ischemic population, there is less initial damage but a greater potential for further destruction. Findings that signal an increased risk of early death include a higher CPK in the absence of thrombolysis, symptoms of congestive heart failure, electrocardiographic evidence of large or multiple Q-waves, right or left bundle branch block, LV hypertrophy with strain, and chest film abnormalities of pulmonary edema (Table 1). In patients considered to be at high risk, it is imperative to ascertain whether or not the infarct-related artery has reperfused.

**TABLE 1.** *Electrocardiographic and clinical markers of poor prognosis following acute myocardial infarction*

| |
| --- |
| Indication of extensive myocardial damage[a] |
|   Cardiogenic shock |
|   Pulmonary edema or other chest film abnormalities |
|   Congestive heart failure |
|   Elevated creatinine phosphokinase release (in absence of thrombolysis) |
|   Left ventricular hypertrophy with strain |
|   Right ventricular infarction |
|   Complete heart block |
|   Large and/or multiple Q waves |
|   Left or right bundle branch block |
| Indication of extensive myocardium remaining ischemic[b] |
|   Continued ischemic chest pain and ST changes |
|   Resting ST depression |

[a]High risk of early death.
[b]Lower risk of early death but higher likelihood of reinfarction and angina.

Commonly, this may be appreciated on clinical grounds such as pain relief, ST-segment normalization, and reperfusion arrhythmias. A prospective evaluation of these factors found that rapid onset of reperfusion arrhythmias identified patients with patent infarct-related arteries 95% of the time. A reduction of 50% or more in ST-segment elevation predicted successful reperfusion in 97% of cases (25). Moss and Benhorin showed that patients with a first infarction can expect a better initial outcome than those who previously had suffered an infarction (21). Sixty percent to 80% of all infarctions are first infarctions. Sudden death rather than recurrent infarction accounts for approximately 50% of all cause mortality, but whether these deaths are mediated by ischemia versus an underlying arrhythmic mechanism remains unknown.

## RESTING ST DEPRESSION

Resting ST depression appears to increase the risk of an adverse outcome in patients. Miranda and associates evaluated the prognostic significance of resting ST depression, exercise test results, and coronary angiographic data (26). The prevalence of severe coronary artery disease defined as three-vessel disease or left main artery disease was two and one-half times greater in AMI patients with resting ST depression than in patients without resting ST depression (43% and 17%, respectively). Other studies indicate that patients with non-Q-wave infarction and resting ST depression have a markedly increase risk of reinfarction and death. The occurrence of silent ischemia on the ECG is also associated with a high incidence of reinfarction.

## MYOCARDIAL INFARCTION TYPE AND LOCATION

With the proliferation of potential therapeutic options and risk stratification, prognosis appears to be affected by the type and location of the infarction. While most first-year postinfarction deaths are attributed to Q-wave infarcts, deaths after year 1 are associated with non-Q-wave ECG findings. Patients with non-Q-wave infarctions suffer less damage but a greater amount of myocardium remains at risk compared to those with Q-wave infarctions. Non-Q-wave infarctions are more common in patients having a second or third infarction which compounds the comparative risk. The incidences of heart failure and death rates in the first year are higher in patients with Q-wave infarctions, although patients with non-Q-wave infarcts have more angina symptoms. Infarct-free survival rate after 4 to 5 years is comparable in patients with both Q- and non-Q-wave infarcts (27). Long-term survival may depend more on severity of coronary artery disease than on Q-wave status.

Mortality of the first Q-wave infarction is higher among those with anterior wall infarctions than those with an inferior lateral type. In inferior wall infarcts, the presence of complete heart block and/or associated right ventricular infarct increases mortality. However, infarction location may be less important than infarct size. In some studies, the location of infarction does not have an independent predictive value once the analysis is adjusted for the effect of infarct size (28). The observation that early reperfusion of patent infarct-related arteries in 25% of Q-wave infarctions compared with patency rates of 54% to 74% in non-Q-wave infarctions indicates less myocardial damage and early reperfusion in survivors of non-Q-wave infarctions (29). Persisting viable muscle may be important in maintaining regional contractility and preventing infarct expansion. After non-Q-wave infarcts, patients manifest evidence of postinfarction ischemia during noninvasive evaluation such as exercise testing and thallium scintigraphy. More extensive evaluation may be necessary in this population. Thallium scintigraphic studies by Gibson and colleagues have shown that greater cardiac complications (reinfarction, unstable angina, sudden death) occur after non-Q-wave infarction due to a larger residual mass of jeopardized myocardium within the perfusion zone of the infarct-related vessel (30). Although several studies suggest that non-Q-wave infarctions have a frequent recurrence rate with an ominous prognosis, the apparent difference in prognosis between Q-wave and non-Q-wave infarction lessens when larger, prospective studies are examined.

## EFFECTS OF MEDICATIONS

Approximately 25% of patients with AMI have received thrombolytic therapy. Although little information exists on how patients given thrombolytic therapy respond to exercise testing, most clinicians believe that risk stratification for patients given thrombolytics can be interpreted in a similar fashion to that for other postinfarction populations. In evaluating the patient response to exercise testing, the contributing role of nitrates, beta-blockers, calcium-blockers, and other vasodilators must be considered. In these patients, valid prognostic statements cannot be made from blood pressure response alone. The goal of medical therapy after infarction is to reduce myocardial oxygen demand by decreasing the afterload, heart rate, or both. This strategy can ultimately lower the ischemic threshold, thereby affecting the exercise-induced ST-segment response. However, most of these drugs do not appear to effect exercise test performance characteristics such as sensitivity and specificity, but rather can actually improve exercise capacity.

## TECHNOLOGY: IDENTIFYING PATIENTS AT RISK

In the postinfarction population, a definitive noninvasive method for detection of myocardial viability within the potential ischemic risk area is required. Diagnostic and prognostic testing must be performed to establish the high-, moderate-, and low-risk level for future cardiac events. Establishing ischemia often leads to cardiac catheterization to define high-risk anatomy and plans for interventional strategies. Coronary angiography alone cannot be used to identify viable myocardium within an ischemic risk area. The focus of interest has shifted from infarct size as a prognostic and therapeutic end point to the noninvasive determinants of the functional correlation of myocardial viability. Angiographic evidence of reperfusion, either spontaneous or postthrombolysis, when correlated with noninvasive markers of myocardial perfusion, metabolism, and regional function, provides the most thorough description of myocardial salvage post-AMI. Of the widely available noninvasive techniques besides ECG stress testing, thallium scintigraphy, radionuclide ventriculography, and two-dimensional echocardiography, can be used to provide valuable insights into tissue viability in the postinfarction setting and determine prognosis.

Combination of noninvasive assessment for residual ischemia with quantification of LV function allows more accurate prediction of first-year postinfarction complications. Although the exercise ECG test is the most feasible, cost-effective, noninvasive test presently available in clinical practice for prognostication, a major limitation of the stress test is that it cannot be interpreted in many patients because of either abnormalities in the baseline ECG or the inability for patients to reach the level of exercise required for near-maximum effort, due to coexisting noncardiac diseases, severe ventricular dysfunction, or angina at rest. Accordingly, certain groups of patients who undergo stress testing may be selective patients at lower risk for subsequent death.

Since the risks of infarction are related to total myocardial damage, including degree of previous infarct damage, imaging techniques that delineate global and regional function provide a comprehensive assessment of myocardial damage. The measurement of global EF by echocardiography or radionuclide ventriculography and delineation of coronary anatomy via contrast ventriculography give an estimate of in-hospital and late prognosis of AMI and the possible need for revascularization.

The ability to detect the presence and location of ischemic myocardium is more important than establishing the presence of anatomic coronary artery disease since anatomic pathology does not necessarily imply myocardial ischemia. Supplementing nuclear imaging techniques to pre–hospital discharge stress testing enhances sensitivity for the diagnosis of myocardial ischemia. Thallium stress scintigraphy helps define patients at low risk even if the exercise ECG is abnormal. Silverman and colleagues, employing resting thallium scintigraphy to stratify patients into high- and low-risk groups on the basis of extent of infarction, showed that

high-risk patients had both an increased in-hospital mortality rate and a mortality rate greater than 80% at 9 months, in contrast to the mortality rate in patients judged to be at low risk on the basis of thallium studies (31).

Exercise radionuclide ventriculography enhances the predictive value for cardiac complications compared to exercise ECG alone, especially for death and recurrent infarcts. Significant differences between patients with and without a major cardiac event are lower resting EFs, lower peak exercise EF, greater number of regional wall motion abnormalities, high resting end-diastolic and end-systolic volumes, and a subnormal increase in contractility with exercise.

In patients with high risk who often are unable to exercise, risk remains high even if the exercise test is negative. Radionuclide perfusion scanning with dipyridamole-thallium, radionuclide EF at rest and with exercise, or echocardiography postexercise enhances the sensitivity of exercise testing to identify ischemic myocardium. For postinfarction patients unable to exercise due to musculoskeletal problems, pulmonary disease, or clinical heart failure, pharmacologic stress testing using dipyridamole, dobutamine adenosine, and thallium has assisted in defining the myocardium at risk. These techniques have similar predictive capabilities to exercise testing. Pierard and colleagues studying pre–hospital discharge low-dose dobutamine stress echocardiography in AMI patients receiving thrombolysis found a potential role for dobutamine in differentiating stunned from necrotic myocardium (32). Detection of myocardial ischemia and assessment of the reversibility of myocardial damage can occur by charting the changes to titrated doses of dobutamine. Available limited studies suggest that low-dose dobutamine may be equivalent to delayed thallium scintigraphy and superior to sestamibi scintigraphy (32, 33). One could hypothesize that due to dobutamine's reliance on the presence of myocardial contractile reserve, it may be a better predictor of the viability of the heart after an acute infarct.

The ECG obtained at discharge cannot accurately estimate the extent of myocardial damage aborted by thrombolytic therapy or acute PTCA. The inability to predict the extent of myocardial damage is due to the inherent deficiencies in the surface ECG, the effect of collaterals to the infarcted region, as well as anatomic variations in the coronary arteries themselves. This limitation emphasizes the importance of assessing both jeopardized and salvaged myocardium after an infarction. Recent application of $^{99m}$Tc-sestamibi, a nonredistributing radionuclide agent in the evaluation of thrombolytic and interventional therapy with infarctions, can provide an estimate of salvaged myocardium (34). Imaging with $^{99m}$Tc-sestamibi accurately estimates infarct size, quantitates the extent of salvage myocardium after coronary reperfusion, and is helpful in establishing prognosis. Serial sestamibi studies clearly offer a more objective and discriminatory approach to management of patients after thrombolytic therapy.

Myocardial salvage achieved by thrombolytic therapy or PTCA can be determined by comparing pre-reperfusion studies with that obtained prior to hospital discharge. A predischarge study of greater than 30% reduction in infarct size suggests a significant salvaged myocardium and correlates with continued patency of the infarct-related vessel, a good predictor of late recovery of myocardial function. The presence of extensive myocardium at risk as demonstrated by relatively small, persistent defects on serial sestamibi studies may identify a subgroup who might benefit from revascularization of the residual stenosis in the infarct-related vessel. The $^{99m}$Tc-sestamibi should yield beneficial information regarding the efficacy of various treatment strategies for acute infarction.

## ECHOCARDIOGRAPHY

Echocardiography can assess a spectrum of complications related to infarctions and provide useful prognostic information in the postinfarction phase. Semiquantitative Doppler echocardiography has evolved and now supplements standard two-dimensional echocardiography. Studies using EF or wall motion indexes from two-dimensional studies have demonstrated predictive value for risks of early complications that are superior to that provided by historical, ECG analysis, and clinical risk stratification (35, 36). Several indices have been formulated that assign a score on the basis of a given myocardial segment's motion. This scoring index estimates the extent of MI. Such indices have been used to predict in-hospital complications of early infarction and identify those at high risk for LV failure, malignant ventricular arrhythmias, or death. Evaluating prognosis is an important measure in the convalescent phase following an infarction. Applegate and co-workers showed that in those patients with uncomplicated infarction low-level exercise echocardiography during the recovery phase was highly predictive of subsequent cardiac events (37). Specifically, patients in whom a wall motion defect at rest worsened with exercise or in those in whom a wall motion defect developed with exercise were at high risk over a mean follow-up of 11 months. In this study and others, exercise ST-segment deviation on a modified Naughton treadmill protocol did not prove to be prognostically important. A decline in EF with exercise has also been used to predict cardiac events but is not as reliable as an indicator as is regional wall motion abnormalities. Exercise two-dimensional echocardiography has been shown to have an overall sensitivity of 75% to 80% and a specificity of 90% to 95%, which compares favorably with a predictive value and diagnostic accuracy of radionuclide scintigraphy (38). Furthermore, exercise echocardiography is less costly and involves no radiation exposure. It has great value in the diagnosis and guidance of therapeutic interventions and establishment of both short- and long-term prognosis.

Studies combining submaximal stress echocardiography with myocardial perfusion imaging or radionuclide ventriculography predict future cardiac events with highest accuracy. Due to the declining incidence of cardiac events over time and the selection bias produced by including lower risk patients, studies performed long after occurrence of the index infarctions have shown less dramatic results. Clearly, the earlier the risk stratification is used, the greater the impact. Noninvasive predischarge functional imaging techniques to unmask patients with potentially jeopardized myocardium does identify high-risk patients who may need further invasive studies and/or surgical or other interventional therapy. Postdischarge risk stratification via nuclear imaging may provide vital prognostic information in high- and low-risk patients, allowing for appropriate allocation of medical resources.

## THROMBOLYTIC THERAPY AND PTCA

The pragmatic consideration of infarction management revolves around risk assessment and the development of a treatment strategy. Extensive investigations support the use of reperfusion therapy in the early phase of infarction. Thrombolytic therapy is expected to reopen about 75% of thrombosed arteries with a reocclusion rate of approximately 10% to 15% (39). Salvage angioplasty successfully employed on arteries that remain occluded postthrombolysis appear to achieve similar short- and long-term mortality rates as successful thrombolysis alone. However, there is an associated procedural morbidity and high reocclusion rate. Abbottsmith and co-workers observed a mortality rate of 39% in patients in whom rescue PTCA was unsuccessful compared with a 5.9% mortality rate when successful (40). The reocclusion rate in initially successful procedures was 21%. Evaluation of invasive salvage procedures must consider morbidity of diagnostic catheterization undertaken in patients who do not quality for PTCA and morbidity in patients where PTCA will fail. The increased risk of procedures in the elderly along with a frequently unfavorable coronary anatomy may suggest an attempt to limit PTCA in this population. The PTCA could be relevant in the context of infarction in high risk where reperfusion and myocardial salvage is expected to be essential for survival. However, the potential for increasing morbidity dictates that each patient be individually assessed as to the risk and potential benefit of intervention. At present, it seems reasonable that only patients with large infarcts usually related to occlusion of a single major artery with persistent angina and/or hemodynamic instability be considered for PTCA after thrombolytic therapy. The role of PTCA after thrombolysis to ensure patency of infarct-related arteries in patients with otherwise small or uncomplicated infarctions remains to be clarified. Invasive investigations are usually necessary in this time period for those patients who develop recurrent angina, persistent CHF, and complex arrhythmias. In those patients who remain asymptomatic, predischarge risk assessment should be considered. For example, of 100 postinfarct patients who remain asymptomatic at discharge, 20% to 30% will have inducible ischemia upon noninvasive testing and 50% to 60% will have absolutely no symptoms (41). Regular exercise stress testing remains the test of choice for most of these patients. If results are very positive, coronary angiography will need to be considered. Evidence of postinfarction ischemia on noninvasive testing indicates a high risk in addition to the overall risk resulting from residual LV dysfunction and coronary anatomy. Controversy exists on whether the decision for angiography is to be established on the presence of ischemia, independent of ventricular dysfunction.

In the prethrombolytic era, the 1- and 6-year mortality rates were 14% and 42%, respectively, for AMI patients discharged from the hospital. In the era of thrombolytic therapy the mortalities have fallen in the range of 3% to 5% for the first year and 11% to 13% for 6 years, contributing to a 60% to 75% reduction in mortality since the 1960s (42). The decrease in MI mortality has been shown for both early and late mortality. This decline in mortality is related to the reduction in arrhythmic deaths and the use of beta-blocking agents and thrombolytic therapy. Mortality still remains high in patients not undergoing thrombolytic therapy, in the elderly (greater than 70 years), in patients with multiple infarctions and/or severe LV dysfunction, and in those with ventricular arrhythmias. Thrombolysis has been shown to be effective in reducing the incidence of life-threatening in-hospital arrhythmias and of improving ventricular function. Several recent studies indicate that reperfusion following thrombolysis modulates late potentials and consequently reduces the prevalence of ventricular late potentials.

Few studies have evaluated the predictive power of risk stratification in patients who have undergone reperfusion therapy. A study of the predictive power of exercise testing suggests that exercise testing provides limited prognostic information in the patients who had reperfusion therapy during the acute phase of infarction. Thirty percent of patients with either a positive exercise test or positive thallium perfusion response to exercise had a cardiac event at 1 year follow-up, compared with 49% of patients who did not receive thrombolytics but had a positive test (43). The TIMI II study suggested that the lack of provoked ischemia on predischarge exercise tests predicts a good result with continued medical therapy in those patients without spontaneous ischemia (44). This suggests that angiography may be deferred until ischemia occurs either spontaneously or under provocation. Further investigation is necessary to specifically define high-risk groups. An algorithm for predischarge risk evaluation for MI patients receiving reperfusion therapy has been developed by the ACC/AHA Joint Task Force (45). Essentially,

predischarge evaluation of a jeopardized myocardium should be undertaken on all reperfused patients and, in most circumstances, patients with clinical features suggesting high risk should have angiography unless there are procedural risks. In low-risk patients, predischarge low-level exercise testing or symptom-limited exercise testing soon after discharge is recommended.

One concept that may significantly impact stratification in the postthrombolytic area is that of the patent infarct-related artery. The TIMI I trial demonstrated that the patency rate achieved with thrombolysis was 31% initially but increased to 73% prior to hospital discharge (46). Schröder and colleagues observed improvement in EF to be greater in patients in whom initial thrombolysis was incomplete but in whom patency was subsequently achieved compared to those with a persistently occluded vessel (47). In the situation of delayed thrombolysis, patients having an infarction with a patent infarct-related artery are less likely to have EP findings associated with an increased risk for sudden death compared to patients with an occluded infarct artery. Such findings have significant implications for the routine management of postinfarction patients, including justifying attempts to open infarct-related arteries even after infarction has occurred with PTCA. Risk stratification can help identify those patients for whom this aggressive approach is probably beneficial.

## CORONARY ANGIOGRAPHY

Coronary angiography appears to be the most direct approach for evaluating for jeopardized myocardium and spontaneous ischemia. Angiographic criteria for high risk are related to both the number of vessels involved and the EF. The anterior descending artery disease has been shown to have important prognostic significance. However, conclusions derived from angiographic analysis in patients who have undergone angiography on at least two occasions suggest that coronary atherosclerosis progression is unpredictable. High-grade lesions not infrequently may be found to be unaltered over years while total occlusion may be observed within a short term in regions which had been previously normal or minimally diseased at the time of the initial study (48). Consequently, coronary angiography is best recognized as a technique for evaluating the anatomic status of the coronary vasculature at a given point in time. It is of limited value as a predictive variable in determining either site or rate of disease progression.

## RISK STRATIFICATION: EMERGENCY DEPARTMENT

Risk stratification for MI begins within the emergency department, based on evidence or suspicion of the likelihood of a jeopardized myocardium. Patients at high risk for massive infarctions need to be identified early so that thrombolytic therapy or other interventions can be undertaken early if thrombolytic therapy is unsatisfactory or contraindicated. Additional stratification after admission is performed based on evidence or suspicion of large areas of jeopardized myocardium. Patient outcome with thrombolytic therapy depends entirely on getting the treatment to appropriate candidates within the first several hours of AMI symptoms. To maximize the effectiveness of thrombolytic therapy in clinical practice, an approach that specifically identifies those patients most likely to benefit from thrombolytic therapy in the clinical setting needs to evolve. A set of outcome predictors actually adjusted for risk is needed to objectively monitor thrombolytic effectiveness and provide useful performance feedback. Furthermore, there is currently a great need for validating clinically based predictors of important outcomes of care for acute infarction. Over the past decade, Selker and associates have developed a predictive instrument for MI, the Thrombolytic Predictive Instrument (TPI) (49). The TPI consists of a set of predictive models developed primarily using multivariate logistic regression to indicate a measure of acute infarction severity, determine probabilities of acute and long-term mortality, evaluate complications of thrombolytic therapy, assess the likelihood of cardiac arrest postinfarction, and judge physician and hospital performance. Multicenter trials are now underway employing this predictive model to assess its applicability.

One of the first predictive models, employed by Pozen and co-workers utilizing multiple logistic regression modeling, attempted to enhance the emergency room clinicians' diagnostic decisions so that fewer patients without ischemia would be admitted to CCUs. The model provided a numerical probability of a patient's likelihood of having acute cardiac ischemia (50).

## MEDICAL TREATMENT

Specific medical and/or other interventional treatment decisions for MI can be guided by findings on risk stratification. Studies investigating the role of beta-blocker therapy for prevention of recurrent infarction and reducing sudden death found reduced morbidity and mortality in patients on beta-blockers, independent of thrombolysis (51). Approximately 20% fewer deaths occurred in patients receiving therapy than in patients receiving placebo. Although the consistent results of a vast number of patients studied provide a strong basis for beta-blocker therapy postinfarction, the benefits of therapy appear only to be within the first year after infarction. No study has documented a reduction in morbidity, mortality, or reinfarction with calcium channel blocker therapy as compared with placebo therapy. Though routine use of calcium channel blockers postinfarction has not yet been recommended, a post hoc analysis of the diltiazem trial did document a reduction in incidence of unstable angina in patients with non-Q-wave infarcts without signs of heart failure (52).

Recent trials with angiotensin-converting enzyme (ACE) inhibitors have established preservation of LV function and an increase in functional capacity independent of thrombolytics, beta-blockers, or aspirin (53). In a trial involving 2,200 patients who have had an AMI resulting in a left ventricular EF of 40% or less, patients who were assigned to receive ace inhibitors or placebo beginning 3 to 16 days after an AMI were followed 2 to 5 years after randomization. The ACE inhibitor group showed a 17% reduction in mortality from all causes, although not evident until 10 months after randomization, and at the median follow-up interval of 3.6 years, the mortality benefit was still increasing. Hospitalization for congestive heart failure symptoms were decreased 19% and reinfarction rates decreased 24% in the ACE inhibitor group.

The Cardiac Arrhythmia Suppression Trial (CAST) was designed to assess whether suppression of asymptomatic or mildly symptomatic ventricular arrhythmia postinfarction in low-risk patients reduced sudden death, cardiovascular mortality, and total mortality. The CAST indicated that type I antiarrhythmic agents significantly elevated the relative risk of death and cardiac arrest in patients with both non-Q-wave and Q-wave infarcts (54). An important result of CAST I is the possibility that antiarrhythmics were responsible for late proarrhythmic effects, since patients receiving either agent had higher death rates from all causes, including from arrhythmias, than did placebo. This study emphasizes the potential hazards of antiarrhythmic drugs in low-risk populations. Therefore, the risks and benefits of such therapies must be considered in postinfarction patients with ventricular arrhythmias. It would be premature to extend the results of CAST to all drugs and all postinfarction patients. No conclusions can be drawn about type I antiarrhythmic agents in postinfarction patients with symptomatic or complex arrhythmia.

Cardiac rehabilitation has been formally evaluated for its impact on morbidity and mortality postinfarction. The role of exercise or multidisciplinary cardiac rehabilitation after infarction has been evaluated by two large meta-analyses (55, 56). These studies have established that cardiac rehabilitation provides up to 25% reduction in total and cardiovascular-related mortality rates. In the Multiple Risk Factor Intervention Research Trial, intense risk factor modification was associated with a decreased cardiac mortality of 57% in asymptomatic high-risk patients with an abnormal exercise test compared with those receiving usual care. Current recommendations for infarct survivors include low doses of aspirin (160 mg/day or 325 mg every other day). Studies with aspirin have shown reduction of death and nonfatal reinfarction by 13% and 31%, respectively (51).

## TREATMENT STRATEGIES

Likelihood ratios can be generated from various studies to help physicians select the type and sequence of diagnostic tests to be performed in assessing the risk of sudden death in post-AMI. This ratio demonstrates the probability that a diagnostic test result would be anticipated in a patient with a particular disorder (ventricular dysfunction, VEA) as opposed to the absence of this target disorder in another patient. This method can be used to determine the posttest probability of having a disorder and can index patients into high, intermediate, or low likelihood ratios (Table 2). Probability theory should play a major role in both the selection of treatment and determining the benefit-risk ratio of therapy.

It is self-evident that noninvasive testing can be used to identify a low likelihood ratio of postinfarction patients who require no further diagnostic evaluation. This low likelihood ratio group is characterized by having well-preserved LV function (EF > 40%), no significant ventricular ectopy on EP study, and no ST depression on exercise testing. The majority of patients surviving acute infarcts fall into this group. In the presence of multiple risk factors, the specificity and positive predictive value for development of life-threatening arrhythmia are greatest. It is reasonable to estimate that patients with poor LV function, frequent or complex ventricular ectopy, and an abnormal signal-averaged ECG have a 30% risk of sudden cardiac death within 2 years. Accordingly, signal-averaged ECG and an EP study should be considered in postinfarction patients who have a high likelihood ratio for sudden death. If the results are negative, no further

therapy or intervention appears to be essential. However, in patients with inducible sustained ventricular tachyarrhythmias, survival may be improved with a suppressive antiarrhythmic drug regimen or an automatic implantable defibrillator (Fig. 2).

Economic reasons increasingly are prompting clinicians to study outcome and its determinants. While an incorrect decision not to start therapy might result in an avoidable death, inappropriate diagnostic studies may cause meaningless suffering to a patient who is unlikely to benefit from such care. Furthermore, when attempting to provide good care for the fewest dollars, we must be cognizant of not only the charges of each test itself, but also the expense of the studies for evaluating each test or procedure. Consequently, since randomized control trials for every test or procedure become inordinately expensive, ethical consideration may preclude the use of controlled trials for many tests or procedures that are established as acceptable medical practice.

## LIMITATIONS TO POST-MI RISK STRATIFICATION:

Risk stratification is predicated by the hypothesis that a specific study parameter when measured at some defined point in time defines subgroups with varying risks for certain predetermined end points. In contrast to ICU severity models which have a probability of hospital mortality as an end point, coronary risk stratification studies employ broader terms of high, moderate, and low risk. Interpretation of these broad categories can vary depending on the time period (peri-infarct, predischarge, postdischarge) and the end point being evaluated. Additionally, few studies have incorporated multivariate techniques to compare relative risks of one potential variable to another. An illness severity scoring system can combine the relative ease of collection of data with a description of illness severity across a wide range of disorders and an excellent correlation with outcome.

It remains uncertain whether present concepts regarding risk stratification need to be modified in the thrombolytic era. Furthermore, the patient population in some of the studies have been analyzed by a retrospective post hoc analysis of a database obtained from infarction patients studies from some other protocol. Attempts to validate risk stratification investigations presume that the populations studied are homogeneous. If the population is heterogeneous, the statistical variations raised by such heterogeneity may not be counterbalanced by studying large populations and determining the mean. Indeed, these populations represent pooled databases of patients of diverse ages, disease states and therefore prognosis. Death, reinfarction, angina, or need for revascularization are frequently employed as end points in postinfarction risk stratification studies. Defining these end points postulates

---

**TABLE 2.** *Likelihood ratios for cardiac mortality and sudden death*

Low ratios
  Ejection fraction > 40%
  No inducible ventricular tachycardia on electrophysiologic study
  No ST depression on exercise testing
Intermediate ratios
  Abnormal signal-averaged electrocardiogram
  ST depression during stress testing
  Ejection fraction < 40%
High ratios
  ≥ 100 ventricular premature beats per hour
  Inducible ventricular tachycardia on electrophysiologic study
  Presence of three clinical factors: ST depression, cardiomegaly, prior myocardial infarction

Data derived from the following studies: Bigger JT, et al. *Am J Cardiol* 1981;48:815. Kostis JB, et al. *J Am Coll Cardiol* 1987;10:231. Richards DAB, et al. *Circulation* 1991;83:756. Theroux P, et al. *N Engl J Med* 1979;301:341.

that a particular end point either results from or is directly caused by the injury which causes the patient to be entered into the study in the first place. A methodologic dilemma arises due to the progression of coronary artery disease. Such progression is not necessarily limited to the infarct-related artery of the index infarct and the progression in non-infarct-related arteries can also result in death, reinfarct, angina development, or need for revascularization. The strong end point of the study becomes ambiguous since it cannot be definitely considered as a complication of the original infarct. Finally, the recent study by Frasure-Smith and colleagues found that major depression in hospitalized patients following an AMI is an independent risk factor for mortality at 6 months and at least equivalent to that of ventricular dysfunction, and a history of a previous infarction complicates the heterogeneity of the patient population studied (57).

## CONCLUSION

This review has attempted to analyze the current status of post-MI risk stratification. The goal of research is not only to prolong the lives of patients with MI but, more importantly, to identify the characteristics of healthy postinfarction populations who will experience early morbidity and mortality. This is of vital importance since the majority of patients with early postinfarction complications are classified as low risk according to stratifying variables. The development of better risk stratification will enhance postinfarction care and diminish morbidity and mortality by targeting therapies and/or diagnostic techniques to populations likely to benefit from them. Importantly, the ability to make an estimate of the probability of death or survival for the individual patient can be more important than merely categorizing the patient into a high- or low-risk group. Finally, the development of guidelines for patient subsets based upon risk stratification will alleviate some of the dogmatic mechanisms utilized by third-party payors and regulatory agencies.

## ACKNOWLEDGMENTS

The authors thank Suzanne Allen, Maureen Harbilas, and Mark Kennedy.

## REFERENCES

1. Moss AJ, Bigger JT Jr, Odoroff CL. Post-infarct risk stratification. *Prog Cardiovasc Dis* 1987;29(6):389.
2. The Multicenter Postinfarction Research Group. Risk stratification and survival after myocardial infarction. *N Engl J Med* 1983;309(6): 331.
3. Willems JL, Willems RJ, Willems GM, et al. Significance of initial ST segment elevation and depression for the management of thrombolytic therapy in acute myocardial infarction. *Circulation* 1990;82: 1147.
4. Bär FW, Vermeer F, de Zwaan C, et al. Value of the admission elec-
trocardiogram in predicting outcome of thrombolytic therapy in acute myocardial infarction. *Am J Cardiol* 1987;59:6.
5. Schulze RA Jr, Strauss HW, Pitt B. Sudden death in the year following myocardial infarction: relation to ventricular premature contractions in the late hospital phase and left ventricular ejection fraction. *Am J Med* 1977;62:192.
6. White HD, Norris RM, Brown MA, et al. Left ventricular end systolic volume as the major determinant of survival after recovery from myocardial infarction. *Circulation* 1987;76:44.
7. Bigger JT Jr, Weld FM, Rolnitzky LM. Prevalence, characteristics, and significance of ventricular tachycardia (three or more complexes) detected with ambulatory electrocardiographic recording in the late hospital phase of acute myocardial infarction. *Am J Cardiol* 1981;48: 815.
8. Moss AJ, Davis HT, DeCamilla J, et al. Ventricular ectopic beats and their relation to sudden and nonsudden cardiac death after myocardial infarction. *Circulation* 1979;60:998.
9. Steinberg JS, Regan A, Sciacca RR, et al. Predicting arrhythmic events after acute myocardial infarction using the signal-averaged electrocardiogram. *Am J Cardiol* 1992;69(1):13.
10. Kostis JB, Byington R, Friedman LM, et al. Prognostic significance of ventricular ectopic activity in survivors of acute myocardial infarction. *J Am Coll Cardiol* 1987;10:231.
11. Bigger JT Jr, Fleiss JL, Kleiger RE, et al. The Multicenter Postinfarction Research Group: the relationship between ventricular arrhythmias, left ventricular dysfunction and mortality in the two years after myocardial infarction. *Circulation* 1984;69:250.
12. Simpson MB. Use of signals in the terminal QRS complex to identify patients with ventricular tachycardia after myocardial infarction. *Circulation* 1981;64:235.
13. Kuchar DL. Role of the signal-averaged ECG in patients at risk for sudden cardiac death. In: Luceri RM, ed. *Sudden cardiac death: strategies for the `90s.* Mt. Kisco, NY: Futura; 1992:29.
14. Pedretti R, Etro M, Laporta A, et al. Prediction of late arrhythmic events after acute myocardial infarction from combined use of noninvasive prognostic variables and inducibility of sustained monomorphic ventricular tachycardia. *Am J Cardiol* 1993;71:1131.
15. Richards DAB, Byth K, Ross DL, et al. What is the best predictor of spontaneous ventricular tachycardia and sudden death after myocardial infarction. *Circulation* 1991;83:756.
16. Roy D, Marchard E, Theroux P, et al. Programmed ventricular stimulation in survivors of an acute myocardial infarction. *Circulation* 1985;72:487.
17. Herlitz J, Hjalmarson A, Holmberg S, et al. Variability, prediction and prognostic significance of chest pain in acute myocardial infarction. *Cardiology* 1986;73:13.
18. Kleiger RE, Miller JP, Bigger JT Jr, et al. The Multicenter Postinfarction Research Group: decreased heart rate variability and its association with increased mortality after acute myocardial infarction. *Am J Cardiol* 1987;59:256.
19. Silva P, Galli M, Campolo L, for the IRES (Ischemia Residual Study Group). Prognostic significance of early ischemia after acute myocardial infarction in low-risk patients. *Am J Cardiol* 1993;71:1142.
20. Froelicher VF, Perdue S, Pewen W, et al. Application of meta-analysis using an electronic spread sheet to exercise testing in patients after myocardial infarction. *Am J Med* 1987;83:1045.
21. Moss AJ, Benhorin J. Prognoses and management after a first myocardial infarction. *N Eng J Med* 1990;322:743.
22. Theroux P, Waters DD, Halphen C, et al. Prognostic value of exercise testing soon after myocardial infarction. *N Engl J Med* 1979;301:341.
23. Roubin GS, Harris PJ, Bernstein L, et al. Coronary anatomy and prognosis after myocardial infarction in patients 60 years of age and younger. *Circulation* 1983;67:743.
24. Krumholz HM, Pasternak RC, Weinstein MC, et al. Cost effectiveness of thrombolytic therapy with streptokinase in elderly patients with suspected acute myocardial infarction. *N Engl J Med* 1992;327: 7.
25. Hohnloser SH, Zabel M, Kasper W, et al. Assessment of coronary artery patency after thrombolytic therapy: accurate prediction utilizing the combined analysis of three noninvasive markers. *J Am Coll Cardiol* 1991;18:44.
26. Miranda CP, Lehmann KG, Froelicher VF. Correlation between resting ST-segment depression, exercise testing, coronary angiography, and long-term prognosis. *Am Heart J* 1991;122:1617.

27. Miranda CP, Herbert WG, Dubach P, et al. Post-myocardial infarction exercise testing: non Q-wave versus Q-wave correlation with coronary angiography and long-term prognosis. *Circulation* 1991;84:2357.

28. Buja LM, Willerson JT. Infarct size—can it be measured or modified in humans? *Prog Cardiovasc Dis* 1987;29:271.

29. Gibson RS. Clinical, functional, and angiographic distinctions between Q-wave and non-Q-wave myocardial infarction: evidence of spontaneous reperfusion and implications for intervention trials. *Circulation* 1987;75(Suppl 5):V-128.

30. Gibson RS, Beller GA, Gheorghiade M, et al. The prevalence and clinical significance of residual myocardial ischemia 2 weeks after uncomplicated non-Q-wave infarction: a prospective natural history study. *Circulation* 1986;73:1186.

31. Silverman KJ, Becker LC, Bulkley BH, et al. Value of early thallium-201 scintigraphy for predicting mortality in patients with acute myocardial infarction. *Circulation* 1980;61(5):996.

32. Pierard LA, DeLandsheere CM, Berthe C, et al. Identification of viable myocardium by echocardiography during dobutamine infusion in patients with myocardial infarction after thrombolytic therapy: comparison with positron emission tomography. *J Am Coll Cardiol* 1990;15:1021.

33. Marzullo P, Parodi O, Reisenhofer B, et al. Value of rest thallium-201/technetium-99m sestamibi scans and dobutamine echocardiography for detecting myocardial viability. *Am J Cardiol* 1993;71:166.

34. Christian TF, Clements IP, Gibbons RJ. Noninvasive identification of myocardium at risk in patients with acute myocardial infarction and nondiagnostic electrocardiograms with technetium-99m-sestamibi. *Circulation* 1991;83(5):1615.

35. Horowitz RS, Morganroth J. Immediate detection of early high-risk patients with acute myocardial infarction using two-dimensional echocardiographic evaluation of left ventricular regional wall motion abnormalities. *Am Heart J* 1982;103(5):814.

36. Sabia P, Afrookteh A, Touchstone DA, et al. Value of regional wall motion abnormality in the emergency room diagnoses of acute myocardial infarction: a prospective study using two-dimensional echocardiography. *Circulation* 1991;84(3 Suppl):185.

37. Applegate RJ, Dell'Italia LJ, Crawford MH. Usefulness of two-dimensional echocardiography during low-level exercise testing early after uncomplicated acute myocardial infarction. *Am J Cardiol* 1987;60(1):10.

38. Ryan T. Vasey CG, Feigenbaum H, et al. Exercise echocardiography: detection of coronary artery disease in patients with normal left ventricular wall motion at rest. *J Am Coll Cardiol* 1988;11:993.

39. Topol EJ, Califf RM, George BS, et al. A randomized trial of immediate versus delayed elective angioplasty after intravenous plasminogen activator in acute myocardial infarction. *N Engl J Med* 1987;317:581.

40. Abbottsmith CW, Topal EJ, George BS, et al. Fate of patients with acute myocardial infarction with patency of the infarct-related vessel achieved with successful thrombolysis versus rescue angioplasty. *J Am Coll Cardiol* 1990;16:770.

41. TIMI Group. Comparison of invasive and conservative strategies after treatment with intravenous tissue plasminogen activator in acute myocardial infarction. *N Engl J Med* 1989;320:618.

42. Yusuf S, Sleight P, Held P, McMahon S, et al. Routine medical management of acute myocardial infarction: lessons from overviews of recent randomized controlled trials. *Circulation* 1990;82(Suppl II):II-117.

43. Tilkemeier PL, Guiney TE, LaRaia PJ, Boucher CA. Prognostic value of predischarge low-level exercise thallium testing after thrombolytic treatment of acute myocardial infarction. *Am J Cardiol* 1990;66:1203.

44. Comparison of invasive and conservative strategies after treatment with intravenous tissue plasminogen activator in acute myocardial infarction. Results of the thrombolysis in myocardial infarction (TIMI) Phase II Trial. *New Engl J Med* 1989;320:618.

45. ACC/AHA Task Force on Assessment of Diagnostic and Therapeutic Cardiovascular Procedures. Guidelines for the early management of patients with acute myocardial infarction: a report of the ACC/AHA Task Force on Assessment of Diagnostic and Therapeutic Cardiovascular Procedures. *Circulation* 1990;82:664.

46. Chesebro JH, Knatterud G, Roberts R, et al. Thrombolysis in myocardial infarction (TIMI) Trial Phase I: a comparison between intravenous tissue plasminogen activator and intravenous streptokinase. Clinical findings through hospital discharge. *Circulation* 1987;76:142.

47. Schröder R, Neuhaus KL, Linderer T, et al. Impact of late coronary artery reperfusion on left ventricular function one month after acute myocardial infarction (results from the ISAM study). *Am J Cardiol* 1989;64:878.

48. Davies MJ. A macro and micro view of coronary vascular insult in ischemic heart disease. *Circulation* 1990;82(Suppl II):II38.

49. Selker HP, Griffith JL, D'Agostino RB. A time insensitive predictive instrument for acute myocardial infarction mortality: a multicenter study. *Med Care* 1991b;29:1196.

50. Pozen MW, D'Agostino RB, Laks MM. A predictive instrument for acute ischemic heart disease to improve coronary care unit admission practices in acute ischemic heart disease. *New Engl J Med* 1984;310:1273.

51. Yusuf S, Wittes J, Friedman L. Overview of results of randomized clinical trials in heart disease. I. Treatments following myocardial infarction. *JAMA* 1988;260(14):2088.

52. Gibson RS, Boden WE, Theroux P, et al. Diltiazem and reinfarction in patients with non Q-wave myocardial infarction: results of a double-blind, randomized, multicenter trial. *New Engl J Med* 1986;315 (7):423.

53. Pfeffer MA, Braunwald E, Moye LA, et al. Effect of captopril on mortality and morbidity in patients with left ventricular dysfunction after myocardial infarction: results of the Survival and Ventricular Enlargement Trial. *New Engl J Med* 1992;327:669.

54. Echt DS, Liebson PR, Mitchell LB, et al. Mortality and morbidity in patients receiving encainide, flecainide or placebo. The Cardiac Arrhythmia Suppression Trial. *New Engl J Med* 1991;324:781.

55. O'Connor GT, Buring JE, Yusuf S, et al. An overview of randomized trials of rehabilitation with exercise after myocardial infarction. *Circulation* 1989;80(2):234.

56. Oldridge NB, Guyatt GH, Fisher ME, et al. Cardiac rehabilitation after myocardial infarction: combined experience of randomized clinical trials. *JAMA* 1988;260(7):945.

57. Frasure-Smith N, Lespérance F, Talajic M. Depression following myocardial infarction. Impact on 6 month survival. *JAMA* 1993;270:1819.

# Subject Index

ISBN 0-397-51465-4